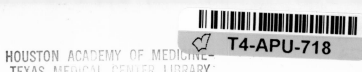

VOLUME 2

PHYSIOLOGY OF THE PERINATAL PERIOD

VOLUME 2

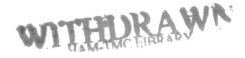

PHYSIOLOGY OF THE PERINATAL PERIOD
Functional and Biochemical Development in Mammals

Edited by

UWE ⌊STAVE • Fels Research Institute
Yellow Springs, Ohio

Foreword by A. ASHLEY WEECH
Professor Emeritus of Pediatrics,
University of Cincinnati College
of Medicine

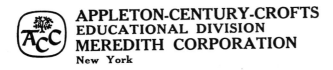
APPLETON-CENTURY-CROFTS
EDUCATIONAL DIVISION
MEREDITH CORPORATION
New York

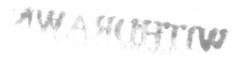
PRINTED IN THE UNITED STATES OF AMERICA
390-84067-x

List of Contributors

F. J. Ballard
CSIRO Kintore Avenue, Adelaide, Australia

William H. Bergstrom
Department of Pediatrics, State University of New York Upstate Medical Center, 766 Irving Avenue, Syracuse, New York 13210

Kurt Brück
Institute of Physiology, University of Marburg, Deutschhausstrasse 2, 355 Marburg, Germany

George W. Brumley
Department of Pediatrics, Duke University Medical Center, Durham, North Carolina 27706

José Cara
Department of Pediatrics, Maimonides Medical Center, 4802 Tenth Avenue, Brooklyn, New York 11219

Jean Claude Dreyfus
Institut de Pathologie Moléculaire, 24 Rue Du Faubourg-Saint-Jacques, Paris 14, France

J. Gleiss
Kinderabteilung St. Josef-Hospital, 42 Oberhausen-Sterkrade, Germany

Peter Gruenwald
Veterans Administration Hospital, Philadelphia, Pennsylvania 19104

Peter Hahn
Department of Gynecology, University of British Columbia, Vancouver General Hospital, Vancouver 8, British Columbia, Canada

Herbert S. Harned, Jr.
Department of Pediatrics, The University of North Carolina School of Medicine, Chapel Hill, North Carolina 27514

Robert T. Herrington
Department of Pediatrics, The University of North Carolina School of Medicine, Chapel Hill, North Carolina 27514

Williamina A. Himwich
Thudichum Psychiatric Research Laboratory, Galesburg State Research Hospital, Galesburg, Illinois 61401

David Yi-Yung Hsia
Department of Pediatrics, Loyola University Stritch School of Medicine, Hines, Illinois 60141

Tryphena Humphrey
Department of Anatomy, University of Alabama in Birmingham, The Medical Center, Birmingham, Alabama 35233

Lubor Jílek
Institute of Physiology, Albertova 5, Praha 2, Czechoslovakia

Emanuel Kauder
Barney Children's Medical Center 1735 Chapel Street Dayton, Ohio 45404

Edmund Kerpel-Fronius
Department of Pediatrics No. II, University Medical School, Tuzolto utca 7-9, Budapest IX, Hungary

Enno Kleihauer
Department of Pediatrics, Universität Ulm, 79 Ulm, Germany

Leonard I. Kleinman
Department of Pediatrics, Physiology and Environmental Health, Kettering Laboratory, University of Cincinnati College of Medicine, Cincinnati, Ohio 45229

Otakar Koldovský
The Children's Hospital of Philadelphia, 18th and Bainbridge Streets, Philadelphia, Pennsylvania 19146

v

John Lind
Department of Pediatrics, Karolinska Hospital and Wenner-Gren Cardiovascular Research Laboratory, Stockholm 60, Sweden

James F. Marks
Department of Pediatrics, University of Texas Southwestern Medical School, 5323 Harry Hines Boulevard, Dallas, Texas 75235

Alvin M. Mauer
Children's Hospital Research Foundation, Elland and Bethesda Avenues, Cincinnati, Ohio 45229

Gaspard de Muralt
Department of Neonatology, University of Berne and The Central Laboratory of the Blood Donor Service of the Swiss Red Cross, Effinger Strasse 39, 3008 Berne, Switzerland

Eduardo Orti
Department of Pediatrics, State University of New York Downstate Medical Center, 450 Clarkson Avenue, Brooklyn, New York 11203

Sergio Porto
Department of Pediatrics, Loyola University Stritch School of Medicine, Hines, Illinois 60141

Julius B. Richmond
Department of Pediatrics, State University of New York Upstate Medical Center, 766 Irving Avenue, Syracuse, New York 13210

K. P. Riegel
Universitäts-Kinderklinik, Lindwurmstrasse 4, 8 Munich 15, Germany

Fanny Schapira
Institut de Pathologie Moléculaire, 24 Rue Du Faubourg-Saint-Jacques, Paris 14, France

F. J. Schulte
Universitäts-Kinderklinik, Humboldtalle 38, 34 Göttingen, Germany

Thomas R. C. Sisson
Department of Pediatrics, Temple University School of Medicine, Philadelphia, Pennsylvania 19140

Selma E. Snyderman
Department of Pediatrics, New York University School of Medicine, 550 First Avenue, New York, New York 10016

Uwe Stave
The Fels Research Institute, Yellow Springs, Ohio 45387

Alfred Steinschneider
Department of Pediatrics, State University of New York Upstate Medical Center, 766 Irving Avenue, Syracuse, New York 13210

G. Stüttgen
Hautklinik der Freien Universität, Berlin, Germany

James R. Tiernan
Department of Child Health, University of Queensland, St. Lucia, Brisbane, Queensland, Australia

Eliana Trávníčková
Institute of Physiology, Albertova 5, Praha 2, Czechoslovakia

Stanislav Trojan
Institute of Physiology, Albertova 5, Praha 2, Czechoslovakia

S. Zoe Walsh
Department of Pediatrics, Karolinska Hospital and Wenner-Gren Cardiovascular Research Laboratory, Stockholm 60, Sweden

David S. Walton
Massachusetts Eye and Ear Infirmary, 243 Charles Street, Boston, Massachusetts 02114

Helmut Wolf
Universitäts-Kinderklinik, Humboldtallee 38, 34 Göttingen, Germany

Preface

Developmental physiology is a relatively new area of biologic and medical science. Frequently this large area has been divided into the developmental physiology of the embryo, fetus, perinatal, or neonatal individual and infant. Knowledge of fetal physiology is needed for a thorough understanding of the functional and metabolic situation of the newborn. The physiology of the perinatal period comprises the most important developmental period that climaxes with parturition of the fetus from its protective intrauterine environment. In these two volumes the contributors have focused on the final preparation for birth, the process of birth, the impact of parturition on the biologic functions of the newborn infant, and an establishment of homeostasis in the early postnatal period.

The prime concern in this text is with human beings, but important information on mammals has been included. Advances in obstetric and pediatric knowledge are dependent not only upon clinical observation, but also on studies of animal development by physiologists, biochemists, geneticists, and others. Pediatric research is concerned primarily with the physiology of normal and abnormal individuals with the direct aim to improve the diagnosis and management of patients. Studies of the developmental physiology of animals are oriented towards analyzing the effects of precisely controlled factors. The presentation of data from human beings together with results from animal experiments may lead to premature or erroneous conclusions concerning the applicability of animal findings to human beings. Some contributors have formulated principles and hypotheses, often by generalizations from the findings of animal experiments. Such generalizations and hypotheses may accelerate the progress of developmental research, but they should not be accepted as applicable to human beings without direct supporting evidence.

Developmental physiology differs from adult physiology in important ways. In adults, the range of functional capacity is fixed. By contrast, the functional capacities of developing organisms and, consequently, the methodology of their measurement, change with the developmental level. For example, the fetus and the newborn differ in metabolism. In this respect, then, they should be considered separately and in relation to other changes which occur between these two developmental levels.

The rates of change in size and functional capacity in individuals are regulated by both genetic and environmental factors. Furthermore, information about the genotypes of individuals would permit more reliable predictions of attained values and rates of change. Among nongenetic factors involved are, for example, the degree of physical and functional derangement during parturition and the rate and extent of postnatal adaptation.

Originally it was intended that this work would survey the entire field of prenatal and postnatal developmental physiology. Owing to the scarcity of relevant data, some omissions, especially those for the fetal period, were unavoidable. I hope, however, that the material included will stimulate research and help to bridge the gaps among the specialized disciplines concerned with perinatology and developmental physiology.

I am most grateful for the cooperation of the contributors; their enthusiasm and helpfulness have made this publication possible. My sincere thanks are due to the publishers, especially to Mr. Richard Van Frank, who helped tremendously with his valuable advice, skill, and patience. I am grateful also to my assistant, Miss Rose Stoltzfus, for her kind and efficient help; to my wife, who prepared numerous drawings; and to Mrs. Dorothy Clark, Mrs. Alice Rockway, and Mrs. Donna Tipton, who typed the manuscripts. Throughout, I have been encouraged and assisted by Dr. L. W. Sontag, Director of the Fels Research Institute, and I have been supported by funds made available from the Samuel S. Fels Fund of Philadelphia.

May 1970   UWE STAVE

Contents

VOLUME 1

Part I GROWTH AND PHYSIOLOGIC CHANGES AT BIRTH

Part II RESPIRATION, CIRCULATION, AND BLOOD

VOLUME 2

CONTENTS

Foreword

Living Nature, not dull Art
Shall plan my ways and rule my heart

CARDINAL NEWMAN:
Nature and Art
1868

One of the ineluctable consequences of growth in any field of science is that subjects of inquiry once established tend to give birth to sub-subjects and that the sub-subjects once established will in time undergo further mitotic division. Not so many years ago problems surrounding the fetus and newly born infant lay in a realm almost to be described as "a no-man's land." Obstetricians properly gave major consideration to understanding and learning about processes and disorders concerned with maternal health and safety. The welfare of the infant was regarded as of secondary importance. Pediatricians on their part hesitated to invade the nursery, a sanctum regarded as belonging to the domain of the accoucheur. And the pathologist, enveloped in the mysteries of life and death in the adult, found scant time for the neonate and the placenta.

Within little more than a score of years all of these things have changed. Obstetricians led by Nicholson Eastman, pediatricians guided by Clement Smith, pathologists represented by Sydney Farber and Edith Potter, the anesthesiologist Virginia Apgar, and many others have recognized the reward to be gained by exploring a previously neglected field. Numerous treatises are now available for the clinician who must supervise the treatment of disorders of this period of life. Compendiums on pathology are readily found. For the student bent on exploring the physiologic happenings of perinatal life, the volume entitled *The Physiology of the Newborn Infant* by Clement A. Smith has been a bible. With so much material now in convenient reference form, one may wonder why still another book. The answer lies in an expansion of methodology in a way now permitting the utilization of new biochemical techniques in unraveling the entangled threads of perinatal physiology. This compilation is not just another book. Nor is it a treatise for the clinician. But, for the investigator dedicated to understanding the genesis of what takes place at the very start of life, the volume will be a "must."

This foreword would be devoid of purpose if it failed to furnish an introduction to the physician who conceived of the need for the volume and at once devoted energy and talent to selecting appropriate authors for each of the 35 chapters, to the writing of three of these chapters himself, to a labor of love involving self-discipline and sacrifice in the careful reading and editing of the other chapters. Dr. Uwe Stave was singularly suited for the task. His medical education began in November of 1945 at the University

xiii

of Hamburg. It is significant that this doctoral thesis was on a subject that presaged future interests. It was (in English translation) entitled "Studies of the Physiology and Pharmacology of the Phrenic-Diaphragm Preparation of the Rat." After an internship he joined the Department of Pharmacology where he became engrossed in investigating the reactions of smooth muscle to various newly synthesized drugs. In April, 1953, he accepted an invitation to become a staff member in the University of Marburg an der Lahn. Here he was associated with a pediatrician with collateral experience in the field of chromatographic chemistry. This was Horst Bickel. Studies of amino acid metabolism ensued. There followed an opportunity to become associated with Theodor Buecher and associates in the Department of Biochemistry where the young Private-Dozent became acquainted with the technics of enzyme chemistry. Published articles over a period of eight and a half years in Marburg reveal a maturing interest in problems of developmental physiology. And, even more important from the standpoint of this foreword, our editor was learning—through his writings and by personal contacts at scientific meetings —to know the scientists of Europe who were making important contributions to the subjects of his interest.

In October 1961, Stave emigrated to the United States in order to join the staff of the Fels Research Institute for the Study of Human Development in Yellow Springs, Ohio. Here he was able to carry on his investigations in an exceedingly stimulating and hospitable environment. In the immediate reaches of a single building he was associated with colleagues in the fields of anthropology, genetics, psychology, psychiatry, psychophysiology, and biochemistry—all of them men with a dedicated interest in the overall study of growth. Once again through writing and travel to scientific meetings he came to know the productive students in a land over the seas from where his work began.

Enough has been said to justify the statement that the editor of this book was "singularly suited for the task." It is appropriate that in his Preface, Doctor Stave himself should say more about his carefully selected contributors. Perhaps also the writer of this foreword, who for many years has been a member of the Scientific Advisory Committee of the Fels Research Institute, is justified in recording his own pleasure in having known Uwe Stave both personally and under circumstances that have permitted familiarity with his work.

A. Ashley Weech, M.D.
*Professor Emeritus of Pediatrics
University of Cincinnati College of Medicine;
Editor-in-Chief
American Journal of Diseases of Children*

VOLUME 2

PHYSIOLOGY OF THE PERINATAL PERIOD

Part IV

BODY FLUIDS AND RENAL FUNCTION

20

Electrolyte and Water Metabolism

EDMUND KERPEL-FRONIUS ● Department of Pediatrics No. II, University Medical School, Budapest, Hungary

The Fetal Fluids

AMOUNT AND COMPOSITION OF INTRAUTERINE FLUIDS

According to measurements during the last trimester of pregnancy, fluid retention is associated with a mean increase of 756 mEq exchangeable sodium and of 171 mEq potassium (MacGillivray and Buchanan, 1958). In this review we are concerned with the fraction of retained water and electrolytes which accumulates during fetal development in the uterine cavity. The intrauterine water content in the primate may be divided into three compartments: fetal, placental, and amniotic fluid. Estimates of the water, sodium, and potassium content of these compartments are shown in Table 1.

In a comparison of the data of Table 1 with the total amount of electrolytes retained during pregnancy it is obvious that the increase of sodium is divided equally between the intrauterine fluid pools and the expanding maternal extracellular fluid space, while most of the retained potassium is used for the formation of fetal tissues.

TABLE 1. Water, Sodium, and Potassium Content of Intrauterine Fluids[a]

Compartment	Water g	Sodium mEq	Potassium mEq
Fetus (3.5 kg)	2,400	243	150.0
Placenta (0.5 kg)	433	49	20.0
Amniotic fluid (0.7 kg)	700	88	2.8
Total	3,533	380	172.8

[a]From Widdowson and Dickerson. 1964. *Mineral Metabolism.* Vol. 2, Part A. Courtesy of Academic Press, Inc.

TABLE 2. Comparison of Maternal and Fetal Fluids in the Lamb[a]

	Ewe, arterial blood		Fetal umbilical blood		Fetal tracheal fluid		Amniotic fluid		Allantoic fluid		Fetal urine	
Osmolality mOsm/liter	302 ±	6.0[b]	300 ±	6.0	300 ±	6.0	275 ±	14.0	278 ±	14.0	264	7.6
Sodium mEq/liter	143 ±	4.9	140 ±	3.4	142 ±	4.6	110 ±	2.0	35.0 ±	27.0	—	
Chloride mEq/liter	108 ±	3.1	105 ±	4.9	144 ±	7.1	94.0 ±	9.6	39.0 ±	21.0	—	
Potassium mEq/liter	4.7		4.4		6.6		10.7		51.4		—	
Total CO$_2$ mEq/liter	22.6 ±	3.6	22.1 ±	1.9	4.4 ±	1.6	18.4		16.9		18.8	
pH	7.44 ±	0.55	7.34 ±	0.65	6.43 ±	0.13	7.07 ±	0.22	6.9 ±	0.25	6.84	0.4
Urea mg/100 ml	—		—		46.0		118		112		—	
Sugar mg/100 ml	135		152		113		304		300		—	
Protein mg/100 ml	6,509		4,439		327		699		1,691		—	

[a]From Adams, et al. 1963a. *J. Pediat.*, 63:881-888; Adams, et al. 1963b. *Biol. Neonat.*, 5:151-158.
[b]Mean ± standard deviation.

The composition of fetal fluids has been thoroughly studied in many mammalian species. One of the aims of these studies was to compare the composition of these fluids with that of the maternal blood plasma. It was hoped that similarities and deviations in composition and the study of concentration gradients between maternal and fetal fluids might reveal clues for the understanding of the mechanisms and principles of intrauterine fluid accumulation. In Table 2 a survey of data of such a comparative study in the lamb is presented.

FETOMATERNAL RELATIONSHIP OF TOTAL OSMOLARITY AND OF SOLUTE CONCENTRATIONS

Total osmolar concentrations. Some authors found a higher osmolar concentration in fetal than in maternal blood plasma. Meschia et al. (1957) have shown that when sampling of fetal and maternal blood was performed with a minimum of interference with placental circulation, the osmotic pressure was the same in both fluids. Delayed sampling, that is, clamping of the cord, caused a rise in osmolar concentration of the fetal plasma. The data in Table 2 show the same osmolar concentration in the blood plasma of the ewe and the fetal lamb. The same holds true for the human. Battaglia (1960) found average values for maternal and fetal plasma of 289.1 mOsm/liter and 292.7 mOsm/liter, respectively.

Plasma sodium concentration. In the ewe and the fetal lamb at term these levels are equal (Table 2). However, data assembled in Table 3 show that it is somewhat embarrassing to take a firm stand with regard to the human fetus and newborn.

The range of variations was found to be even greater for measurements performed in plasma of young fetuses: 134 to 188 mEq/liter (Westin et al., 1959). This big range conveys the impression that extremely high values may be due to shortcomings of the sampling technique or to pathology. On the other hand, very low values may reflect maternal hyponatremia, a condition that is frequently found in mothers treated with a low-sodium diet, diuretics, and glucose solutions prior to delivery. In brief, we agree with Battaglia et al. (1960), Crawford (1965), and others that the concentration of sodium in the blood plasma of the human fetus near term is practically the same as in the maternal plasma. The latter is frequently a few milliequivalents lower and occasionally is much lower than the accepted normal values for older infants or adults.

TABLE 3. Plasma Sodium Concentration in Cord Blood in mEq/liter

Sources	No.	Mean	Range	S.D.
Acharya and Payne (1965)	14	146.8	126-166	±8.1
Oliver et al. (1961)	19	139.0	130-158	±8.0
Battaglia et al. (1960)	10	140.1	137-145	—
Pincus et al. (1956)	12	135.0	127-142	±5.0
Crawford (1965)	62	135.0	—	±6.1

Concentration of plasma potassium. This level in the newborn is a much discussed problem ever since Widdowson and McCance (1956) reported very high values in the human fetus and in the fetal pig. The relevant information serving as a base for discussion is summarized in Table 4.

In early fetal life very high plasma potassium concentrations were reported. In the previable fetuses of Westin et al. (1959) the range was 8.0 to 12.8 mEq/liter, and Widdowson and McCance (1956) found a mean value of 10.2 mEq/liter in the human and 17.5 mEq/liter in the pig fetus. Before evaluating the somewhat contradictory data presented, some pitfalls of methodology must be discussed. The conceivable causes for real or apparently high potassemia are the following: 1, intrauterine hypoxia and acidosis; 2, escape of potassium from the red cells, since the cells of the newborn and fetus give up their potassium with great speed in vitro (Keitel, 1959); 3, hemolysis, occurring easily during sampling of blood from fetal vessels; 4, delayed sampling of cord blood, causing potassium gain from the hypoxic placental tissue; 5, a genuine ability of the fetus to maintain an uphill gradient for potassium between maternal and fetal circulation. Hyperpotassemia in the first condition is pathologic, while a sampling technique which is open to criticism may also have caused artifacts; finally, an uphill gradient would imply some form of active potassium transport from mother to fetus.

A critical inspection of the values shown in Table 4 leads to the suggestion that some authors may have included in their material some severely acidotic cases, or

TABLE 4.   **Plasma Potassium Concentration in Cord Blood and During the First Hours of Life in mEq/liter**

Sources	Species	No.	Mean	Range	S.D.	Mean in maternal plasma
Oliver et al. (1961)	Human, term	40	9.10	6.8-14.3	±2.0	—
Widdowson and McCance (1956)	Human, term	5	8.00	4.8-12.9	—	—
Acharya and Payne (1965)	Human, term	14	7.79	5.6-12.0	±2.0	—
Battaglia et al. (1960)	Human, term	7	4.47	3.1- 5.8	—	3.85
Crawford (1965)	Human, term	62	4.50	—	±0.61	3.50
Pincus et al. (1956)	Human, term	12	5.40	4.5- 6.8	±0.7	—
Pincus et al. (1956)	Most premature		6.10	5.6- 7.2	±0.6	—
Nicolopoulos and Smith (1961)	Premature	12	5.80	—	±0.35	—
Nicolopoulos and Smith (1961)	Most premature	4	7.50	—	±0.97	—
Kerpel-Fronius et al. (1964)	Guinea pig	32	4.31	—	±0.18	5.00
Kerpel-Fronius et al. (1964)	Dog	32	5.14	—	±0.66	4.15
Kerpel-Fronius et al. (1964)	Rat	164	6.13	—	±0.32	4.31
Serrano et al. (1964)	Dog	6	5.30	—	—	4.10
Widdowson and McCance (1956)	Pig	11	8.60	5.3-11.8	—	6.00
Adams et al. (1963a, b)	Lamb		4.40			4.70

that their sampling technique was not absolutely perfect. However, we agree with the conclusion of Widdowson and Dickerson (1964) in their excellent review when they state that "it seems unlikely that this is the whole cause of the high values." The means of all authors were found to be 0.5 to 1 mEq/liter higher than the corresponding maternal values, and concentrations certainly are increasing with decreasing maturity of the fetus. This thesis is also supported by evidence from comparative physiology. The somatic immaturity at birth of certain species of animals is reflected by a higher potassemia. The immaturely born rat, pig, and dog exhibit consistently higher plasma potassium concentrations relative to maternal plasma, in contrast to more mature newborns such as the guinea pig and the lamb. The dog is a particularly suitable animal for such studies since the sodium and not the potassium is the dominant cation in canine erythrocytes. This excludes the possibility of a high plasma potassium concentration from being an artifact in this species. The conclusive proof that the fetus can maintain a transplacental uphill gradient against maternal blood was brought by experiments of Serrano et al. (1964). In potassium-deficient pregnant bitches plasma potassium concentration fell from 4.1 mEq/liter to 2.7 mEq/liter, while the fetal concentration remained unchanged and was 5.3 mEq/liter in controls and 5.4 mEq/liter in newborns of potassium-deficient mothers. The uphill gradient of striking proportions in the experimental group, and the important fact that carcass potassium did not decrease in these newborns, strongly suggest some form of active transport for this ion through the placental barrier.

Plasma magnesium concentration. Knowledge on magnesium has lagged behind that of other electrolytes, largely due to methodologic difficulties. The results of the literature are contradictory. Economou-Mavrou and McCance (1958) found higher values in the fetal pig: 3.79 mEq/liter with a range of 3.5 to 4.2, against 2.60 mEq/liter with a range of 2.2 to 4.42 in the sow. In the human fetus magnesiemia was also found to be somewhat higher than in adults. In the term infant opinions are divided about the possibility of a gradient for plasma magnesium between maternal and fetal plasma. Recently Anast (1964) reported identical values in newborns on the first day of life—1.94 mg/100 ml (range: 1.36 to 2.9) —and in older children—1.94 mg/100 ml (range: 1.51 to 2.58).

Plasma calcium and phosphorus concentrations are discussed in Chapter 22.

Plasma chloride and total CO_2 concentrations. According to unanimous opinion there are only slight differences in the *plasma chloride* concentrations between term infants and adults (Pincus et al., 1956; Graham et al., 1951; and others). In premature infants the range of variation is greater and the mean chloride concentration is higher. The *total carbon dioxide* content is low at birth, which reflects a variable degree of metabolic acidosis. The range of variations increases immediately after birth. A detailed analysis of this problem is presented in Chapter 3. Twenty-four hours after birth healthy full-term infants exhibit an average value of 21 mEq/liter, with a range of 16.1 to 24.9 (Graham et al., 1951; and others), the corresponding concentrations for adults being 24 mEq/liter, with a range between 21.4 and 26.4 mEq/liter.

Plasma pH: According to in-utero measurements by the new scalp-sampling technique developed by Saling (1966), the pH in fetal blood is only a couple of hundredth units lower than that in maternal blood before onset of labor. With labor in progress the fetal pH very slowly decreases. Values below 7.2 are generally considered to reflect intrauterine asphyxia (Saling, 1966; Kubli, 1966). Premature infants, as shall be discussed later, exhibit a conspicuous tendency to acidosis.

THE ORIGIN OF INTRAUTERINE FLUID ACCUMULATION

During fetal development a net quantity of 3.5 liters of water, 380 mEq of sodium, and 173 mEq of potassium must have been transferred from the mother to the intrauterine cavity (as shown in Table 1). The mechanism of this transfer still remains obscure. Isotope studies revealed exchange rates which by far exceeded the net transfer rates; the latter are defined as the transfer of water or of electrolytes in one direction in excess of the transfer in the reverse direction. The two-directional transfer rates appear to be enormously high (Table 5) as shown by Plentl (1959). Exchange rates for water between mother and fetus increase ten times between midpregnancy and term, while the initially high exchange rates between mother and amniotic fluid and between fetus and amniotic fluid increase at a much slower rate as term approaches. The turnover rates for sodium and potassium were found to be much smaller than those for water.

The reported isotope studies are interesting and important, but they do not solve the problem of the driving forces of the net transfers, which result in the accumulation of intrauterine fluids. Since no appreciable gradients were observed for total osmotic pressure or for plasma sodium concentration, the search was extended as to whether differences in colloid osmotic or hydrostatic pressure on both sides of the placental membrane could be responsible. The colloid osmotic pressure depends primarily on plasma protein concentration and therefore must necessarily be lower in fetal than in maternal blood. The fetal plasma protein concentration increases with maturity from 2.5 percent found in previable fetuses (Westin et al. 1959), to 5 to 6 percent at term; these fetal values are considerably lower than the maternal values. The gradient in colloid osmotic pressure, if unopposed by any other force, would, thus, favor the movement of water from the fetus

TABLE 5. Transfer Rates for Water Between Mother and Fetus (in ml per hour)[a]

	Weeks of pregnancy	
	20	40
I. Mother—fetus	302	3,657
Fetus—mother	259	3,682
II. Mother—amniotic fluid	79	265
Amniotic fluid—mother	107	247
III. Fetus—amniotic fluid	70	149
Amniotic fluid—fetus	37	165

[a]From Plentl. 1959. *Ann. N.Y. Acad. Sci.*, 75:746-761.

to the mother, and it certainly could not explain the net transfer of fluids from the mother to the intrauterine cavity. The same holds true for the hydrostatic pressure. Seeds (1965) reviewed the available data on hydrostatic pressure in the intervillous space, in the umbilical artery, and in the umbilical vein and concluded that "if a hydrostatic pressure gradient exists in the steady state, it appears to favor an exchange from fetus to mother and does not explain the fluid accumulation within the uterus in pregnancy." In summing up we can conclude that the net fluid transfer from the mother to the intrauterine fluid pools cannot be explained simply by osmotic, colloid osmotic, or hydrostatic pressure differences between fetal and maternal blood.

For the time being we must be satisfied with Seeds' (1965) assumption that gradients which are too small or infrequent for accurate measurements by present techniques may supply small daily fluid amounts which are necessary for the normal intrauterine development. Temperature differences within the vascular beds of the placenta may also be considered as a possible driving force. As for potassium and probably also for magnesium some hitherto unknown mechanism for active transport must be searched for.

EFFECTS OF CHANGES IN VOLUME AND COMPOSITION OF MATERNAL EXTRACELLULAR FLUID ON THE FETUS

Although the problem of the mechanism of net fluid transfer across the placenta remains unsolved, it has been shown that acute changes in maternal extracellular fluid volume and composition lead to predictable changes in the fetal fluids. In a series of impressive experiments Battaglia et al. (1960) created osmotic gradients between human maternal and fetal blood by infusion of mannitol, hypertonic saline, or isotonic glucose solutions into the maternal circulation. The hypertonic expansion of maternal extracellular fluid was accompanied by a similar but smaller rise in osmolarity in the fetal blood plasma, while increasing plasma protein concentration indicated net movement of fluid from the fetus to the mother. Dilutional hyponatremia was induced in the mother by injecting 5 percent glucose solution, and it resulted in a decrease of the osmolar concentration in fetal blood. This indicated a transfer of water from the mother to the fetus and/or a transfer of sodium in the opposite direction. These observations in the human were supplemented by similar experiments in animals. Burns et al. (1963) induced water depletion in rabbit fetuses by an intravenous infusion of hypertonic mannitol solution into pregnant rabbits. The resulting decrease in fetal extracellular fluid was 18 percent, and the loss of cell fluid was calculated to be 15 percent. These high amounts of fluids were transferred from the fetus to the mother through the placenta. The increase in osmotic pressure in the fetal blood was less marked than in the maternal, and about half of the increase in osmolarity in the fetal fluids could be ascribed to the transfer of mannitol. Osmotic gradients which were experimentally produced among fetal, maternal, and amniotic fluid pools by injection of sucrose solution into the amniotic sac of pregnant monkeys also led to fetal dehydration; the placental water content remained unchanged in these experiments (Burns et al., 1964).

In addition to such experiments of short duration it was shown that chronic salt depletion also affects the fetal fluid pools. Phillips and Sundaram (1966) induced sodium depletion in pregnant ewes by draining the saliva from one parotid gland for a period of six days. Fetal sodium concentration showed a smaller reduction than either maternal or amniotic sodium concentration. The authors assumed that some still unidentified mechanism must have provided some degree of independence to the fetal sodium plasma level from the maternal plasma level. Furthermore it was presumed that these fetuses responded to sodium deficiency by restricting their renal sodium loss.

These assumptions need to be verified, but they seem to hold true only for the type of hyponatremia that is accompanied by dehydration of some days' duration. In Altstatt's (1965) clinical cases, in which iatrogenic transplacental hyponatremia was caused by a low-salt diet and by administrating large amounts of 5 percent glucose solutions to the mother, changes in fetal sodium concentration exhibited a close parallelism to maternal concentrations. In the four cases observed, maternal sodium concentrations of 119, 118, 117, and 119 mEq/liter were accompanied by the following neonatal values: 120, 119, 122, and 114 mEq/liter. In experimental dialysis maternal and fetal plasma sodium concentration changes were also practically identical.

For potassium a genuine independence of fetal from maternal plasma concentration was shown to exist. As mentioned above (Serrano et al., 1964), hypopotassemia induced in bitches decreased neither the fetal plasma potassium level nor the total carcass potassium of the fetus.

Concerning hydrogen ion concentration, an increasing maternal acid accumulation during labor is reflected by a parallel increase in fetal negative base excess as shown by studies carried out with the fetal scalp sampling technique. In fetal asphyxia, however, base excess in fetal blood decreases out of proportion to maternal values (Kubli, 1966). From these experiments and observations the following conclusions can be drawn: osmotic gradients can be maintained for an appreciable time on both sides of the placenta; solutes move at a slower rate than water; chemical gradients between mother and fetus or fetus and amniotic fluid effectuate considerable shifts of water between fetal and maternal fluid pools; the fetus may be dehydrated or overhydrated by fluid shifts due to osmotic gradients, and parallel to maternal changes, such as sodium concentrations, the fetal fluids may become hyper- or hypotonic. Furthermore, the knowledge gained from these experiments helps to explain clinical observations on fetal damage due to the altered composition of maternal fluids; for example, fetal water intoxication was observed in connection with inappropriate or overzealous fluid administration to the mother.

VOLUME, COMPOSITION, ORIGIN, AND DISPOSAL OF AMNIOTIC FLUID

Amniotic fluid appears in all mammalian species early in pregnancy. In the human a few milliliters of this fluid have been found as early as in the eighth week of gestation. Figure 1 shows the rate of accumulation of this fluid during pregnancy.

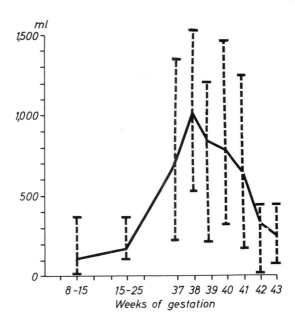

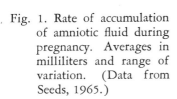

Fig. 1. Rate of accumulation of amniotic fluid during pregnancy. Averages in milliliters and range of variation. (Data from Seeds, 1965.)

The peak value of 1,000 ml is reached at about two weeks before term. Thereafter the amount of fluid slowly diminishes until the fortieth week. This decrease is accelerated as soon as normal term is passed; the average fluid volume decreases to about one quarter of its peak value after 43 weeks of gestation. This decrease in fluid volume may occur in consequence of diminishing functional efficiency of the placenta, which begins after the normal term is passed.

The individual variations of fluid volume are large even in normal pregnancies. Extreme values, however, surpassing 1.5 to 2 liters (hydramnios) or volumes below 0.5 liter (oligohydramnios) are frequently associated with fetal pathology.

Progressive distension of the uterus is thought to be necessary for normal uterine, placental, and fetal development. The removal of amniotic fluid at about mid-pregnancy causes death of the fetuses; however, very near to term survival without amniotic fluid is possible (Adolph, 1967).

In the first half of gestation the *composition* of amniotic fluid is similar to that of extracellular fluid. Later in pregnancy osmolarity and sodium concentration fall below the fetal or maternal levels in blood plasma (Table 2). Other conspicuous changes are the increase in potassium, urea, uric acid, creatinine, and acidity.

The composition of early amniotic fluid, which is practically identical with extracellular fluid, speaks for its provenance from the maternal blood plasma. Later in pregnancy the problem becomes more complicated since the secretions of the fetal kidneys and lungs appear to participate to a large extent in the formation of this fluid. The convincing proof that amniotic fluid is being modified by a steadily increasing admixture of fetal urine is, in addition to the decreasing osmolarity and sodium concentration, the accumulation of fetal waste products in the amniotic fluid. Table 2 shows that fetal urine is hypotonic and that the amniotic fluid of the lamb has a high urea and potassium content. In the human, urea concentration in amniotic fluid at term varies between 24 and 44 mg/100 ml, creatinine levels are between 2 and 3.7 mg/100 ml, and uric acid reaches a value of 6.8 mg/100 ml. These values are considerably higher than those in fetal plasma.

The important role of the fetal kidneys in the *formation* and regulation of amniotic fluid is supported by clinical observations. Bain and Scott (1960) reviewed 50 cases of fetal urinary tract malformations with the common feature that no fetal micturition could have occurred. Among these cases bilateral renal agenesis was present in 28, severe cystic dysplasia in 17, and congenital urethral atresia in 5 cases. In all but 1 case fluid was recorded as being absent, deficient, or suggestive of liquor deficiency. Liquor was present in 1 anencephalic case, in which malformation no amniotic fluid could have been swallowed. The extensive literature on the relation of renal agenesis and oligohydramnios permits the general conclusion that if the mechanisms for the disposal of amniotic fluid are operating normally, the absence of fetal urination is associated with oligohydramnios. Thus, the absence of fetal micturition disturbs the steady state of amniotic fluid formation and disposal.

The same conclusions can be drawn when the problem of amniotic fluid formation is evaluated from available data on fetal urine formation. In general, fetal urine flow was found to be surprisingly high. Alexander et al. (1958) measured amounts of 1.9 ml/min/kg at 61 days of gestation and 0.04 ml at term in sheep, the latter value being still twice as high as in adults. The authors concluded that the rate of urine formation is more than enough to account for the total volume of fetal fluids observed. It was, of course, admitted that several factors are involved in the formation of fetal fluids (Alexander and Nixon, 1961). Wright and Nixon (1961) have calculated that the total volume of fluid that is absorbed by the gut of fetal sheep between 80 days of gestation and term was about 32 liters, which is in the same range as the volume of urine produced during this time (about 40 liters).

Another source of amniotic fluid is the *fetal tracheal fluid*. This fluid has the same total osmolar and sodium concentration as fetal blood plasma (see Table 2), and it appears to be an ultrafiltrate of the latter. The reason for certain differences in composition, such as the very low pH and total CO_2 content and the high chloride concentration, remains at present unexplained, but the origin of the fetal tracheal fluid and its direction of flow is known. The fluid produced by the fetal airways flows out of the trachea and pharynx into the esophagus, and part of it enters the amniotic cavity. The rate of flow was found to be to 1 to 2 ml/minute in fetal lambs at term (Adams et al., 1963a), and such an amount should contribute appreciably to the volume of amniotic fluid.

Filtration and diffusion through the fetal membranes and also their secretions may be additional sources of amniotic fluid. Adolph (1967) attributes great significance to the fetal membranes as far as the formation of early amniotic fluid is concerned.

In the *disposal of amniotic fluid* the gut of the fetus is believed to play an important role. According to Scott and Wilson (1957) in 54 out of 169 cases of hydramnios the excessive accumulation of amniotic fluid could be ascribed to conditions in which there had probably been a failure of the fetal swallowing mechanism, or where the fetus was mechanically incapable of swallowing. All cases of esophageal atresia are accompanied by hydramnios except those in which both segments of the esophagus communicate with the trachea, thus providing a route for swallowing. Anencephaly and other severe neurologic anomalies frequently interfere with swallowing, and, therefore, they are associated with hydramnios.

The inability to swallow is certainly one of the causes of hydramnios, but Moya et al. (1960) reviewed 1,745 cases from the literature and found esophageal malformations in 26.7 percent and other pathologic conditions interfering with swallowing in 17.7 percent of all cases. Fluid exchange relies on a finely tuned system of production and removal. There are many sites for interference. An imbalance of only a few milliliters per hour in transfer rates could result in the formation of hydramnios.

THE REGULATION OF VOLUME AND COMPOSITION OF FETAL FLUIDS

By studying the data on the chemical composition and the rate of formation of amniotic fluid, tracheal fluid, and fetal urine on one hand, and the estimated rate of swallowing of amniotic fluid on the other, the present knowledge can be summarized as follows: Early in pregnancy the amniotic fluid seems to be like a dialysate of maternal and/or fetal blood plasma. As gestation proceeds, the volume and composition of amniotic fluid is increasingly altered by large admixtures of fetal urine and tracheal fluid and by the swallowing and absorption of this fluid. Fetal waste products and probably a certain amount of the swallowed water must finally enter the maternal circulation.

The placenta, the fetal and maternal kidneys, and the fetal lung and intestine may play a certain role in maintaining the volume and composition of the fetal fluids. How these multiple processes are ultimately integrated still eludes our full understanding. Osmolarity and sodium concentrations are evidently in equilibrium with maternal concentrations, but no convincing results are available which prove that the regulation of electrolyte levels could be absolutely independent from the mother. It is not fully known how much the fetal kidney function contributes to the regulation of these concentrations. A decreasing sodium concentration in fetal urine during gestation speaks for a sodium-saving ability of the fetal kidneys. Whether the fetal urine volumes vary with changing sodium concentrations in fetal plasma remains to be investigated. Similarly, potassium regulation remains problematic.

Normal potassium concentration can be maintained in fetal fluids in spite of maternal potassium depletion.

Changes in Body Water Compartments and Electrolyte Contents During Growth

FLUID SPACES DURING GROWTH

It has been known for many years that progressive decrease in water and chloride content of the body are characteristics of growth and development. In the light of more recent knowledge these processes are understood to occur in consequence of the decrease in extracellular body fluid volume and of the increase in fat and in proteins. Figure 2 is based on analytic data from Iob and Swanson (1934) which reflect the impressive extent of these changes during intrauterine development and how they continue through early infancy. The developmental changes in electrolyte contents and in the size of the fluid spaces have been studied in detail by dilution methods. Values obtained with deuterium oxide or antipyrine, which are both frequently used to measure total body water (TBW), agree with those obtained by direct postmortem analysis.

The measurement of extracellular fluid volume is a more controversial problem. The substances used for this purpose measure different spaces. According to the size of space as measured in adults, two groups can be distinguished: 1, chloride, bromide, and thiocyanate; and 2, inulin, mannitol, and thiosulfate. The volume of extracellular water (ECW) measured with substances of group 1 is about 25 percent of the body weight, while the volume of ECW measured with the second group (inulin) is considerably smaller; it is about 16 percent of the body weight. The "battle of the boundaries," as Gamble (1956) called the discussion on the significance of parameters measured by the various substances, is of importance, since intracellular water (ICW) is usually calculated by subtracting ECW from TBW. If the calculation is based on ECW measured by any substance of group 2, ICW is considerably greater, and consequently the calculated concentration of intracellular solutes is considerably lower than if substances of group 1 are used. In the first case large amounts of exchangeable sodium and chloride would be assigned to the intracellular fluid compartment. Since inulin only partially penetrates dense connective tissue water, bone water, and transcellular fluid, and since these compartments of the sodium- and chloride-containing fluids evidently have to be assigned to the extracellular system, in praxi, the "inulin space" refers only to the "mobile" fraction of ECW. We agree with those authors (Cheek, 1961; Forbes, 1962) who consider the corrected bromide space (i.e., the space corrected for intracellular chloride) in the adult as the extracellular fluid space.

The foregoing discussion has less bearing on the newborn period since at this

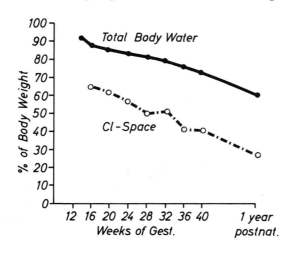

Fig. 2. Changes in total body water and chloride space during intrauterine development in man. (Data from Iob and Swanson, 1934.)

age the spaces measured with any of the substances of either group 1 or group 2 are more similar than in adults (Fig. 3).

In searching for the reason for this age-dependent difference, that is, the inequality of the inulin and chloride spaces in the adult, we agree with Friis-Hansen (1961) that it reflects the increasing heterogeneity of the extracellular fluid during development, i.e., the increasing proportion of dense connective tissue water in total ECW with growth. An additional comment is necessary regarding the volume of ECW measured with substances belonging to either group 1 or group 2 in the newborn. Friis-Hansen (1961) found a mean value for ECW of 44.5 percent of the body weight; this was measured with thiosulfate, and it is appreciably higher than the corrected bromide space of the newborn. For the latter Fink and Cheek (1960) gave a mean value of 35.8±6 percent, and Clapp et al. (1962) measured 38.7±3.4 percent on the first day of life. The correction factor used for intracellular chloride might thus be either somewhat too high or, which seems to be more likely, the exclusion of the brain from the volume of distribution of bromide introduces a larger error in the measurement of ECW in the newborn than in the adult. This assumption is supported by the fact that the brain of the newborn contains 11.2 percent of the TBW, while that of the adult accounts for only 2.2 percent. Furthermore, the chloride concentration is higher in the brain of the newborn than in adults.

It appears reasonable to conclude that in the adult the difference between the corrected bromide space and the inulin space should be ascribed to that part of the extracellular fluid system that has an organized structure. Hence, for the calculation of the volume of intracellular fluid in the adult the difference between TBW and corrected bromide space (and certainly not the difference between TBW and inulin or thiosulfate space) should be used, while for the calculation of the ICW in the newborn the difference between TBW and thiosulfate space seems to be more appropriate. Table 6 summarizes some data on the size of the fluid compartments obtained by current methods.

If fluid volumes are calculated on a fat-free basis, differences in ECW between

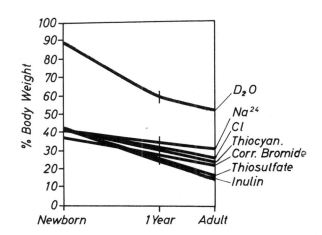

Fig. 3. Comparison between the relative volumes of distribution of various substances used for measuring fluid spaces in the human newborn, at one year of age, and in adults. (Adapted from Friis-Hansen. 1961. *Pediatrics,* 28:169–181.)

TABLE 6.   **TBW, ECW, and Calculated Volume of ICW in the Human Newborn and Adult (in percent of body weight)**

Sources	Age	TBW D₂O space	ECW	ICW	ECW measured by
Parker et al. (1958)	23-54-year old males	54.3	23.4	30.9	Corrected bromide space
Parker et al. (1958)	0-11 days	76.4	41.6	34.8	Thiosulfate
Friis-Hansen (1961)	1 day term	78.4	44.5	33.9	Thiosulfate
Clapp et al. (1962)	1 day term	77.4	38.7	39.8	Corrected bromide space
Fink and Cheek (1960)	1 day term	—	35.8	—	Corrected bromide space
Fink and Cheek (1960)	Prematures 1-6 days	85.8	40.5	44.8	Corrected bromide space

the newborn and the adult appear to be smaller, and the ICW in the adult is higher than in the newborn (Table 7).

ELECTROLYTE CONTENT OF THE BODY DURING GROWTH

Developmental changes in the total electrolyte content of the body are summarized in Table 8.

CHANGES IN COMPOSITION OF ORGANS AND TISSUES DURING GROWTH

The great changes in total body electrolyte composition that occur during maturation invite study of the correlations of changes in organ proportions and in organ composition.

The typical developmental changes in water content and size of fluid spaces in the peripheral muscle are illustrated in Figure 4. The peculiarities of the immature human muscle compared with the adult muscle are the high proportion of ECW per 100 g of dry substance and the much less expanded ICW. In the fresh *muscle*

TABLE 7.   **Fluid Spaces of the Adult Compared with Those of a Newborn Expressed (in g per kg of fat free body weight)**

	TBW	ECW	ICW
Adult	720	305	415
Newborn	823	448	375

[a]ECW and ICW recalculated from the data of Parker et al. as shown in Table 6.

TABLE 8. Chloride, Sodium, and Potassium Content of the Fetus and Newborn Compared with Values Found in Adult Man (in mEq per kg)

Age	Chloride	Sodium	Potassium	Method	Sources
Fetus (271 g)	76.0	96.0	46.0	Chemical analysis	Widdowson and Dickerson (1964)
Newborn	49.7 (56.6)[a]	73.7 (84)	40.4 (46)	Chemical analysis	Camerer and Söldner (1900)
Adult man	33.2 (42.8)	62.3 (80)	51.5 (64.8)	Chemical analysis	Forbes and Lewis (1956)
Newborn	48.0	—	—	Bromide	Cheek (1954)
Newborn	—	80.0	40.0	Na^{24} K^{42}	Corsa et al. (1956)
Adult man	31.6	—	—	Bromide	Dunning et al. (1951)
Adult man	—	41.9 (+30%)[b]	—	Na^{24}	Forbes and Lewis (1956)
Adult man	—	—	46.3 (+5%)[c] K^{42}		Corsa et al. (1956)

[a]Figures in parentheses indicate values per kilogram of fat-free body matter.
[b]Amount of nonexchangeable sodium.
[c]Amount of nonexchangeable potassium.

of the premature infant the ECW accounts for about half of the weight of the muscle, while the content in dry matter and in ICW is smaller than in the newborn. A very similar order of increasing maturity is seen when the fluid spaces of the very immaturely born rat are compared with those of the more mature puppy and the maturely newborn guinea pig. The composition of the muscle of the newborn rat shows a considerably less mature pattern than that of the human premature of 1.6 kg. The upper columns show that differences in maturity, as first pointed out by Widdowson and Dickerson (1960), are reflected to a much lesser degree in the myocardium of the three species of newborn animals.

The changes in the electrolyte content of various organs and tissues during growth and development were extensively studied by Widdowson and Dickerson (1960, 1964). From the wealth of information summarized in their review of 1964, Table 9 presents an excerpt of some basic data. These data demonstrate the maturational trends for some organs.

TABLE 9. Developmental Changes of the Electrolyte Content of Some Organs[a]

	Fetus (20-22 weeks)				Newborn				Adult			
	H_2O	Na	K	Cl	H_2O	Na	K	Cl	H_2O	Na	K	Cl
Muscle[b]	887	90.6	57.6	65.6	804	60.1	57.7	42.6	792	36.3	92.2	22.1
Heart[b]	860	46.1	81.1	41.0	841	64.2	54.3	49.3	827	57.8	66.5	45.6
Skin[c]	901	120.0	36.0	96.0	828	87.1	45.0	66.9	694	79.3	23.7	71.4
Brain[b]	922	91.7	52.0	72.6	897	80.9	58.2	66.1	774	55.2	84.6	40.5

[a]From Widdowson and Dickerson. 1964. *Mineral Metabolism.* Vol. 2, Part A. Courtesy of Academic Press, Inc.
[b]In g or mEq per kg of fresh tissue.
[c]In g or mEq per kg of fat-free skin.

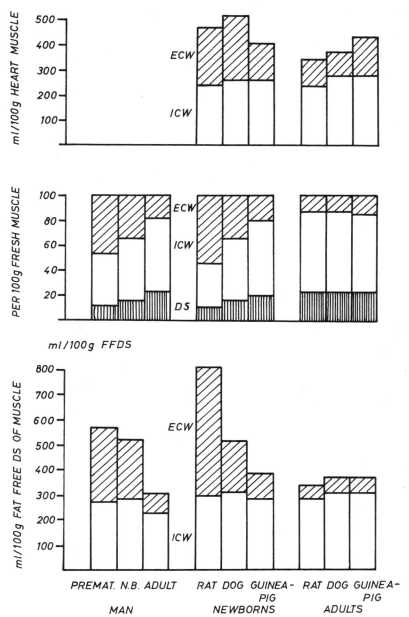

Fig. 4. Changes in the volume of water compartments in the skeletal muscle and cardiac muscle during growth in man and in newborn animals. Premature infant weighing 1.6 kg; NB, newborn full-term infant. ECW, ICW, extracellular and intracellular water; DS, dry substance; FFDS, fat free dry substance. (Adapted from Kerpel-Fronius. 1937. *Z. Kinderheilk.*, 58:726–738; Kerpel-Fronius et al. 1964. *Biol. Neonat.*, 6:177–196.)

The composition of the human skeletal muscle reflects exactly the maturational changes described for the total body. Widdowson and Dickerson (1960) point out that among animals born at different stages of maturity, the muscle of the immaturely born rat exhibits the highest water, chloride, and sodium content.

The water and chloride content of the *heart,* in contrast with the great changes occurring in skeletal muscle, shows only minor changes with age. Widdowson and Dickerson (1960) related this difference in chemical maturation to variations in the speed of functional maturation; the heart matures functionally earlier than the skeletal muscle.

The decrease in the water content of the *skin* is due to an increase in collagen; it is associated with an increase of the connective tissue water fraction of total ECW. Parallel with these changes the Na:Cl ratio falls, indicating an increase in connective tissue chloride. The proportion of ICW is low in all age groups, as could be suggested from the low potassium content. The skin certainly is the main depot of ECW of the body. The decrease of the water and chloride content of the *brain* is a characteristic phenomenon of growth.

Another important depository for ECW is the *skeleton.* The water content of bone decreases, while its sodium content rises during growth. The diminishing exchangeability of bone sodium with age is a further interesting feature of the growth process (Forbes et al., 1957). As already mentioned the radiosodium space in the newborn is of about the same size as the thiosulfate space, while in the adult the amount of sodium found by chemical analysis is approximately 30 percent higher than the exchangeable sodium and much higher than the fraction of sodium allocated to ECW. These changes indicate that during maturation a rising amount of bone sodium is bound in a rather inaccessible form in the crystalline bone structure.

ROLE OF CHANGING ORGAN PROPORTIONS IN THE DECREASE OF EXTRACELLULAR FLUID VOLUME DURING GROWTH

That proportion of the body weight that accounts for major tissues and organs undergoes great changes during growth and maturation. The relative contribution of those tissues to TBW and total ECW and ICW in each stage of maturation depends on both the changing size in relation to body weight and the changes in composition.

Organs rich in ECW, such as skin and brain, account for a much higher percentage of body weight, and hence of TBW, in the newborn than in the adult, while the muscle mass is not only less in the newborn but also contains a much higher percentage of ECW. The differences of those three organs, which represent more than 60 percent of TBW, and the higher water content of the skeleton easily explain the higher ECW content of the immature body (Fig. 5). The decrease in ECW during growth obviously results from two maturational processes—firstly, the decreasing proportion of body weight that accounts for tissues rich in ECW, and secondly, the decrease in the percentage of ECW in the skeletal muscle.

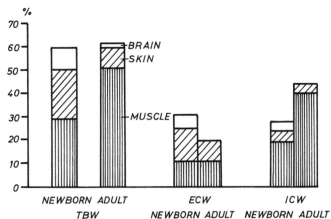

Fig. 5. Contribution of the muscles, the skin, and the brain to total body water (TBW), extracellular water (ECW), and intracellular water (ICW), respectively, in the newborn and the adult. Data in percent of TBW (TBW = 100%). (Adapted from Kerpel-Fronius. 1937.)

INTRACELLULAR SOLUTES DURING GROWTH

The potassium concentration in the ICW space of the muscle of the human embryo was found to be very high; in the newborn it appeared to be somewhat lower compared with the adult (Widdowson and Dickerson, 1964). The differences of intracellular potassium concentrations between newborn and adult animals are insignificant. Intracellular fluid volume and potassium content expressed per 100 g of fat-free dry matter (FFDM) decrease in a parallel manner in the rat during development, and intracellular potassium concentration remains practically unchanged (Fig. 6).

The high ICW volume (expressed per unit of FFDM in the newborn) is partially due to the low concentration of intracellular protein. It was calculated that the concentration of intracellular protein increases in muscle per kilogram of intracellular water during extrauterine growth from 32.2 g in the newborn to 44.4 g in the adult (Widdowson and Dickerson, 1964). Accordingly, the ratio mEq K/g protein-N in muscle tissue is higher in the newborn than in the adult. This ratio is of some importance for clinical investigations since it is used in balance experiments to calculate a loss or gain of intracellular potassium above or below the amount derived from protoplasmic catabolism or anabolism, respectively.

In summary, the main features of the maturational processes are a considerable decrease in TBW, ECW, and chloride content, a smaller decrease in sodium content, and an increase in potassium, nitrogen (protein), and fat contents; these are the main differences between the newborn and adult when compared on the basis of body weight. The main change in the composition of ECW is its increasing heterogeneity, as judged by the increasing difference between the chloride space

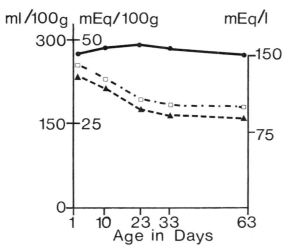

Fig. 6. Changes in intracellular fluid volume per 100 g fat-free dry matter (FFDM, dot dash line), in potassium content per 100 g FFDM (broken line), and in potassium concentration per liter intracellular water (solid line) during the development of the rat. Ordinate, left outside, ICW in ml/100g FFDM; left inside, potassium content in mEq/100g FFDM; right, potassium concentration. (Adapted from Jelinek., 1961.)

and the inulin space. Plasma potassium concentration shows a moderate decrease and total CO_2 a small increase.

The age-dependent difference in the exchangeable fraction of total sodium is due to the increasing amounts of sodium that are deposited in the bone crystalline structures. In ICW a considerable increase in intracellular protein concentration takes place, while no such differences seem to occur in the potassium concentration during postnatal development.

Body Fluid Homeostasis in the Newborn

OVERALL EFFICIENCY AND MATURATION PATTERNS OF HOMEOSTATIC DEFENSE MECHANISMS

Disturbances in the volume and composition of body fluids occur more frequently in infancy than at other ages. This is due partially to the high incidence of diseases which primarily endanger the body fluid homeostasis and partially to a less efficient defense mechanism. The latter can be illustrated by the observation that diets, such as milk evaporated to one quarter of its original volume, or salt- and protein-free food, produce extreme changes in the osmolarity and volume of the body fluids within a very short time. After the first challenge osmolarity of the

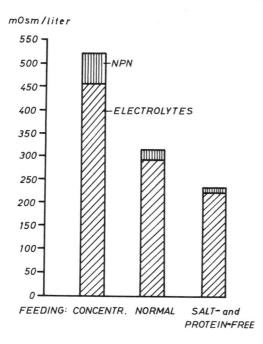

Fig. 7. Lability of osmotic regulation in plasma of 10-day-old puppies after feeding concentrated milk, normal diet, or a salt- and protein-free diet. (Adapted from Kerpel-Fronius, 1958.

blood plasma in puppies rose to 526 mOsm/liter; after the second it decreased to 232 mOsm/liter. Dehydration occurred in the first experiment while in the second an increase of the water content of all organs was observed (Fig. 7).

The newborn has a limited capacity to excrete a water, electrolyte, or hydrogen-ion load, a limited ability to produce a concentrated urine or to react to antidiuretic and aldosterone hormones, and a small glomerular filtration rate. In a stress situation the functional immaturity of these performances will be fully exposed. Serial studies of these functions during growth yield so-called maturation curves. These curves reveal that the various functions mature at quite individual rates and that a low initial performance does not allow one to predict the later speed of maturation. Figure 8 shows that the capacity to excrete a water load, which in the newborn is

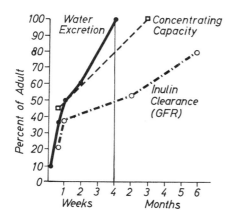

Fig. 8. Maturation of some renal functions. Data in percent of adult values. Water excretion according to Ames, 1953; GFR in the newborn from Strauss, 1965; remaining data from Kerpel-Fronius, 1959.

only 10 percent of that of adults, reaches maturity within 1 month, while the concentrating mechanism matures at 3 months and the glomerular filtration rate at 12 to 18 months of age (see also Ch. 21).

Such timetables of maturation may be of assistance to the clinician, since these data expose the weak points of the defense mechanisms in each age group.

WATER OUTPUT

RENAL WATER EXPENDITURE

The ability of the newborn to excrete excess water or to save water when the intake is low is less efficient than in the adult. Both maximum and minimum urine volumes are dependent on the amount of solutes that requires excretion by the kidneys. When the solute load is small, only a limited diuretic response to a water load is possible, while high solute loads increase the obligatory urine volume. The solute load is an inseparable determinant of renal water expenditure, and the latter is integrated with the infant's metabolic rate, nutritional state, and stage of development. The spectacular effects of nutrition and growth on water expenditure were demonstrated in experiments by the Cambridge group (McCance, 1961). Newborn puppies were fed with an amount of water equivalent to the water that their normal supply of milk contains. Without the milk solids no cell growth was possible, and the kidneys of these puppies were unable to excrete the water that was not incorporated into growing tissues.

Water retention causes dilutional hyponatremia, a condition that is not uncommon in early infancy. On the other hand, in fast growing animals, such as the piglet or the rabbit, a high fraction of electrolytes and nitrogen from food is incorporated into the structures of growing tissues. Assuming a failure of growth without a reduction in food intake, the totality of the molecules derived from food would burden the excretory mechanisms. We calculated from the data of Davies et al. (1964) that under such circumstances the osmolar load that requires excretion would be fourfold compared to that in the normally growing animal. Such an enormous solute load would either greatly increase urine volume and lead to dehydration, or, if entirely retained, increase NPN by 318 mg/100 ml. The way this problem is presented here is, of course, hypothetical and suitable only to point out the powerful homeostatic effect of growth.

In the slowly growing human premature the effect of the growth failure would be much smaller. Assuming a daily incorporation of 10 g of isotonic fluid and of 250 mg N/kg, the failure to thrive would increase the load to be excreted by 40 percent when cow's milk providing an intake of 4.4 g of protein (per kg in 24 hours) is fed. The load of solutes presented to the kidneys by feeding cow's milk is higher than the load in an equal amount of human breast milk. With an intake of 200 ml/kg/day the solute load in the first case is 60.9 mOsm/kg and in the second only 14.0 mOsm/kg (American Academy of Pediatrics, 1957).

The ability of the newborn to economize the renal water expenditure during hydropenia is a much discussed question. Until the recent observations of Edelman and Barnett (1960) it was axiomatic that the maximum concentration of the urine in young infants does not exceed 700 mOsm/liter, that is, about half of the value observed in adults. Low concentrating ability was attributed to a target organ insensitivity to antidiuretic hormone due to functional or anatomic immaturity. Newborn rats certainly do not respond to the injection of pitressin by raising the urine/plasma (U/P) ratio of inulin until the age of about 28 days, and the response to pitressin in the human newborn is also smaller than in the adult (Heller and Lederis, 1959).

The newborn infant, however, is able to respond to an injection of hypertonic saline with a decrease in urine flow rate and an increase in urinary osmolarity. Following the infusion of isotonic dextran the reverse changes consistent with ADH inhibition were observed (Fisher et al., 1963). Such observations indicate that the newborn has a certain potential for ADH release and renal response. It is interesting to note, however, that in spite of the application of stimuli known to mobilize ADH, antidiuretic activity in blood plasma can be detected only rarely during the first two months of life, while it is found regularly during the third month following the same stimuli (Martinek et al., 1963). Some new ideas on possible causes for the apparent immaturity of the concentrating mechanism of young infants were offered by Edelman and Barnett (1960). Assuming in terms of the countercurrent multiplier mechanism that the young infant may not achieve a satisfactory gradient of urea between cortex and papilla, the authors studied the effect of high-protein feeding on the ability to concentrate the urine. In fact, after an initial period of feeding 9 g protein/kg/day they observed during thirsting that a 25-day-old infant concentrated his urine up to 1,139 mOsm/liter. The effect of high-protein intake on the renal concentrating mechanism was enhanced by a low volume diet providing 115 ml water/kg/24 hours (Fig. 9).

Working with young and newborn rabbits Yaffe and Anders (1960) and Fleishaker et al. (1960) provided experimental evidence that the cortex-to-papilla gradient of urea is markedly different between hydropenic newborn and adult animals. The low urea content of the primary urine and of the papilla is due to

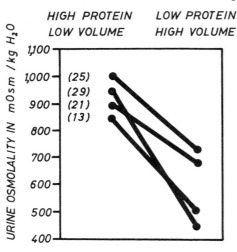

Fig. 9. Concentrating ability of young infants as influenced by various diets. High-protein diet provided 9 g protein, and low-protein diet 2.5 g protein per kg body weight per day. High-volume diet provided 220 ml and low-volume diet 115 ml per kg body weight per day. Numbers in parenthesis, age in days. (Adapted from Edelman and Barnett, 1960.

the large retention of nitrogen for growth. However, premature infants between one and three days of age were found to be unable to increase urinary osmolarity above 552 mOsm/liter after fasting, thirsting, or high-protein diet (Strauss, 1960). The author attributed this failure to achieve a higher concentration to the fact that the loop of Henle had not reached its mature length at that stage of development and thus impaired the efficient function of the countercurrent mechanism. Although it has to be admitted that the osmolarity in the urine of young infants can be raised to higher levels than previously thought, it must be emphasized that this increase can only be achieved by an amount of protein intake that is never used in practice.

In conclusion, it seems to be proven that the renal concentrating mechanism in infancy is dependent on nutritional and developmental factors.

EXTRARENAL WATER EXPENDITURE

Extrarenal water losses vary with total metabolic rate, food intake, motoric activity, ambient temperature, environmental humidity, and respiratory minute volume.

Under usual environmental conditions at rest the insensible perspiration reflects the level of the basal metabolic rate. According to the higher value of the latter in young infants, Levine et al. (1930) calculated a mean value of water loss by the skin and lungs of 1 g of water (kg/hour), that is, about twice as much as in adults. However, immediately after birth the mean extrarenal loss was found to be considerably lower—0.7 ml/kg/hour (Little et al., 1955). This finding is in concordance with recent data that oxygen consumption in the human infant is rather low immediately after birth and increases considerably during the first few days of life (Hill and Rahimtulla, 1965; Scopes, 1966; see also Ch. 16). High caloric feeding may double the insensible losses (De Rudder, 1928), and so does the rise in ambient temperature from 21°C to 34°C (American Academy of Pediatrics, 1957). According to Hungerland (1954) motoric activity increases insensible perspiration more in infants than in adults. During normal perspiration pulmonary water loss alone accounts for about one third of the total insensible loss, i.e., 0.35 ml/kg/hour (Hooper et al., 1954).

Hyperventilation increases pulmonary water loss to a great extent. In a severe case of primary hyperventilation Kerpel-Fronius (1959) measured a loss of 4.5 ml/kg/hour, that is, a more than tenfold increase above the basal value measured by Hooper et al. (1954). Pulmonary water loss may be almost completely prevented by keeping infants in an atmosphere of 100 percent relative humidity (O'Brien et al., 1954).

EFFECT OF WATER AND FOOD DEPRIVATION

The first challenge imposed on the body fluid homeostasis of the neonate, neglecting here early acidosis, is the low water intake. The weight loss of 5 to 6 percent of the initial body weight during the first few days of life is accompanied by the loss of some sodium, chloride, and potassium, but most probably it is due to the correction of initial overhydration and not to real dehydration (Fisher et al., 1963; Visser et al., 1964). Some additional arguments support this thesis. Cheek et al. (1961) made serial measurement of the bromide space in newborn infants. On the fifth day of life the weight loss reached its maximum of 50 g/kg, and the ECW loss was 20 ml/kg. The decrease of the ECW volume continued during the following days and reached 40 g/kg at about 10 days of age, at which time the weight loss was already restored. The comment of the authors seems to be justified in that with the acceleration of tissue growth, the loss of ECW is replaced by new tissue protein, ICW, and possibly some fat. Thus, the initial loss of some ECW and sodium appears to be part of the physiologic maturation in that the decrease of ECW proceeds most rapidly during the first 10 days of life and continues at a slower rate during early infancy.

In spite of an observed weight loss of 6 percent during the first three days of life, Fisher et al. (1963) found a mean urinary osmolarity of only 187 mOsm/kg. If this weight loss were due to dehydration, it would have been expected to stimulate the secretion of ADH with a subsequent rise of the urinary solute concentration. Most interesting observations on "neonatal hyperosmolarity" (Gautier, 1964; Davis et al., 1966) can be reconciled with the hypothesis (Fisher et al., 1963; Visser et al., 1964) that weight and ECW loss in *early fed infants* is mostly not due to dehydration in sensu stricti. Furthermore, we like to speculate that the rise in osmolarity that occurs during the first few days of life may in some cases be due to a correction of an initial hypotonic expansion of the ECW compartment. This assumption is supported by the fact that the mean value of maternal osmolarity and the corresponding osmolarity in cord blood in Gautier's (1964) material were rather low (280 mOsm/liter), while the osmolarity after 48 hours rose to about 294 mOsm/liter and was in correspondence with normal values of older infants. The same conclusions can be drawn if we scrutinize the changes in plasma osmolarity and in plasma sodium values found by Davis et al. (1966) during the first days of life in early fed, term infants (Fig. 10).

The range of variation of the initial values is 108 to 142 mEq/liter, and we suggest that some cases of transplacental hyponatremia must have been included in this material; 48 hours later the mean value reached 142 mEq/liter, with a range of 130 to 151, while at 168 hours of life, at a time when the ascending weight

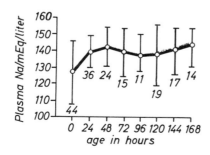

Fig. 10. Plasma sodium concentration in the normal human newborn. Mean of the normal and range of variation (± 2 S. D.) are shown. Numbers indicate the number of estimations on each day. (Adapted from Davis et al., 1966.)

curve excludes dehydration, plasma sodium is stabilized at a mean level of 140 mEq/liter, which is definitely higher than the initial value and is very close to the value found at 48 hours. Of course, it must be admitted that a number of the newborns in this series must have suffered from genuine hyperosmolarity probably due to low fluid intake in these cases. This hyperosmolarity might be due not only to hypernatremia but also to an increase of other blood constituents as pointed out by Davis et al. (1966). We also suggest that the increase observed in mean plasma osmolarity and in mean plasma sodium concentration results from a certain heterogeneity of the population studied, i.e., cases with transplacentally acquired hyponatremia, and some others with water depletion due to low fluid intake might have been included in the same group.

In term or premature infants, withholding of food and water results in a considerable increase in weight loss in excess of that noted in early fed infants. This dehydration is accompanied by hypernatremia. In term infants studied by Hansen and Smith (1953) the weight loss was 10 to 15 percent and in premature infants 14 to 19 percent of the initial weight after 72 hours of fasting and thirsting. In term infants the ensuing dehydration was not accompanied by a substantial increase in sodium excretion. In these cases it might be surmised that a rapidly progressing dehydration has stimulated the secretion of mineralocorticoids, which effected the tubular reabsorption of sodium in spite of a rising plasma sodium concentration. The same effect can be observed in adults during water deprivation that leads to dehydration of comparable severity. The response of the aldosterone secretion rate to a low-sodium diet, although smaller in the first days of life, was found to be normal between 8 and 15 days of age (Weldon et al., 1967). The assumption of Visser et al. (1964), that physiologic weight loss in early fed and *not* dehydrated infants will not stimulate the secretion of aldosterone during this period seems to be likely. Such an effect could be expected only in the case of the stimulus of a more severe water depletion. The important role of aldosterone in neonatal sodium homeostasis is supported by observations in infants with salt-losing syndrome due to adrenal hyperplasia. According to Visser et al. (1964) the onset of symptoms as late as the second week of life may be due to the fact that this is the age when the sodium balance should become positive in the normal infant. The delayed onset of renal salt excretion may also be associated with the initially very low GFR, which increases sharply during the first week of life.

Water depletion due to water deprivation proceeds at a faster rate in the newborn than in the adult. An apparently equal rate of loss was found only when body surface was used as a basis of comparison. Since the newborn's TBW content expressed per unit of surface area is, compared with that of the adult, very low, this basis of comparison leads to erroneous conclusions with regard to the magnitude of water loss (Fig. 11).

Equal losses of, for instance, 5 liters referred to the body surface of the adult turn out to be of a very different order of magnitude if it is calculated in percent of individual total water content. The premature would lose about one third, the newborn more than one quarter of his total body water, but an adult person would lose only 10 percent of his total water.

Dehydration due to water deprivation occurs faster in infants than in adults since

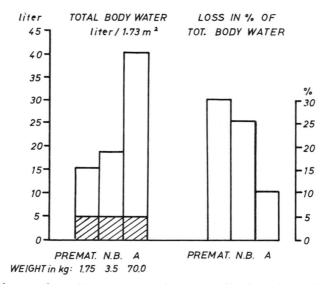

Fig. 11. Significance of equal losses expressed per unit of body surface. NB, newborn; A, adult. Water loss ▨ = 5 liter/1.73 m². (Adapted from Kerpel-Fronius, 1958.)

water reserves in the former are low in relation to the metabolic rate and consequently to obligatory urine volume and to dermal and pulmonal losses of water. Talbot and Richie (1958) calculated that infants develop a similarly serious degree of water depletion within one and a half days as adults do in the course of five days of thirsting.

EFFECT OF ELECTROLYTE LOADS

In the case of a salt load the adjustment of output and intake will require a time interval during which retention will ensue. This retention after a salt load is greater in newborn infants than in adults. Gamble et al. (1951) found in older infants that the accumulation of surplus electrolytes in the body continued through almost eight days and amounted to about 15 percent of the initial body content of electrolytes.

McCance and Widdowson (1957) observed that under certain conditions the relation of sodium to water intake may be such that a hypertonic expansion of extracellular fluid ensues. According to those authors: "Hypertonic expansion of the extracellular fluid must take place: (1) An intake of sodium chloride greater than excreted by the kidneys; (2) An intake of water greater than that required to maintain the normal volume of extracellular fluid, but insufficient to meet the amounts being excreted by all channels and the maintenance of a normal internal concentration of electrolytes." The authors observed this type of disturbance in piglets fed with evaporated cow's milk, which contained more sodium chloride than sow's milk; furthermore, in piglets and in premature infants fed with a rather large addition of sodium chloride to their milk mixture. The sodium concentration of the blood plasma rose, and there was an increase in body weight. Most probably an intracellular dehydration must accompany the rise in extracellular sodium concentration. McCance and Widdowson (1963) also studied the excretion of sodium chloride and of sodium and potassium bicarbonate loads in newborn piglets. During the 40 hours of the experiment the sodium was not excreted when administered as chloride, and sodium retention was accompanied by water retention. If the sodium was given as bicarbonate, about half of the sodium was excreted; however, hypokalemia, hypochloremia, and severe alkalosis ensued. More than 90 percent of the potassium was excreted, together with a great amount of sodium and chloride. The observed disturbances in homeostasis were dehydration, hyperkalemia, and moderate alkalosis.

Potassium is readily excreted by prematures; however, a higher intake increases the plasma potassium concentration. This was found to be directly correlated with the potassium intake (Keitel, 1959).

EFFECTS OF DIET ON BODY COMPOSITION

The question of whether body composition can be changed by varying the intake of electrolytes is still under discussion. In prolonged balance experiments Rominger et al. (1929) found a considerably larger retention of electrolytes in infants fed cow's milk than in those fed human milk, which has a considerably lower ash content. The retention of sodium per kg of retained water also appeared to be higher. However, Wallace et al. (1958) were skeptical about the validity of data obtained in long-term balance experiments. They point to the inherent errors of this method, "The errors in doing a balance are not randomly plus or minus, but systematically positive. The higher the intake of a constituent the greater the apparent retention; eventually absurd artifacts may result." According to these authors, the determination of the composition of the whole body by direct chemical analysis is the more reliable method of approach to characterize the effects of high- and low-mineral intakes. Applying this method in weanling rats, Wallace et al. (1958) found that the composition of the fat-free bodies per unit of weight was essentially the same, that is, independent of the variations of intake. Differences were found to occur only in the amounts of skeletal constituents and in fat. In conclusion, the intracellular electrolytes cannot be changed except by feeding of extreme diets. However, Widdowson (1958) showed that variations in food intake during the *early suckling* period can accelerate the chemical maturation of the tissues in terms of an earlier replacement of certain amounts of the extracellular fluid by protein and intracellular fluid. Forbes (1962) discussed the same problem in an excellent review and emphasized the importance of the reference basis for expressing electrolyte composition. He promoted the thesis that with the exception of fat and calcium no striking differences in the percentage composition can be produced by diet. Differences may be noted, however, when values are expressed on a per animal basis. Animals fed with a high-protein and electrolyte diet may become larger, and thus, accumulate more protein and solids over a period of time than if they were fed a diet that contained less of these constituents.

EFFECT OF HYDROGEN ION LOADS

THE INFLUENCE OF FOOD AND GROWTH ON ACID EXCRETION

McCance and Widdowson (1960) emphasize in their work on natural development of acid-base control in the newly born that the results of such studies are "in keeping with what is known about the integration of food, growth and renal function in maintaining the stability of the internal environment in the first day of life." Data assembled in Table 10 bear on some of these points.

In all age groups the hydrogen ion excretion of breast-fed infants is less than that of infants fed cow's milk. Under the stimulus of the higher acid load generated by cow's milk feeding the one-week-old newborn infant, and to a lesser degree even the premature infant, is capable of increasing hydrogen ion excretion above the level observed in the breast-fed term infant. The lower phosphate excretion of the breast-fed infant accounts for the higher percentage of hydrogen ions excreted as ammonium salt as compared with infants of all age groups fed cow's milk.

The renal defense response to induced acidosis was compared in studies with a seven-day-old newborn term infant and an adult person by administering a single dose of an acidifying drug (Hatemi and McCance, 1961). The percentage of the hydrogen ions that were excreted by the newborn within eight hours after the administration of 54 mEq NH_4Cl per m^2 was about one fifth of that excreted by the adult. The hydrogen ion clearance index was calculated from the hydrogen

TABLE 10.   Acid Excretion in Full-Term Newborns, a Prematurely Born Infant, Older Infants, and Adults

Age	pH	Averages of titratable acidity + ammonia	Percentage of titratable acidity + NH4 excreted as NH4	Sources
Full term, day 1	6.4	0.76 mEq/kg/24 hr	76	McCance and Widdowson (1960)
Full term, day 7 (breast fed)	6.2	0.71 mEq/kg/24 hr	82	
Full term, day 7 (on cow's milk)	5.9	1.73 mEq/kg/24 hr	42	
1.5 kg, premature, day 7 (on cow's milk	6.2	0.96 mEq/kg/24 hr	44	Kerpel-Fronius et al. (1970)
2-6 months, infants (breast fed)	6.4	10.0 (m^2/12 hr)[a]	70	Fomon et al. (1959)
2-6 months, infants (on cow's milk)	5.3	58.0 (m^2/12 hr)[a]	45	
Adult	5.8	1.44 mEq/kg/24 hr	56	

[a] Averages per m^2/12 hr.

ion excretion and the carbon dioxide content in the blood plasma (Elkinton et al., 1960) and was found to be considerably lower; it was 0.35 in newborns against 1.70 in the adult. The ability to deal with such a stress of an acid load, as assessed by the value of the hydrogen ion clearance index, seems to mature at a fast rate, since adult levels were achieved within three months (Peonides et al., 1965). Although the newborn term infant fails to excrete hydrogen ions as rapidly as adults following an acute acid load, he is fully capable of maintaining an average pH value of 7.41, with a range of variation of only 7.35 to 7.46, and a total carbon dioxide content of 21 mEq/liter, with a range between 16.0 and 22.4 mEq/liter (Graham et al., 1951). The corresponding values for adult controls (Graham et al., 1951) are pH 7.42 (range: 7.38 to 7.44) and total carbon dioxide content 24 mEq/liter (range 21.4 to 26.4 mEq/liter). Most premature infants, in contrast to healthy, full-term newborns, fail to achieve such adjustment. As known since the pioneer work of Ylppö (1916), many infants with low birth-weight exhibit abnormalities in their parameters which define the acid-base balance. Not counting pathologic conditions which occur mostly within the first few days of life, a number of apparently healthy prematures exhibited a range of variation in blood pH extending from 7.19 to 7.53 until the third or fourth week of life (Reardon et al., 1950; Blystad, 1956; Goldman et al., 1961; Chernick et al., 1964; Kildeberg, 1964; Kerpel-Fronius et al., 1964; Ballabriga, 1965; Bucci et al., 1965; Ungari et al., 1965; Ranlow and Siggaard-Andersen, 1965; Shain et al., 1967). In spite of the fact that most of these infants were acidotic when judged by adult standards, they appeared to be normal when judged by clinical appraisal. Following the description of Ranlow and Siggaard-Andersen (1965) the characteristic course of acidosis in these infants is the following: After initial acidosis during the first few hours of life, the pH and base excess values are stabilized at a level which is similar to the low normal level of adults. After the third day of life, the level of base excess indicates an increasing acidosis which reaches its maximum during the second week of life. For this type of acidosis Kildeberg (1964) coined the term "late metabolic acidosis."

The incidence of late metabolic acidosis is high. Shain et al. (1967) found in 33 percent of their infants with birth weights below 2,500 g a blood pH below 7.29, and Ranlow and Siggaard-Andersen (1965) measured a base excess below -5 mEq/liter in 11 out of 12 infants with birth weights below 1,750 g.

Acidosis results from the interaction of many factors. The acidogenic type of diet, the slowing down of growth, a certain sluggishness in the respiratory response to acidosis, and the limited capacity of the kidneys to excrete hydrogen ions are believed to be of importance for the formation of acidosis. The young premature infant is certainly handicapped in his defense against acidosis by a deficiency of the renal function. Net acid excretion at low levels of total CO_2 in blood was found to be considerably lower in premature than in older infants (Kerpel-Fronius et al., 1970).

These observations are suggestive of a maturation of the capacity to excrete hydrogen ions; late metabolic acidosis appears at an age when this function is small and it disappears spontaneously with its improvement. In accordance with this opinion is the observation of Rubin et al. (1961) that premature infants at four weeks of age, following a prolonged loading with $CaCl_2$, excrete less ammonium salts per kg body weight than six- to eight-week-old infants; there was also a considerable difference in the hydrogen ion clearance indices.

A certain sluggishness of respiratory compensation may play a contributory role in the genesis of acidosis. It appears that relatively slight changes in base deficit do not elicit consistent respiratory responses in young premature infants. However, with increasing stimulation and with base excess values below -10.0 mEq/liter, the effort for respiratory compensation in premature infants of two weeks of age is already comparable with the regulatory mechanisms observed in older infants (Kerpel-Fronius and Heim, 1964).

Since the extent of metabolic acid production may also vary with the rate of growth, it was assumed that failure of growth by increasing the hydrogen ion load imposed on the kidneys would be a contributory factor in the origin of late metabolic acidosis. According to recent balance experiments by Kildeberg (1968, 1969), however, the growth of the skeleton, i.e. the apposition of bone minerals, increases hydrogen ion production. It may, thus, be assumed that failure of growth, frequently observed in young acidotic premature infants, results at least in two opposite effects: the smaller apposition of protoplasmic tissue increases, while inhibited skeletal growth decreases metabolic acid production.

Conclusions

The volume and the composition of fetal fluids are regulated by the integrated functions of the placenta, the fetal and maternal kidneys, the fetal lung and gut, and the fetal anabolic metabolism. Changes in the volume and composition of the maternal fluids, maternal acidosis, dehydration, or hyper- or hypoosmolarity affect and may eventually damage the fetus. Potassium deficiency of the mother, however, does not decrease fetal plasma potassium nor the total body potassium of the fetus. Body composition changes during pre-and postnatal growth. The main factors of this maturation are the decrease in extracellular fluid volume and the increase in cell fluid, cell protein, and fat content of the body. The protein content of the intracellular fluid increases during growth, while the intracellular potassium concentration does not change significantly during extrauterine growth.

In spite of marked functional and compositional differences between adults and newborns, these factors are well balanced in each age group. The defense mechanism of the newborn is fully capable of meeting normal demands. However, under stress conditions the fragility and instability of the system for maintaining body fluid homeostasis is exposed.

The ability of the newborn to excrete excess water or to save water when the intake is low is less efficient than that of the adult, and in the case of salt loads the adjustment of output to intake is sluggish. Hypertonic expansion of extracellular fluid is frequently observed. Variations in food intake during the early suckling period can accelerate the chemical maturation of the soft tissues only in terms of an earlier replacement of certain amounts of ECW by protein and ICW, while intracellular electrolytes remain unchanged.

Premature infants exhibit a conspicuous tendency to late metabolic acidosis during the second week of life.

REFERENCES

Acharya, P. T., and W. W. Payne. 1965. Blood chemistry of normal full-term infants in the first 48 hours of life. Arch. Dis. Child., 40:430-441.

Adams, F. H., T. Fujiwara, and S. Rowshan. 1963a. The nature and origin of the fluid in the fetal lamb lung. J. Pediat., 63:881-888.

———— A. J. Moss, and L. Fagan. 1963b. The tracheal fluid in the fetal lamb. Biol. Neonat., 5:151-158.

Adolph, E. F. 1967. Ontogeny of volume regulations in embryonic extracellular fluids. Quart. Rev. Biol., 42:1-38.

Alexander, D. P., and D. A. Nixon. 1961. The fetal kidney. Brit. Med. Bull., 17:112-117.

———— D. A. Nixon, W. F. Widdas, and F. X. Wohlzogen. 1958. Renal function in the sheep foetus. J. Physiol. (London), 140:14-22.

Altstatt, L. B. 1965. Transplacental hyponatremia in the newborn infant. J. Pediat., 66:985-988.

American Academy of Pediatrics. 1957. Report, Committee on Nutrition: Water requirement in relation to osmolar load as it applies to infant feeding. Pediatrics, 19:339-341.

Ames, R. G. 1953. Urinary water excretion and neurohypophyseal function of full term and premature infants shortly after birth. Pediatrics, 12:272-282.

Anast, C. S. 1964. Serum magnesium levels in the newborn. Pediatrics, 33:969-974.

Bain, A. D., and J. S. Scott. 1960. Renal agenesis and severe urinary tract dysplasia. A review of 50 cases with particular reference to the associated anomalies. Brit. Med. J., 1:841-846.

Ballabriga, A. 1965. Study of the acid-base balance of the premature infant during various diets. Helv. Paediat. Acta, 20:527-543.

Battaglia, F., et al. 1960. Fetal blood studies. XIII. The effect of administration of fluids intravenously to mothers upon the concentration of water and electrolytes in plasma of human fetuses. Pediatrics, 25:2-10.

Blystad. W. 1956. Blood gas determinations on premature infants. I. Investigations of premature infants without respiratory complications. Acta Paediat., 45:13-23.

Bucci, G., A. Scalamandre, P. G. Savignoni, and M. Mendicini. 1965. Acid-base status of normal premature infants in the first week of life. Biol. Neonat., 8:81-103.

Burns, P. D., R. O. Linder, V. E. Drose, and F. Battaglia. 1963. The placental transfer of water from fetus to mother following the intravenous infusion of hypertonic annitol to the maternal rabbit. Amer. J. Obstet. Gynec., 86:160-167.

———— et al. 1964. Effects of osmotic gradients across the primate placenta upon fetal and placental water contents. Pediatrics, 34:407-411.

Camerer, W., and Söldner. 1900. Die chemische Zusammensetzung des Neugeborenen. Z. Biol., 39:173-192.

Cheek, D. B. 1954. Observations on total body chloride in children. Pediatrics, 14:5-10.

————— 1961. Extracellular volume: Its structure and measurement and the influence of age and disease. J. Pediat., 58:103-125.

————— T. G. Maddison, M. Malinek, and J. H. Coldbeck. 1961. Further observations on the corrected bromide space of the neonate and investigation of water and electrolyte status in infants born of diabetic mothers. Pediatrics, 21:861-869.

Chernick, V. F. Heldrich, and M. E. Avery. 1964. Periodic breathing of premature infants. J. Pediat., 64:330-341.

Clapp, W. M., L. J. Butterfield, and D. O'Brien. 1962. Body water compartments in the premature infant with special reference to the effects of the respiratory distress syndrome and of maternal diabetes and toxemia. Pediatrics, 29:883-889.

Corsa, L., Jr., D. Gribetz, C. D. Cook, and N. B. Talbot. 1956. Total body exchangeable water, sodium, potassium in "hospital normal" infants and children. Pediatrics, 17:184-191.

————— et al. 1950. The measurement of exchangeable potassium in man by isotope dilution. J. Clin. Invest., 29:1280-1295.

Crawford, J. S. 1965. Maternal and cord blood at delivery. IV. Glucose, sodium, potassium, calcium and chloride. Biol. Neonat., 8:222-237.

Davies, J. S., E. M. Widdowson, and R. A. McCance. 1964. The intake of milk and the retention of its constituents while the newborn rabbit doubles its weight. Brit. J. Nutr., 18:385-392.

Davis, J. A., D. R. Harvey, and J. F. Stevens. 1966. Osmolality as a measure of dehydration in the neonatal period. Arch. Dis. Child., 41:448-450.

De Rudder, B. 1928. Die Perspiratio insensibilis beim Säugling. II. Ihre Abhängigkeit von der Calorienzufuhr. Z. Kinderheilk., 46:384-390.

Dunning, M. F., J. M. Steele, and A. Y. Bergen. 1951. The measurement of total body chloride. Proc. Soc. Exp. Biol. Med., 77:854-858.

Economou-Mavrou, C., and R.A. McCance. 1958. Calcium, magnesium and phosphorus in foetal tissues. Biochem. J., 68:573-580.

Edelman, C. M., Jr., and H. L. Barnett. 1960. Role of the kidney in water metabolism in young infants. J. Pediat., 56:154-179.

Elkinton, J. R., E. J. Nuth, G. D. Webster, and R. A. McCance. 1960. The renal excretion of hydrogen ion in renal tubular acidosis. I. Quantitative assessment of the response to ammonium chloride as an acid load. Amer. J. Med., 29:554-575.

Fink, C. W., and D. B. Cheek. 1960. The corrected bromide space [extracellular volume] in the newborn. Pediatrics, 26:397-401.

Fisher, D. A., et al. 1963. Control of water balance in the newborn. Amer. J. Dis. Child., 106:137-146.

Fleishaker, G. H., O. J. Gesink, and W. W. McCrory. 1960. Effect of age on distribution of urea and electrolyte in kidneys of young rabbits. Amer. J. Dis. Child., 100:558.

Fomon, S. J., D. M. Harris, and R. L. Jensen. 1959. Acidification of the urine by infants fed human milk and whole cow's milk. Pediatrics, 23:113-120.

Forbes, G. B. 1962. Methods for determining composition of the human body: With a note on the effect of diet on body composition. Pediatrics, 29:477-494.

————— and A. M. Lewis. 1956. Total sodium, potassium and chloride in adult man. J. Clin. Invest., 35:596-600.

————— G. L. Mizner, and A. Lewis. 1957. Effect of age on radiosodium exchange in bone [rat]. Amer. J. Physiol., 190:152-156.

Friis-Hansen, B. 1961. Body water compartments in children: Changes during growth and related changes in body composition. Pediatrics, 28:169-181.

Gamble, J. L. 1956. Personal communication.

———— et al. 1951. Effects of large loads of electrolytes. Pediatrics, 7:305-320.

Gautier, E. 1964. Neonatal hyperosmolarity, an instance of unresponsiveness to anti-diuretic hormone. *In* Jonxis, J. H. P., H. K. A. Visser, and J. A. Troelstra, ed. The Adaptation of the Newborn Infant to Extra-uterine Life. Leiden, H. E. Stenfert Kroese, pp. 83-94.

Goldman, H. G., et al. 1961. Acidosis in premature infants due to lactic acid. Pediatrics, 27:921-931.

Graham, B. D., et al. 1951. Development of neonatal electrolyte homeostasis. Pediatrics, 8:68-78.

Hansen, J. D. L., and C. A. Smith. 1953. Effects of withholding fluid intake in immediate postnatal period. Pediatrics, 12:99-113.

Hatemi, N., and R. A. McCance. 1961. Renal aspects of acid-base control in the newly born. III. Response to acidifying drugs. Acta Paediat. Scand., 50:603-616.

Heller, H., and K. Lederis. 1959. Maturation of the hypothalamoneurohypophysial system. J. Physiol. (London), 147:299-314.

Hill, J., and K. A. Rahimtulla. 1965. Heat balance and the metabolic rate of newborn babies in relation to environmental temperature; and the effect of age and of weight on basal metabolic rate. J. Physiol. (London), 180:239-265.

Hooper, J. M. D., I. W. Y. Evans, and T. Stapleton. 1954. Resting pulmonary water loss in the newborn infant. Pediatrics, 13:206-210.

Hungerland, H. 1954. Wasserhaushalt. *In* Brock, J., ed. Biologische Daten für den Kinderarzt, 2nd ed. Berlin, Springer-Verlag, pp. 480-542.

Iob, V., and W. W. Swanson. 1934. Mineral growth of the human fetus. Amer. J. Dis. Child., 47:302-306.

Jelinek, J. 1961. Changes in water and electrolyte distribution in the body of rats during development. *In* The Development of Homeostasis. Prague. Publishing House of the Czechoslovak Academy of Sciences, pp. 267-278.

Keitel, H. G. 1959. The concentration of potassium in the plasma. Amer. J. Dis. Child., 97:583-590.

Kerpel-Fronius, E. 1937. Über die Besonderheiten der Salz-und Wasserverteilung im Säuglingskörper. Z. Kinderheilk., 58:726-738.

———— 1958. Clinical consequences of the water and electrolyte metabolism peculiar to infancy. *In* Wolstenholme, G. E. W., and M. O'Connor, ed. CIBA Foundation Colloquia on Aging. London, Churchill, Ltd. Vol. 4.

———— 1959. Pathologie und Klinik des Salz-und Wasserhaushaltes. Budapest, Publishing House, Hungarian Academy of Sciences.

———— and T. Heim. 1964. Efficiency of respiratory compensation for metabolic acidosis in premature infants. Biol. Neonat., 7:203-213.

———— T. Heim, and E. Sulyok. 1970. The development of the renal acidifying processes and their relation to acidosis in low-birth-weight infants. Biol. Neonat., 15:267-278.

———— L. Nagy, and B. Magyarka. 1964. Volume and composition of fluid compartments in peripheral and cardiac muscles of animals born at different stages of maturity. Biol. Neonat., 6:177-196.

Kildeberg, P. 1964. Disturbances of hydrogen ion balance occurring in premature infants. II. Late metabolic acidosis. Acta Paediat. Scand., 53:517-526.

———— 1968. Clinical Acid-Base Physiology. Studies in neonates, infants, and young children. Copenhagen, Munksgaard.

———— K. Engel, and R. W. Winters. 1969. Balance of net acid in growing infants. Acta Paediat. Scand., 58:321-329.

Kubli, F. 1966. Fetale Gefahrenzustände und ihre Diagnose. Stuttgart, Thieme.

Levine, S. Z., M. Kelly, and J. R. Wilson. 1930. Insensible perspiration in infancy and childhood. II. Proposed standards for infants. Amer. J. Dis. Child., 39: 917-929.

Little, J. A., W. A. Brodszky, and R. Greathouse. 1955. The insensible weight loss of newborns and of older infants. Amer. J. Dis. Child., 90:630-631.

MacGillivray, I., and T. J. Buchanan. 1958. Total exchangeable sodium and potassium in nonpregnant women and in normal and preeclamptic pregnancy. Lancet, 2:1090-1093.

Martinek, J., M. Janovsky, and V. Stanincova. 1963. Concentration mechanism in young infants. Excerpta Medica International Congress Series No. 78:647-652.

McCance, R. A. 1961. Mineral metabolism of the fetus and the newborn. Brit. Med. Bull., 17:132-136.

———— and E. M. Widdowson. 1957. Hypertonic expansion of the extracellular fluids. Acta Paediat. Scand., 46:337-353.

———— and E. M. Widdowson. 1960. Renal aspects of acid base control in the newly born. I. Natural development. Acta Paediat. Scand., 49:409-414.

———— and E. M. Widdowson. 1963. The effect of administering sodium chloride, sodium bicarbonate, and potassium bicarbonate to newly-born piglets. J. Physiol. (London), 165:569-574.

Meschia, G. F. C., F. Battaglia, and D. H. Barron. 1957. A comparison of the freezing points of fetal and maternal plasmas of sheep and goat. Quart. J. Exp. Physiol., 42:163-170.

Moya, F., V. Apgar, L. St. James, and C. Berrien. 1960. Hydramnios and congenital anomalies. J.A.M.A., 173:1552-1556.

Nicolopoulos, D. A., and C. A. Smith. 1961. Metabolic aspects of idiopathic respiratory distress (hyaline membrane syndrome) in newborn infants. Pediatrics, 28:206-222.

O'Brien, D., J. D. L. Hansen, and C. A. Smith. 1954. Effect of supersaturated atmospheres on insensible water loss in the newborn infant. Pediatrics, 13:126-132.

Oliver, F. K., Jr., J. A. Dennis, and G. D. Bates. 1961. Serial blood-gas tensions and acid-base balance during the first hour of life in human infants. Acta Paediat. Scand., 50:346-360.

Parker, H. W., K. H. Olesen, J. McMurrey, and B. Friis-Hansen. 1958. Body water compartments throughout the life span. In Wolstenholme, G. E. W., and U. O'Connor, ed. CIBA Foundation Colloquia on Aging. London, Churchill, Ltd. Vol. 4.

Peonides, A., B. Levin, and W. F. Young. 1965. The renal excretion of hydrogen ions in infants and children. Arch. Dis. Child., 40:33-39.

Phillips, G. D., and S. K. Sundaram. 1966. Sodium depletion of pregnant ewes and its effect on foetuses and foetal fluids. J. Physiol. (London), 184:889-897.

Pincus, J. G., I. F. Gittleman, M. Saito, and A. E. Sobel. 1956. A study of the plasma values of sodium, potassium, chloride, CO_2-tension, sugar, urea, the protein base-binding power, pH and hematocrit in prematures on the first day of life. Pediatrics, 18:39-49.

Plentl, A. A. 1959. The dynamics of amniotic fluid. Ann. N. Y. Acad. Sci., 75: 746-761.

Ranlow, P., and O. Siggaard-Andersen. 1965. Late metabolic acidosis in premature infants. Acta Paediat. Scand., 54:531-540.

Reardon, H. S., et al. 1950. Studies of acid-base equilibrium in premature infants. Pediatrics, 6:753.

Rominger, E., H. Berger, and E. Meier. 1929. Klinisch-experimentelle Untersuchungen zwischen Wasser und Kochsalz beim gesunden Säugling. Z. Kinderheilk., 48: 43-66.

Ruben, B. L., P. L. Calcagno, M. I. Rubin, and D. H. Weintraub. 1956. Renal defense response to induced acidosis in premature infants:Ammonia production and titratable acid excretion. Amer. J. Dis. Child., 92:513.

Rubin, M. I., P. L. Calcagno, and B. L. Ruben. 1961. Renal excretion of hydrogen ions: A defense against acidosis in premature infants. J. Pediat., 59:848-860.

Saling, E. 1966. Das Kind in der Geburtshilfe. Stuttgart, Thieme.

Schain, R. J., and K. O. O'Brien. 1957. Longitudinal studies of acid-base status in infants with low birth weight. J. Pediat., 70:885-890.

Scopes, J. W. 1966. Metabolic rate and temperature in the human baby. Brit. Med. Bull., 22:88-91.

Scott, J. S., and L. K. Wilson. 1957. Hydramnios as an early sign of oesophageal atresia. Lancet, 2:569-572.

Seeds, A. E., Jr. 1965. Water metabolism of the fetus. Amer. J. Obstet. Gynec., 92: 727-745.

Serrano, C. V., L. M. Talbert, and L. G. Welt. 1964. Potassium deficiency in the pregnant dog. J. Clin. Invest., 43:27-31.

Strauss, J. 1960. Urinary concentration in newborn premature infants. Amer. J. Dis. Child., 100:635.

——— K. Adamsons, Jr., and L. S. James. 1965. Renal function of normal full-term infants in the first hours of extrauterine life. I. Infants delivered naturally and given a placental transfusion. Amer. J. Obstet. Gynec., 91:286-290.

Talbot, N. B., and R. Richie. 1958. The effect of age on the body's tolerance for fasting, thirsting and for overloading with water and certain electrolytes. In Wolstenholme, G. E. W., and U. O'Connor, ed. CIBA Foundation Colloquia on Aging. London, Churchill, Ltd. Vol. 4, pp. 139-149.

Ungari, S., A. Donath, E. Rossi, and R. Tobler. 1965. The influence of the acidification of the milk on the acid-base balance of prematures. Z. Kinderheilk., 92:105-112.

Visser, H. K. A., H. J. Degenhart, W. S. Cost, and W. Croughs. 1964. Adrenocortical control of renal sodium and potassium excretion in the newborn period. In Jonxis, J. H. P., H. K. A. Visser, and J. A. Troelstra, eds. Nutricia Symposium on The Adaptation of the Newborn Infant to Extra-uterine Life. Leiden, H. E. Stenfert Kroese, pp. 45-123.

Wallace, W. W., W. B. Weil, and A. Taylor. 1958. Effect of variable protein and mineral intake upon the body composition of the growing animal. In Wolstenholme, G. E. W., and M. O'Connor, eds. CIBA Foundation Colloquia on Aging. London, Churchill, Ltd. Vol. 4.

Weldon, V. V., A. Kowalski, and C. J. Migeon. 1967. Aldosterone secretion rates in normal subjects from infancy to adulthood. Pediatrics, 39:713-723.

Westin, B., et al. 1959. Some constituents of umbilical venous blood of previable fetuses. Acta Paediat. Scand., 48:609-613.

Widdowson, E. M. 1958. Discussion. In Wolstenholme, G. E. W., and M. O'Connor, eds. CIBA Foundation Colloquia on Aging. London, Churchill, Ltd. Vol. 4, p. 136.

———— and J. W. T. Dickerson.   1960.   The effect of growth and function on the chemical composition of soft tissues.   Biochem. J., 77:30-43.

———— and J. W. T. Dickerson.   1964.   Chemical composition of the body.   *In* Connor, C. F., and F. Bronner, ed.   Mineral Metabolism.   New York, London, Academic Press, Inc., Vol. 2, Part A.

———— and R. A. McCance.   1956.   The effect of development on the composition of the serum and extracellular fluid.   Clin. Sci., 15:361-371.

Wright, G. H., and D. A. Nixon.   1961.   Absorption of amniotic fluid in the gut of foetal sheep.   Nature (London), 190:816.

Yaffe, S. J., and T. F. Anders.   1960.   Renal solute content in young rabbits.   Amer. J. Dis. Child., 100:558-559.

Yllpö, A.   1916.   Neugeborene, Hunger und Intoxicationsacidosis in ihren Beziehungen zueinander.   Z. Kinderheilk., 14:268.

21

Physiology of the Perinatal Kidney

LEONARD I. KLEINMAN ● **Departments of Pediatrics, Physiology, and Environmental Health, University of Cincinnati College of Medicine, Ohio**

Introduction

In the mammalian kidney urine is formed by ultrafiltration of plasma through the glomerulus and by alteration of this filtrate by the renal tubules. The principles of glomerular and tubular function are basically similar in the perinatal and adult animal. In this chapter perinatal renal function will be discussed in terms of these basic principles. Further, emphasis will be placed on comparison of renal function between the adult and perinatal animal. An attempt will be made not only to describe the similarities and differences between the adult and the perinate but to explain them in terms of modern concepts of renal physiology.

Embryology of the Mammalian Kidney

The kidneys of most vertebrates develop through three successive but overlapping stages—the pronephros, the mesonephros, and the metanephros. The functional significance of the three stages of renal development is not the same in all animals. The mesonephros, for example, is a functional organ in cattle, sheep, pigs, cats, opossum, and rabbits (McCance, 1962; Smith, 1951). In rodents and man, on the other hand, the mesonephros never becomes functional. Moreover, the mesonephros persists for varying periods of time in different mammalian species. In the pig degeneration occurs in the first half of gestation, whereas in the rabbit degeneration takes place in the second half.

The definitive mammalian kidney, the metanephros, develops from the union of the cranial part of the ureteral bud with the metanephric blastema. The ureteral bud arises from an offshoot of the mesonephric duct and ultimately forms the ureters, renal pelves, major and minor calyces, and collecting ducts. The nephroblastic cells of the metanephric blastema, upon contact with the ureteral bud, eventually develop into the glomerulus, proximal convoluted tubule, loop of Henle, and distal convoluted tubule.

The development of the glomerular capillary tuft has been a subject of considerable controversy in recent years. Vernier and Birch-Andersen (1962) suggest that glomerular capillaries form in situ in the endothelial cell mass of the metanephric blastema rather than from an ingrowth of capillaries from afferent arterioles. Branches of the afferent arterioles then connect with capillaries formed in the glomerulus to establish continuity of the circulation. Potter (1965), on the other hand, presents evidence that the capillaries of the glomeruli originate as direct outgrowths from adjacent vessels, and the cells they contain come from the general circulation. The glomerular capillaries do not originate in situ, but once they have infiltrated into the metanephric blastema they continue to grow and differentiate in this area.

The first glomeruli to develop are those which will be found in the juxtamedullary region of the mature kidney. Potter (1965) has shown that at 22 weeks' gestation all the glomeruli in the human fetus are juxtamedullary glomeruli. Since glomerular development starts in the juxtamedullary region and progresses toward the capsule, at any time during development there is a greater percentage of mature nephrons in the juxtamedullary region than there is in the outer cortex.

In *man* the number of nephrons increases continually from 6 weeks' gestation (origin of the metanephros) until 36 weeks' gestation. From then until about 12 years of age growth of the kidney consists of maturation of those nephrons already present (MacDonald and Emery, 1959). In the rat, glomerular differentiation is not complete before birth and continues until the second or third month of life (Arataki, 1926).

There is abundant evidence that glomeruli and tubules of various species are functioning early in gestation. Cameron and Chambers (1938) demonstrated secretion of phenol red by a 3.5-month-old human fetus. Fetal lambs demonstrate both glomerular and tubular function by 60 days' gestation (term at about 145 days) (Alexander and Nixon, 1963). Fetal pigs have been observed to excrete urine as early as at 44 days' gestation (total gestation time is 120 days) (Perry and Stanier, 1962).

In those animals with a functional allantoic sac the fetal urine first passes into the allantois and later (during gestation) passes into the amniotic sac. In rodent and man the urine always passes into the amnion (McCance, 1962). It should be emphasized that the composition of the allantoic fluid of the fetal rabbit and pig is altered by the chorioallantoic membrane (McCance and Stanier, 1960; Crawford and McCance, 1960). Thus, the fluid found in the allantoic sac is not necessarily the same as that excreted by the kidney.

Glomerular Function

PHYSIOLOGIC PRINCIPLES OF GLOMERULAR FILTRATION

The glomerular filtration rate (GFR) is a function of certain forces which act on the plasma in the glomerular capillaries. These forces can be summarized as follows for uncharged particles:

(1) $$GFR = K_F(\Delta P - \bar{\pi})$$

K_F is the filtration coefficient, ΔP is the hydrostatic pressure difference between the glomerular capillary and capsular space, and $\bar{\pi}$ is the mean colloid osmotic pressure of the plasma in the glomerular capillary.

K_F is a function of the permeability of the walls of the glomerulus as well as of the surface area available for filtration. Pressure in the glomerular capillary depends on flow through the glomerulus and on the relative resistance to flow of the afferent and efferent glomerular arterioles. For example, flow through the glomerulus may be normal or low, but if efferent arteriolar resistance is much greater than afferent arteriolar resistance, glomerular capillary pressure will be high and filtration may be increased. $\bar{\pi}$ is a function of the concentration of proteins in arterial plasma as well as of glomerular blood flow. The latter is important since protein-free water is constantly being removed throughout passage through the glomerulus. If flow is high relative to filtration (a low filtration fraction), a smaller increase in colloid osmotic pressure of plasma will result from a given filtration rate, and the mean colloid osmotic pressure will be lower than if flow were low, even though the initial osmotic pressure were the same in the two cases.

Glomerular filtration rate is usually measured using a substance which is freely filterable and not reabsorbed or secreted by the tubules. Clearance of this substance, defined as $\dfrac{UV}{P}$ where U is the concentration of the substance in urine, P is the concentration of the substance in plasma, and V is the rate of urine flow, is equal to the GFR. Inulin fulfills the criteria mentioned above and is widely used. Creatinine may be used in certain species and has the advantage of being an endogenous substance, thus removing the necessity for continuous infusion.

GLOMERULAR FILTRATION IN THE PERINATAL KIDNEY

As mentioned in the previous section, glomerular filtration rate is measured indirectly using a substance which is freely filterable and not altered in any way by the tubules. Inulin has been shown in adult species to fulfill these requirements (Smith, 1951; Gutman et al., 1965). The assumption is usually made that inulin clearance represents glomerular filtration rate in the newborn animal as it does in the adult. It must be emphasized, however, that although there is some indirect evidence that there is no reabsorption of inulin by the tubules of premature infants (Barnett et al., 1948), there are no direct studies comparable to those done in adult animals (Gutman et al., 1965) which indicate that inulin is a purely glomerular substance in the perinatal animal. The problem becomes even more complicated when a substance other than inulin is used as a glomerular marker. For example, endogenous creatinine clearance is often measured to determine glomerular filtration rate. Dean and McCance (1947) showed that the creatinine clearance of babies was essentially the same as inulin clearance. However, Calcagno et al. (1954) demonstrated that while this may be so in the hydropenic state, under conditions of osmotic diuresis (with mannitol), the creatinine clearance rose to almost twice the level of the simultaneous inulin clearance. These studies suggest that there may be tubular secretion of creatinine which becomes apparent under conditions of osmotic diuresis. Moreover, during osmotic diuresis in infants, the inulin clearance rose about 50 percent over hydropenic conditions whereas the inulin clearance remains relatively constant under similar conditions in the adult. This is probably due to the increased lability of glomerular filtration in the neonate but may also be due to the presence of tubular reabsorption of inulin under hydropenic conditions which is decreased under conditions of osmotic diuresis.

Another problem involved in discussing perinatal renal function arises from the difficulty of deciding what parameter to use as the basis of comparison with the adult of the species. A more detailed discussion of this problem is presented in Chapter 20 on water and electrolyte metabolism. In this chapter comparison will be made on the basis of body surface area or body weight because most of the data in the literature are presented in those terms.

Values for glomerular filtration rates (inulin and creatinine clearance) for various species of differing gestational and postnatal ages are presented in Table 1 (see also Fig. 8, Ch. 20). It is clear from these data that the perinatal animal has a markedly lower inulin or creatinine clearance than does the adult whether compared on a surface area or body weight basis. In addition, there is a great amount of variability in the reported values. This is true even when tests were performed on the same individual. Calcagno and Rubin (1963), on the same day and on the same patient (a one-week-old infant), reported inulin clearances ranging from 18 to 34 ml/minute/1.73 m². This may be due to the marked lability of glomerular filtration in the newborn or to the technical difficulty of estimating glomerular filtration accurately in the neonate.

The data of Alexander and Nixon (1963) in Table 1 indicate that no improvement occurs in glomerular function (reported as creatinine clearance) with maturation of the fetal lamb. In fact, there appears to be a slight decrease in the creatinine clearance. Moreover, in an earlier study, Alexander et al. (1958) measured simultaneous urea, fructose, and creatinine clearances in lambs ranging from 117 to 142 days' gestation and simultaneous urea and fructose clearances in lambs from 61 to 104 days of age. They found no significant differences in the clearance as measured by either of these techniques and so assumed that they all measured filtration rate. They noted that filtration rate, as measured by these clearances, actually declined (per unit body weight of the animal) from 61 days' gestation to 142 days. However, it is possible that the clearances measured were not equal to the glomerular filtration rates. For example, Smith et al. (1966) found the inulin clearance on fetal lambs aged 130 to 145 days of gestation to be significantly greater than simultaneous creatinine clearances. Moreover, inulin clearances measured by Smith et al. (1966) (Table 1) were *lower* than the creatinine clearances measured by Alexander and Nixon (1963) on fetuses of the same age, suggesting that there may be technical as well as physiologic variables affecting measurement of filtration rates in the fetus.

The reasons for the decreased glomerular filtration rate in the perinatal animal

TABLE 1. Glomerular Filtration Rates in Fetal and Neonatal Animals

Species	Age Fetal	Postnatal	Filtration rate	Sources
Lamb	60 days		0.4 ml/min/kg[a]	Alexander and Nixon (1963)
	70 days		2.0 ml/min/kg	
	77 days		2.4 ml/min/kg	
	127 days		1.3 ml/min/kg	
	132 days		1.7 ml/min/kg	
		12 hours	4.0 ml/min/kg	
		7 days	1.5 ml/min/kg	
		Adult	2.6 ml/min/kg	
	130-145 days		0.75 ml/min/kg[b]	Smith et al. (1966)
		Adult	2.4 ml/min/kg	
Guinea pig	40 days		0.011 ml/min/100 g[a]	Boylan et al. (1958)
	60 days		0.025 ml/min/100 g	
	70 days (term)		0.008 ml/min/100 g	
		Birth	0.042 ml/min/100 g	
		0-4 days	0.125 ml/min/100 g	
		4-7 days	0.180 ml/min/100 g	
		Adult	0.250 ml/min/100 g	
Rat		2 days	0.12 ml/min/100 g[b]	Falk (1955)
		4 days	0.23 ml/min/100 g	
		12 days	0.36 ml/min/100 g	
		Adult	0.63 ml/min/100 g	
Dog		1 day	0.40 ml/min/kg[b]	Heller and Capek (1965)
		7 days	1.22 ml/min/kg	
		13 days	1.84 ml/min/kg	
		30 days	3.33 ml/min/kg	
		60 days	3.80 ml/min/kg	
		Adult	4.29 ml/min/kg[a]	Smith (1951)
Pig		1-2 days	1.44 ml/min/kg[a] (fed sow's milk) 0.85 ml/min/kg (fasted)	McCance and Widdowson (1956)
Monkey	150 days		2.4 ml/min/kg[a,c]	Chez et al. (1964)
		Adult	3.1 ml/min/kg[b,c]	Sweet et al. (1961)
Man		Premature	45 ml/min/1.73m^2[b]	Weil (1955)
		Full-term newborn	40 ml/min/1.73m^2[b]	Weil (1955)
		Adult	125 ml/min/1.73m^2[b]	Weil (1955)

[a]Creatinine clearance.

[b]Inulin clearance.

[c]Creatinine clearances in adult monkeys (Smith and Clark, 1938) have been shown to be significantly higher than simultaneous inulin clearances. Therefore, the creatinine clearance by Chez et al. (1964) may overestimate glomerular filtration rate and the fetal glomerular function may not be as close to that of the adult as it appears to be in the chart.

will be discussed in terms of the factors involved in equation 1. These factors, however, are not easily measured directly, nor have they been studied in the perinatal animal. Colloid osmotic pressure is slightly lower in arterial blood of the perinatal animal than in that of the adult (Smith, 1959), but nothing is known of mean colloid osmotic pressure of the plasma in the glomerular capillaries. As mentioned earlier, the mean colloid osmotic pressure in the glomerular capillary is a function of the filtration fraction as well as of the arterial colloid osmotic pressure.

Arterial pressure is lower in the perinatal animal than in the adult animal. Yet, this does not necessarily mean that the driving pressure in the glomerular capillary is also lower in these animals. In adult animals the glomerular filtration rate remains relatively constant over a wide range of arterial pressures due to autoregulation of the resistance of the glomerular arterioles. Recent evidence (Lubbe and Kleinman, 1969), however, reveals that over the low blood pressure ranges found in the newborn animal, autoregulation of glomerular filtration rate with changes in arterial pressure does not occur in newborn puppies. In addition, the glomerular filtration rate correlated excellently with the mean arterial blood pressure in the developing puppy. This correlation was found to exist both as a function of age and independent of age. Thus, older puppies had both higher blood pressure and higher glomerular filtration rates than younger ones, but in those cases in which blood pressure differed in similarly aged puppies, the animals with the higher blood pressure had the larger glomerular filtration rate. In addition, acute increases in blood pressure in puppies resulted in acute increases in glomerular filtration rate. It appears likely, therefore, that the low glomerular filtration rate found in the newborn animal is largely related to the low arterial blood pressure.

Blood flow through the kidney of the perinatal animal is lower than through that of the adult. Renal plasma flow through the kidney is usually measured as the clearance of para-aminohippurate (PAH) on the assumption that almost all of this substance is removed from the blood on one passage through the kidney. This assumption is essentially valid in the adult animal where 90 to 95 percent is removed but may not be valid in the perinatal animal.

Weil (1955) calculated that the PAH clearances of newborn infants measured by a number of investigators prior to 1955 averaged 200 ml/minute/1.73 m². This is in contrast to the figure of 650 ml/minute/1.73 m² in the adult human. Thus the renal plasma flow of the neonatal animal appears to be as severely limited as the glomerular filtration rate. The filtration fraction in the neonate averaged 0.4 in the studies of both West et al. (1948) and Strauss et al. (1965) as compared with the value of 0.15 to 0.20 in the adult (Smith, 1951). It must be emphasized, however, that the filtration fraction is based on the ratio inulin clearance divided by PAH clearance (or mannitol clearance divided by PAH clearance in the studies of West et al., 1948) and assumes that these clearances accurately measure glomerular filtration rate and renal plasma flow. That this assumption is not valid for PAH clearance was demonstrated by Calcagno and Rubin (1963). They found that less than 60 percent of the PAH was extracted during passage through the kidneys of infants of less than 3 months of age whereas 91 percent of the PAH was extracted by the kidneys of older children. Thus, the values for renal plasma flow calculated from PAH clearance should be increased by 30 percent in the young infants. Furthermore, the filtration fraction calculated from the corrected values for renal plasma flow averaged 0.23 in the young infants, a value approaching but still greater than that in the adult.

The low renal blood flow in the newborn animal has been confirmed more recently by techniques other than the Fick Principle. Gruskin et al. (1968), using microspheres, and Assali et al. (1968), using electromagnetic flowmeters, found the renal plasma flow to be lower in the newborn than in the older animal. Furthermore, these authors, as well as Lubbe and Kleinman (1969), found the resistance to flow in the vessels of the newborn kidney to be greater than that in the adult. The increased resistance to flow in the newborn kidney may not necessarily contribute to low glomerular filtration, however, unless the large resistance is due primarily to the afferent glomerular arteriole or vessels more proximal to it. If the large resistance is due to the efferent glomerular arteriole or vessels more distal to it, then glomerular filtration rate should not be adversely affected.

Smith (1951) has suggested that the decreased glomerular filtration rate in the perinatal animal may be due to a decreased filtration coefficient (K_F) related to the immaturity of the glomerular epithelium. Gruenwald and Popper (1940) believed that there was rupture of the glomerular epithelial cell layer at birth and that this contributed to the improvement of glomerular filtration after birth. Vernier and Birch-Andersen (1962), on the other hand, found no support for this hypothesis and demonstrated that at five months' gestation many glomeruli histologically appeared to be fully capable of function. In addition, if the filtration coefficient were reduced in the newborn animal, the glomerular filtration rate should be restricted more than renal plasma flow so that the filtration fraction would be low. Filtration fraction, however, has been found to be essentially the same in both the newborn animal and the adult (Calcagno et al., 1963; Lubbe and Kleinman, 1969). A normal filtration fraction with a low filtration coefficient could exist only if the driving force for filtration in the glomerular capillary were higher. This driving force could be increased if glomerular capillary blood pressure were increased or colloid osmotic pressure or capsular pressure were decreased. Arterial blood pressure in the newborn puppy is about 40 mm Hg compared to 110 mm Hg in the adult (Lubbe and Kleinman, 1969). Even if there were no drop in pressure across the afferent arteriole (i.e. no significant resistance at that location), and even if the capsular pressure were zero (a very unlikely possibility), with a mean capillary colloid osmotic pressure of 15 mm Hg (approximately one-half of the adult), the driving force would be less than that of the adult. Thus, a decreased filtration coefficient is unlikely as a major cause for low glomerular filtration in the newborn animal. Moreover, since newborn puppies are able to filter at arterial blood pressures at which adult dogs are unable to filter, it is possible that the filtration coefficient may be even greater in the newborn animal than in the adult.

Tubular Function

PHYSIOLOGIC PRINCIPLES OF TUBULAR FUNCTION

The function of the kidney tubules is to alter the glomerular filtrate by transporting solutes and water across the tubular cells. Transport from the tubular lumen to interstitial fluid or peritubular capillaries is termed *reabsorption* and transport from capillary to tubular lumen is called *secretion*. Transport can be either passive (along an electrochemical gradient) or active (against an electrochemical gradient and requiring metabolic energy). Examples of passive transport in the kidney are movement of water, certain organic acids, and some of the urea. Recent studies suggest active urea transport by tubules of rat (Lassiter et al., 1966) and dog (Goldberg et al., 1967). Examples of active reabsorption are movement of sodium, glucose, and amino acids; examples of active secretion are movement of organic bases and PAH.

There are two types of active transport systems in the kidney—systems which are limited by a transport maximum (T_m) and those which apparently cannot be saturated. Examples of the former are provided by glucose, bicarbonate, and PAH transport; an example of the nonsaturable system is sodium transport. A characteristic of the first kind of transport is that all of the substance is reabsorbed or secreted until the maximum amount which can be transported, the T_m, is reached. In the second kind of transport a relatively constant fraction of the substance is transported and excreted. For example, in any nephron all of the glucose that is filtered is reabsorbed and none is excreted until the T_m for glucose of that nephron is reached, while a certain amount of sodium is always excreted.

The T_m of a substance (glucose, for example) must be distinguished from the term "plasma threshold." The plasma threshold for glucose is that plasma concentration of glucose at which glucose first appears in the urine, whereas the T_m for glucose is the maximum amount of glucose (mg/minute) which the tubules can reabsorb. The threshold is, of course, a function of the T_m since glucose will be excreted in the urine at low filtered glucose loads if the tubules cannot reabsorb glucose well. Since the filtered glucose load is dependent upon the plasma glucose concentration (filtered load = GFR × plasma concentration), in the case of impaired reabsorption glucose will be excreted in the urine at low plasma glucose concentrations. In other words, the plasma threshold for glucose will be low in this case. However, threshold is also a function of heterogeneity of tubular transport ability. If one group of nephrons has a low transport ability and another has a high transport ability, glucose will be excreted in the urine at relatively low plasma concentrations due to the glucose escaping reabsorption from the first group of nephrons before the more efficient tubules become saturated. $T_{m_{glucose}}$ for the kidney as a whole will depend on the relative proportion of well and poorly functioning nephrons. Similarly, even when tubular function in all the tubules is the same, if the filtered load presented to some tubules is greater than that to others due to different filtration rates among the nephrons, then the saturation will be reached at lower plasma concentrations in those nephrons with the larger filtration rates than in the nephrons with low filtered loads. The plasma threshold for the whole animal will, therefore, be decreased.

PERINATAL TUBULAR FUNCTION

Tubule cells, from a human fetus of 3 months' gestation, growing in tissue culture, have been observed to transport phenol red from the environment into the tubular lumen (Cameron and Chambers, 1938). Perry and Stanier (1962)

tion, the puppies excreted 56 percent of the test dose whereas the adult dogs excreted 85 percent of the dose in four hours. These authors felt that two-day-old puppies responded to a water load as well as a two-week-old rat but less well than a one- to two-week-old human infant.

The ability to excrete a water load is a function of route of administration, glomerular filtration rate, solute load, and diluting ability. Hoy (1966) has shown that water loads given by vein to newborn rats induced twice as much water diuresis as water administered intraperitoneally or by gastric tube. The glomerular filtration rate of the newborn is markedly lower than that of the adult, as discussed in a previous section, and this will limit the excretion of a water load. Edelmann and Barnett (1960) feel that the limitation in handling a water load is also related to the fact that newborn infants excrete a small solute load. Therefore, even though the newborn kidney can dilute the urine well, without adequate solute excretion water excretion will be decreased.

An adult man excretes a urine of about 1,000 mOsm/liter and is able to increase the concentration of solutes to 1,400 to 1,500 mOsm/liter under conditions of dehydration. A newborn animal excretes urine either hypotonic or slightly hypertonic to plasma, and a newborn human can concentrate his urine to only 600 to 700 mOsm/liter under conditions of water deprivation. Falk (1955) found that an adult rat excretes a urine with a concentration of 1,500 mOsm/liter on a normal diet. A 1-day-old baby rat has a urine osmolarity of 600 mOsm/liter, and not until 3 weeks of age does it excrete urine of 1,500 mOsm/liter. Upon water deprivation the adult rat can concentrate its urine to 1,900 mOsm/liter whereas 12-day-old rats were able to produce a urine of only 1,000/mOsm/liter. Studies on young puppies revealed that they could not concentrate their urine as well as could adult dogs (McCance, 1948).

The reasons for the poor ability of the newborn animal to concentrate urine can probably best be discussed on the basis of those physiologic factors which determine the concentrating ability of the animal.

ACTIVE TRANSPORT OF SODIUM OUT OF THE ASCENDING LIMB OF THE LOOP OF HENLE

There have been no direct investigations of the ability of the cells of Henle's loop to actively transport sodium against an electrochemical gradient. However, since the newborn animal is capable of excreting a very dilute urine, and since dilution of urine is also dependent upon sodium transport in Henle's loop this may not be a primary factor in the newborn animal's inability to excrete a concentrated urine.

LENGTH OF THE LOOP OF HENLE

It has been shown in rats (Boss et al., 1963) and man (Peter, 1927) that the loops of Henle of the perinatal kidney are immature and shorter than those in adult animals of the same species. This would indicate that the newborn animal ought not to be able to develop as large a concentration gradient of sodium from papilla to cortex. However, Yaffe and Anders (1960) found that the gradient for sodium from papilla to cortex in one-week-old rabbits deprived of water was the same as that for adults. The reason for the discrepancy may be due to species difference or to the fact that the section from the papilla was not sufficiently thin to include just the tip of the papilla where maximal concentration would occur.

IMPERMEABILITY OF COLLECTING TUBULES TO WATER DUE TO INSUFFICIENT ADH OR ADH INSENSITIVITY

Heller and Ledreis (1959) found that the amount of antidiuretic hormone in the pituitary of one-day-old rats was only one sixth of that found in adult rats when compared on a body weight basis. However, guinea pigs and human newborns have antidiuretic activity in the pituitary comparable to that in adults when compared on a body weight basis although there is a decreased concentration of this hormone in human infants per gram of pituitary tissue. Janovsky et al. (1965) were unable to detect antidiuretic activity (greater than 0.5 μU per ml plasma) in plasma from infants aged 16 days to 5 months. When these infants were loaded with sodium chloride, antidiuretic activity was noted in the infants aged 2½ to 5 months but not in younger babies. Plasma from infants older than 5 months contained antidiuretic activity with or without an osmotic stimulus. Thus, the poor ability of the newborn animal to concentrate his urine may be related, in part, to the diminished ability of the pituitary gland to secrete ADH.

Barnett and Vesterdal (1953) measured the response in well-hydrated adults and infants to ADH injection and found the increase in urinary osmolality to be greater in the adult than in the infant. However, this is not conclusive proof of insensitivity to ADH since a decreased medullary solute concentration in the infant could account for the difference. Edelmann et al. (1960) calculated that during hydropenia the amount of osmotically free water reabsorbed by the collecting tubules would have to be only 2 ml per 1.73 m² if the urine flow were 0.5 ml per 1.73 m² to produce a urine with a concentration of 1,500 mOsm/liter. Under conditions of mannitol diuresis infants were able to reabsorb 3 to 4 ml of free water per 1.73 m², indicating that the factor limiting maximal urinary osmolarity at low rates of urine flow is not the maximal rate at which water can be reabsorbed by the collecting tubule nor the permeability of the collecting tubule to water under the influence of ADH.

UREA EXCRETION

As mentioned earlier urea plays an important role in the concentrating ability of the kidney. Although the protein intake of newborn infants is about the same as that for adults when compared on a body surface basis the infant excretes much less urea. The reason for this is that the infant has a greater anabolic rate, and it excretes less nitrogen. Further, the fraction of the excreted nitrogen present as urea is lower in the infant than in the adult.

Although the total concentration of solutes in the urine of an infant is much lower than that of an adult (Edelmann, 1967), there is not much difference in the nonurea solute concentration in the two groups. When infants were given high-protein feedings they were able to increase their urine osmolarity to values above 900 mOsm/liter due entirely to increased concentration of urea. Newborn infants, however, differed from adult mammals (rats and dogs) and were not able to increase their nonurea solute concentration with increased urea load (Edelmann et al., 1967). Further evidence of the importance of the low urea output as a factor in the reduced concentrating ability can be found in the experiments of Yaffe and Anders (1960) and Fleishaker et al. (1960). Fleishaker et al. (1960) found that the concentration of urea in the papilla of rabbits increased progressively with age from just before birth to adult life. Furthermore, the gradient of urea concentration from papilla to cortex also increased with age. Yaffe and Anders (1960) similarly found that at one week of age rabbits had a smaller papillary-to-cortex concentration gradient for urea than did adult rabbits.

It thus appears that an important factor in the reduced concentrating ability of the newborn animal is the low urea load to the kidney which results in a diminished urea concentration in the medulla of the kidney and therefore a low total solute concentration in the urine.

MEDULLARY BLOOD FLOW

Anatomic studies by Ljundqvist (1963) revealed that, in the human fetus, post-glomerular vessels in the cortex do not appear after the eighth fetal month, and up to that time the lobar circulation is primarily medullary. Although there have been no physiologic studies to date which have measured intrarenal blood flow distribution in the perinatal animal, the low extraction of PAH suggests that the proportion of renal medullary blood flow may be higher in the kidney of the perinatal animal than it is in the adult. A relatively large blood flow through the vasa recta could dissipate the medullary solute concentration gradient and thus decrease the concentrating ability of the kidney.

PHYSIOLOGIC PRINCIPLES OF ACID EXCRETION

The kidney compensates for the body's production and ingestion of acid in two ways. 1, It excretes hydrogen ions, and 2, it retains the buffer bicarbonate so there will not be a large change in the free hydrogen ion concentration, or pH, of the blood.

BICARBONATE REABSORPTION

Under normal circumstances all of the bicarbonate which is filtered by the adult animal is reabsorbed by the tubules. If the rate of filtration of bicarbonate exceeds 28 m moles of bicarbonate per liter of glomerular filtrate in man (or 26 m moles in the dog) then the excess will be excreted in the urine. This maximum value can be altered by changing the P_{CO_2} of plasma (an increase in P_{CO_2} increases bicarbonate reabsorption), by variations in body stores of potassium (increased potassium decreases bicarbonate reabsorption), by variations in body stores of chloride (increased chloride decreases bicarbonate reabsorption), and by the activity of carbonic anhydrase (EC 4.2.1.1) in the kidney.

Briefly, the mechanism of bicarbonate reabsorption involves the following events. Within the tubular cell carbon dioxide is converted to hydrogen and bicarbonate ions. This reaction is accelerated by carbonic anhydrase. The hydrogen ion is actively pumped out of the cell into the tubular lumen in exchange with sodium. (Both potassium and hydrogen compete for the exchange with sodium in the distal tubule so that the more potassium ions there are the less hydrogen ions will be secreted.) Once in the tubular lumen the hydrogen ions combine with the bicarbonate to form CO_2 which then diffuses back into the cell. In the cell the CO_2 is converted to hydrogen and bicarbonate ions. The bicarbonate ions diffuse into the peritubular blood, and the hydrogen ions are resecreted into the tubular lumen. The net effect, therefore, is the reabsorption of bicarbonate.

ACID SECRETION

The kidney is able to actively transport hydrogen ions from the tubular cell to the lumen as mentioned in the previous paragraph. The maximum amount of hydrogen ions that can be transported is limited by the maximum gradient of hydrogen ions that can be maintained between the tubular lumen and the tubular cell. In man the maximum urinary free hydrogen ion concentration, or minimum, urinary pH, is 4.8. If the kidney had to excrete all its hydrogen ions in the free ionic form then the normal adult kidney would be able to excrete less than one percent of the body's normal acid production. Therefore, most of the hydrogen ions excreted by the kidney need to be buffered. There are two primary buffers in the urine—the buffers that are filtered by the glomerulus, the most important one being phosphate, and the buffer produced by the tubular cells, which is ammonia. Therefore the ability of the kidney to excrete acid will depend in part on the load of phosphate presented to the tubules and on the ability of the tubular cells to synthesize ammonia. The amount of acid excreted as free hydrogen ions plus the hydrogen ions bound to the filtered buffers is known as the *titratable acid*.

Ammonia is synthesized in the tubular cells from a nitrogen pool of amino and amide groups contributed to by tubular intracellular as well as renal arterial glutamine and amino acids. The ammonia synthesized from this nitrogen pool passively diffuses across the tubular cell membrane into the tubular lumen, and there it combines with the free hydrogen ion to form ammonium ion. The charged ammonium ion cannot diffuse back into the cell because the cell membrane is impermeable to it in contradistinction to the high membrane permeability to the noncharged ammonia molecule. The ability of the tubular cells to secrete ammonia, therefore, depends upon the ability of the kidney cells to synthesize ammonia and upon the amount of free hydrogen ions present in the tubular lumen to trap the ammonia there as ammonium ions. Synthesis of ammonia by the cells will depend upon availability of substrate, enzyme activity, and intracellular pH. Since the amount of hydrogen ions in the tubules is a function of both hydrogen ion concentration and urine volume, ability of tubular fluid to trap the ammonia will depend on the pH of this fluid as well as on urine flow.

ACID EXCRETION BY THE PERINATAL KIDNEY

The allantoic fluid of the fetal pig at 46 days' gestation has a pH of 6. Most of the acid exists in the form of carbonic acid but, in addition, there is a significant amount of ammonium ions present. In addition the pig mesonephros, metanephros, chorioallantoic membrane, and amniotic membrane have carbonic anhydrase activity (McCance and Widdowson, 1960a). The newborn human has a bladder filled with a urine of pH of about 6.3 (McCance and Widdowson, 1960b). Thus the fetus, at least in the later part of gestation, is able to secrete hydrogen ions into the tubular lumen.

Although the perinatal animal is clearly able to excrete an acid urine, measurement of renal acidifying ability is usually ascertained by determining the ability of the kidney to respond to an acid load. Vaughn et al. (1968) studied the fetal and neonatal response to acid loading in sheep. They infused HCl into near term and newborn lambs and produced a decrease in blood pH, bicarbonate, and base excess. However, total acid excretion (titratable acid plus ammonia) did not change significantly until the acid dose per unit body weight was three times that required to effect such a change in adult animals. They felt that the *placenta* played a large role in excreting the acid load in the fetus since there was a marked decrease in uterine venous blood pH after the fetus had been infused with acid (see Ch. 3).

Cort and McCance (1954) infused ammonium chloride or sulfate into two-day-old puppies and adult dogs and found that the puppies were able to lower their urinary pH to the same extent as were the adults (to about pH 4.8), but it took a longer time to reach maximal acidification. There was, however, a marked difference in the total hydrogen ion excreted between the adult and the puppies. The puppies excreted less titratable acid due to the small amount of phosphate in the urine, and they excreted practically no ammonia.

The human fetus and newborn infant during the first week of life lives in a state of mild metabolic acidosis. His arterial pH is between 7.34 and 7.37, and his plasma bicarbonate concentration is slightly reduced. In spite of this, the newborn infant during the first week of life usually does not excrete a urine of pH less than 5.4 and averages a urinary pH closer to 6 (Edelmann, 1967).

McCance and Widdowson (1960b) found that the urine of newborns at one week of age averaged pH 6.2 for breast-fed infants and pH 5.9 for infants fed cow's milk formula. At birth babies excreted 0.41 mEq/liter titratable acid and 4.55 mEq/liter ammonia so that the ammonia accounted for approximately 90 percent of the buffered hydrogen ions. On the first and second days of life before the onset of feeding these same babies excreted about 11 mEq/liter titratable acid and 32 mEq/liter ammonia. Although the percentage of buffered hydrogen ions due to ammonia dropped to 75, this was due to the increase in titratable acid being larger than the increase in ammonia (McCance and Widdowson, 1960b).

At one week of age the acid constituents of the urine are dependent upon the diet (McCance and Widdowson, 1960b). Breast-fed babies excrete about 50 percent of the amount of acid per kilogram body weight compared with adults whereas babies fed cow's milk formula excrete more acid than does the adult. In breast-fed babies more than 80 percent of the buffered acid is due to ammonia, in the cow's milk-fed babies about 40 percent is due to ammonia, and in the adult 56 percent is due to ammonia. The reasons for the marked difference in acid excretion between breast-fed and cow's milk-fed babies is due primarily to the larger amounts of phosphorus and protein in the cow's milk formula. The increased phosphorus permits more hydrogen ions to be buffered as titratable acid. The higher protein in the diet provides more sulphur-containing amino acids than the infant can assimilate. Thus there is an increase in the amount of acid produced by the body (in the form of sulfuric acid) and an increased acid load to the kidney. The kidney must therefore excrete more hydrogen ions and ammonia to form ammonium sulfate. The newborn's kidney is, therefore, apparently able to adapt quite well to this increased sulfate since he does indeed excrete a large amount of ammonium sulfate in the urine.

Although the newborn human's kidney is able to handle the small acid loads from the diet he is not able to respond as well as the adult to large acid loads. Hatemi and McCance (1961) and McCance and Hatemi (1961) gave ammonium or calcium chloride to one-week-old newborn infants and measured their response to this acid load over an eight-hour period. An equivalent procedure was performed on adults. They found that, although the infants lowered their urinary pH from 6.2 to 5.4 at eight hours, the drop was not as rapid nor as pronounced as that of the adults who dropped their urine pH from 6.2 to 4.8 in three hours. Moreover, the rise in titratable acid and ammonia excretion was negligible in the infants while both of these measures of acid excretion were increased markedly in the adult. If the babies were loaded with phosphate before they were given the ammonium or calcium chloride they responded to the acid load with a marked increase in titratable acid, but their ammonia excretion was not different from those infants who were not loaded with phosphate. The relevance of phosphate availability to excretion of acid was evidenced by the fact that without phosphate the infants were able to excrete only 4 percent of the acid load in eight hours whereas those babies who were given phosphate excreted almost 10 percent of the acid in the same time (adults excreted 20 percent of the acid load without phosphate and 30 percent with phosphate in that time).

Edelmann et al. (1967) gave ammonium chloride to infants between 1 month and 1 year of age who were on a cow's milk formula and found that they were able to lower their urinary pH to 4.9 and excrete more titratable acid per unit body surface area than a group of older children between 3 and 12 years given an equivalent dose of acid. This was attributed to the high phosphate load in the diet of the infants. However, the younger infants were not able to excrete as much ammonia per unit body surface area as were the older children. Ammonia excretion, when compared on the basis of ammonia excreted per milliliter glomerular filtration rate, however, was similar in the two age groups.

Tudvad et al. (1954) measured bicarbonate reabsorption in premature infants ranging in age from 8 to 37 days. They found that the T_m for bicarbonate reabsorption was 2.60 mEq per 100 ml of glomerular filtration rate. This is about the same as the value of 2.74 mEq/100 ml obtained by Pitts et al. (1949) on adults. However, since the filtration rate is decreased in the infants, the maximal reabsorption of bicarbonate per body weight or surface area is comparably reduced. A decreased amount of carbonic anhydrase in the tubules could decrease bicarbonate reabsorption. Carbonic anhydrase activity has been shown to be low in the kidneys of fetal and newborn animals (Maren, 1967). The extent of the enzyme inactivity, however, may not be sufficient to interfere with bicarbonate reabsorption. Maren (1967) states that enzyme activity must be less than 1 percent of that found in the adult before significant interference with physiologic function can be noticed, and the enzyme activity reported in the perinatal kidney is much higher than that. Moreover, when the carbonic anhydrase inhibitor, acetazolamide, was administered to newborn infants bicarbonate reabsorption was markedly reduced, indicating that carbonic anhydrase activity was present in these infants (Tudvad et al., 1954). It is still possible, however, that bicarbonate reabsorption, and hydrogen ion secretion, might be more efficient with a higher level of enzyme activity.

The plasma threshold for bicarbonate was found to be between 22 and 24 m moles/liter (Tudvad et al., 1954). This is lower than the 28 m moles/liter threshold for bicarbonate found in adults by Pitts et al. (1949). Since the newborn kidney apparently has the ability to reabsorb as much bicarbonate per unit filtration rate as does that of the adult, why does the newborn spill bicarbonate before the adult does? Edelmann et al. (1967) believe this is so because of a greater heterogeneity in the ratio of glomerular surface area to proximal tubular volume (Fetterman et al., 1965). Nephrons with a low ratio of glomerular surface area to proximal tubular volume would be expected to present a small bicarbonate load to the tubules, and bicarbonate would not be spilled in the urine until the plasma bicarbonate rises to relatively high levels. Those nephrons with a high glomerular surface area to proximal tubular volume ratio would present a high bicarbonate load to the tubules and would spill bicarbonate at a lower plasma bicarbonate level. Thus, with a great deal of heterogeneity there would be excretion of bicarbonate from the high glomerular to tubular ratio nephrons, and the plasma threshold for bicarbonate would be low. This would explain, at least in part, the low plasma bicarbonate concentration found in newborn infants.

In summary, the newborn infant has a decreased ability to secrete hydrogen ions against a concentration gradient, and he is unable to provide enough phosphate or ammonia buffer. By one week of age the ability of the kidney to excrete free and titratable acid is improved in the presence of enough dietary phosphate, but there still remains a marked impairment in ammonia excretion. The reasons for the decreased ability to secrete ammonia are not clear. There may be less availability of free hydrogen ions necessary to trap the ammonia. This in turn may result from low urine flow rates due to diminished glomerular filtration. Or there may be decreased presentation of amino acid substrate because of low peritubular blood flow. Finally, there may be low enzyme activity in the tubular cells, accounting for a low synthesis of ammonia. The question, however, remains unanswered.

Bicarbonate reabsorption per unit glomerular filtration rate in a one-week-old newborn is the same as in the adult, but bicarbonate will be excreted in the urine more rapidly, possibly due to glomerular tubular heterogeneity. The result of all these factors is that the newborn animal is less well able to cope with a metabolic acidosis than is the adult but can maintain acid-base homeostasis if the acid load is not too great.

Conclusions

The perinatal kidney does not function as efficiently as the adult kidney. Both glomerular and tubular function are low, and in most cases both these functions are diminished proportionately. In some respects, such as PAH and glucose transport, tubular function appears to be more severely restricted than glomerular function.

The reasons for both the low glomerular filtration rate and the poor tubular function are still unclear. Low arterial blood pressure probably plays a major role in limiting glomerular filtration in the perinatal animal although other factors may also be operative. Diminished renal blood flow in the perinatal animal is probably related both to the low blood pressure and the increased renal vascular resistance. Intrarenal blood flow distribution may be different in the perinatal animal in that a greater fraction of the total blood flow may go to the medulla and bypass cortical tubular transport sites. Studies of intrarenal blood flow distribution may shed light on the diminished PAH and glucose transport by the proximal tubule, as well as the poor ability of the perinatal kidney to excrete ammonia or a concentrated urine.

The newborn animal is not as well able as is the adult to excrete a sodium load, and this appears to be due to its low glomerular filtration rate and inability to invoke those compensatory mechanisms which decrease fractional sodium reabsorption. Although the newborn animal is able to dilute its urine as well as is the adult it cannot excrete as concentrated a urine. Inability to excrete a concentrated urine is related, in part at least, to the low urea load to the kidney and the low level of circulating ADH. The role of high medullary blood flow, short loops of Henle, and limited sodium transport by the ascending limb of Henle's loop still needs to be evaluated.

The neonatal animal cannot respond as well as an adult to acid loads by excreting ammonia. Bicarbonate reabsorption per unit surface area is less in the newborn animal than in the adult, but bicarbonate reabsorption per unit glomerular filtrate is the same. However, the plasma threshold for bicarbonate in the newborn animal is lower than in the adult, thus accounting for greater bicarbonate excretion, a lower plasma bicarbonate, and perhaps the mild metabolic acidosis seen in the newborn infant.

ACKNOWLEDGMENT

Preparation of this chapter was supported in part by federal grant number U.S.P.H. ES-00159.

REFERENCES

Alexander, D. P., and D. A. Nixon. 1961. The foetal kidney. Brit. Med. Bull., 17:112-117.
———— and D. A. Nixon. 1963. Reabsorption of glucose, fructose, and mesoinositol by the foetal and post-natal sheep kidney. J. Physiol. (London), 167:480-486.
———— D. A. Nixon, W. F. Widdas, and F. X. Wohlzogen. 1958. Renal function in the sheep foetus. J. Physiol. (London), 140:14-22.
Ames, R. G. 1953. Urinary water excretion and neurohypophysial function in full term and premature infants shortly after birth. Pediatrics, 12:272-281.
Arataki, M. 1926. Post-natal growth of kidney with special reference to number and size of glomeruli (albino rat). Amer. J. Anat., 36:399-436.
Assali, N. S., G. A. Bekey, and L. Morrison. 1968. Fetal and neonatal circulation. In Assali, N. S., ed. Biology of Gestation. New York, Academic Press, Inc., Vol. 2.
Barnett, H. L., and J. Vesterdal. 1953. The physiologic and clinical significance of immaturity of kidney function in young infants. J. Pediat., 42:99-117.
———— W. R. Hare, H. McNamara, and R. S. Hare. 1948. Measurement of glomerular filtration rate in premature infants. J. Clin. Invest., 27:691-699.
———— J. Vesterdal, H. McNamara, and H. D. Lauson. 1952. Renal water excretion in premature infants. J. Clin. Invest., 31:1069-1073.
Boss, J. M. N., H. Dlouha, M. Kraus, and J. Krecek. 1963. The structure of the kidney in relation to age and diet in white rats during the weaning period. J. Physiol. (London), 168:196-204.
Boylan, J. W., E. P. Colbourn, and R. A. McCance. 1958. Renal function in the foetal and new-born guinea-pig. J. Physiol. (London), 141:323-331.
Calcagno, P. L., and M. I. Rubin. 1963. Renal extraction of PAH in infants and children. J. Clin. Invest., 43:1632-1639.
———— M. I. Rubin, and D. H. Weintraub. 1954. Studies on the renal concentrating and diluting mechanisms in the premature infant. J. Clin. Invest., 33:91-96.
Cameron, G., and R. Chambers. 1938. Direct evidence of function in kidney of an early human fetus. Amer. J. Physiol., 123:482-485.
Capek, K., H. Dlouha, J. Fernandez, and M. Popp. 1968. Regulation of proximal tubular reabsorption in early post-natal period of infant rats: Micropuncture study. In Proc. Int. Union Physiol. Sciences. Washington, D. C. Abstracts of Volunteer Papers, Vol. 7, p. 72.

Chasis, H., et al. 1945. The use of sodium p-aminohippurate for the functional evaluation of the human kidney. J. Clin. Invest., 24:583-588.

Chez, R. A., F. G. Smith, and D. L. Hutchinson. 1964. Renal function in the intrauterine primate fetus. I. Experimental technique; rate of formation and chemical composition of urine. Amer. J. Obstet. Gynec., 90:128-131.

Cort, J. H., and R. A. McCance. 1954. The renal response of puppies to an acidosis. J. Physiol. (London), 124:358-369.

Crawford, J. D., and R. A. McCance. 1960. Sodium transport by the chorioallantoic membrane of the pig. J. Physiol. (London), 151:458-471.

Dean, R. F. A., and R. A. McCance. 1947. Inulin, diodone, creatinine and urea clearances in newborn infants. J. Physiol. (London), 106:431-439.

——— and R. A. McCance. 1949. The renal responses of infants and adults to the administration of hypertonic solutions of sodium chloride and urea. J. Physiol. (London), 109:81-97.

Edelmann, C. M., Jr. 1967. Maturation of the neonatal kidney. In Proc. Third Int. Congr. Nephrol., Washington, 1966. Vol. 3, pp. 1-12.

——— and H. L. Barnett. 1960. Role of the kidney in water metabolism in young infants: Physiologic and clinical considerations. J. Pediat., 56:154-179.

——— H. L. Barnett, and V. Troupkov. 1960. Renal concentrating mechanisms in newborn infants: Effects of dietary protein and water content, role of urea and responsiveness to antidiuretic hormone. J. Clin. Invest., 39:1062-1064.

——— H. L. Barnett, and H. Stark. 1966. Effect of urea on concentration of urinary non-urea solute in premature infants. J. Appl. Physiol., 21:1021-1025.

——— et al. 1967. Renal bicarbonate reabsorption and hydrogen ion excretion in normal infants. J. Clin. Invest., 46:1304-1317.

Falk, G. 1955. Maturation of renal function in adult rats. Amer. J. Physiol., 181:157-170.

Fetterman, G. H., N. A. Shuplock, F. J. Philipp, and H. S. Gregg. 1965. Growth and maturation of human glomeruli and proximal convolutions from term to adulthood: Studies by microdissection. Pediatrics, 35:601-619.

Fleishaker, G. H., O. J. Gesink, and W. W. McCrory. 1960. Effect of age on distribution of urea and electrolytes in kidneys of young rabbits. Amer. J. Dis. Child., 100:557.

Goldberg, M., A. J. Wotczak, and M. A. Ramirez. 1967. Uphill transport of urea in the dog kidney: Effects of certain inhibitors. J. Clin. Invest., 46:388-399.

Gordon, H. H., H. McNamara, and H. R. Benjamin. 1948. The response of young infants to ingestion of ammonium chloride. Pediatrics, 2:290-302.

Gruenwald, J., and H. Popper. 1940. Histogenesis and physiology of renal glomerulus in early post-natal life: Histological examinations. J. Urol., 43:452-458.

Gruskin, A. B., C. M. Edelmann, Jr., and S. Yuan. 1968. Maturational changes in renal blood flow in piglets. Fed. Proc., 27:630.

Gutman, Y., C. W. Gottschalk, and W. E. Lassiter. 1965. Micropuncture study of inulin absorption in the rat kidney. Science, 147:753-754.

Hatemi, N., and R. A. McCance. 1961. Renal aspects of acid base control in the newly born. III. Response to acidifying drugs. Acta Paediat. Scand., 50:603-616.

Heller, H., and K. Ledreis. 1959. Maturation of the hypothalamoneurohypophyseal system. J. Physiol. (London), 147:299-314.

Heller, J., and K. Capek. 1965. Changes in body water compartments and inulin and PAH clearance in the dog during post natal development. Physiol. Bohemoslov., 14:433-438.

Hoy, P. A. 1966. Diuresis in newborn rats given intravenous water or salt solution. Proc. Soc. Exp. Biol. Med., 122:358-361.

Janovsky, M., J. Martinek, and V. Stanincova. 1965. Antidiuretic activity in the plasma of human infants after a load of sodium chloride. Acta Pediat., 54:543-549.

Lassiter, W. E., M. Mylle, and C. W. Gottschalk. 1966. Micropuncture study of urea transport in rat renal medulla. Amer. J. Physiol., 210:965-970.

Ljundgvist, A. 1963. Fetal and postnatal development of intrarenal pattern in man. Acta Pediat., 52:443-454.

Lubbe, R., and L. I. Kleinman. 1969. Relationship between GFR and blood pressure in newborn puppies. Physiologist, 12:289.

MacDonald, M. S., and J. L. Emery. 1959. The late intrauterine and postnatal development of human renal glomeruli. J. Anat., 93:331-340.

Maren, T. H. 1967. Carbonic anhydrase: Chemistry, physiology and inhibition. Physiol. Rev., 47:595-781.

McCance, R. A. 1948. Renal function in early life. Physiol. Rev., 28:331-348.

———— 1962. Age and renal function. In Black, D. A. K., ed. Renal Disease. Oxford, Blackwell Scientific Publications, pp. 157-170.

———— and N. Hatemi. 1961. Control of acid-base stability in the newly born. Lancet, 1:293-297.

———— and E. M. Widdowson. 1955. The response of puppies to a large dose of water. J. Physiol. (London), 129:628-635.

———— and E. M. Widdowson. 1956. Metabolism, growth and renal function of piglets in the first days of life. J. Physiol. (London), 133:373-384.

———— and M. W. Stanier. 1960. The function of the metanephros of foetal rabbits and pigs. J. Physiol. (London), 151:479-483.

———— and E. M. Widdowson. 1960a. The acid base relationships of the foetal fluids of the pig. J. Physiol. (London), 151:484-490.

———— and E. M. Widdowson. 1960b. Renal aspects of acid base control in the newly born. I. Natural development. Acta Paediat. Scand., 49:409-414.

———— and E. M. Widdowson. 1963. Effect of administering sodium chloride, sodium bicarbonate and potassium bicarbonate to newborn piglets. J. Physiol. (London), 165:569-574.

———— N. S. B. Naylor, and E. M. Widdowson. 1954. The response of infants to a large dose of water. Arch. Dis. Child., 29:104-109.

Perry, J. S., and M. W. Stanier. 1962. The rate of flow of urine of foetal pigs. J. Physiol. (London), 161:344-350.

Peter, K. 1927. Die Entwicklung der menschlichen Niere nach Isolationspräparaten. In Peter, K., ed. Untersuchungen über Bau und Entwicklung der Niere. Jena, Fischer, Vol. 2, Sect. 5.

Pitts, R. F. 1963. Physiology of the Kidney and Body Fluids. Chicago, Year Book Medical Publishers, Inc.

———— J. L. Ayer, and W. A. Schiess. 1949. The renal regulation of acid base balance in man. III. The reabsorption and excretion of bicarbonate. J. Clin. Invest., 28:35-44.

Potter, E. L. 1965. Development of the human glomerulus. Arch. Path. (Chicago), 80:241-255.

Rubin, M. I., E. Bruch, and M. Rapoport. 1949. Maturation of renal function in childhood: Clearance studies. J. Clin. Invest. 28:1144-1162.

———— P. L. Calcagno, and B. L. Ruben. 1961. Renal excretion of hydrogen ions: A defense against acidosis in premature infants. J. Pediat., 59:848-860.

Smith, C. A.   1959.   Physiology of the Newborn Infant. Springfield, Ill., Charles C Thomas, Publisher.

Smith, F. G., F. H. Adams, M. Borden, and J. Hilborn.   1966.   Studies of renal function in the intact fetal lamb. Amer. J. Obstet. Gynec., 96:240-246.

Smith, H. W.   1951.   The Kidney. New York, Oxford University Press.

————— and R. W. Clark.   1938.   The excretion of inulin and creatinine by the anthropoid apes and other infrahuman primates. Amer. J. Physiol., 122:132-142.

Strauss, J., K. Adamsons, and L. S. James.   1965.   Renal function of normal full term infants in the first hours of extrauterine life. I. Infants delivered naturally and given a placental transfusion. Amer. J. Obstet. Gynec., 91:286-290.

Sweet, A. Y., M. F. Levitt, and H. L. Hodes.   1961.   Kidney function, body fluid compartments and water and electrolyte metabolism in the monkey. Amer. J. Physiol., 201:975-979.

Tudvad, F.   1949.   Sugar reabsorption in prematures and full term babies. Scand. J. Clin. Lab. Invest., 1:281-283.

————— and J. Vesterdal.   1953.   The maximal tubular transfer of glucose and para-aminohippurate in premature infants. Acta Paediat. Scand., 42:337-345.

————— H. McNamara, and H. L. Barnett.   1954.   Renal response of premature infants to administration of bicarbonate and potassium. Pediatrics, 13:4-16.

Vaughn, D., et al.   1968.   Fetal and neonatal response to acid loading in the sheep. J. Appl. Physiol., 24:135-141.

Vernier, R. L.   1965.   Current concepts of renal development. Pediat. Clin. N. Amer., 11:759-766.

————— and A. Birch-Andersen.   1962.   Studies of the human fetal kidney. I. Development of the glomerulus. J. Pediat., 60:754-768.

Weil, W. B., Jr.   1955.   Evaluation of renal function in infancy and childhood. Amer. J. Med. Sci., 229:678-694.

West, J. R., H. W. Smith, and H. Chasis.   1948.   Glomerular filtration rate, effective renal blood flow and maximal tubular excretory capacity in infancy. J. Pediat., 32:10-18.

Yaffe, S. J., and T. F. Anders.   1960.   Renal solute content in young rabbits. Amer. J. Dis. Child., 100:558.

22

Perinatal Calcium and Phosphorus Metabolism

WILLIAM H. BERGSTROM ● Department of Pediatrics, State University of New York Upstate Medical Center, Syracuse, New York

Our understanding of antenatal calcium and phosphorus metabolism is derived chiefly from animal data and from a distressingly small number of analyses of human material. The common laboratory animals have rates of maturation so different from our own (and from each other) that the amount of information transferable from species to species is quite limited. Systematic antenatal chemical descriptions of the primates are not yet available.

In human embryos prior to the appearance of the skeleton, calcium and phosphorus together comprise about 0.2 percent of the total body mass. Figure 1 shows their accretion rates during gestation. At birth more than 90 percent of the total body content of calcium and phosphorus is in the form of hydroxyapatite, or "bone salt" (Shohl, 1939). Bone at term is relatively undermineralized, having approximately half of the adult normal ash weight: dry weight ratio.

Factors governing antenatal osteogenesis are probably similar to those operative

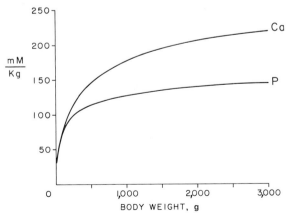

Fig. 1. Accretion rates of calcium and phosphorus during gestation. (Data from Fee and Weil, 1963; Kelly et al., 1951.)

after birth, which are poorly understood. Prerequisites include orderly cartilage growth, calcification of cartilage, osteoclastic remodeling, osteoid synthesis, and final mineralization. The work of Abdul-Karim et al. (1966, 1967) indicates that estrogen may be essential to normal fetal bone growth. These authors were able to inhibit orderly cartilage growth and osteoid synthesis by administering an antiestrogenic compound (ethamoxytriphetol) to pregnant ewes and to prevent these adverse effects by simultaneous estrogen therapy.

Disorders of antenatal osteogenesis are for the most part related to substrate synthesis rather than to calcium and phosphorus metabolism. Thus, in achondroplasia, dyschondroplasia, osteogenesis imperfecta, and osteopetrosis the skeleton may be grossly deformed or the total bone mass much larger or smaller than usual, but the concentrations of calcium and phosphorus in body fluids are normal, and such bone as is present is normally mineralized. In hypophosphatasia, unmineralized osteoid may simulate rickets both grossly and microscopically, but serum calcium and phosphorus are characteristically normal at birth. The disorder is thought to result from the synthesis of an abnormal, uncalcifiable organic matrix. Among the infectious diseases, syphilis and rubella affect bone in utero, producing characteristic diaphyseal and periosteal lesions without influencing mineral metabolism (Reed, 1969). Intrauterine hyperparathyroidism with bone lesions established at birth was reported by Aceto et al. (1966) in the child of an untreated hypoparathyroid mother. This rare and instructive case is discussed further below.

Congenital rickets has been seen only in association with severe maternal osteomalacia. In the series reported by Maxwell (1930) from north China, mothers of the affected infants were multiparous, had bone pain, and had been almost totally deprived of calcium and calciferol by dietary and cultural patterns. Elsewhere, very wide variations in maternal nutrition have had little or no effect on fetal skeletal development (Booher and Hausmann, 1931; Jackson, 1961). Drastic alterations in the Ca and P intake of pregnant rats produce only minor changes in the bones of the offspring (Sontag et al., 1936). From these clinical and laboratory findings it has been inferred that fetal calcium and phosphorus requirements may be met, if necessary, almost entirely at the expense of maternal stores. The newborn at term contains approximately 30 g of calcium and 24 g of phosphorus, representing only three to four percent of his mother's normal skeletal content. The amounts of calcium and phosphorus normally supplied to the fetus from the mother's diet as compared to those contributed by her skeleton and soft tissues are not well defined.

In postnatal life at least five factors affect calcium and phosphorus homeostasis; there may well be others as yet undefined. Those recognized include diet, calciferol, parathyroid hormone, thyrocalcitonin, and cortisol. Calciferol facilitates intestinal absorption of calcium and secondarily of phosphate. It enhances bone mineralization and renal tubular phosphate transport; these effects are reversed at very high dose levels. Parathyroid hormone (PTH) also mediates intestinal transport, though to a much lesser degree. By regulating the rate of osteoclastic reabsorption of bone PTH stabilizes serum calcium concentration. Serum phosphorus is the resultant of intestinal absorption, bone deposition and reabsorption, and renal tubular transport. The latter is the principle locus of PTH phosphorus homeostasis.

Thyrocalcitonin (TCT), secreted by the interstitial "c" cells of the thyroid, has an effect on osteoclastic activity opposite to that of PTH. Although its hypocalcemic efficacy is established, its physiologic significance is undefined. Cortisol also inhibits osteoclasis and is thus a PTH antagonist.

The amounts of calcium and phosphorus available for diffusion or transport across the placenta depend upon maternal regulatory factors. It is, therefore, very difficult to assess fetal homeostatic mechanisms; indeed, it is possible that the fetus is normally passive. Disturbances in maternal parathyroid function can evoke appropriate responses in the fetal glands. Independent operation of the other regulatory factors has not yet been shown in the fetus.

Many investigators feel that pregnancy induces functional maternal hyperparathyroidism (Ludwig, 1962). Much of the evidence for this opinion is indirect, although Hamilton et al. (1936) isolated increased amounts of a substance with bioassay characteristics of parathyroid hormone from the serum of pregnant women. During the last trimester maternal serum calcium concentration is slightly decreased; renal tubular phosphate reabsorption is unchanged (Kerr et al., 1962). Both of these findings are inconsistent with hyperparathyroidism. Bodansky and Duff (1941) showed that rats on low calcium diets regularly lost skeletal calcium and phosphate during pregnancy. Parathyroidectomy prevented maternal demineralization and resulted in poorly calcified fetuses. However, on high calcium diets maternal skeletons were unchanged during pregnancy, and neither mothers nor fetuses were affected by parathyroidectomy. Evidently the parathyroids are essential for the transfer of calcium and phosphate from mother to fetus when dietary calcium is restricted. No transfer is necessary when calcium is abundant. However, it is not clear how the low and high calcium intakes selected for these studies correspond to those of rats in their natural state, and the data are therefore hard to interpret in terms of human nutrition. Normal bone structure and composition are maintained by populations whose calcium intake varies from 200 to 1,200 mg/day, suggesting a wide range in proportionate intestinal absorption. This has been confirmed by balance studies. Adaptation to low-calcium diets is achieved over a period of several months by most individuals; a few are unable to increase their intestinal absorption appropriately and remain in negative balance, presumably at the expense of skeletal mineral (Malm, 1963). In the chick, adaptive enhancement of calcium absorption involves synthesis of a specific calcium-binding protein (CaBP) found only in the intestinal mucosa and in the kidney (Wasserman and Taylor, 1968; Wasserman et al., 1968). Mammals also possess this protein; its physiologic regulation in the higher forms has not yet been studied but is probably consistent throughout the vertebrates as are the other known factors in calcium homeostasis. CaBP synthesis is calciferol-dependent but seems not to require estrogen or parathyroid hormone. The laying hen, whose calcium requirement is high, has more CaBP than the pullet. A similar adaptive increase in maternal CaBP during mammalian pregnancy has not yet been established.

The incomplete data presently available thus suggest that mothers who are provided adequate calciferol can adapt to a wide range of calcium intakes so as to assure normal fetal mineralization. When dietary calcium is inadequate the fetus is supplied at the expense of the maternal skeleton; this process is parathyroid-dependent. Ideal allowances of calcium and calciferol during pregnancy have not been defined; both almost surely lie below the present United States averages. It is thus difficult to evaluate calcium phosphate supplementation during pregnancy in terms of maternal or fetal benefit; animal data do not support the practice, and controlled studies in human beings are not available.

Maternal parathyroid disease induces transient functional changes in the offspring after delivery. Tetany lasting for several weeks has been seen in the infants of hyperparathyroid mothers (Hartenstein and Gardner, 1966; Ertel et al., 1969). Whether this is due to suppression of the fetal parathyroids or to stimulation of TCT secretion has not been determined; the former possibility is more consistent with the observed hyperphosphatemia. Conversely, hyperparathyroidism has been reported in the offspring of a hypoparathyroid mother (Aceto et al., 1966). This circumstance is rare, since hypoparathyroidism is a less common disease, and untreated mothers rarely carry babies to term. Fetal response in both disorders is probably evoked by abnormal calcium ion concentrations rather than by placental transfer of maternal hormone, although the latter factor cannot be excluded. Thus, continuous exposure to excessive calcium ion concentration in utero may suppress fetal parathyroid function, whereas calcium lack may serve as a stimulus. This hypothesis is based on the presumption that fetal parathyroids, at least near term, respond in the same fashion as do those of postnatal subjects and explants in tissue culture. Scothorne's (1964) studies of human parathyroid explants suggest that the glands are functional by the twelfth week of gestation. Sinclair (1942) was able to alter fetal parathyroid size in the rat by manipulating the maternal diet. It is likely that during normal pregnancy fetal parathyroids are minimally stimulated, since the calcium and phosphorus concentrations of their circumambient fluids are regulated by maternal parathyroid and renal function and possibly by the placenta as well. Widdowson et al. (1962) found that urine collected immediately after birth contained very little phosphorus (0.24 mg/100 ml). Since these samples were formed in utero, it may be inferred that prenatal parathyroid activity was minimal.

It has long been known that Ca and P concentrations in human cord blood at term exceed those of simultaneously taken maternal venous samples (Economu-Mavrou and McCance, 1958). In the very large series assembled by Todd et al. (1939) calcium averaged 10.7 mg/100 ml and phosphorus 5.6 mg/100 ml. This phenomenon, confirmed in other mammalian species (Fuchs and Fuchs, 1956), has led to the general conclusion that the placenta actively transports calcium and phosphorus. Studies in a few previable fetuses, however (Westin et al., 1959), have shown no transplacental gradient for calcium in the fetal weight range from 50 to 750 g.

Such measurements of ultrafiltrable calcium as are available indicate that this moiety, which corresponds quite closely to the ionized calcium in interstitial fluid, is equal in fetal and maternal plasma (Andersch and Oberst, 1936). Plasma albumin concentration is the principal determinant of the proportions of bound and diffusible calcium. Albumin in previable fetuses is low; at term it is 3.1 g/100 ml as compared with the average maternal level of 2.6 g/100ml (Smith, 1959). These variations have not been systematically correlated with the transplacental gradients noted above; without such data it is difficult to estimate the magnitude of placental transport. In the case of phosphorus no such considerations apply, and the gradient strongly suggests active transport.

It is well known that the intestinal mucosa and the renal tubules discriminate between strontium and calcium in postnatal life. Strontium is absorbed less readily by both these epithelia, resulting in a proportionately smaller uptake from the intestine and a greater urinary excretion. These phenomena have been shown to be present in utero by Widdowson et al. (1962). On the other hand, Lough et al. (1963) found that the capacity of newborns to discriminate against strontium was very low compared with that of adults.

As was noted above, the normal ranges of fetal serum calcium and phosphorus concentrations are defined by very sparse data. Abnormalities or deviations during this period have not been described. Nevertheless, there is indirect evidence that intrauterine hypercalcemia may occur. The characteristics of idiopathic hypercalcemia (elfin facies, mental retardation, and failure to thrive) were first described in infants who had received calciferol supplements now considered excessive. Individual variation in susceptibility to the effects of this vitamin has been postulated to explain the fact that relatively few children so treated were affected (Taussig, 1966; Fanconi, 1962). In some patients stenotic lesions of the aorta and other large arteries suggested an antenatal onset of the disorder. Beuren et al. (1966) found the typical stigmata and vascular lesions in the offspring of mothers who had received massive doses of calciferol (12.5 mg or 500,000 units) repeatedly during pregnancy. It has since been possible to reproduce the vascular lesions in the offspring of calciferol-treated rabbits (Friedman and Mills, 1969). These findings strongly suggest that intrauterine hypercalcemia may have been present.

Neonatal Period

Within a few hours after birth, serum phosphorus concentration begins to increase from its initial average of 5.6 mg/100 ml, reaching 7 to 8 mg/100 ml within a week, and remaining at this relatively high level for most of the first month of life. During the onset of hyperphosphatemia urinary phosphate is low, and such data as are available suggest that most of the filtered phosphate is reabsorbed, as is apparently the case in utero. By the third day tubular phosphate conservation decreases (Connelly et al., 1962) and serum phosphorus concentration achieves a plateau. In normal full-term infants samples from the cord or fontanelle have an average serum calcium concentration of 10.7 mg/100 ml. Within a day or two this level decreases to the range characteristic of older children and adults (Bakwin, 1939).

Connelly et al. (1962) compared the responses of newborns to parathyroid hormone given on the first and third days of life. They found enhancement of renal phosphate excretion at both ages with an increase in the proportion C_p/C_{cr}. The change at three days was greater than that seen at one day. Untreated infants also showed a decrease in TRP during the period of study. They concluded that both endogenous parathyroid activity and renal tubular responsiveness increased within the first three days. Their data define a transient state of hypoparathyroidism in early infancy. McCrory et al. (1952), studying somewhat older neonates, found that the proportion of excreted P to filtered P was as high by six days of age as that in fasting adults. The response of their subjects to exogenous parathyroid hormone was also similar to that of adults. They concluded that the higher serum phosphate and intolerance of phosphate loading exhibited by infants as compared with older children or adults could be attributed to the lower glomerular filtration rates of the younger subjects. These two viewpoints can be reconciled by assuming that the parathyroid glands and renal tubules are hypoactive during the first two to three days of postnatal life, during which time hyperphosphatemia is established. Thereafter, the relatively low GFR of early infancy may maintain serum P above the later normal level and render the subject more susceptible to phosphorus loading.

Decreased renal phosphorus excretion, whatever its cause, has the clinical correlate of susceptibility to tetany in the presence of excessive dietary phosphate. Cow's milk contains approximately five times as much phosphorus as human milk and has a Ca/P ratio of 1:1 instead of 2:1. Most commonly used dilutions of whole or evaporated milk therefore impose a phosphate load on the formula-fed infant, as was pointed out by Rohmer and Woringer (1923), Bakwin (1939), Gardner (1952), and Gardner et al. (1950). Gardner (1952) demonstrated parathyroid hyperplasia, hyperphosphatemia, and an increased incidence of neonatal tetany in formula-fed as compared with breast-fed infants. The composition of commercial formulas has since been altered to decrease phosphorus and increase the calcium: phosphorus ratio, with the result that tetany is now uncommon in normal full-term, formula-fed infants.

It is possible that the relative hypoparathyroidism of the neonate results as much from lack of stimulation of phosphate excretory mechanisms as from immaturity of the parathyroids and kidneys. In the studies cited above, McCrory et al. (1952) found that tubular phosphate reabsorption was increased when intestinal phosphate absorption was reduced by oral aluminum hydroxide gel. The ability of an infant so treated to excrete exogenous phosphate was markedly reduced, since tubular reabsorption established during phosphate deprivation persisted throughout the acute loading period. Adult rats kept on a low-phosphorus diet for two weeks showed fatal tetany following parenteral phosphate loads well tolerated by animals on the standard high-phosphate ration. Injection of parathyroid hormone prior to loading was protective, and phosphate tolerance was reestablished by five days on the standard diet (Bergstrom, 1968). It seems likely that this experiment was analogous to that of McCrory et al. (1952). The rapidly growing fetus exists in a relatively low-phosphorus environment established by maternal homeostasis. Teleologic reasoning suggests that phosphorus conservation is appropriate to the circumstances and that neither parathyroids or renal tubules receive stimuli to increase phosphorus excretion. The demonstration by Aceto et al. (1966) of intrauterine hyperparathyroidism in the infant of an untreated hypoparathyroid mother is consistent with this speculation, as is the functional capacity of fetal parathyroid explants shown by Scothorne (1964).

The skeleton at birth is relatively undermineralized, with an ash weight:dry weight ratio approximately half of that found in adult bone. It is probable that this circumstance increases the risk of tetany by providing abundant receptor sites for calcium. An analogous situation is that of the older rachitic infant who has abundant unmineralized osteoid and is notoriously susceptible to tetany.

Hypocalcemia resulting from excessive dietary phosphate is usually seen when food intake is well established after the first week of life and is associated with hyperphosphatemia. Symptomatic hypocalcemia in premature infants, in the off-spring of diabetic mothers, and in association with maternal hyperparathyroidism may occur on the first day of life. A few instances of congenital idiopathic hypo-parathyroidism have also been reported (Lobdell, 1959; Taitz et al., 1966; Huber et al., 1967), but these comprise only a small fraction of the total incidence of neonatal hypocalcemia. Curtis et al. (1962) reported an instance of neonatal hypoparathyroidism associated with cytomegalic inclusion disease.

In a series of 111 premature infants Gittleman et al. (1956) found 55 whose serum calcium concentration was less than 8.0 mg/100 ml at some time during the first week of life. Many of these patients were asymptomatic. The incidence of hypocalcemia was inversely correlated with birth weight within the group, ranging from 75 percent in 1,080- to 1,470-g infants to 41 percent in those weighing 1,920 to 2,475 g. The authors mention two factors besides functional immaturity which may be operative. The first is the elevated level of cortisol characteristic of maternal serum at term. This steroid is known to oppose parathyroid hormone in calcium homeostasis, i.e., it tends to cause hypocalcemia through inhibition of bone resorption (Cañas et al., 1967). Klein et al. (1954) have shown that cortisol crosses the placenta and that cord serum levels after delivery may exceed those of normal adults. There is then a precipitous drop; infants two to five days old have essentially no measurable serum cortisol (see Ch. 30). It would therefore seem that hypocalcemia could be attributed to cortisol only within the first day or two of life. Even at this time its effect is doubtful, since infants delivered by cesarean section have low cord serum cortisol levels but an increased incidence of hypocalcemia (14 percent in the study of Gittleman et al., 1956). The second factor discussed is that of starvation, presumably common in prematures who are slow to establish adequate caloric intake. Fasting releases endogenous phosphate from protein catabolism and has in fact been shown to bring about healing of active rickets in both human and animal subjects. Deposition of bone calcium in infants with minimal calcium intake and abundant undermineralized osteoid could establish hypocalcemia by the same mechanism as that in rapidly healing rickets. The skeleton of the premature is much less mineralized than that of the full-term infant, since the majority of calcium and phosphate accretion occurs during the last trimester. This phenomenon is readily appreciated by cursory inspection of radiographs.

Bruck and Weintraub (1955) found hypocalcemia, that is, less than 8.0 mg/100 ml, in 66 percent of 51 premature infants and emphasized the correlation between postnatal fasting and hypocalcemia, stating that, "After 33 or more hours, no calcium level above 8.0 mg/100 ml was observed, whereas all levels taken during the first 12 hours of life were above 8 mg." It is interesting that these authors found no corresponding hyperphosphatemia in their premature group as compared with normal newborns. Craig and Buchanan (1958) reported 26 babies who had hypocalcemic tetany within the first 36 hours of life. Of these, 22 were premature, including 10 whose mothers were diabetic. Serum phosphorus, measured in 16 patients, was not over 7.4 mg/100 ml at the onset of symptoms. Impairment of neonatal calcium-phosphorus homeostasis in the offspring of diabetic mothers was also described by Zetterström and Arnhold (1958). Craig (1958) pointed out that the clinical signs of early hypocalcemia are not those of classic tetany (i.e., carpopedal spasm, inspiratory stridor, and seizures) and that Chvostek's and Trousseau's signs are not often present. Instead, the clinical picture is one of rapid, shallow respirations, apneic intervals, and poor color, followed by increasing hyperexcitability, wild agitation, and tachycardia. Later, episodes of flaccidity and apparent complete exhaustion supervene. Vomiting was a frequent finding in the series discussed by Dodd and Rapoport (1949).

Smith (1959) suggests that prematures can absorb dietary calcium as well as full-term infants. Defective fat absorption, with the corollary of decreased uptake of vitamin D, is probably not an important factor within the first 48 hours of life.

Evidence summarized by Silverman (1964) indicates that prematures have an absolute calciferol requirement greater than that of full-term infants. The data relate to the prophylaxis of rickets and thus do not pertain strictly to the neonatal period. However, the author has seen several instances of hypocalcemia during the second and third weeks of life in prematures receiving 200 to 300 units of calciferol per day.

With the possible exception of relatively prolonged postnatal fasting, the factors predisposing to early hypocalcemia in prematures are exaggerations of tendencies present in all neonates, comprising functional immaturity of the parathyroids, kidneys, and bones.

An association between maternal diabetes and early neonatal tetany has been noted by Craig (1958) and others. However, so many of the patients reported were also premature that it is difficult to assess the etiologic significance of diabetes.

Gittleman et al. (1956) found an increased incidence of hypocalcemia on the first day of life in infants born by cesarean section: 14 percent when the indication for section was cephalopelvic disproportion and 37 percent when section was done for placenta previa, abruptio placentae, diabetes, or eclampsia. In normal full-term deliveries the incidence was 1.2 percent, whereas it was 100 percent in 14 infants following "abnormal pregnancy or labor or both." Unfortunately, the nature of the maternal complications was not specified. All three of these groups showed higher serum phosphorus concentrations than did the normal controls, but the difference (6.5 and 6.2 mg/100 ml as compared with 5.7 mg/100 ml) is so small that its physiologic significance seems doubtful. Although it is tempting to ascribe hypocalcemia in these patients to maternal overproduction of cortisol, no confirmatory data are available.

In summary it appears that the neonate is functionally hypoparathyroid from either immaturity or lack of intrauterine stimulation of parathyroids and kidneys. This tendency is exaggerated by prematurity and by maternal hyperparathyroidism. cesarean section, maternal distress preceding or during labor, and possibly maternal diabetes predispose to early hypocalcemia by means which are presently obscure. The incidence of hypocalcemia is high among the special groups discussed, and the clinical signs are nonspecific. Since response to therapy is prompt, a high index of suspicion is appropriate.

REFERENCES

Abdul-Karim, R.   1967.   Fetal endocrinology—a review. J. Med. Liban., 20:201.
———— R. E. L. Nesbitt, Jr., and J. T. Prior.   1966.   Study of the effects of experimentally induced endocrine insults upon pregnant and non-pregnant ewes. Fertil. Steril., 17:637.
Aceto, T., Jr., R. E. Batt, and E. Bruck.   1966.   Intrauterine hyperparathyroidism: A complication of untreated maternal hypoparathyroidism. J. Clin. Endocr., 26:487.
Andersch, M., and F. W. Oberst.   1936.   Filterable serum calcium in late pregnant and parturient women, and in newborns. J. Clin. Invest., 15:131.
Bakwin, H.   1939.   Tetany in newborn infants: Relation to physiologic hypoparathyroidism. J. Pediat., 14:1.
Bergstrom, W. H.   1968.   Unpublished data.
Beuren, A. J., et al.   1966.   Vitamin-D-hypercalcämische Herz-und Gefässerkrankung. Deutsch. Med. Wschr., 91:881.
Bodansky, M., and V. B. Duff.   1941.   Dependence of fetal growth and storage of calcium and phosphorus on the parathyroid function and diet of pregnant rats. J. Nutr., 22:25.
Booher, L. E., and G. H. Hausmann.   1931.   Studies on the chemical composition of the human skeleton. I. Calcification of the tibia of the normal newborn infant. J. Biol. Chem., 94:195.
Bruck, E., and D. H. Weintraub.   1955.   Serum calcium and phosphorus in premature and full-term infants. Amer. J. Dis. Child., 90:653.
Cañas, F. M., W. H. Bergstrom, and S. J. Churgin.   1967.   Effects of the adrenal on calcium homeostasis in the rat. Metabolism, 16:670.
Connelly, J. P., J. D. Crawford, and J. Watson.   1962.   Studies of neonatal hyperphorus in foetal tissues. Biochem. J., 68:573.
Craig, W. S.   1958.   Clinical signs of neonatal tetany: With especial reference to their occurrence in newborn babies of diabetic mothers. Pediatrics, 22:297.
———— and M. F. G. Buchanan.   1958.   Hypocalcemic tetany developing within 36 hours of birth. Arch. Dis. Child., 33:505.
Curtis, J. C., W. F. Dodge, and C. W. Daeschner.   1962.   Cytomegalic inclusion disease associated with hypoparathyroidism. Pediatrics, 29:52.
Dodd, K., and S. Rapoport.   1949.   Hypocalcemia in the neonatal period. Amer. J. Dis. Child., 78:537.
Economu-Mavrou, C., and R. A. McCance.   1958.   Calcium, magnesium, and phosphorus in foetal tissues. Biochem. J., 68:573.
Ertel, N. H., J. S. Reiss, and G. Spergel.   1969.   Hypomagnesemia in neonatal tetany associated with maternal hyperparathyroidism. New Eng. J. Med., 280:260.
Fanconi, G.   1962.   Physiology and pathology of calcium and phosphorus metabolism. Advances Pediat., 12:307.
Fee, B. A., and W. B. Weil.   1963.   Body composition of infants of diabetic mothers by direct analysis. Ann. N. Y. Acad. Sci., 110:869.
Friedman, W. F., and L. F. Mills.   1969.   The relationship between vitamin D and the craniofacial and dental anomalies of the supravalvular aortic stenosis syndrome. Pediatrics, 43:12.

Fuchs, F., and A. Fuchs. 1956. Studies on the placental transfer of phosphate in the guinea pig. I. The transfer from mother to fetus. Acta Physiol. Scand., 38:379.

Gardner, L. I. 1952. Tetany and parathyroid hyperplasia in the newborn infant: Influence of the dietary phosphate load. Pediatrics, 9:534.

———— et al. 1950. Etiologic factors in tetany of newly born infants. Pediatrics, 5:228.

Gittleman, I. F., J. B. Pincus, E. Schmerzler, and M. Saito. 1956. Hypocalcemia occurring on the first day of life in mature and premature infants. Pediatrics, 18:721.

Hamilton, B., L. Daref, W. J. Highman, Jr., and C. Schwartz. 1936. Parathyroid hormone in blood of pregnant women. J. Clin. Invest., 15:323.

Hartenstein, H., and L. I. Gardner. 1966. Tetany of the newborn associated with maternal parathyroid adenoma. New Eng. J. Med., 274:266.

Huber, J., P. Cholnoky, and H. E. Zoethout. 1967. Congenital aplasia of parathyroid glands and thymus. Arch. Dis. Child., 42:190.

Jackson, W. P. U. 1961. Effects of altered nutrition on the skeletal system: The requirement of calcium in man. In Brock, J. S., ed. Recent Advances in Human Nutrition. New York, Little, Brown and Company, p. 293.

Kelly, H. J., R. E. Sloan, W. Hoffman, and C. Saunders. 1951. Accumulation of nitrogen and six minerals in the human fetus during gestation. Human Biol., 23:61.

Kerr, C., et al. 1962. Calcium and phosphorus dynamics in pregnancy. Amer. J. Obstet. Gynec., 83:2.

Klein, R., J. Fortunato, and C. Papadatos. 1954. Free blood corticoids in the newborn infant. J. Clin. Invest., 33:35.

Lobdell, D. H. 1959. Congenital absence of the parathyroid glands. Arch. Path. (Chicago), 67:412.

Lough, S. A., J. Rivera, and C. L. Comar. 1963. Retention of strontium, calcium, and phosphorus in human infants. Proc. Soc. Exp. Biol. Med., 112:631.

Ludwig, G. D. 1962. Hyperparathyroidism in relation to pregnancy. New Eng. J. Med., 267:637.

Malm, O. J. 1963. Adaptation to alterations in calcium intake. In Wasserman, R. H., ed. The Transfer of Calcium and Strontium across Biological Membranes. New York, Academic Press, Inc., pp. 143-173.

Maxwell, J. P. 1930. Further studies in osteomalacia. Proc. Roy. Soc. Med., 23:19.

McCrory, W. W., C. W. Forman, H. McNamara, and H. L. Barnett. 1952. Renal excretion of inorganic phosphate in newborns. J. Clin. Invest., 31:357.

Reed, G. B., Jr. 1969. Rubella bone lesions. J. Pediat., 74:208.

Rohmer, P., and P. Woringer. 1923. L'action du phosphate de soude sur la calcémie du nourisson. C. R. Soc. Biol. (Paris), 89:575.

Schmitz, E. 1924. Untersuchungen über den Kalkgehalt der wachsenden Frucht. Arch. Gynaek., 121:1.

Scothorne, R. J. 1964. Functional capacity of fetal parathyroid glands with reference to their clinical use as homografts. Ann. N. Y. Acad. Sci., 120:669.

Shohl, A. T. 1939. Mineral Metabolism. New York, Reinhold Publishing Corp.

Silverman, W. A. 1964. Dunham's Premature Infants, 3rd ed. New York, Hoeber Medical Division, Harper & Row, Publishers.

Sinclair, J. G. 1942. Fetal rat parathyroids as affected by changes in maternal serum calcium and phosphorus through parathyroidectomy and dietary control. J. Nutr., 23:141.

Smith, C. A. 1959. The Physiology of the Newborn Infant, 3rd ed. Springfield, Ill., Charles C Thomas, Publisher, p. 266.

Sontag, L. W., P. Munson, and E. Huff. 1936. Effects on the fetus of hypervitaminosis D and calcium and phosphorus deficiency during pregnancy. Amer. J. Dis. Child., 51:302.

Taitz, L. S., C. Zarate-Salvador, and E. Schwartz. 1966. Congenital absence of the parathyroid and thymus glands in an infant. Pediatrics, 38:412.

Taussig, H. B. 1966. Possible injury to the cardiovascular system from vitamin D. Ann. Intern. Med., 65:1195.

Todd, W. R., E. G. Chuinard, and M. T. Wood. 1939. Blood calcium and phosphorus in the newborn. Amer. J. Dis. Child., 57:1278.

Wasserman, R. H., and A. N. Taylor. 1968. Vitamin D-dependent calcium-binding protein: Response to some physiological and nutritional variables. J. Biol. Chem., 243:3987.

————— R. A. Corradino, and A. N. Taylor. 1968. Vitamin D-dependent calcium-binding protein: Purification and some properties. J. Biol. Chem., 243:3978.

Westin, B., et al. 1959. Some constituents of umbilical venous blood of previable human fetuses. Acta Paediat. Scand., 48:609.

Widdowson, E. M., R. A. McCance, G. E. Harrison, and A. Sutton. 1962. Metabolism of calcium, strontium, and other minerals in the perinatal period. Lancet, 2:373.

Zetterström, R., and R. G. Arnhold. 1958. Impaired calcium-phosphorus homeostasis in newborn infants of diabetic mothers. Acta Paediat. Scand., 47:107.

Part V

NEUROMUSCULAR SYSTEM

23

Physiology of the Neonatal Central Nervous System

WILLIAMINA A. HIMWICH ● Thudichum Psychiatric Research Laboratory, Galesburg State Research Hospital, Galesburg, Illinois

Introduction

The maturity of the neonatal animal of any species is the product of its rate of development in utero and requires additional development and integration of behavior before reaching the adult state. The growth and development of the brain, including the attainment of the adult levels of the various chemical constituents as well as of metabolism, proceed in all species of animals from the time of appearance of the neural streak until maturity. The chronologic relation of this maturation to physiologic events, such as implantation, birth, opening of the eyes, and so forth, varies in the different species of animals. The problems of comparison and the difficulties of drawing generalizations from one species to another have been considered by Himwich (1962). Among the mammalian species, at the time of birth, the young may be deemed either relatively mature, such as lamb and guinea pig, or relatively immature, such as rat, mouse, and man. In general, such a classification describes the behavior of the entire animal rather than that of an individual system. In the mammals born relatively mature, not only the central nervous system (CNS), but also the muscular and bony structures, are sufficiently matured to allow the young to subsist with a minimum of maternal care.

It has been pointed out by Anokhin (1964) in his elegant studies of systemogenesis that even in the young born immature some CNS nuclei have reached relative maturity at birth. Which nuclei these are depends upon which parts of the CNS are necessary for the survival of the young. Other areas of less importance to the survival of the neonate may be less mature at the same chronologic age. One of the big problems in attempting to relate human development to that of young animals from other species is the impossibility of fitting the total human organism logically into the scale of development of any other species. In some ways, the human infant is born more mature than a baby rabbit; for example, the visual system is more mature with the eyes open and beginning to function. On the other hand, the brain of the baby rabbit develops at a much faster rate after birth (Bishop, 1950). It becomes exceedingly important for these reasons that we consider the maturity of the young of one species as compared with another in terms of specific functions and systems, such as the visual system, the auditory system, and so forth. In this chapter, we shall attempt to examine what is known of the physiology of the CNS of the human newborn, as indicated by biochemical and electrophysiologic analyses.

Brain Constituents

There is widespread interest in the biochemical development of the human brain, but, unfortunately, the data are scarce. The outstanding difficulty in biochemical studies of the human newborn is the fact that the brain can be sampled only after death. While certain parameters may show little or no change, the influence of anoxia upon such relatively simple measures as brain weight and moisture content have been well documented in experimental animals (Edstrom and Essex, 1956). It is necessary in this field to scrutinize carefully all the data available, especially at any points at which they do not conform to values or trends obtained on the newborn of experimental animals. Where the data on human beings diverge, we are faced always with the question of whether the divergence is a true species difference, a difference in developmental rate, or an artifact due to the condition of the neonate. This problem becomes increasingly complex, since except for those who lose their lives suddenly in an accident, most persons suffer from a longer or shorter period of deranged metabolism, anoxia, or other complicating factors before death. These factors are especially difficult to pinpoint in the case of the neonate since it is impossible to document how long an infant may have been in distress before birth or how abnormal his condition may have been. Nonetheless, we can only proceed to examine what data are available on the human brain, keeping these doubts firmly in mind.

Data on the growth of the brain, its water content, and changes in lipid and protein can be found in the literature (MacArthur and Doisy, 1918-19, Tilney and Rosett, 1931). The picture in general is similar to that seen in other animals. At the time of birth, the brain is growing rapidly in weight, is losing water, and is accumulating lipids and proteins (Fig. 1). The data on myelination suggest that little myelin is laid down before the second month of postnatal life, after which time it accumulates rapidly. Cellular differentiation, however, has been well underway from approximately 15 weeks before birth. Cellular multiplication, which started with conception, will continue in the brain at least during the first year, as judged by changes in DNA concentration of the brain during fetal life and to the end of the first year of life (Mandel and Bieth, 1952).

Potassium, sodium, and chloride have been determined on some of the samples obtained of human fetal brain. The data suggest for most brain parts an increase with age in potassium and little change in sodium or chloride (Himwich et al., 1963). The only other values we have been able to locate in the literature are those of Kimitsuki (1955), who determined the electrolyte content of cerebral hemispheres of fetuses. Kimitsuki's data are similar to those of the author except for chloride content.

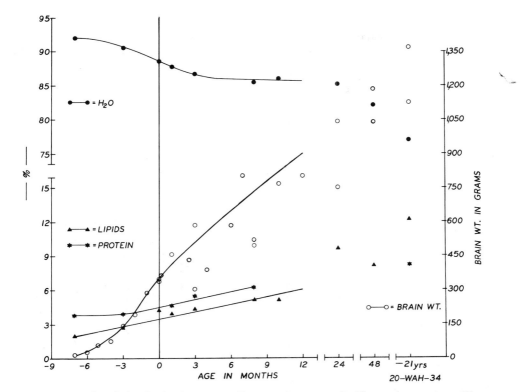

Fig. 1. Growth of the brain in man. Changes in water, lipids, and protein. (From Himwich et al. 1963. *Advances Biol. Psychiat.*, 5:263–278.)

Lipids have, of course, been studied more extensively than other brain constituents since an abnormal lipid metabolism seems to occur in many types of mental deficiency and also because the lipids change slowly after birth. Because of the great importance of these compounds, a table of classification taken from the work of Rossiter (1962) is included (Table 1). Although older workers (Koch and Mann, 1907; MacArthur and Doisy, 1918-19) did not find appreciable amounts of cerebrosides in fetal brain, more recent studies with better methods have made it possible to study these compounds during development. The brains of fetuses show a distinctive cerebroside pattern by the eighth fetal month. Cerebrosides and phosphatidyl ethanolamine increase during gestation while phosphatidyl choline decreases. The relation of these changes is well discussed by Clausen et al. (1965) (Figs. 2 and 3). By the third fetal month, the gangliosides show an adult type of pattern (Svennerholm, 1964) (Table 2) which may be changed by birth trauma such as anoxia. From the fourth fetal month until term, the concentration of gangliosides doubles. Analyses indicate that these lipids occur in the axons as well as in the cell bodies of the neurons.

In general, in infant and fetal brain the majority of the lipid-soluble hexoses are glycolipids other than cerebrosides and sulfatides. In these brains, the hydroxy

TABLE 1.   Classification of Lipids Found in the Nervous System[a]

A. *Phosphatides* (phospholipids)
    1. *Glycerophosphatides* (phosphoglycerides)
        Phosphatidyl cholines (lecithins)
        Phosphatidyl ethanolamines
        Phosphatidyl serines
        Plasmalogens (phosphatidal ethanolamines)
        Cephalin B
    2. *Inositol phosphatides* (phosphoinositides)
    3. *Sphingomyelins* (phosphosphingosides)
B. *Glycolipids*
    1. *Cerebrosides* (glycosphingosides)
    2. *Cerebroside sulfate esters* (sulfatides)
    3. *Mucolipids*
        Gangliosides
        Strandin
                             } Sphingolipids
C. *Nonsaponifiable lipids*
    1. *Sterols*
    2. *Hydrocarbons*
D. *Neutral fat* (triglycerides)
E. *Protein-bound lipids*
    1. *Proteolipids*
    2. *Phosphatidopeptides*
    3. *Lipoproteins*

[a]From Rossiter. 1962. *Neurochemistry*, 2nd ed. Courtesy of Charles C Thomas, Publisher.

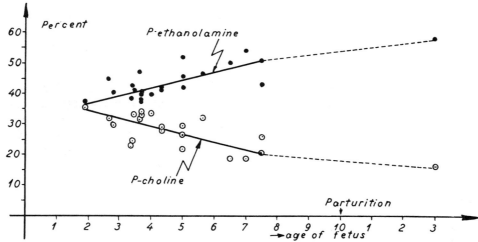

Fig. 2. Phosphocholine and phosphoethanolamine as percentage of the total polar lipids from human brain as a function of age of fetus. Ordinate, phosphocholine or phosphoethanolamine as percentage of the total extractable polar lipids from human brain. (From Clausen et al. 1965. *J. Neurochem.*, 12:599–606.)

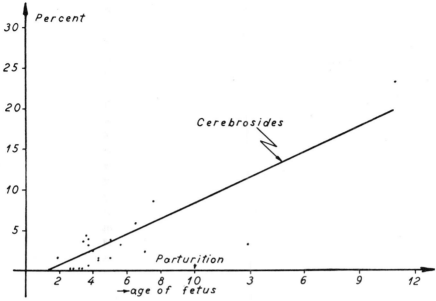

Fig. 3. Cerebrosides in percentage of the total extractable glycerophosphatides from human brain as a function of age of fetus. Ordinate, cerebrosides in percentage of the total extractable glycerophosphatides from human brain. (From Clausen et al. 1965. *J. Neurochem.*, 12:599–606.)

fatty acids are low in concentration, but in all specimens C_{24} is the principal hydroxy fatty acid just as in adult brain. Menkes et al. (1966) suggest that before myelination 16:0, 18:0, and 18:1 fatty acids predominate, while after myelination long-chain and hydroxy fatty acids predominate. O'Brien and Sampson (1965b)

TABLE 2. Lipid Composition of Human Premature and Full-Term Infant Brain[a]

| | Premature | | | | | Full-term | | |
	24 weeks	28 weeks	33 weeks	33 weeks	35 weeks	1	2	3
Water[b]	90·5	90·2	90·8	91·1	90·7	90·1	91·1	89·6
Total nitrogen	10·4		9·5	9·1		9·3	9·3	9·7
Total hexosamine	0·64		0·56	0·72	0·67	0·67	0·70	0·79
Total lipids	24·6	26·5	26·1	28·5	30·3	29·9	27·8	29·1
Cholesterol	4·6	5·4	5·1	5·1	6·6	6·3	5·4	5·2
Phospholipids	18·8	21·2	20·6	21·6	22·5	21·8	20·5	21·1
Kephalins	8·8	8·9	9·8	10·8	10·3	10·1	9·6	9·6
Lecithins	9·5	10·0	9·0	10·6	11·1	10·7	10·7	10·7
Sphingomyelins	0·60	0·63	0·65	0·60	0·70	0·60	0·65	0·75
Gangliosides								
Lipid hexosamine	0·120	0·115	0·107	0·141	0·136	0·155	0·125	0·145
Lipid N-acetyl-neuraminic acid	0·33	0·32	0·32	0·38	0·38	0·44	0·35	0·38

[a]From Svennerholm. 1964. *J. Neurochem.*, 11:839-853.
[b]Percentage of fresh weight. (All other values are expressed in percentage of dry weight.)

believe that myelin is apparently the same irrespective of age. They say, "Since myelin is 'chemically mature' at an early age . . . a specific composition must be reached before myelin can be formed; one in which saturated glycerophosphatides and long-chain sphingolipids predominate." In human myelin, the ratio of protein amino acids to polar lipids is 2.38:1 (O'Brien and Sampson, 1965a). (For additional information on brain lipid metabolism, see Ch. 15.)

The amino acids of the proteolipids of human brain show the presence of two main compounds (Tables 3, 4). The one present in gray matter is unaffected by maturation. The proteolipid in the fetal white matter resembles that in gray matter. However, with maturation a protein accumulates which is present in the bulk of the proteolipids of white matter and is a constituent of myelin (Prensky and Moser, 1967). Cystathionine has a high concentration in white matter as compared with γ-amino butyric acid (GABA) which is present largely in gray matter (Gjessing and Torvik, 1966).

The histochemistry of the developing human cerebellum has been studied by Meyer (1963). Alkaline phosphatases are actively present in the vessel endothelium, as might be expected from their role in transport of substances such as glucose. The acid phosphatases occur parallel to cytoplasmic basophilia suggesting, according to Meyer, a role in RNA synthesis. The highest content is in Purkinje cells and in the large cells of the dentate nucleus.

The developing basal ganglia have also proved to be fertile areas for the study of histochemistry (Duckett and Pearse, 1967) (Fig. 4). By the seventh week of embryonic life, oxidative enzymes are present in the diencephalic germinal layer.

TABLE 3. Amino Acid Composition of Proteolipids of Human Gray Matter at Different Ages[a,b]

Amino acid	33-week fetus	39-week fetus	14 days	25 days	18 months	23 months	8 yr	55 yr	79 yr
Aspartic acid	—	7·8	7·1	7·4	7·2	7·3	7·2	7·4	4·1
Threonine	6·5	15·7[c]	6·8	6·3	6·9	5·9	6·6	5·7	6·0
Serine	12·7		8·3	7·9	8·2	7·9	8·9	6·8	7·2
Glutamic acid	7·1	5·4	5·7	5·8	6·0	5·6	5·5	5·8	5·0
Proline	4·5	6·7	4·4	4·4	5·2	5·1	6·0	4·9	4·0
Glycine	11·9	9·2	9·3	8·2	10·3	9·0	9·6	10·9	10·4
Alanine	13·1	15·8	11·9	12·9	12·6	12·9	12·9	12·2	10·9
Valine	6·8	6·3	7·0	8·0	7·4	7·8	6·5	7·7	7·6
Half-cystine	<0·5	<0·5	0·9	1·8	1·0	1·0	0·4	—	<0·6
Methionine	1·9	2·4	2·4	2·4	2·8	2·2	2·9	—	3·2
Isoleucine	6·6	3·8	4·8	3·7	5·8	4·9	4·8	5·8	7·9
Leucine	12·8	11·7	13·9	13·9	14·2	13·5	12·5	13·5	12·7
Tyrosine	2·2	2·4	2·2	1·9	2·1	1·4	2·7	—	2·7
Phenylalanine	6·3	5·6	6·5	5·7	7·3	6·1	5·9	7·3	6·7
Lysine	2·9	3·5	4·0	4·4	3·6	4·6	3·6	2·9	4·0
Histidine	1·5	1·8	2·4	2·5	—	2·5	1·4	1·3	1·3
Arginine	3·3	2·6	2·5	2·7	2·7	2·5	2·5	1·8	5·3

[a]From Prensky and Moser. 1967. *J. Neurochem.*, 14:117-121.
[b]Results are expressed as moles recovered per 100 moles of total amino acid. No determinations were made of tryptophan or amide nitrogen.
[c]Separation of threonine and serine was incomplete.

TABLE 4. Amino Acid Composition of Proteolipids of Human White Matter at Different Ages[a,b]

Amino acid	33-week fetus	4 days	14 days	25 days	18 months	23 months	24 months	8 yr	43 yr	79 yr
Aspartic acid	6·9	6·9	5·9	5·4	4·5	3·8	4·3	4·4	4·3	3·6
Threonine	6·3		7·6	6·9	8·2	8·3	8·2	7·1	8·0	8·5
Serine	10·1	19.0[c]	7·3	7·1	6·2	6·1	6·3	4·1	6·8	6·0
Glutamic acid	6·7	5·5	5·9	6·4	5·8	6·1	5·4	6·1	5·3	3·9
Proline	5·6	5·0	3·9	4·6	2·5	2·9	2·8	3·2	2·9	2·4
Glycine	9·0	10·7	9·0	9·7	10·3	10·9	12·6	11·0	10·4	10·3
Alanine	12·4	12·3	13·1	12·2	12·0	12·1	12·5	12·4	12·6	12·2
Valine	6·4	5·6	7·4	7·6	7·1	7·1	8·9	8·0	7·5	7·3
Half-cystine	0·8	—	1·9	2·6	3·4	3·9	—	2·7	3·5	3·9
Methionine	2·1	1·5	2·2	2·2	1·8	1·7	1·8	1·8	1·4	1·8
Isoleucine	5·1	5·9	5·0	5·3	5·0	4·7	5·4	5·2	5·0	5·1
Leucine	12·6	13·1	13·0	13·3	12·1	11·8	12·3	12·2	12·0	11·9
Tyrosine	2·3	2·8	2·8	3·3	4·3	4·2	3·5	4·9	4·8	5·2
Phenylalanine	5·3	6·2	7·0	7·3	8·7	8·5	8·9	9·1	8·5	8·7
Lysine	3·6	2·5	3·7	4·2	4·0	3·9	3·3	3·9	3·7	4·2
Histidine	2·0	0·6	1·9	2·4	1·6	1·5	1·1	1·4	0·7	2·2
Arginine	2·7	2·4	2·4	2·7	2·5	2·4	2·2	2·6	2·6	2·7

[a]From Prensky and Moser. 1967. *J. Neurochem.*, 14:117-121.
[b]Results are expressed as moles recovered per 100 moles of total amino acid. No determinations were made of tryptophan or amide nitrogen.
[c]Separation of threonine and serine was incomplete.

The enzymatic individuality of different nuclei as reported in the rat by Friede (1959) was also found in human studies. By the sixth month of gestation, acetylcholinesterase activity appears (Duckett and Pearse, 1967). Similar data have been presented by Youngstrom (1941) (Fig. 5).

Bertler (1961) found both norepinephrine and dopamine in the five-month-old fetus, although dopamine was not present at the end of the first trimester (Fig. 6). At five months of fetal life, dopamine was very low. By eight months, dopamine had increased nearly to the level found in the adult human brain. Although norepinephrine had also increased, its rate of increase was not as high as that for dopamine. These data suggest a different maturation pattern for norepinephrine and dopamine. Hornykiewicz (1964) has suggested that the relative development of the hypothalamus and related autonomic functions at birth in the human infant as compared with the extrapyramidal motor functions might account for the difference in the patterns of maturation for norepinephrine and dopamine.

The esterases in young infants in the first half year of life have been compared with those of adult human brain (Barron and Bernsohn, 1968). The zymograms of the free esterases are qualitatively similar at both ages. The esterases characteristic of adult white matter did not appear in the infant until about four months of age. The acetylcholinesterase and butyrylcholinesterase in infants one to four months of age were identical to the adult patterns. In general, the bound esterase increased in cortex and cerebellar cortex, but in white matter the proportion of free to bound esterase did not change during development.

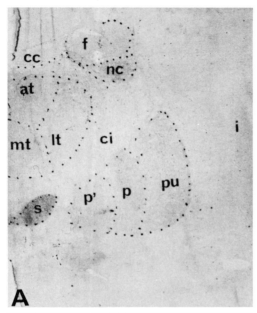

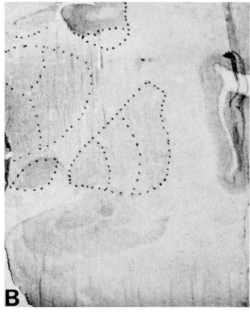

Fig. 4. Coronal sections through the basal ganglia of a 20-week-old fetus. A. The sites of NADH diaphorase activity are in the subthalamic nucleus (s), putamen (pu), pallidum (p', p), nucleus caudatus (nc), and anterior (at), medial (mt), and lateral (lt), thalamic nuclei. Other surrounding areas present little if any of this activity. ×3. B. The sites of NADH diaphorase activity are the subthalamic nucleus (s), the fountains of Hortega (f), the insular cortex, and the hippocampal region. ×3. (From Duckett and Pearse. 1967. *Histochemie,* 8:334–341.)

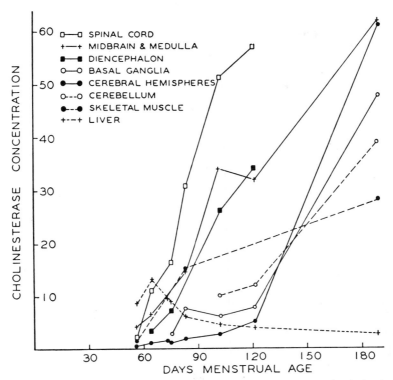

Fig. 5. Acetycholinesterase activity of various parts of human fetal brain. (From Youngstrom. 1941. *J. Neurophysiol.*, 4:473–477.)

Blood-Brain Barrier

The whole area of interpretation of hematoencephalic exchange is fraught with difficulty because we do not understand the mechanisms involved. Certainly no generalization can be drawn, and data cannot be assumed to apply to any species except the one studied and only under the *specific* experimental conditions observed.

The chief clinical observations upon which the condition of the blood-brain barrier in human infants can be based are cases of kernicterus (Zachau-Christiansen and Vollmond, 1965; Zuelzer, 1960). The lesions in the brain associated with this condition have been well documented (Fig. 7). Attempts to reproduce this syndrome in experimental animals suggest that anoxia may be necessary for the entrance of bilirubin into the brain (Chen et al., 1965, 1967; Rozdilsky and Olszewski, 1960, 1961). In man the work of Gröntoft (1954) also supports this thesis.

Many reviews of the blood-brain barrier phenomena (Dobbing, 1961; Lajtha, 1968) as they apply to animals of all ages have been published. In general the younger the animal the greater is the hematoencephalic exchange. Among the best animal studies have been those of Roth and his colleagues (Roth et al., 1959) in the Department of Pharmacology, University of Chicago, and of Lajtha (Lajtha

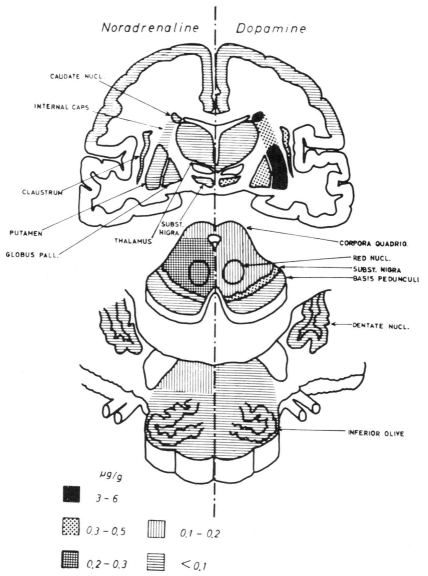

Fig. 6. Noradrenaline and dopamine in the human brain. (From Bertler. 1961. *Acta Physiol. Scand.*, 51:97–107.)

et al., 1963). The latter have studied the penetration of individual amino acids in young and adult animals (Lajtha, 1961). Although again each amino acid must be considered individually, the general rule of better penetration in the younger animals held. The most exciting finding is that one amino acid can inhibit the entry of others (Guroff and Udenfriend, 1962).

Domek et al. (1960) demonstrated that myelin offers a barrier to the entrance

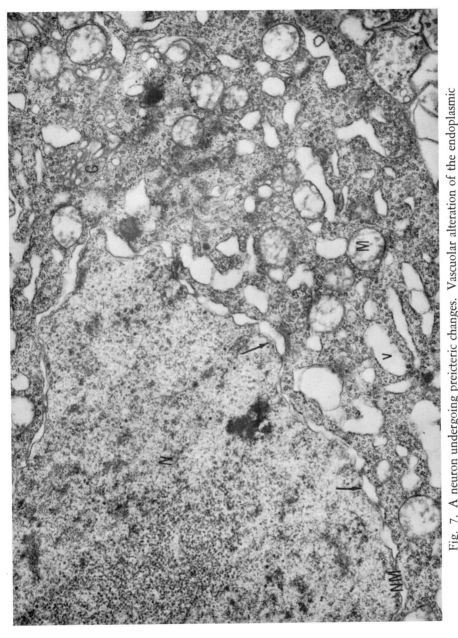

Fig. 7. A neuron undergoing preicteric changes. Vascuolar alteration of the endoplasmic reticulum is conspicuous. The mitochondria are swollen, and their interiors have become electron-lucid. The inner and outer nuclear membranes are separated, showing a tendency to vacuole formation (arrow). ×14,000. (From Chen et al. 1966. *Amer. J. Path.*, 48:683–711.)

of phenobarbital into the brain. The same probably applies to urea (Schoolar et al., 1960) and thiopental (Domek et al., 1960), but not to acetazolamine-S[35] (Roth et al., 1959). The lack of myelin in young brains may explain the relatively faster penetration of some materials. Barlow et al. (1959) state: "It would seem that a series of factors can and do affect the distribution of compounds in brain. Consideration of the physical properties of the substance (fat or water solubility, dissociation, etc.), the blood-brain barrier, water compartmentation of brain tissues, and probably local biochemical and metabolic factors in specific anatomical units of brain is necessary."

Metabolism

Himwich et al. (1959) attempted to duplicate on human babies studies of the oxygen consumption of animal brains for purposes of comparison with similar data from experimental animals. The data have been reported on more than 50 babies who showed no marked pathology and whose mothers were free of complications of pregnancy. Obviously, these infants could not have been normal since they all died either at birth or shortly thereafter. The actual data on the oxygen consumption of the parts were widely scattered, so regression equations were prepared using the method of least square and lines drawn on the graph from these equations (Fig. 8). These lines suggest that at 140 days of gestation, that is, at approximately the twentieth week, the oxygen consumption of the medulla oblongata is well above that of the other brain parts. The oxygen consumption of this part remained at approximately the same level as the fetus matured, whereas the oxygen consumption

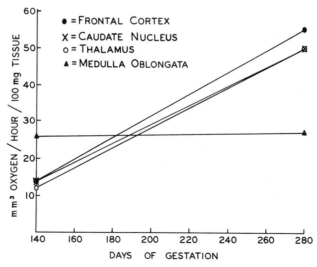

Fig. 8. Oxygen consumption of human brain parts at various periods of gestation. Values for 140 days and 280 days calculated from regression equations. (From Himwich et al. 1959. *J. Appl. Physiol.,* 14:873–877.)

of other areas increased markedly. The pathway of glucose metabolism in the human fetal cortex appears to be mainly the Embden-Meyerhof glycolytic pathway (Villee and Loring, 1961) as in the rabbit (Villavicencio et al., 1958) and in counter distinction to the rat where the pentose phosphate shunt is of importance (Guerra et al., 1967).

One of the enzymes involved in the aerobic metabolism of the brain is succinic dehydrogenase. This enzyme is necessary for the complete oxidation of pyruvic acid via the Krebs or citric acid cycle. Cassin and Herron (1961) found that in rabbits this enzyme reached its adult level in the cortex at the same time that the mature picture of intolerance to anoxia became evident in brain. Succinic dehydrogenase activity persists for a long period of time after death. Determinations of succinic dehydrogenase show the changes in activity of this enzyme in the various brain parts as the human fetus matures (Himwich et al., 1963). These data indicate that, with the exception of the spinal cord and the medulla oblongata, there is a tendency for succinic dehydrogenase activity to increase with age, and, therefore, they support the results obtained on oxygen consumption of the brain parts.

In the adult brain (rat) isotopic carbons present in glucose rapidly become incorporated into amino acids. This characteristic pattern appears first at the critical period of development when enzymes are developing rapidly and probably is dependent upon changes in the enzyme systems controlling glycolysis and the oxidation of glucose. These changes are accompanied by a threefold increase of decarboxylic amino acids (Gaitonde and Richter, 1966) (Fig. 9). Some labeled glutamate may go via the oxoglutarate shunt into fatty acids. However, even in developing brain this pathway appears to be of little quantitative significance (D'Adamo and D'Adamo, 1968).

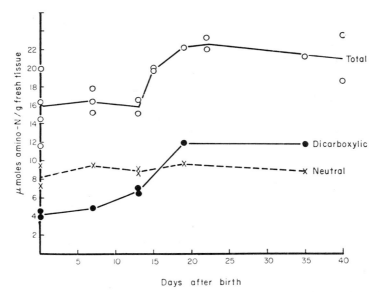

Fig. 9. Amino acid content of the developing rat brain. (From Gaitonde and Richter. 1966. *J. Neurochem.*, 13:1309–1318.)

All of these rapidly changing metabolic patterns in the brain during development are dependent upon enzyme changes. The lack of data on human infants and the various species of animals used with their different rates of maturation make it difficult to predict exactly what is the metabolic pattern in the human brain in the perinatal period. Nonetheless, a knowledge of what is happening in general in developing brain is necessary for an understanding of the period.

The development of the theory of compartmentation of glutamic acid metabolism (Waelsch, 1961) has contributed greatly to our understanding of amino acid metabolism. In the cortex of the cat, at least, this compartmentation follows a developmental pattern (Berl, 1965) appearing between the third and sixth weeks of life. As the pattern becomes definitive the pool available for glutamine formation contracts, and the other pool or pools enlarge. In kittens the glutamine synthetase activity (Berl, 1966) of the neocortex correlates well with the compartmentation data. In other areas the correlation is poor. Possibly as suggested by Salganicoff and De Robertis (1965) the subcellular distribution of the enzyme may be of more importance than total concentration.

Our understanding of the enzymes related to glutamic acid and its metabolic relatives is greater than for any other single metabolic group. Glutamate decarboxylase (GD) and γ-aminobutyrate transaminase (GABA-T) have been extensively studied. The ratio between these two enzymes remains constant during development (van den Berg and van Kempen, 1964). Sims et al. (1968) have reported GABA-T on whole brain taking into consideration not only the changes in enzyme activity with age but also the increase in brain weight (Fig. 10). It is of interest that this curve is very similar to but smoother than that based on a unit of fresh weight. In monkey a fivefold increase in hexosephosphate aminotransferase (GTF) occurs after birth, and glutamate dehydrogenase (GDH) and

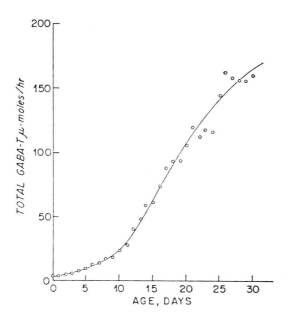

Fig. 10. Total brain amino butyrate transaminase (GABA-T) and rat age in days. Rates in μ moles per hour. (From Sims et al. 1968. *J. Neurochem.*, 15:667–672.)

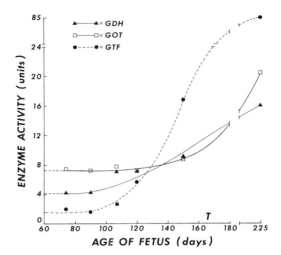

Fig. 11. Development of brain enzymes in the fetal monkey. Each point represents an average of values obtained from four different fetuses. See text for abbreviations. (From Jolley and Labby. 1960. *Arch. Biochem.* 90:122–124.)

aspartate aminotransferase (formerly glutamate-oxaloacetic transaminase, GOT) increase less rapidly (Jolley and Labby, 1960) (Fig. 11). Pitts and Quick (1967) in a systematic study of succinate semialdehyde dehydrogenase found abrupt changes in the rate of increase at two and six days of age. At day two, there was a similar rate change in weight and at day ten in protein. The largest increase in the enzyme just preceded the critical period. A synthesis of these enzyme changes with the concentration changes of both substrates and products during development should give an interesting new perspective on the biochemical changes during development.

The LDH isoenzymes (lactate dehydrogenase) show in one case (E in Fig. 12) an increase with age whereas the isoenzyme B in Figure 12 decreases and A in Figure 12 shows little change. The definitive isozymatic composition of LDH, however, is reached only after 20 days in the rat at which time the brain is fully organized and well along in the development of mature integration (Bonavita et al., 1962). In fetal animals Lagnado and Hardy (1967) have found that the electrophoretic distribution of A type esterases varies with age. In all animals studied, including man, a fetal type of enzyme is replaced by a more mature type during maturation (Fig. 13). In man the period of most rapid transition is from one month before birth to one year after birth. The exact function of these enzymes is unknown, but the authors (Lagnado and Hardy) suggest they may be concerned with tissue growth or with the numerous instances of cell death that occur during early growth.

Although most studies have been made on enzymes involved in amino acid or carbohydrate metabolism, some workers have dealt with those responsible for lipid metabolism. D(-)-β-hydroxybutyric dehydrogenase activity is greatest during the period of rapid growth and maturation of the brain (Klee and Sokoloff, 1967). The enzyme activity rises at the same time as does cytochrome c oxidase activity but then falls while cytochrome c oxidase maintains its high level (Fig. 14). The distribution of the enzyme (D(-)-β-hydroxybutyric dehydrogenase) suggests that it may be concentrated more in glia than in neurons and may be linked with lipid

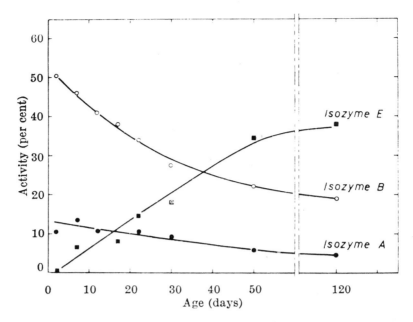

Fig. 12. Changes in the percentage activity of three LDH isozymes from the whole rat brain during the postnatal development. Each experimental point represents the mean of at least three determinations. (From Bonavita et al. 1962. *Nature* [*London*], 196:576–577).

and myelin synthesis. Glycerol-3-phosphate dehydrogenase also shows a developmental pattern of change, with its peak activity in the rat forebrain appearing after 30 days and the greatest rate of increase being found during the period of active myelinization (Laatsch, 1962). Glyceraldehyde phosphate dehydrogenase, on the other hand, shows less change with development and has the greatest increase in activity between the fourth and twenty-first days of age (Fig. 15). Two other enzymes with probable relationship to myelinization have been studied in rabbits at various ages: namely, phosphocholine-glyceride transferase and choline phosphokinase. The former shows maximum activity during the period of active myelinization. As would be expected, this maximum activity appears in the cortex at later times than in the medulla (McCaman and Cook, 1966).

The relation between the development of the brain and the ability to resist anoxia will not be considered here since the whole topic of anoxia will be considered in detail in Chapter 34.

Electrophysiologic Activity

SPONTANEOUS

Since Lindsley (1939) published his historic paper of the EEG of the fetus, there has been no doubt that the fetus as well as the newborn does show spontaneous

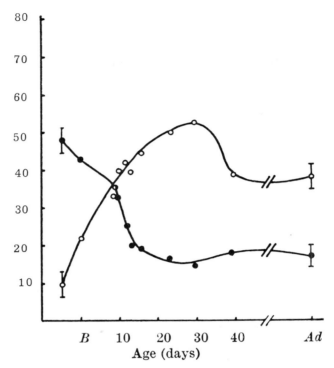

Fig. 13. Effects of age on the relative distribution of A type esterases from rabbit brain. ○, fraction A₁, ●, fraction A₂. B, birth. Ad, adult. Most values represent means of at least three determinations on different animals (S.D. 2 to 5 percent). Standard deviations are shown for extreme ages. (From Lagnado and Hardy. 1967. *Nature* [*London*], 214:1207–1210).

electric activity from the brain. One physiologic measurement that can be made readily on the newborn infant is the electric activity of the brain both spontaneous and evoked. It is no wonder, therefore, that a great volume of data is available. Ellingson (1958) and Kellaway and Petersén (1964) and recently Parmelee et al. (1967a, b, 1968) in this country, Dreyfus-Brisac et al. (1962), Mound and Pajot (1965), and Passouant (1964) in France, and Arshavsky et al. (1966) in Russia have published much excellent material on this subject (Fig. 16). In the normal, full-term child the EEG appears to be of little diagnostic value as far as future evidence of neurologic damage is concerned. This point is thoroughly discussed by Ellingson (1967). As he points out, in the absence of pathology of the nervous system, the importance of an abnormal EEG can only be determined by a longitudinal study. Such studies unfortunately are few. Investigations of epilepsy in the newborn have been conducted by Passouant and Cadilhac (1962), of cerebral palsy by Lesný (1964). Ellingson (1964) has followed up a number of children for as long as seven years, his records extending as far into fetal life as the twenty-fourth week of conceptual age. Records of the premature infants have also been made by Parmelee et al. (1967a, 1968) and Dreyfus-Brisac et al. (1962).

The current surge of interest in paradoxic sleep and its function (Roffwarg

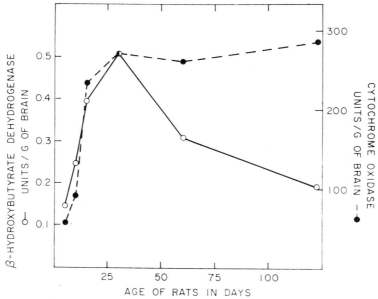

Fig. 14. β-hydroxybutyric dehydrogenase and cytochrome oxidase activities in rat brain as a function of age. One unit of β-hydroxybutyric dehydrogenase activity is defined as the amount of enzyme activity catalyzing the formation of 1 μMol of acetoacetate per minute. Cytochrome oxidase was assayed by the method of Cooperstein and Lazarow; 1 unit is the amount of enzyme activity causing a change in the logarithm of the ferrocytochrome c concentration of 1.0 per minute at room temperature. The values for both enzyme activities represent the mean of two assays done with two different enzyme concentrations. (From Klee and Sokoloff. 1967. *J. Biol. Chem.*, 242:3880–3883.)

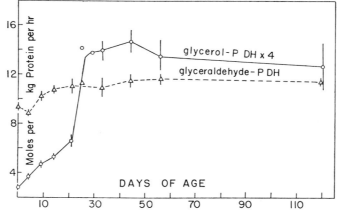

Fig. 15. Glycerol-3-phosphate and glyceraldehydephosphate dehydrogenases of whole rat forebrain as a function of age. Each point represents the mean for at least six animals except that the 25 and 29 points are each the mean of two animals. The bars represent ± one standard error. (From Laatsch. 1962. *J. Neurochem.*, 9:487–492.)

et al., 1966) has led to a reexamination of young infants, both premature and full-term (Figs. 17 and 18). Dreyfus-Brisac (1968) has even collected records from a group of previable infants of 24 to 28 weeks of gestational age. Monod et al. (1967) have followed sleep patterns in the young suffering from pathology. Newborn mongols appear to have longer periods of nonREM (rapid eye movement) sleep than do normal infants. Tracings during sleep show more low amplitude slow activity (Goldie et al., 1968).

Shepovalnikov (1962) believes that alpha activity is present in newborns and is an intrinsic activity of the brain. Lindsley (1939) as well as Ellingson and Lindsley (1949) believes that it develops from the slow waves of infancy. Churchill et al. (1966) in studying the effects of birth conditions (such as presentation or drug administration) on the newborn EEG came to the conclusion that Shepovalnikov's thesis should be further investigated before a decision is made.

Parmelee et al. (1968) have coded with a 3-digit code the EEG patterns between 28 and 40 weeks of conceptional age and find these codes useful, for example, in differentiating the premature from the infant small-for-dates (Table 5). Attempts at quantifying the EEG data in the neonate have also been made by Bartoshuk (1964) and Bartoshuk and Tennant (1964). Quiet sleep increases as the infant matures while active (REM) sleep decreases. Quiet sleep, which is 10 percent of the total at 31 to 32 weeks of gestational age, increases to approximately 50 percent at 3 months of age, while active sleep decreases from 68 percent at 33 to 34 weeks of gestational age to 36 percent at 3 months. These data apply to records visually scanned. Dreyfus-Brisac (1968) in a study of previable infants (24 to 27 weeks of gestational age) showed that such infants had neither quiet nor active sleep patterns.

There appear to be differences in the EEG during development in various ethnic groups (Pampiglione, 1965). Alpha activity developed earlier in African Negro children than in European and Indian children. Before alpha, there appeared a well-defined sinusoidal rhythmic activity at 5 to 6 cycles/second in the occipital area on eye closure. This pattern also is seen earlier in African Negro children than in others.

TABLE 5. **Percentage of Each Sleep State at Each Gestational Age as Obtained by Computer Sorting of Coded Data from Polygraphic Recordings.**[a]

Gestational age (weeks)		N	Active sleep		Transitional sleep		Quiet sleep	
			Mean %	Range	Mean %	Range	Mean %	Range
Premature Infants	30	2	15	14-17	67	63-70	18	15-20
	31-32	5	27	7-44	63	43-83	10	4-17
	33-34	4	45	36-57	46	35-53	10	6-14
	35-36	7	42	29-61	46	38-60	11	8-24
	37-38	8	32	15-55	43	30-66	24	9-47
	39-40 (term) ...	9	32	12-46	38	21-63	31	21-48
	53 (3 months past term)	8	25	15-37	29	13-36	45	30-59
Term Infants	39-40 (term) ...	6	38	19-48	34	24-42	28	18-40
	53 (3 months past term)	6	23	15-34	30	19-37	47	38-59

[a]From Parmelee et al. 1967a. *Develop. Med. Child. Neurol.*, 9:70-77.

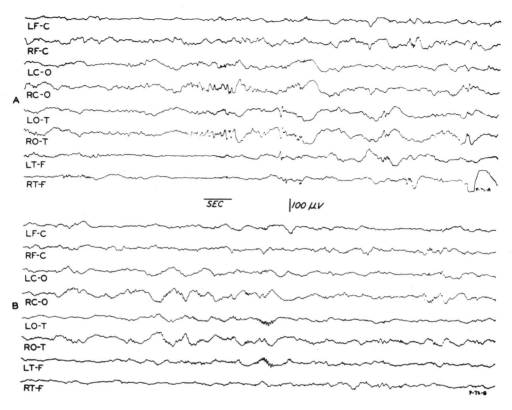

LF-C
RF-C
LC-O
RC-O   A
LO-T
RO-T
LT-F
RT-F

$\overline{SEC}$ |$100\,\mu V$

LF-C
RF-C
LC-O
RC-O   B
LO-T
RO-T
LT-F
RT-F

Fig. 16. EEGs of a premature newborn. Gestational age at birth 30 weeks. Birth weight 1,558 g. A. EEG No. 1: 65 hours after birth; weight 1,490 g. Note asynchrony and sporadic sharp transients. B. EEG No. 2: gestational age 31 weeks; weight 1,500 g. There has been a striking change in the 7 days since EEG No. 1; the pattern is that typically seen several weeks later.

EVOKED POTENTIAL

The evoked potential offers means of evaluating the status of the various sensory systems in the neonate. It has even been proposed as a means of determining the degree of prematurity. Engel and Butler (1963) found the latency of the visual evoked potential as good a criterion of conceptual age as was birth weight. The auditory evoked potential has similarly been evaluated by Graziani et al. (1968). In general, the evoked responses in the infant are simple in wave form with a longer latency, a great fatigability, and a more discrete topographic localization than in the adult. The visual evoked potential can always be seen in the neonate although averaging techniques may be required (Ellingson, 1966; Ferriss et al., 1966; Hrbek and Mareš, 1964). Responses have been recorded at 24 weeks (Engel, 1964) and 28 weeks of gestational age (Ellingson, 1960). The wave form may be adult in shape as early as the first month of postnatal life or maturation may be delayed

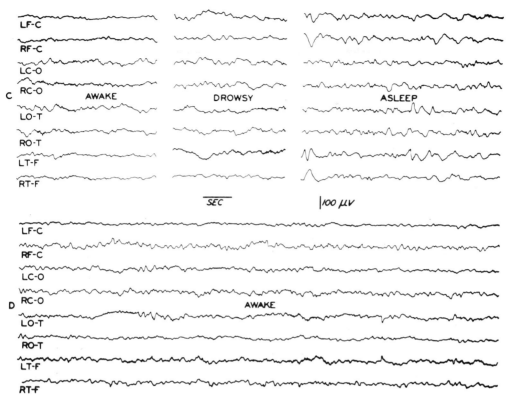

Fig. 16, cont. C. EEG No. 7: gestational age 36 weeks; weight 2,268 g. The transition from wakefulness to sleep, seen for the first time, is characterized by an increase in the prominence of the slower components. D. EEG No. 8: gestational age 37 weeks; weight 2,590 g. The pattern is typical of the full-term infant. (From Ellingson. 1964. *Progr. Brain Res.,* 9:26–53.)

until two to three years of age (Ellingson, 1967). There appears to be little agreement on the incidence of responses in normal as compared to neurologically abnormal infants. Hrbek and Mareš (1964) obtained differences, but neither Engel and Butler (1963) nor Ellingson (1964) could confirm this.

The following response has been studied with many divergent results, but under suitable conditions Ellingson (1967) found a high incidence of following in infants. The optimum frequency appears to be 3 per second. With age the following response can be elicited at higher frequencies, and the optimum frequency seems to be close to the dominant rhythm during wakefulness (Glaser and Levy, 1965).

The auditory and somesthetic responses have been less thoroughly studied than the visual. The auditory responses are probably nonspecific responses to auditory stimuli and not primary ones. The nonspecific character of the response makes it difficult to relate it to maturation. Dreyfus-Brisac and Blanc (1956) have found

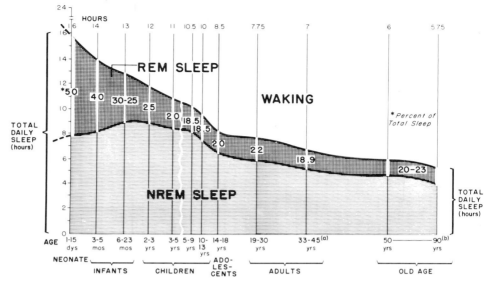

Fig. 17. Graph showing changes (with age) in total amounts of daily sleep and daily REM sleep and in percentage of REM sleep. Note sharp diminution of REM sleep in the early years. REM sleep falls from 8 hours at birth to less than 1 hour in old age. The amount of nonREM sleep (NREM) throughout life remains more constant, falling from 8 hours to 5 hours. In contrast to the steep decline of REM sleep, the quantity of nonREM sleep is undiminished for many years. Although total daily REM sleep falls steadily during life, the percentage rises slightly in adolescence and early adulthood. This rise does not reflect an increase in amount; it is due to the fact that REM sleep does not diminish as quickly as total sleep. Work in progress in several laboratories indicates that the percentage of REM sleep in the 50- to 85-year group may be somewhat higher than represented here. (Adapted from Roffwarg et al. 1966. *Science,* 152:604–619.)

such responses only after 8 months of conceptual age. Graziani et al. (1968), however, obtained responses from 30-week-old prematures which correlated well with estimated postconceptual age but not with birth weight or postnatal age.

Somesthetic responses have been little studied. Desmedt et al. (1967) report interesting differences in adult and newborn responses to stimulation of the hand. The extension of such studies will increase our ability to interpret the maturation of the CNS in the neonate.

Effects of Drugs

GENERAL

In considering the effects of drugs upon the neonate, we must evaluate not only the effects of drugs which have been given to the mother during the period of pregnancy, which may or may not influence the baby at birth, but also the responses

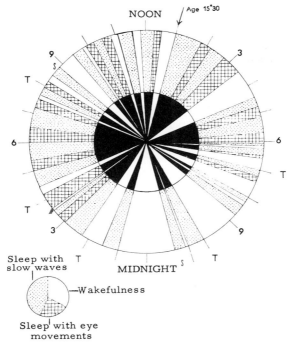

Fig. 18. Cycles in the course of a night and a day (24 hours) in a newborn, recorded from 15 hours and 30 minutes to 39 hours and 30 minutes after birth. Inner circle, periods of sleep (black) and wakefulness (white). Outer circle, calm sleep (dotted area), sleep with eye movements (hatched area). Lower circle, total duration of wakefulness, of sleep with slow waves (calm or slow sleep), and of sleep with eye movements (during the 24-hour period). (From Passouant. 1964. *J. Psychol. Norm. Path.*, 3:257–279.)

of the young organism to drugs administered directly to it. These reactions may be quite different from those of the fully mature individual. In an excellent review on drug administration in the neonatal period, Nyhan (1961) points out that the response to a drug is the result of the interaction of a number of factors, any or all of which may vary with age. In some cases, the response is related directly to the weight and surface area of the animal or patient, and, since surface area is so much larger in proportion to weight in the young infant than in the adult, the simple difference in size may make a significant difference in the response. Other factors are the absorption and excretion of drugs as well as their distribution in the body.

Once the drugs have been absorbed, differences in metabolism or in detoxication may be evident. Some of these differences are due to the low activity of specific enzyme systems of the neonate. The enzyme systems require time to mature just as do other physiologically and biochemically important parameters. As one example, the toxicity of chloramphenicol in newborn and premature infants is probably due to an immature stage of enzymatic development which does not allow the efficient removal of the drug. Tolbutamide is another drug which is very slowly metabolized in the newborn (Nitowsky et al., 1966). After the first few days of life, the rate of metabolism of this compound approaches that of the adult. Among the anesthetic agents, sodium-4-hydroxybutyrate appears to cross the placenta at least in the guinea pig and to produce depression in the fetus (Cosmi et al., 1968). Such depression, however, has not been noted in human infants whose mothers were given this compound before birth, a fact which underlines the hazards of extrapolating data from one species to another. The newborn rat has been reported to be more susceptible to pentobarbital than the adult (Homburger et al., 1947). An excellent review on the effects of drugs commonly used in obstetrics on fetuses and newborns has been written by Shnider (1966). He points out that almost any drug given to a pregnant woman and consequently found in her blood

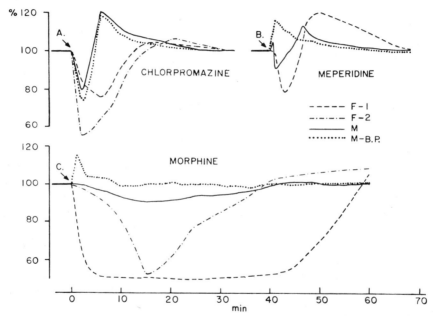

Fig. 19. Effects of drugs on fetal and maternal brain aO$_2$ and maternal blood pressure in three experiments. In each experiment, brain aO$_2$ was recorded simultaneously from two fetuses (F-1 and F-2) and the mother (M). Blood pressure (M-BP) was recorded from maternal carotid artery. Drugs were injected, intravenously, at arrow. The curves were plotted from continuous recordings. Abscissa, time in minutes. Ordinate, blood pressure and aO$_2$ in percent (100 percent represents average during control period).

Control averages (μA = diffusion current = oxygen availability) for experiment with:

Chlorpromazine	Meperidine	Morphine (0.15 mg/kg)
F-1: 0.27 μA ($\pm$5%)	F-1: 0.20 μA ($\pm$0%)	F-1: 0.75 μA ($\pm$7%)
F-2: 0.115 μA ($\pm$0%)	M: 0.15 μA ($\pm$3%)	F-2: 0.026 μA ($\pm$8%)
M: 0.28 μA ($\pm$5%)	M-BP: 60 mm Hg ($\pm$3%)	M: 0.144 μA ($\pm$3%)
M-BP: 70 mm Hg ($\pm$0%)		M-BP: 68 mm Hg ($\pm$3%)

(From Misrahy et al. 1963. *Anesthesiology,* 24:198–202.)

must be assumed to pass into the infant's circulation. Our knowledge is only fragmentary as to what effects these drugs may have on the baby. Some information has been obtained from animal experimentation. The effect of drugs during pregnancy upon fetal cerebral oxygen has been studied in guinea pigs (Misrahy et al., 1963) (Fig. 19) and upon response to anoxia and resuscitation in rabbits (Campbell et al., 1968). In interpreting such results, however, it must be remembered that the fetal guinea pig just before birth is relatively mature, and whether or not these data can be generalized for use in human beings is difficult to say. Nyhan (1961) and Nyhan and Lampert (1965) point out that the responses to drugs in the very young are sufficiently novel to warrant establishment of a systematic developmental pharmacology. Even when quantitative adjustments are made for the size of the patient, impressive qualitative differences still occur. It is never safe to extrapolate to the neonate pharmacologic results obtained in later life, and fetal effects in particular are completely unpredictable. Optimally the therapeutic responses to drugs of the newborn and of the fetus should be determined experimentally before the drug is used clinically. Alcohol has different effects on the young animal than on the adult or the fetus, the young being more resistant to the toxic effects (Chesler et al., 1942a). The same relative resistances were shown by the animals to morphine (Chesler et al., 1942b). Divergent results were found by Kupferberg and Way (1963), who noted the greatest toxicity to morphine in the young animals and ascribed this difference to greater brain permeability in the young.

Immature or newborn mice and guinea pigs showed a marked inability to metabolize many drugs, being particularly unable to form glucuronides as a means of detoxication. It is of interest that the newborn guinea pig, which is in many ways quite mature, nevertheless shows an immature pattern of drug metabolism. In this respect, the degree of immaturity of an enzyme system in the guinea pig seems to equal that in the newborn mouse, an animal born at a very immature stage (Jondorf et al., 1958-59). Young rabbits show a marked lack in enzymes necessary to metabolize hexabarbital, pyramidon, and amphetamine, among other drugs. Fouts and Adamson (1959) suggest in this regard that in the young animal some inhibitors may be present.

EEG EFFECTS

The ease of recording the EEG in the newborn has led to many investigations of the effects on the infant's EEG of drugs given either to the mother or to the child in the neonatal period. Children whose mothers had received barbiturate have been reported by Ellingson (1958) to show a transient depression of the EEG. Borgstedt and Rosen (1968) also found transient behavioral and electroencephalographic changes in newborns at birth which could be correlated with the sedative-hypnotic or narcotic medications given to their mothers during labor. These effects, however, were transient.

Thalidomide given to the pregnant guinea pig causes changes in the EEG of the fetus—largely electric silence (Bergström et al., 1963). These data suggest

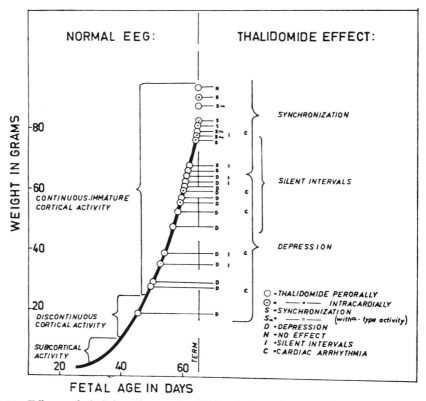

Fig. 20. Effects of thalidomide on the EEG of the guinea pig fetus at different fetal stages. (From Bergström et al. 1963. *Med. Exp.,* 11:119–127.)

that thalidomide is a sedative, being narcotic in the younger fetuses and neurotoxic in the youngest ones (Fig. 20). Bleyer and Rosen (1968) found that in the guinea pig meperidine had a convulsant effect in the mother and a depressant effect in the fetus. The effect in the mother was short-lived but continued longer in the fetus (Fig. 21).

An extensive study of the sleep cycle in the developing kitten and rabbit and of the effects of various drugs administered to the young animal has been completed by Shimizu and Himwich (1969) (Table 6). The drugs include LSD which diminishes REM sleep in the kitten (Shimizu and Himwich, 1968a). However, in animals younger than six to eight days of age, the decrease was less than in the older animal. Similar data were found on the phenothiazines, imipramine and haloperidol (Shimizu and Himwich, 1968b, 1969; Shimizu et al., 1968). The reasons for these differences may be found in the absorption, excretion, and metabolism of the drugs or in the fact that in the younger animal the cerebral structures involved in sleep are still too immature to respond to the drugs. With amphetamine (Shimizu and Himwich, 1968c), the period of wakefulness in the kitten was increased with a concomitant diminution in activated (REM) sleep. As with the other drugs,

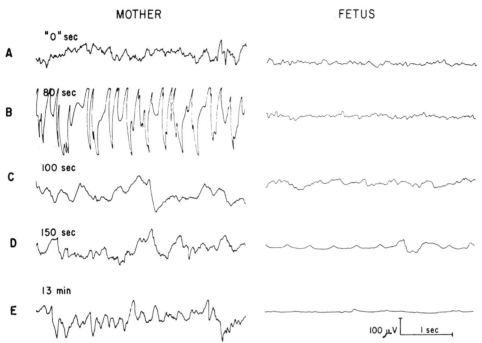

Fig. 21. Convulsive-depressive response to meperidine (17 mg/kg). A. control EEGs of mother (left) and fetus (right) sampled during the minute before injection of the drug into a maternal vein. B. 80 seconds after the injection, the maternal EEG shows sharp waves. Fetal EEG changes are not yet apparent. C. At 100 seconds the maternal epileptiform activity has ceased and the fetal EEG shows increased voltage and slowing. D. At 150 seconds the maternal EEG shows increased activity and the fetal EEG shows flattening. E. At 13 minutes the maternal EEG has begun to return to the preinjection pattern; the fetal EEG continues flat. (From Bleyer and Rosen. 1968. *Electroenceph. Clin. Neurophysiol.*, 24:249–258.)

TABLE 6.   Effect of Drugs on the Durations of Single Episodes of Both Phases of Sleep in Growing Kittens[a]

Age in days		Control	Imipramine (5 mg/kg)	Chlorpromazine (10 mg/kg)	Propériciazine (3 mg/kg)	Haloperidol (5 mg/kg)
1-3	Slow wave sleep	0.6 ± 0.2	0.9 ± 0.1[a]	1.1 ± 0.4[a]	1.2 ± 0.2[b]	0.8 ± 0.3
	Activated sleep	2.4 ± 0.3	0.5 ± 0.2[b]	1.4 ± 0.4[b]	1.8 ± 0.2[b]	2.7 ± 0.7
6-8	Slow wave sleep	1.2 ± 0.3	1.4 ± 0.5	2.2 ± 0.6[a]	1.8 ± 0.1[a]	1.2 ± 0.3
	Activated sleep	3.1 ± 0.6	0.5 ± 0.5[b]	1.4 ± 0.5[b]	1.9 ± 0.5[a]	2.3 ± 0.6
11-13	Slow wave sleep	1.6 ± 0.3	4.2 ± 1.5[b]	4.3 ± 0.7[b]	3.0 ± 0.7[b]	1.8 ± 0.4
	Activated sleep	4.4 ± 0.5	0.8 ± 1.1[b]	1.5 ± 1.1[b]	2.9 ± 1.1[a]	3.2 ± 1.1
16-18	Slow wave sleep	2.3 ± 0.6	9.2 ± 1.9[b]	9.1 ± 1.7[b]	5.2 ± 1.9[a]	4.2 ± 0.5[a]
	Activated sleep	5.2 ± 1.3	0.2 ± 0.4[b]	2.1 ± 1.1[b]	3.1 ± 1.1[a]	6.2 ± 1.5
21-23	Slow wave sleep	3.2 ± 0.6	11.3 ± 3.5[b]	18.2 ± 8.6[b]	6.5 ± 1.0[b]	9.2 ± 2.9[b]
	Activated sleep	5.5 ± 1.5	0 ± 0[b]	2.7 ± 1.3[b]	4.0 ± 1.5	6.3 ± 2.0
26-28	Slow wave sleep	4.7 ± 1.2	22.3 ± 9.0[b]	21.0 ± 6.7[b]	10.6 ± 2.7[b]	9.0 ± 2.2[b]
	Activated sleep	6.4 ± 1.4	0 ± 0[b]	3.9 ± 1.9[a]	4.2 ± 1.5[a]	7.2 ± 1.0

[a]From Shimizu and Himwich. 1969. *Develop. Psychol.*, 13:161-169.
[b]Each figure indicates the mean value in minutes ± S.D. In the control study 6-7 kittens were used, in each age group, and 5 kittens in each age group for each of the drug studies. Letters show that the differences are statistically significant ([a]: P < 0.05; [b]: P < 0.005) as calculated with the Student's T Test.

these effects became more significant after the kittens were two weeks old. Propériciazine did not affect the percentage of wakefulness in the kittens as chlorpromazine did. The propériciazine animals were also more playful than were those receiving chlorpromazine.

Few studies have yet been made on the effects on postnatal behavior of the young of drugs given to the mother. Monod (1967) has noted differences in sleep-wakefulness patterns in neonates whose mothers received chlorpromazine during the latter part of pregnancy. Chlorpromazine given to pregnant rats has also been reported to influence postnatal behavior (Jewett and Norton, 1966).

REFERENCES

Anokhin, P. K. 1964. Systemogenesis as a general regulator of brain development. Progr. Brain Res., 9:54-86.

Arshavsky, I. A., M. Akhundki, and S. S. Solomatin. 1966. Characteristics of electrical activity and steady potential of the brain cortex in children under three months of age during sleep and wakefulness. Biull. Eksp. Biol. Med., 9:8-12.

Barlow, C. F., et al. 1959. Observations on isotype-labeled drugs in the central nervous system. *In* Proceedings of the Second International United Nations Conference on the Peaceful Uses of Atomic Energy, Geneva, September, 1958. New York, Pergamon Press, Inc. pp. 243-247.

Barron, K. D., and J. Bernsohn. 1968. Esterases of developing human brain. J. Neurochem., 15:273-284.

Bartoshuk, A. K. 1964. Human neonatal EEG: Frequency analysis of awake and asleep samples from four areas. Psychon. Sci., 1:281-282.

———— and J. M. Tennant. 1964. Human neonatal EEG correlates of sleep-wakefulness and neural maturation. J. Psychiat. Res., 2:73-83.

van den Berg, J. C., and G. M. J. van Kempen. 1964. Glutamate decarboxylase and γ-aminobutyrate transaminase in developing rat brain: Maturational changes in cerebral cortex IV. Experientia, 20:1-3.

Bergström, R. M., L. Bergström, P. Putkonen, and K. Sainio. 1963. The effects of thalidomide on the electrical activity of the brain in the intrauterine guinea-pig foetus. Med. Exp., 11:119-127.

Berl, S. 1965. Compartmentation of glutamic acid metabolism in developing cerebral cortex. J. Biol. Chem., 240:2047-2054.

———— 1966. Glutamine synthetase. Determination of its distribution in brain during development. Biochemistry, 5:916-922.

Bertler, A. 1961. Occurrence and localization of catechol amines in the human brain. Acta Physiol. Scand., 51:97-107.

Bishop, E. J. 1950. The strychnine spike as a physiological indicator of cortical maturity in the postnatal rabbit. Electroenceph. Clin. Neurophysiol., 2:309-315.

Bleyer, W. A., and M. G. Rosen. 1968. Meeperidine-induced changes in the maternal and fetal electroencephalograms of the guinea pig. Electroenceph. Clin. Neurophysiol., 24:249-258.

Bonavita, V., F. Ponte, and G. Amore. 1962. Lactate dehydrogenase isozymes in the developing rat brain. Nature (London), 196:576-577.

Borgstedt, A. D., and M. G. Rosen. 1968. Medication during labor correlated with behavior and EEG of the newborn. Amer. J. Dis. Child., 115:21-24.

Campbell, A. G. M., J. E. Milligan, and N. S. Talner. 1968. The effect of pretreatment with pentobarbital, meperidine, or hyperbaric oxygen on the response to anoxia and resuscitation in newborn rabbits. J. Pediat., 72:518-527.

Cassin, S., and C. S. Herron, Jr. 1961. Cerebral enzyme changes and tolerance to anoxia during maturation in the rabbit. Amer. J. Physiol., 201:440-442.

Chen, H.-C., I.-N. Lien, and T.-C. Lu. 1965. Kernicterus in newborn rabbits. Amer. J. Path., 46:331-343.

———— C.-S. Lin, and I.-N. Lein. 1966. Ultrastructural studies in experimental kernicterus. Amer. J. Path., 48:683-711.

———— C.-S. Lin, and I.-N. Lien. 1967. Vascular permeability in experimental kernicterus: An electron-microscopic study of the blood-brain barrier. Amer. J. Path., 51:69-99.

Chesler, A., G. C. LaBelle, and H. E. Himwich. 1942a. The relative effects of toxic doses of alcohol on fetal, newborn and adult rats. Quart. J. Stud. Alcohol, 3:1-4.

———— G. C. LaBelle, and H. E. Himwich. 1942b. A study of the comparative toxic effects of morphine on the fetal, newborn and adult rats. J. Pharmacol. Exp. Ther., 75:363-366.

Churchill, J. A., J. Grisell, and J. D. Darnley. 1966. Rhythmic activity in the EEG of newborns. Electroenceph. Clin. Neurophysiol., 21:131-139.

Clausen, J., H. O. Christensen Lou, and H. Andersen. 1965. Phospholipid and gly-colipid patterns of infant and foetal brain: Thin-layer chromatographic studies. J. Neurochem., 12:599-606.

Cosmi, E. V., H. O. Morishima, S. S. Daniel, and L. S. James. 1968. Effect of sodium-4-hydroxybutyrate (Gamma-OH) on fetal and newborn guinea pigs. Amer. J. Obstet. Gynec., 100:72-75.

D'Adamo, A. F., Jr., and A. P. D'Adamo. 1968. Acetyl transport mechanisms in the nervous system: The oxoglutarate shunt and fatty acid synthesis in the developing rat brain. J. Neurochem., 15:315-323.

Desmedt, J. E., J. Manil, H. Chorazyna, and J. Debecker. 1967. Potentiel évoqué cérébral et conduction corticipète pour une volée d'influx somesthesique chez le nouveau-né normal. C. R. Soc. Biol. (Paris), 161:205.

Dobbing, J. 1961. The blood-brain barrier. Physiol. Rev., 41:130-188.

Domek, N. S., C. F. Barlow, and L. J. Roth. 1960. An ontogenetic study of pheno-barbital-C^{14} in cat brain. J. Pharmacol. Exp. Ther., 130:285-293.

Dreyfus-Brisac, C. 1968. Sleep ontogenesis in early human prematurity from 24 to 27 weeks of conceptional age. Develop. Psychobiol., 1:162-169.

———— and C. Blanc. 1956. Electro-encéphalogramme et maturation cerebrale. Ence-phalé, 45:205-241.

———— J. Flescher, and E. Plassart. 1962. L'électroencéphalogramme: Critère d'âge con-ceptionnel du nouveau-né à terme et prématuré. Biol. Neonat., 4:154-173.

Duckett, S., and A. G. E. Pearse. 1967. Histoenzymology of the developing human basal ganglia. Histochemie, 8:334-341.

Edstrom, R. F. S., and H. E. Essex. 1956. Swelling of the brain induced by anoxia. Neur-ology, 6:118-124.

Ellingson, R. J. 1958. Electroencephalograms of normal, full-term newborns immediately after birth with observations on arousal and visual evoked responses. Electroenceph. Clin. Neurophysiol., 10:31-50.

———— 1960. Cortical electrical responses to visual stimulation in the human infant. Electroenceph. Clin. Neurophysiol., 12:663-677.

———— 1964. Studies of the electrical activity of the developing human brain. Progr. Brain Res., 9:26-53.

———— 1966. Development of visual evoked responses in human infants recorded by a response averager. Electroenceph. Clin. Neurophysiol., 21:403-404.

———— 1967. The study of brain electrical activity in infants. In Lipsitt, L. P., and C. C. Spiker, eds. Advances in Child Development and Behavior. New York, Academic Press, Inc., Vol. 3, pp. 53-97.

———— and D. B. Lindsley. 1949. Brain waves and cortical development in newborns and young infants. Amer. J. Physiol., 4:248-249.

Engel, R. 1964. Electroencephalographic responses to photic stimulation, and their cor-relation with maturation. Ann. N.Y. Acad. Sci., 117:407-412.

———— and B. V. Butler. 1963. Appraisal of conceptual age of newborn infants by electroencephalographic methods. J. Pediat., 63:386-393.

Ferriss, G. S., G. D. Davis, E. R. Hackett, and M. M. Dorsen. 1966. Maturation of visual evoked responses in human infants. Electroenceph. Clin. Neurophysiol., 21:404.

Fouts, J. R., and R. H. Adamson. 1959. Drug metabolism in the newborn rabbit. Science, 129:897-898.

Friede, R. L. 1959. Histochemical investigations on succinic dehydrogenase in the central nervous system. I. The postnatal development of rat brain. J. Neurochem., 4:101-110.

Gaitonde, M. K., and D. Richter. 1966. Changes with age in the utilization of glucose carbon in liver and brain. J. Neurochem., 13:1309-1318.

Gjessing, L. R., and A. Torvik. 1966. Distribution of cystathionine in human brain. Scand. J. Clin. Lab. Invest., 18:565.

Glaser, G. H., and L. L. Levy. 1965. Photic following in the EEG of the newborn. Amer. J. Dis. Child., 109:333-337.

Goldie, L., J. A. H. Curtis, U. Svendsen, and N. R. C. Roberton. 1968. Abnormal sleep rhythms in mongol babies. Lancet, 1:229-230.

Graziani, L. J., E. D. Weitzman, and M. S. A. Velasco. 1968. Neurologic maturation and auditory evoked responses in low birth weight infants. Pediatrics, 41:483-494.

Gröntoft, O. 1954. Intracranial haemorrhage and blood-brain barrier problems in the new-born. Acta Path. Microbial. Scand., Suppl. 100: 5-109.

Guerra, R. M., E. Melgar, and M. Villavicencio. 1967. Alternative pathways of glucose metabolism in fetal rat brain. Biochim. Biophys. Acta, 148:356-361.

Guroff, G., and S. Udenfriend. 1962. Studies on aromatic amino acid uptake by rat brain in vivo: Uptake of phenylalanine and of tryptophan; inhibition and stereoselectivity in the uptake of tyrosine by brain of muscle. J. Biol. Chem., 237:803-806.

Himwich, W. A. 1962. Biochemical and neurophysiological development of the brain in the neonatal period. Int. Rev. Neurobiol., 4:117-158.

———— D. K. Pennelle, and B. E. Tucker. 1963. Comparative biochemical development of fetal human, dog, and rabbit brain. Recent Advances Biol. Psychiat., 5:263-278.

———— et al. 1959. Metabolic studies on perinatal human brain. J. Appl. Physiol., 14: 873-877.

Homburger, E., B. Etsten, and H. E. Himwich. 1947. Factors influencing the susceptibility of rats to barbiturates. Fed. Proc., 6:131.

Hornykiewicz, O. 1964. The distribution and metabolism of catecholamines and 5-hydroxytryptamine in human brain. In Richter, D., ed. Comparative Neurochemistry, Proc. of the 5th Int. Neurochemical Sympos., 1962. Oxford, Pergamon Press, Inc., pp. 379-386.

Hrbek, A., and P. Mareš. 1964. Cortical evoked responses to visual stimulation in fullterm and premature newborns. Electroenceph. Clin. Neurophysiol., 16:575-581.

Jewett, R. E., and S. Norton. 1966. Effect of tranquilizing drugs on postnatal behavior. Exp. Neurol., 14:33-43.

Jolley, R. L., and D. H. Labby. 1960. Development of brain enzymes concerned with glutamic acid metabolism in fetal monkey and pig. Arch. Biochem., 90:122-124.

Jondorf, W. R., R. P. Maickel, and B. B. Brodie. 1958-59. Inability of newborn mice and guinea pigs to metabolize drugs. Biochem. Pharmacol., 1:352-355.

Kellaway, P., and I. Petersén. 1964. Neurologic and Electroencephalographic Correlative Studies in Infancy. New York, Grune & Stratton, Inc.

Kimitsuki, M. 1955. Studies on inorganic substances in cerebrum. Fukuako Acta Med., 46:998-1005.

Klee, C. B., and L. Sokoloff. 1967. Changes in D(-)-β-hydroxybutyric dehydrogenase activity during brain maturation in the rat. J. Biol. Chem., 242:3880-3883.

Koch, W., and S. A. Mann. 1907. A comparison of the chemical composition of three human brains at different ages. J. Physiol. (London), 36:36.

Kupferberg, H. J., and E. L. Way. 1963. Pharmacologic basis for the increased sensitivity of the newborn rat to morphine. J. Pharmacol. Exp. Ther., 141:105-112.

Laatsch, R. H. 1962. Glycerol phosphate dehydrogenase activity of developing rat central nervous system. J. Neurochem., 9:487-492.

Lagnado, J. R., and M. Hardy. 1967. Brain esterases during development. Nature (London), 214:1207-1210.

Lajtha, A. 1961. Exchange rates of amino acids between plasma and brain in different parts of the brain. *In* Kety, S. S., and J. Elkes, eds. Regional Neurochemistry. Oxford, Pergamon Press, Inc., pp. 19-24.

———— S. Lahiri, and J. Toth. 1963. The brain barrier system. IV. Cerebral amino acid uptake in different classes. J. Neurochem., 10:765-773.

———— and D. Ford. 1968. Conclusions. Progr. Brain Res., 29:535-537.

Lesný, I. 1964. Electroencephalographic study of infantile cerebral palsy with special regard to electroclinical correlations. Acta Univ. Carol. [Med.] (Praha), Monographia 15.

Lindsley, D. B. 1939. A longitudinal study of the occipital alpha rhythm in normal children: Frequency and amplitude standards. J. Genet. Psychol., 55:197-213.

MacArthur, C. G., and E. A. Doisy. 1918-19. Quantitative chemical changes in the human brain during growth. J. Comp. Neurol., 30:445-486.

Mandel, P., and R. Bieth. 1952. Comparative study of the biochemical development of the brain. C. R. Soc. Biol. (Paris), 235:485-486.

McCaman, R. E., and K. Cook. 1966. Intermediary metabolism of phospholipids in brain tissue. J. Biol. Chem., 241:3390-3394.

Menkes, J. H., M. Philippart, and M. C. Concone. 1966. Concentration and fatty acid composition of cerebrosides and sulfatides in mature and immature human brain. J. Lipid Res., 7:479-486.

Meyer, P. 1963. Histochemistry of the developing human brain. I. Alkaline phosphatase, acid phosphatase and AS esterase in the cerebellum. Acta Neurol. Scand., 39:123-138.

Misrahy, G. A., A. V. Beran, and E. J. Prescott. 1963. Effects of drugs used in pregnancy on availability of fetal cerebral oxygen. Anesthesiology, 24:198-202.

Monod, N. J. 1967. Personal Communication.

———— J. Eliet-Flescher, and C. Dreyfus-Brisac. 1967. The sleep of the full-term and premature infant. III. The disorders of the pathological newborn sleep organization: Polygraphic studies. Biol. Neonat., 11:216-247.

———— and N. Pajot. 1965. Le sommeil du nouveau-né et du prématuré. I. Analyse des études polygraphiques (mouvements oculaires, respiration et E.E.G.) chez le nouveau-né à terme. Biol. Neonat., 8:281-307.

Nitowsky, H. M., L. Matz, and J. A. Berzofsky. 1966. Studies on oxidative drug metabolism in the full-term newborn infant. J. Pediat., 69:1139-1149.

Nyhan, W. L. 1961. Toxicity of drugs in the neonatal period. J. Pediat., 59:1-20.

———— and F. Lampert. 1965. Response of the fetus and newborn to drugs. Anesthesiology, 26:487-500.

O'Brien, J. S., and E. L. Sampson. 1965a. Lipid composition of the normal human brain: Gray matter, white matter, and myelin. J. Lipid Res., 6:537-544.

———— and E. L. Sampson. 1965b. Fatty acid and fatty aldehyde composition of the major brain lipids in normal human gray matter, white matter, and myelin. J. Lipid Res., 6:545-551.

Pampiglione, G. 1965. Brain development and the E.E.G. of normal children of various ethnical groups. Brit. Med. J., 2:573-575.

Parmelee, A. H., et al. 1967a. Sleep states in premature infants. Develop. Med. Child Neurol., 9:70-77.

———— et al. 1967b. The electroencephalogram in active and quiet sleep in infants. Presented at International Symposium on Clinical Electroencephalography in Childhood, Goteborg, Sweden, August 7-9, 1967. Uppsala, Almqvist and Wiksells. In preparation.

——— et al. 1968. Maturation of EEG activity during sleep in premature infants. Electroenceph. Clin. Neurophysiol., 24:319-329.

Passouant, P. 1964. Influence de l'âge sur l'organisation du sommeil de nuit et la période de sommeil avec mouvements oculaires. J. Psychol. Norm. Path., 3:257-279.

——— and J. Cadilhac. 1962. EEG and clinical study of epilepsy during maturation in man. Epilepsia, 3:14-43.

Pitts, F. N., Jr., and C. Quick. 1967. Brain succinate semialdehyde dehydrogenase. II. Changes in the developing rat brain. J. Neurochem., 14:561-570.

Prensky, A. L., and H. W. Moser. 1967. Changes in the amino acid composition of proteolipids of white matter during maturation of the human nervous system. J. Neurochem., 14:117-121.

Roffwarg, H. P., J. N. Muzio, and W. C. Dement. 1966. Ontogenetic development of the human sleep-dream cycle. Science, 152:604-619.

Rossiter, R. J. 1962. Chemical constituents of brain and nerve. In Elliott, K. A. C., I. H. Page, and J. H. Quastel, eds. Neurochemistry. Springfield, Ill., Charles C Thomas, Publisher, pp. 10-54.

Roth, L. J., J. C. Schoolar, and C. F. Barlow. 1959. Sulfur-35 labeled acetazolamide in cat brain. J. Pharmacol. Exp. Ther., 125:128-136.

Rozdilsky, B., and J. Olszewski. 1960. Permeability of cerebral vessels to albumin in hyperbilirubinemia: Observations in newborn animals. Neurology, 10:631-638.

——— and J. Olszewski. 1961. Experimental study of the toxicity of bilirubin in newborn animals. J. Neuropath. Exp. Neurol., 20:193-205.

Salganicoff, L., and E. De Robertis. 1965. Subcellular distribution of the enzymes of the glutamic acid, glutamine and γ-aminobutyric acid cycles in rat brain. J. Neurochem., 12:287-309.

Schoolar, J. C., C. F. Barlow, and L. J. Roth. 1960. The penetration of carbon-14 urea into cerebrospinal fluid and various areas of the cat brain. J. Neuropath. Exp. Neurol., 19:216-227.

Shepovalnikov, A. 1962. Rhythmic components of the infant EEG. Zh. Vyssh. Nerv. Deiat. Pavlov., 12:797-808.

Shimizu, A., and H. E. Himwich, 1968a. Effect of LSD on the sleep cycle of the developing kitten. Develop. Psychobiol., 1:60-64.

——— and H. E. Himwich. 1968b. Effects of phenothiazine derivatives on the sleep-wakefulness cycle in growing kittens. Folia Psychiat. Neurol. Jap., 22:297-305.

——— and H. E. Himwich. 1968c. The effects of amphetamine on the sleep-wakefulness cycle of developing kittens. Psychopharmacologia, 13:161-169.

——— K. Bost, and H. E. Himwich. 1968. Electroencephalographic studies of haloperidol. Int. Pharmacopsychiat., 1:134-142.

——— and H. E. Himwich. 1969. Effects of psychotropic drugs on the sleep-wakefulness cycle of the developing kittens. Develop. Psychobiol., 2:161-167.

Shnider, S. M. 1966. Fetal and neonatal effects of drugs in obstetrics. Anesth. Analg. (Paris), 45:372-378.

Sims, K. L., J. Witztum, C. Quick, and F. N. Pitts, Jr. 1968. Brain 4-aminobutyrate:2-oxoglutarate aminotransferase: Changes in the developing rat brain. J. Neurochem., 15:667-672.

Svennerholm, L. 1964. The distribution of lipids in the human nervous system. I. Analytical procedure: Lipids of foetal and newborn brain. J. Neurochem., 11:839-853.

Tilney, F., and J. Rosett. 1931. The value of brain lipoids as an index of brain development. Bull. Neurol. Inst. N. Y., 1:28-71.

Villavicencio, M., et al. 1958. Pathways of glucose metabolism in rabbit cerebral cortex. Acta Physiol. Lat. Amer., 8:219-229.

Villee, C. A., and J. M. Loring. 1961. Alternative pathways of carbohydrate metabolism in foetal and adult tissues. Biochem. J., 81:488-494.

Waelsch, H. 1961. Compartmentalized biosynthetic reactions in the central nervous system. *In* Kety, S. S., and J. Elkes, eds. Regional Chemistry: Physiology and Pharmacology of the Nervous System. New York, Pergamon Press, Inc.

Youngstrom, K. A. 1941. Acetylcholine esterase concentration during the development of the human fetus. J. Neurophysiol., 4:473-477.

Zachau-Christiansen, B., and K. Vollmond. 1965. 7. The relation between neonatal jaundice and the motor development in the first year. Acta Paediat. Scand. Suppl. 159:26-29.

Zuelzer, W. W. 1960. Neonatal jaundice and mental retardation. Arch. Neurol. (Chicago), 3:127-135.

24

Function of the Nervous System During Prenatal Life

TRYPHENA HUMPHREY • Department of Anatomy,
The University of Alabama in Birmingham, The Medical
Center, Birmingham, Alabama

Introduction

That the nervous system begins to function early during prenatal life is demonstrable only by the movements resulting from its activity. The skeletal muscle reflexes of the fetus are one manifestation of function and constitute its overt behavior (Hooker, 1944). Another way that function is revealed is through visceral reactions, such as cardiac action, intestinal activity due to smooth muscle contraction, or glandular secretion. Probably the neural regulation of the heart is the earliest evidence for function of the nervous system in visceral reactions, for nerve fibers invade the heart at about 16 to 19 mm (Jordan and Kindred, 1942), and electrocardiograms have been secured as early as 9.5 weeks of menstrual age (36.0 mm CR, Hooker fetal series; Heard et al., 1936).

In lower vertebrates like fishes there is evidence that the motor neurons of the spinal cord can function before the reflex arc is completed (Hamburger, 1963). For higher mammals and for man this is not the case. The earliest proof of function of the human nervous system, therefore, is provided by the elicitation of a reflex. What part of the reflex arc matures last is a matter of conjecture as yet.

The function of the neuromuscular system in the development of the overt behavior of the human fetus is the major concern of the present discussion. Although the title of this book mentions only the physiology of the perinatal period, it should be remembered that the functional capacities of the nervous system at that time are dependent upon the morphologic development earlier in fetal life. Far more attention has been given to the capabilities of premature and perinatal infants than to the functional capacities of the fetus before the age of viability is attained. Indeed, until the last 35 to 40 years there had been relatively little reliable objective information available on the reactions of human fetuses during the first half of fetal life.

Historical Background of Human Fetal Activity Investigations

The early comments on human fetal activity, some of which date back to 1885 (Preyer) and even before, are casual notes, not carefully planned observations. These accounts were reviewed in the 1944 and 1952 papers of Hooker. The extensive and detailed investigations of Minkowski (1922, 1923, 1928) also are based on dictated records. Motion picture recording was used by Fitzgerald and Windle (1942) for the few human embryos that they studied, but the methods of stimulation were not uniform, and no photographic documentation has been published. Likewise, as yet no photographic records are available from the observations of the Soviet investigators such as Golubewa et al. (1959). The early literature on human prenatal activity has been treated extensively in the papers of Hooker (1944, 1952, 1958) and will not be considered further. Likewise, the literature concerned with subhuman mammalian prenatal activity was discussed in some detail by Hooker (1944, 1952) and by Hamburger (1963). Reference will be made to it only insofar as it is relevant to the interpretation of human fetal reflex activity.

Basis of Present Account

In the present account, the function of the nervous system, as manifested by the overt activity of the fetus, is based primarily on the work of Hooker and his co-workers, with some ancillary material from the work of other investigators. Consequently brief mention will be made of the methods utilized in his work. Fetuses removed by cesarean section, when the therapeutic termination of pregnancy was deemed necessary by a committee of consulting obstetricians, were placed under a motion picture camera in an isotonic fluid bath as soon as possible (usually normal mammalian saline or Tyrode's solution). The solution was maintained as near to normal body temperature as feasible. The time lapse between beginning placental separation and the initial observations was usually about 1.5 to 2 minutes (Hooker, 1944).

Most of the motion pictures were taken at 16 frames per second. A few records were made at 24 frames per second. Some slow motion recordings were done, but they proved extremely costly and added relatively little to the information provided by the photographs at normal speed. Color film, also an expensive method, was not employed. The motion picture camera used for most of the work was a 35-mm World War I surplus camera, motor driven and operated by a foot switch to leave the hands of the observer free to move the fetus and to stimulate it with the esthesiometers.

The major observations were made by touching the cutaneous surfaces of the fetus with hair esthesiometers similar to the von Frey hairs used by neurologists. These esthesiometers were calibrated to exert a pressure no greater than 10, 25, 50, and 100 mg and 2 g. In order to prevent penetration of the delicate epithelium of the young fetuses and so stimulate the underlying muscles directly, the tips of the hairs were coated with a droplet of smooth, transparent, inert material. Stroking the skin surface provided the more effective stimulation since both spatial and temporal summation resulted, whereas punctate or spot stimuli would seldom elicit reflex activity. Movements caused by unknown stimuli, the so-called spontaneous movements, were photographed when they occurred.

The Effects of Anoxia, Asphyxia, Narcotics, and Anesthetics on Fetal Reflexes

After placental separation reflexes are elicitable from fetuses only until the oxygen supply is depleted. During the first few weeks after activity begins, the movements occur for about 5 to 8 minutes. As the fetus becomes older, the time increases to 10, then 15 to 20 minutes or even more. With depletion of the oxygen supply, anoxia develops and asphyxia takes over as the carbon dioxide and lactic acid accumulate. All overt activity then ceases, although heart action continues for some time (Windle, 1940; Humphrey, 1953). Many anesthetics and various drugs administered to the mother preoperatively cross the placental barrier and influence the activity of the fetus. These include general anesthetics like chloroform, ether, nitrous oxide, and sodium amytol and drugs like morphine, codeine, barbiturates, and tranquilizers. For the limited preoperative period involved, demerol does not affect the fetus. Likewise, neither spinal novocaine nor local anesthetics influence fetal reflexes.

Observations of activity based on mammals that have the fetal circulation maintained and drug and anesthetic effects eliminated vary from those on human fetuses, as is to be expected. The surprising thing, of course, is that there should be so little difference in the sequence of development of activity for the different mammals studied. Nevertheless, at least some of the differences were attributed to the effects of progressive anoxia and asphyxia on the human fetus or to the influence of drugs and anesthetics. Consequently several of the investigators of lower mammalian reflexes considered the activity observed for human fetuses by Hooker and others to be so much affected by asphyxia that it could not be the normal sequence of behavioral development (Fitzgerald and Windle, 1942; Windle and Becker, 1940; Windle, 1944) and that even the reflexes themselves were abnormal (Windle, 1950).

The effects of narcotics and anesthetics on reflex activity are similar to those of anoxia. However, in all instances the reflex is either elicited or suppressed. Because a higher oxygen level is required for newly functioning reflex arcs, the reflexes that become active first in development are the last to disappear when asphyxia arrests all reflexes (Table 1). The most recently functional reflex arcs can be activated only when the conditions are optimal. Consequently, until large amounts of data are collected, it is always possible that any given reflex may not have been elicited at as early an age as it may be demonstrated when more data become available. As demonstrated in the experimental literature, a reflex does not change its character and become abnormal (Humphrey, 1953). *It is not the reflex that is abnormal, but the morphologic and/or functional conditions under which it*

TABLE 1.   Example of the Sequence of Suppression of Fetal Reflexes by Anoxia and Asphyxia[a]

Reflex elicited	Order and time of appearance	Order of suppression
Total pattern contralateral flexion reflexes	Earliest in development 7.5 weeks — beginning 8.5 weeks — fully developed	Last of all of reflexes that disappear with asphyxia
First of local reflex, orbicularis oculi contraction (action not accompanied by trunk and extremity movements)	10.5 weeks — 2 weeks after total pattern contralateral flexion reflexes are fully developed	Before total pattern contralateral flexion reflexes are suppressed by asphyxia
Later developing local reflexes such as tongue movements	12.5 weeks for earliest motion picture evidence — 4 weeks after total pattern reflexes are fully developed	Prior to first local reflex as well as before total pattern reflexes are lost through asphyxia

[a]Note that progressive action of anoxia and asphyxia suppresses the reflexes elicited by cutaneous stimulation in the reverse of the order of their appearance in development.

is obtained (Humphrey, 1969c). Thus the Babinski reflex, for example, indicates abnormality in the nervous system when elicited from an adult but is a part of normal development both prenatally and postnatally.

The Significance of Different Types of Stimuli

Two types of general somatic afferent stimuli may be used to elicit reflexes— exteroceptive and proprioceptive stimuli. The light stroking stimuli with hair esthesiometers used by Hooker and his co-workers are exteroceptive stimulations, although there is a minor amount of superficial pressure. Proprioceptive stimuli result from deep pressure or from stretching a muscle. These types of stimulation were commonly used by Windle and his collaborators in their investigations. Tapping on the amnion, also employed by these observers, produces a considerable amount of diffuse pressure on widely spread areas. Stretching muscles by lifting and releasing a limb also elicits proprioceptive reflexes of a type that is always local in character even in the adult (Humphrey, 1953). It is quite impossible to make comparisons between such proprioceptive reactions and exteroceptive reflexes elicited by light stroking of cutaneous surfaces. Neither the age of origin nor the course of development would be alike, for different neuronal arcs are utilized. Cinematographic recording has been found essential if all—or even most—of the actions of the reflex responses to cutaneous stimuli are seen. Such recording will be even more necessary in evaluating the time of onset and the later developmental history of reflexes evoked by stretch and pressure stimuli.

Theories on the Development of Fetal Behavior

Differences in the sequences observed in the development of motor activity among the different mammals studied produced two major views concerning the manner in which behavior develops. From his studies on *Amblystoma*, Coghill (1929) developed the concept that all of the neuromuscular system capable of responding to the stimulus reacts when a reflex is first elicited during development. When well developed, these reflexes involved head, trunk, and extremity movements. Coghill referred to these reactions of *Amblystoma* as total pattern reflexes and stated that partial patterns like the local movements of a single limb, for example, individuated out of the total pattern reflexes. Coghill found that even mouth opening begins as part of a forward jumping movement following a visual stimulus (Coghill, 1929).

From his observations of early human fetal activity, Hooker (1944) concluded that the exteroceptive stimuli utilized in his studies elicited reflexes of the total pattern type described by Coghill, i.e., a lateral flexion of the head (muscle action in the cervical region) that extended to include the upper extremities, the lower trunk, the rump, and the lower extremities in that general order as the fetus increased in age. He found that the local reflexes elicited by these light stroking stimuli appeared later in development than did the total pattern reflexes. Reference has also been made in these studies to the union of some local reflexes with others later in development or with more generalized body and/or extremity activity in the development of functional combinations of reflexes, some of which are retained in late fetal life and postnatally (Hooker and Humphrey, 1954; Humphrey, 1964a).

Although accepting Coghill's interpretation for tailed amphibians, some workers on mammalian fetuses, including Windle (1944), have considered that the proprioceptive local reflexes, such as those observed on lifting a limb and releasing it, develop first of all in mammals. Consequently they advanced the theory that behavior evolves by the addition and integration of local reflexes to build up complex functional activity.

Other interpretations of the manner of behavioral development have been proposed by the Soviet investigators and by Kuo (1967). In his concept of behavioral gradients Kuo emphasizes that for any given response and in any given stage of development the entire organism is involved in either an active or passive manner (Kuo, 1967). Many Soviet investigators (Golubewa et al., 1959; Anokhin, 1964) stress the importance of heterochronic maturation of individual parts of a functional system in early development and systemogenesis in later fetal life. It could be said for all of these viewpoints that their proponents have concentrated attention on some facets of behavioral development to the relative exclusion of certain other aspects.

Determination of Fetal Age

The age of the human fetus has been expressed in different ways. For the observations made by Hooker and his co-workers from 1932 to 1962 menstrual age based on the data accumulated by Streeter (1920) was used. Since this account is based on the records and publications of Hooker and his co-workers, menstrual age taken from these records is used throughout the discussion unless stated otherwise. Menstrual age was determined from the crown rump length (CR) as compared with the curve constructed from Streeter's data (Graph 1), not from the history secured from the mother, which is often incorrect. The curve for menstrual age given by Mall (1910) has been added to Graph 1 since the ages determined from Mall's data differ from those based on the Streeter data. The most accurate information obtainable is the crown rump length of the fetus, if taken carefully before fixation while the fetus is still immersed in fluid so that the normal curvature of the spine is retained. Fixation changes the size of the fetus, either through swelling of the tissues (as with formalin) or through shrinkage (especially with alcohol).

Because ovulation occurs at about the middle of the menstrual cycle and fertilization takes place within a day or two after ovulation, theoretically fertilization age (or rather presumptive fertilization age, Patten, 1953; Arey, 1965) is approximately two weeks less than menstrual age (Patten, 1953; Arey, 1965). The data from Patten's curve for fertilization age have been added to Graph 1 and extended to the 30-week age level. It is possible to determine the time of ovulation quite accurately with the cooperation of an intelligent mother because of the change in body temperature that occurs at that time, but even when secured this date simply provides a better estimate of fertilization age. "Ovulation age" is sometimes used, but it is an unfortunate term because embryonic development begins with fertilization. "Gestation age," although sometimes erroneously used as synonymous with menstrual age, is the equivalent of fertilization age. It is evident, then, that there is no truly accurate way of determining the exact age of any fetus.

The First Reflexes Elicited by Exteroceptive Stimulation

The first reflex observed consists of bending the head to the side opposite the perioral area stimulated (contralateral head flexion). The muscles involved are limited to the cervical and possibly upper thoracic levels of the trunk (Hooker, 1952, 1958). This reflex was first noted by Hooker for a 20.7-mm embryo and by Fitzgerald and Windle (1942) for a 20.0-mm embryo, i.e., at 7.5 weeks of menstrual age (Graph 1). Although the extent of the muscle contraction in this reflex is restricted to the cervical and upper thoracic regions, the reflex itself meets the requirements for the total pattern reflexes described by Coghill because all of the neuromuscular structures capable of reacting to the stimulus participate.

It has been suggested (Humphrey, 1952, 1953, 1954, 1955, 1964a) that the neuronal arc functioning for this reflex of the human embryo at this time has for its sensory limb the trigeminal nerve fibers transmitting impulses from about the mouth to upper cervical spinal cord levels and for its motor limb the spinal accessory neurons and nerve fibers supplying the sternocleidomastoid muscle and probably the cervical part of the trapezius. Perhaps the upper cervical motor neurons innervating neck muscles also participate, although these nerve cells are less well differentiated. The axons of commissural neurons constitute the internuncial fibers that cross in the ventral white commissure at upper cervical spinal cord levels (Fig. 1).

Maturation of the embryo is rapid, and the lateral flexion reflexes soon extend

Fetal Age
Days Weeks

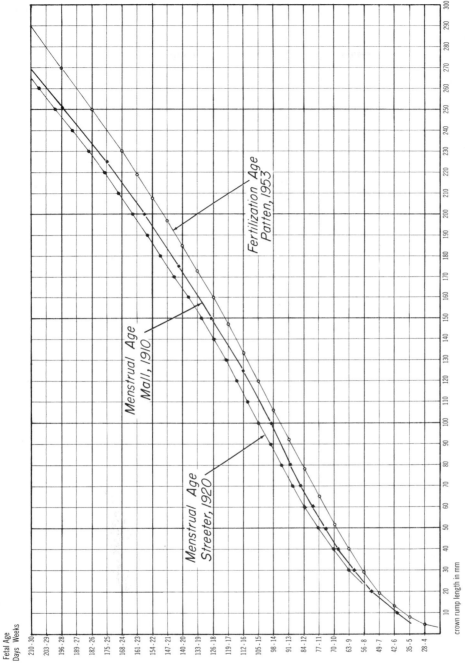

crown rump length in mm

Graph 1. Three curves showing fetal age from 3 to 30 weeks (21 to 210 days) as determined by crown rump measurements expressed in millimeters.

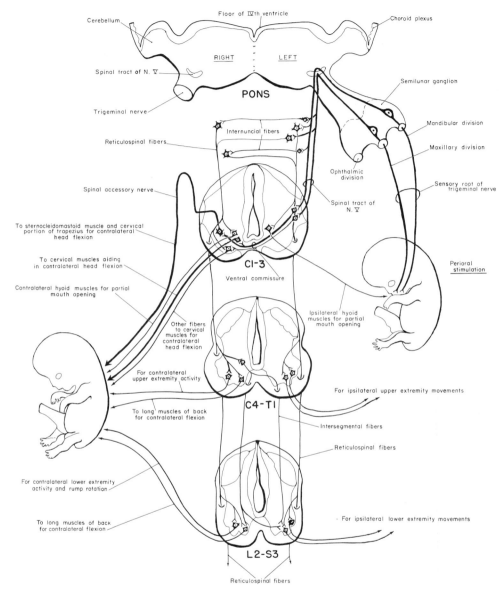

Fig. 1. Diagram to illustrate the fiber pathways involved in the total pattern contralateral
flexion reflexes that include extremity movements bilaterally and active mouth opening like that illustrated in Figure 3 A to C (p. 761). The sensory limb of these
reflexes and the internuncial and motor fibers of the earliest functioning reflex arc
are drawn in *heavy* lines. Other internuncial fibers and the additional efferent fibers
for mouth opening and the other parts of the fully developed contralateral total
pattern reflex are shown by narrower lines. The drawing of the fetus on the right
side of the figure is an enlargement from Figure 3A (27.1 mm fetus) and shows the
position of the fetus at the time of stimulation. On the left side, the drawing is

to the remaining thoracic and the lumbosacral levels so that as early as 25.0 mm (Hooker, 1958) the contralateral flexion reflex following perioral stimulation includes bending the head, trunk, and pelvis to the opposite side. Movements of the extremities are then added to the lateral flexion reflexes, beginning with extension of both arms at the shoulders. The lower extremities soon participate enough in the reflex so that the soles of the feet separate slightly. The extension of the arms is usually sufficient to pull the hands away from over the mouth for two or three motion picture frames before the fetus returns to the resting position. With this increased involvement of the neuromuscular system, the reticulospinal pathways (Barcroft and Barron, 1939) and propriospinal fibers (fasciculus proprius) become active also (Fig. 1).

The Development of Mouth Opening as Part of the Contralateral Flexion Reflexes

At 26.0 mm, some rotation of the pelvis (or rump rotation) is added to the contralateral flexion reflexes. When the more forceful extension of the arms pulls the hands downward to uncover the mouth, the mandible is often actively lowered and the mouth partially opened, that is, opened in the midline region but not all of the way to the corners (Figs. 2A and B). At this time also the lower extremities participate in this reaction and the soles of the feet, facing each other when the fetus is at rest, are pulled apart. For this 26.0-mm fetus, the motion picture records show that mouth opening accompanied 9 of the 16 contralateral total pattern flexion reflexes elicited, or 56.2 percent. One of these reflexes took place when the hair esthesiometer was drawn over the face area while the fetus was still in the amniotic sac. More details about body and extremity movements of these contralateral flexion reflexes are given in the papers of Hooker (1944, 1952, 1954, 1958, 1960). The oral activity is discussed further in the accounts of the author (1968a, 1969c, d).

During the period from 26.0 mm to 28.0 mm CR, the contralateral flexion reflexes increase in frequency and in the extent of the movements. Both the upper and the lower extremities soon begin to move asymmetrically in the reflex, the digits spread apart, and the hands flex, but the mouth still opens only partially (Figs. 3A to C). Rotation of the rump to the contralateral side becomes marked. A week later (Fig. 3D), the movements of the pelvis and the upper and lower extremities are even greater in amplitude, and the mouth opening that constitutes part of the reflex is complete, i.e., the lips are separated at the corners as well as

from Figure 3B and illustrates the position of the fetus at the peak of the reflex action. Probably the muscles that open the mouth in the midline region at this age, but not all of the way to the corners, are supplied by the first three cervical nerves (C_1 to C_3) and indicated in this diagram as hyoid muscles. These include the sternohyoid (Moyers, 1950), the omohyoid, and the thyrohyoid (Moyers, 1950; Root, 1946), which act indirectly, and the geniohyoid which acts directly (see Humphrey, 1954, p. 148). The outlines for the pons and spinal cord levels were drawn from sections of the nervous system of a fetus of the same age.

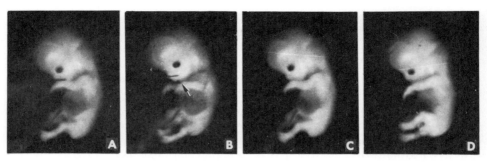

Fig. 2. Contralateral (A and B) and ipsilateral (C and D) total pattern flexion reflexes elicited by stimulating the perioral region of a 26.0-mm human fetus (No. 24, 8.5 weeks menstrual age, Graph 1).

A. The resting position before action begins. B. The contralateral flexion of head, trunk, and pelvis, the arm extension that pulls the hands downward off of the face and separates them, the abduction of the legs that separate the soles of the feet, and the partially open mouth (at *arrow*) $\frac{1}{6}$ second later. The black line passing across the nose to end near the corner of the mouth is the 100-mg hair esthesiometer. The resting position before the ipsilateral reflex is illustrated in C and the height of the action in D. At this time the head, the trunk, and the pelvis are bent ipsilateralward, and the soles of the feet are separated also, but the mouth remains covered by the hands. The marked ipsilateral pelvic flexion shown here took place $\frac{3}{8}$ of a second after the movement began. Photographs at about 1.2 times the size of the fetus.

in the midline (Fig. 3D). The total pattern type of contralateral flexion reflex continues throughout the 10-week age period and may be seen even later as well, but then it is often combined with other movements such as head extension or turning the chin ipsilaterally. In the reflexes that include mouth opening at 11 weeks, the mandible is lowered less far, the mouth does not open so widely, and the lips are separated no farther in the midline than at the corners (Fig. 4B-D). Later on in development, at 11.5 weeks for example, the mouth again opens all of the way to the corners as part of a combined head extension and contralateral flexion reflex (Humphrey, 1969c).

The Relation of Mouth Opening Reflexes to Palatal Closure

Perhaps it is worthy of mention that when the first mouth opening reflexes develop as part of the total pattern contralateral flexion reflexes, the palate has not yet formed to separate the common oral-nasal space into the nasal and oral cavities. These mouth opening reflexes begin concomitantly with the period of change of the palatal processes from the vertical to the horizontal position that is essential for palatal closure. This active lowering of the mandible undoubtedly plays a major role in withdrawing the tongue from between the vertical palatal processes and their immediate change to the horizontal position and closure (Humphrey, 1968b, 1969a). Unless closure takes place, the resulting cleft palate

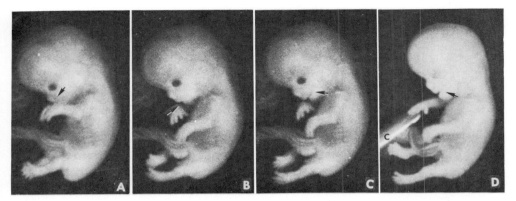

Fig. 3. A, B, and C illustrate a contralateral flexion reflex elicited by stimulating the left perioral area from the corner of the mouth upward across the nose of a 27.1-mm fetus (No. 116, 8.5 weeks menstrual age, Graph 1). A. The curved linear shadow across the nose indicated by the *arrow* is the stimulator as it is being removed before the reflex began. In B. The *arrow* points to the partially open mouth revealed when the arms extend unequally (left more than right), and the soles of the feet separate as the legs abduct. C. The lips are well apart only in the middle, although lateral to this area the beginning separation of the lips is shown by the dark line indicated by the *arrow* at the corner of the mouth. The left hand at this time is rather sharply flexed, and the digits of the hands and feet are spread apart. The photographs are about 1.6 normal size. Six motion picture frames are spanned by the illustrations (16 frames per second). D. A contralateral flexion reflex of a 34.3-mm fetus, CR length (No. 134, 9.5 weeks menstrual age; Graph 1). The mouth is often more widely open with the lips separated as far as the corners. Other parts of the reflex, such as head flexion and rump rotation, are more pronounced than in A, B, and C. The photograph is approximately 1.2 normal size. This single photograph, like that in C, illustrates the peak of activity in the reflex. The right hand and foot are near the clamp on the umbilical cord (c).

interferes with the sucking and swallowing reflexes that are essential for normal feeding postnatally.

Ipsilateral Total Pattern Flexion Reflexes

Ipsilateral responses to stroking the surface of the perioral area with the tip of the stimulator have not been elicited as early in development as have the contralateral reflexes. The first was cinematographically recorded at 22.6 mm, approximately half a week later than the first contralateral total pattern reaction was seen as reported in the papers of Hooker (1952). For this embryo only 1 ipsilateral flexion reflex (limited to cervical levels) was recorded in the motion pictures, whereas 5 more extensive contralateral reflexes (some with beginning arm extension) were photographed. Ipsilateral total pattern reflexes are far less frequent throughout early development than those contralateral to the stimulus. However,

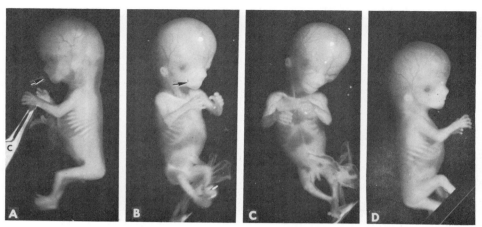

Fig. 4. Photographs showing extension of the head, trunk, and pelvis and oral reflexes of a fetus of 11 weeks of menstrual age (No. 65, 48.5 mm CR length, Graph 1), reproduced at about 0.9 of the true size. The stimulus eliciting the two reflexes in B and C and in D appear to have been along the back as the fetus was pulled over the underlying cloth surface. A. The peak of an extension reflex resulting from touching the midline perioral area with the clamp (c) on the umbilical cord. The lips (at *arrow*) are tightly closed or compressed. B and C. The fetus just before movement began (B) and later (C) at the peak of the reflex when the head, trunk, and pelvis were bent lateralward, the lower extremities extended, one arm extended at the shoulder and the elbow of the other arm flexed, and the mouth open to the corners but with little separation of the lips even at the midline. D. Photograph at the crest of the activity of another mouth opening reflex showing a profile view of the separation of the lips to about the same degree laterally as in the midline. There was little indication of upper extremity movement and the lower extremities are not completely in the field.

2 of the 18 reflexes photographically recorded for a 26.0-mm fetus were ipsilateral to the side stimulated. Both were as vigorous as the contralateral reflexes. One was elicited by a perioral stimulus (Figs. 2C and D), and the other followed a contralateral reflex without an intervening perioral stimulation. Throughout the early period of reflex activity when the total pattern type of reflex is dominant, these ipsilateral reactions constitute only a small percentage (5.4 percent, Table 2) of the total number of lateral flexion reflexes cinematographically recorded (Hooker, 1952, 1958; Humphrey, 1968a, 1969c).

Although mouth opening is frequent as part of the contralateral flexion reflexes, it has not been seen with an ipsilateral response to perioral stimulation until 10 weeks of menstrual age and only once at 10 weeks (38.2 mm CR) (Humphrey, 1968a, 1969c). The ipsilateral reflexes are often less vigorous than the contralateral ones. In connection with the forceful ones, however, where mouth opening would be expected, the face is turned away from the camera so it is not possible to see the mouth adequately, as a rule. In a strong reflex (Fig. 2, compare A and B with C and D) the action is as vigorous as in the contralateral reflexes and includes the

TABLE 2.   Lateral Flexion Reflexes Cinematographically Recorded from Fetuses of 20.7 mm to 40.7 mm CR[a]

CR length in mm	Menstrual age in weeks; no. of fetus	Reflexes contralateral to area of stimulation	Reflexes ipsilateral to area of stimulation
20.7	7.5 (93A)	1	0
22.6	8– (131)	5	1
25.0	8+ (4)	13	0
26.0	8.5 (24)	16	2
27.1	8.5 (99)	7	0
27.1	8.5 (116)	14	4
27.7	8.5 (61)	10	0
28.0	8.5 (29)	20	0
32.7	9+ (94)	7	1
34.3	9.5 (134)	27	0
34.8	9.5 (127A)	13	2
35.0	9.5 (16)	18	0
36.0	9.5 (18)	9	0
37.5	10.0 (105)	18	0
38.2	10.0 (101)	8	1
40.7	10.0 (103)	8	0
	Total	194 (94.6%)	11 (5.4%)

[a]Menstrual age is based on the tables of Streeter (1920) and taken from the records of Hooker.

marked rump rotation and the separation of the soles of the feet that usually are present on mouth opening, but the mouth is completely obscured by the ipsilateral hand when the head bends ipsilateralward.

The Classification of Reflexes as Negative and Positive Reactions

The contralateral flexion reflexes were referred to in the early studies of mammalian fetal activity as avoiding reactions (Coghill, 1916; Angulo y Gonzalez, 1932; Humphrey, 1952; Hooker and Humphrey, 1954; and many others) because the area touched by the stimulator is removed from the stimulating agent. They are known also as "negative" or "nociceptive" reflexes (Kappers et al., 1936; Humphrey, 1964a, b) and are referred to as protective in their functional potential. Ipsilateral responses are classed as positive in character (Humphrey, 1964a, b). They have been considered to be the initial reflexes in the development of reactions related to feeding (Humphrey, 1964a, 1969c) since the perioral area that is touched approaches the stimulator (Table 2).

Like the contralateral and ipsilateral flexion reflexes just mentioned, the more complicated head movements that develop later in fetal life are both negative and positive. The negative reactions again precede the positive ones in their order of appearance. Thus head extension, which quickly moves the face away from the stimulus, develops before ventral head flexion, which brings the fetal face toward the source of stimulation (Humphrey, 1964a, b, 1969c). Likewise rotation of the face, either combined with trunk movements, or later as face rotation alone, is first directed away from the source of stimulation and only later toward it.

After the total pattern types of reflexes have largely disappeared, head movements occur in association with other reflexes to form combinations either protective in their functional potential or related to feeding. Adequate functioning of the full-term newborn infant for nursing depends on turning the face toward the nipple that stimulates the lips, as well as on mouth opening. This reflex occurs whether the lips are touched at the corners of the mouth or at the middle of the upper or the lower lip (Prechtl, 1958; Humphrey, 1969d). For premature infants, the positive response to lip stimulation has not developed as satisfactorily as for normal full-term infants (Humphrey, 1969d for discussion).

As estimated by the number of motion picture frames involved, the contralateral flexion reflexes are executed more rapidly than are the ipsilateral ones. Both the ipsilateral flexion reflex of the 26.0-mm fetus elicited by touching the face (Figs. 2C and D) and that following a contralateral flexion reflex consumed far more time, for example, than did the forceful contralateral flexion reflexes of this fetus (over one second as compared with half a second or less). Thus the avoiding or negative type of lateral flexion reflex is quicker than the positive one. When reflexes appear that are more restricted in their action and when functional combinations are formed, again the protective or avoiding reactions are completed more rapidly than are the positive reflexes of equivalent complexity that are related to feeding (Humphrey, 1968a).

The Pathways and Areas Involved in the Total Pattern Reflexes

The pathway suggested by the author (1952) for the first contralateral flexion reflexes of human fetuses in response to perioral stimulation is illustrated in Figure 1. At the time when flexion is limited to the cervical region (20 to 21 mm), the fibers of the maxillary and mandibular divisions of the trigeminal nerve have been traced through the first cervical levels of the spinal cord (Humphrey, 1952, 1954), and differentiation has begun in this portion of the spinal trigeminal nuclear complex (Brown, 1958). Both the commissural fibers that carry the impulses to the opposite side and the motor root fibers have developed at these levels much earlier. Therefore, these reflexes are probably mediated over a typical three-neuron reflex arc with the major action dependent upon the sternocleidomastoid and the cervical part of the trapezius muscles (Fig. 1). The motor neurons of the spinal accessory nerve that supply these muscles are the best developed motor neurons in the upper cervical region at this time. Undoubtedly the reticulospinal pathways which develop early embryologically and phylogenetically participate in the reflex as soon as it extends farther caudalward. Likewise neurons that connect different segments of the spinal cord through the fasciculus proprius (or propriospinal fibers) must also take part. In addition, the motor neurons at all levels obviously function as soon as the extremities are included in the reflex activity. When the mouth begins to open by lowering the mandible (Fig. 2B), at least part of the muscles supplied by the first two cervical nerves are involved in the mouth opening (Humphrey, 1954, 1968a). Probably the anterior belly of the digastric muscle also participates early, for both this muscle (Gasser, 1967) and the neurons believed by some investigators to supply it also differentiate early (Jacobs, 1970). When the mouth opens completely about a week later in development (Fig. 3D), no doubt all of the muscles that participate in mouth opening are involved to some degree in the action.

During this early period of activity the only cutaneous surface that has been shown to be sensitive to stimulation is the face in the areas innervated by the sensory fibers of the maxillary and mandibular nerves (Table 3). During the

TABLE 3.   Sequence of Development of Sensitivity of Cutaneous Surfaces and Oral Mucosa[a]

Surface areas shown sensitive to stimulation	Menstrual age in weeks[b]
Rima oris (or vermilion border) of the lips and adjacent perioral areas (maxillary and mandibular branches of trigeminal nerve)	7.5
More peripheral perioral areas, including the alae of the nose and the chin	8 to 9.5
Bridge of nose, lower eyelid, and area below it	10.5
Palms of hands	10 to 10.5 (possibly earlier)
Upper eyelid (ophthalmic division of trigeminal nerve)	10.5 (possibly earlier)
Genital areas and genitofemoral sulcus[c]	10.5 (possibly earlier)
Shoulder area	10.5
Soles of the feet	10.5 to 11
Eyebrows and forehead	11
Upper arm and forearm	11
Back (probably)	11
Upper chest	11.5
Thighs and legs	11 to 12
Remaining chest areas	13
Tongue anteriorly	14 (probably earlier)
Back, scapular area, lateral wall of trunk	14
Abdominal wall	15
Buttocks[c]	17
External auditory canal	17.5
Dorsal surface of hand	18.5
Posterior tongue areas (possibly posterior pharyngeal wall)	17 to 18.5 (probably earlier)
Inside of nostrils[d]	24

[a] The data are mainly from Hooker (1952) and Humphrey (1964a) with unpublished supplementary information from the film analysis records of Hooker.
[b] Determined from the tables of Streeter (1920) as recorded by Hooker.
[c] From dictated records only and not cinematographically verified.
[d] Reported by Golubewa, Shulejkina, and Vainstein, 1959.

first 7.5 to 8.5 weeks, no nerve fibers have grown near enough to the surface to touch the basement membrane of the cutaneous epithelium (Hogg, 1941; Humphrey, 1966), although a few have reached it for the oral mucosa (Humphrey, 1966). All of these nerve fibers terminate as naked, growing nerve tips, a few of which touch the basement membrane of the mucosa although none has been identified in cutaneous areas nearer than 5 μ even in the lips (Humphrey, 1966). By 9.5 weeks, however, when the mouth opens widely, some maxillo-mandibular fibers penetrate the mucosal basement membrane inside of the lips and a few touch this membrane in the perioral cutaneous areas. By 10 weeks, more maxillary and mandibular fibers contact the basement membrane periorally. On the mucosal surfaces a few already end on large, basally located epithelial cells to form primitive Merkel's end discs, the first specialized nerve terminations to appear in development (Humphrey, 1966). For the cutaneous surfaces these receptors develop somewhat later, but Hogg (1941) found them at 12 weeks (63.5 mm CR). During this 10- to 12-week age period, also, differentiation is taking place in the subnucleus interpolaris portion of the spinal trigeminal nuclear complex (Brown, 1962) that is especially concerned with the mediation of reflexes over motor cranial nerves (Humphrey, 1969b).

Characteristics of Reflexes from 8.5 to 10 Weeks
(26.0 to 41.0 mm CR)

From the 8.5-week through the 10-week age level, the reflexes elicited by perioral cutaneous stimulation are stereotyped in nature (Hooker, 1944, 1952, 1958), i.e., they vary only in the vigor and in the magnitude of the reaction. Almost identical movements may be seen several times in succession. The reflexes elicited are either contralateral or, more rarely, ipsilateral flexion reflexes. If the contralateral reflex is a strong one even at 8.5 weeks, it usually includes mouth opening (during the time that the hands uncover the mouth), asymmetric upper and lower extremity movements, separation of the soles of the feet, spreading of the digits of both the hands and the feet, and flexion of the hands (Fig. 3). If the reflex elicited is a weak one, it is not accompanied by mouth opening, the upper extremity movements are symmetric and less extensive, and separation of the soles of the feet does not occur. Instead, only head, trunk, and pelvic flexion, with or without rump rotation, may take place. The strength of the stimulus, the excellence of the oxygen supply, the number of times that the area has already been stimulated, and other factors all enter into the determination of the forcefulness and duration of the reflex elicited.

By 9.5 weeks, it is possible to observe stages in opening and closing of the mouth while it is uncovered by the hands during the contralateral flexion reflexes (Humphrey, 1968a, 1969c). Since mouth closure at this age requires more time than lowering the mandible to open it, closure is evidently due to a passive return to position rather than to active muscle contraction. At 10 weeks, the mouth appears to be opening less far as a part of the contralateral flexion reflexes. Head and trunk extension then begin to replace the earlier lateral flexion reflexes and are the dominant action for a brief interval with peak activity at about 11 weeks. The extension reflexes likewise are elicited less often after a brief period of maximum frequency. Mouth opening then occurs as a part of mixed contralateral flexion and head and trunk extension reflexes elicited by perioral stimulation by 11.5 weeks (Humphrey, 1968a, b), but trunk and extremity movements continue to decrease in both extent and frequency during later development.

The Development of Head and Trunk Extension Reflexes

After having attained a peak of development by 9.5 to 10 weeks, the contralateral (and ipsilateral) total pattern reflexes decrease in number and in vigor. By 10.5 to 11 weeks, the responses to stimulation of the maxillomandibular areas of the face are changing to an extension of the head, trunk, and pelvis (Fig. 4) rather than the lateral flexion reflexes elicited earlier. Stimulation at or near the midline is the most effective. When the extension reflex is vigorous, the head is hyperextended. Neither the upper extremities nor the lower extremities always participate in the same manner or to the extent that they act in the contralateral flexion reflexes elicited earlier. When the extremities take part in the extension reflexes, the extension at the proximal joints (shoulder and elbow, hip and knee) is greater for distal joints of the lower extremities (Humphrey, 1968a).

The mouth does not open with the extension reflexes, but at their peak the lips are often compressed. As a result the vermilion borders almost disappear for the very brief interval that the head is maximally extended in this rapidly executed reflex (Fig. 4A).

Except for minor variations in the amplitude of the movement and in its duration, the extension reflexes are essentially alike, or stereotyped. Almost identical movements may be elicited repeatedly. Because not all of the neuromuscular mechanisms that participate earlier in the total pattern lateral flexion reflexes act in these extension reflexes, even when the latter are the most vigorous, these reactions cannot be considered true total pattern reflexes in the sense that the term was used by Coghill (1929).

The essential changes that give rise at this time to the extension reflexes include the contraction of the dorsal longitudinal axial muscles bilaterally instead of unilaterally. The bilateral muscle action is undoubtedly due largely to the development of ipsilateral as well as contralateral connections between the reticulospinal pathways and the spinal cord motor neurons (Fig. 5). A degree of inhibitory effect from higher centers over the neurons acting in the contralateral flexion reflex must be effective by this time also.

When the trunk extension reflexes first appear, there is a period of transition from the contralateral flexion reflexes. Consequently, a reaction may begin with head extension, then go over into flexion at the lower levels of the trunk, and include rump rotation. As development progresses these mixed reactions decrease in frequency and tend to disappear. Sometimes, however, a reflex begins with head extension, then passes over into the contralateral flexion type of reflex, especially if the stimulus is more peripherally applied or the same area has been

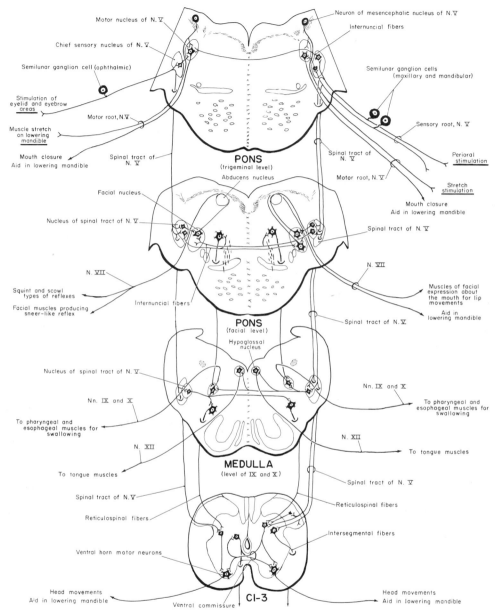

Fig. 5. Diagram to illustrate some of the neuronal pathways involved in the more limited reactions of the combined head, arm, and face movements and in the local reflexes that appear following stimulation of the cutaneous facial areas from 10 to 10.5 weeks onward. The fiber paths for such reflexes as mouth opening and closure, swallowing, tongue movements, and contraction of the eyelid and corrugator muscles are shown. The outlines for the levels through the pons, medulla, and spinal cord were drawn from sections of the brain stem of a fetus of 107.5 mm CR length (15.5 weeks menstrual age).

stimulated several times in succession. Also when the oxygen supply is becoming exhausted, often only the contralateral flexion reflexes can be elicited before all activity is abolished (Table 1). This is an example of reversion to the earlier developed type of reflex when anoxia develops.

The Development of Local Reflexes in Response to Stimulation of the Face

In the papers of Hooker (1952, 1958) and in the earlier ones of the author (1954, 1964a), active mouth opening was given as the first local reflex to be elicited by stimulating facial areas supplied by the trigeminal nerve. However, as now demonstrated, lowering of the mandible develops initially as part of a total pattern contralateral flexion reflex. The orbicularis oculi reflex in response to stimulation of the ophthalmic fibers of the trigeminal nerve is evidently a true local reflex. This reflex was reported by Hooker (1952, 1958) and by Humphrey (1964a) as early as 10 to 10.5 weeks and verified recently from the cinematographic records at 10.5 weeks (46.5 mm CR). According to Hooker (1952) it is not combined with head movements until later. Swallowing was reported at 10.5 weeks by Hooker (1954, 1958) and by Hooker and Humphrey (1954) from dictated records but has not been verified from the motion picture records before 12 to 12.5 weeks (Hooker, 1952). Thus the earliest truly local reflexes from facial stimulation are evidently orbicularis oculi (10 to 10.5 weeks) and corrugator reactions (11 weeks), both set off by stimulation of the ophthalmic fibers of the trigeminal nerve. Because both of these actions are protective in their future potential, the earliest local reflex verified thus far, as well as the first total pattern flexion reflexes, belong in the category of avoiding, or protective (also negative or nociceptive) reflexes. Figure 5 illustrates the neuronal pathways for some of the local reflexes and their combination with head movements.

Mouth Opening and Closing Reflexes at Eleven Weeks and Later

As already mentioned, the character of mouth opening changes from its first appearance at 8.5 weeks through the 10-week period. At 11 weeks, when compression of the lips rather than mouth opening accompanies marked head extension, mouth opening of a different type has been seen (Figs. 4B to D). The lips separated about equally in the midline and at the corners. Closure as well as opening was so rapid that the entire reflex required only about half a second. One reflex accompanied a contralateral body flexion reflex where the head rotated as well as flexed (Figs. 4B and C); another included very little movement aside from quick opening and closing of the mouth (Fig. 4D). These two reflexes, both of which were elicited when the position of the fetus was changed so that its back brushed along the underlying cloth surface, are the earliest mouth opening reflexes elicited by other than perioral stimuli.

As development progresses, stimulation of a wide variety of areas of the body may produce mouth opening at times (Humphrey, 1968a, 1969c). It was observed after touching the volar surface of the forearm at 12.5 weeks (70.0 mm CR) as part of a reflex that included bending of the head toward the forearm stimulated. The fingertips of the two hands moved apart then returned to position. When the mouth was wide open the tongue could be seen between the lips (Fig. 6B).

For this same 70.0-mm fetus, stimulation of the sole of the foot in one instance elicited an extremely rapid mouth opening and closing reflex. It was accompanied only by an exceedingly slight ipsilateral bending of the head at the same time (Fig. 6A) but was followed at once by a kick of the leg on the side stimulated.

In addition to forearm and foot-sole stimulation, mouth opening was elicited from this fetus both by eyelid and by perioral stimuli. None of the reflexes from these four areas were alike. It is evident, then, that by 12.5 weeks oral reflexes already may be elicited from a wide range of cutaneous surfaces and be accompanied by quite different movements. From about 13 weeks onward (Hooker, 1952, 1958) the reflexes become remarkably variable rather than stereotyped.

Stimulation of still other cutaneous areas has been found to evoke oral reflexes for somewhat older fetuses. These areas include the palm of the hand (Fig. 6C) the eyelids, and the back (Fig. 7) at 14 weeks (Humphrey, 1968a, 1969c). The movements that are associated with these oral reflexes are variable. Tongue action accompanied the mouth opening from palmar stimulation (Fig. 6C). Squintlike action from eyelid muscle contraction and sneerlike lip elevation (Figs. 7A and B) were part of a head, trunk, and extremity reflex combination following eyelid stimulation (Hooker, 1939; Humphrey, 1968a). Lip and tongue stimulation elicited mouth opening and closure with the appearance of a groove or furrow in the tongue at 15.5 weeks (Fig. 6D). As the lip and tongue movements that are essential for sucking make their appearance the sensitive area for the elicitation of oral reflexes becomes limited mainly to the tongue, the lips, and the perioral zone adjacent to the lips.

Until 11 weeks, mouth closure has been considered passive because it requires more time than does depression of the lower jaw in opening it. The mouth opening reflexes at 11 weeks (Figs. 4B to D) are followed by a quick closure, one of them described as snaplike in character (Humphrey, 1968a, 1969c). A mouth opening reflex elicited by stimulating the sole of the foot at 12.5 weeks also was followed by an equally rapid closure (Fig. 6A). The quick closure in these instances is active. Undoubtedly it is due to stretching the masticatory muscles like the masseter and so activating the two neuron reflex arcs that mediate stretch reflexes (Humphrey, 1968a, 1969c) over the neurons and fibers of the mesencephalic root of the trigeminal nerve and the motor nerve cells of this nerve (Fig. 5).

Before the earliest sneerlike reflex has been noted at 14 weeks (Figs. 7A and B), mouth closure has been due to elevation of the mandible, at first passively (a relatively slow return to position), then actively (due to muscle contraction set off by stretch stimuli). The sneerlike facial expression results from elevation of the upper lip near the corner of the mouth and may include lifting of the ala of the nose. These actions are mediated over the motor fibers of the facial nerve, like those of the earlier appearing squint and scowl type reflexes. From 14 weeks onward, more and more of the muscles of facial expression participate in the local

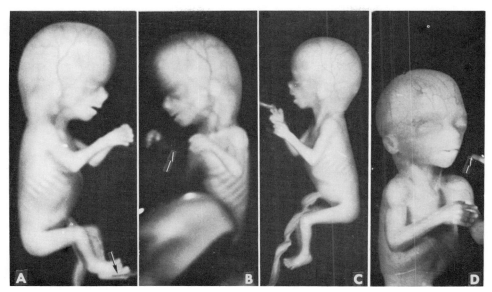

Fig. 6. Photographs of oral area reflex activity of four different fetuses showing different types of mouth opening and, for three of the reflexes, evidence for tongue movements. A and B. No. 110, 12.5 weeks, 70.0 mm CR length, 0.8 natural size; C. No. 37, 14 weeks, 85.5 mm CR length, 0.6 natural size; D. No. 135, 15.5 weeks, 107.5 mm CR length, 0.6 natural size. In each case the photograph illustrates approximately the stage of maximum movement in the reflex. A. Stimulation of the sole of the left foot (*arrow* points to stimulator being removed) followed by a rapid mouth opening and closing reflex in which the separation of the lips lasted only ⅛ of a second. Slight ipsilateral bending of the head accompanied the jaw movement which was followed by a rapid kick of the leg on the side stimulated. B. Stimulation of the volar surface of the right forearm by the observer's finger (at point of *arrow*) followed by ipsilateral bending of the head, extension of the contralateral arm with flexion of the forearm, and mouth opening with the tongue elevated to obscure the lateral part of the space between the lips. C. Stimulation of the left hand resulting in a greater degree of lowering of the mandible than shown in B, accompanied by elevation, protrusion, and then retraction of the tongue. In this photograph the tongue is elevated and is easily noted between the lips laterally. Only finger closure of the stimulated hand and a little head movement accompanied the oral activity. D. Lip and tongue movements elicited by drawing the stimulator (see *arrow*) across the lips and tongue from the midline region lateralward to the corner of the mouth. In addition to the separation of the lips shown here, the dark zone inside the lips at the midline is the longitudinal groove in the tongue formed by lifting of its two sides. At the end of the reflex the lips closed on the stimulator. The lips in this reflex are separated and brought together by the action of the muscles of facial expression and not by depressing of the jaw.

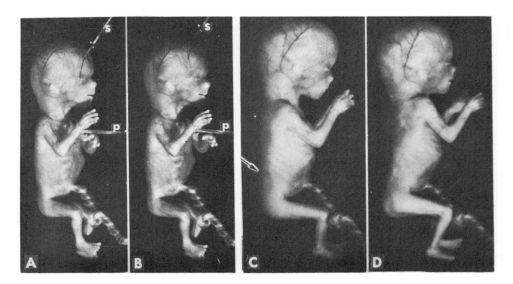

Fig. 7. Photographs illustrating two reflexes elicited by stimulating the cutaneous surfaces of a fetus of 14 weeks of menstrual age (No. 13, 88.5 mm CR, Graph 1). In A and B the fetus is shown at about half size and in C and D at about three fifths of the normal size.

A and B. Simultaneous and eyelid and oral reflexes elicited by drawing the stimulator (s) across the cheek, over the eyelids and off the forehead. With this reflex, the head bent contralateralward. In A the fetus is shown at rest. In B the contraction of the eyelid muscle has flattened the eyeball and obscured the fusion line between the lids. The upper lip has lifted near the corner and the corner pulled lateralward. Neither trunk nor extremity action accompanied this reflex although these movements may be present with such reflexes. The action shown involved about half a second. A pipette (p) squirted hot saline against the fetus at this time, but no specific effect was demonstrable.

C and D. The reaction secured by drawing the stimulator (position of *arrow* in C) upward along the back. The head and trunk extended and the mouth opened, the chest and abdominal muscles contracted to elevate the rib cage and flatten the abdominal wall in an inspiratory gasp accompanied by shoulder and other movements to give a response characteristic for a tickling reaction such as is seen postnatally. The total reflex, including the return to the resting position, consumed about three seconds. Slightly over one second was involved in the part shown.

reflexes such as moving the lips. When tongue movements begin, the hypoglossal nerve constitutes the motor limb of these reflex arcs (Fig. 5). One sensory limb of these reflex arcs continues to be the trigeminal nerve fibers, but other sensory fibers function in these reflexes also as soon as activity in the oral area may be elicited by stimulation of the sole of the foot (Fig. 6A), the palm of the hand (Fig. 6C), and other areas (Figs. 6B, 7C, and 8C).

Both mouth opening and head movements have a dual functional relationship in mammals. Although mouth opening was reported earlier to be an isolated local reflex when it first appears (Hooker, 1954, 1958; Hooker and Humphrey, 1954; Humphrey, 1954, 1964a, b), photographic prints from the motion pictures of these reflexes (Figs. 2 and 3) clearly demonstrate that they begin as part of the total pattern contralateral flexion reflexes (Humphrey, 1968a, 1969c, d). Thus, initially mouth opening develops as part of an avoiding reflex and so belongs with the defense or protective reactions early in development and only later becomes part of the developmental reflex sequence for feeding. When the mouth opening reflex is no longer an integral part of the contralateral flexion reflex, it also becomes associated with ipsilateral head responses, tongue movements, and other oral activity, such as swallowing, all of which are clearly feeding reactions. Postnatally mouth opening and closure continue to serve in both capacities. The fetal reflexes involving oral activity, like those postnatally, are more rapid as part of the avoiding reflexes of protective or negative character than when they are associated with the positive feeding ones, such as swallowing and tongue movements.

Tongue Movements

Until the mouth opens widely there is neither opportunity to see the tongue nor to touch it without stimulating the lips at the same time. Consequently, the exact time that active tongue movements begin has never been determined (Hooker, 1958; Humphrey, 1964a, 1968a, 1969c). Examination of microscopic sections shows that such extrinsic tongue muscles as the genioglossus and hyoglossus of the 11-week fetus are clearly able to contract. However, no photographic proof of tongue movement has been observed until 12.5 weeks, a week and a half later. In the reflex mouth opening of this 12.5-week fetus (Fig. 6B), elevation of the tongue has taken place, for it is visible near the corner of the wide open mouth. As part of a reflex of one 14-week fetus the tongue was not only elevated but thrust forward, then retracted before the mouth closed (Fig. 6C). In the mouth opening and closing reflex of a 15.5-week fetus in Figure 6D there was a longitudinal groove or furrow in the elevated tongue. When the upper lip puckered and the lower lip protruded at 20 weeks (Figs. 9B and C), the tongue was also visible just behind the lips and hence must have both elevated and moved forward. In the crying of a resuscitated nonviable premature infant of 23.5 weeks, the elevated tongue with the tip turned backward has the same position as is usually seen when a newborn infant cries.

Swallowing Reflexes

Reflex swallowing has been observed fairly early in development from stimulation of the lips. It was thought at one time to begin as early as 10.5 weeks (Hooker, 1954, 1958; Hooker and Humphrey, 1954), but no motion pictures were secured and swallowing has not been demonstrated photographically until 12.5 weeks. This difference is mentioned here partly to emphasize the hazards of attempting to interpret fetal movements without motion picture records that can be viewed repeatedly and studied from photographic prints as well. It may be, however, that stimulation of the mucosa might elicit swallowing before it can be elicited by touching the lips.

Inasmuch as amniotic fluid must enter the oral cavity as soon as the mouth opens widely (and be retained when it closes), possibly this fluid in the mouth stimulates the oral mucosa and leads to swallowing earlier in development than the motion picture records have shown it to occur. This concept is supported by the fact that the nerve fibers make contact with the basement membrane of the oral mucosa by 8.5 weeks (27.1 mm), when mouth opening is frequent although partial, and terminate on the basal epithelial cells as primitive Merkel's discs at 10 weeks (37.0 mm CR), after the mouth opens more completely (p. 759·). Therefore, adequate sensory receptors for such reflexes are present before 10.5 weeks (Humphrey, 1966). Indeed, nerve fibers contact the basement membrane of the mucosal epithelium a week earlier than that of the lips, and the primitive Merkel's discs appear two weeks before they have been identified for the cutaneous surfaces at 12 weeks (Hogg, 1941).

The first part of a swallowing reflex at 13 weeks is reproduced in Figures 8A and B. It was accompanied by slight head extension as the larynx elevated and the mouth opened (Fig. 8B), then some ventral head flexion as the mouth partly closed and the larynx descended in completing the swallowing act. In this swallowing reflex the mouth remained partly open. In a swallowing reflex recorded at 14 weeks (Humphrey, 1968a), the mouth closed completely when the head flexed ventralward (88.5 mm CR). Then the mouth reopened again.

Fetal swallowing reflexes normally occur in utero. They were demonstrated at 12 weeks' gestation by Davis and Potter (1946). It has been estimated that as much as 500 ml of amniotic fluid may be swallowed by the normal near term human fetus in 24 hours (Pritchard, 1965; Adams et al., 1967a), although none was swallowed by anencephalic fetuses of a comparable age (Pritchard, 1965). The frequency of fetal swallowing and other factors that influence it in utero are unknown, according to Adams et al. (1967a). Arshavsky (1959) suggested a nutrient function for the substances in the amniotic fluid, a view held by Preyer in 1885. At least these reflexes must strengthen the pharyngeal and esophageal musculature. Adequate strength of swallowing is just as essential for nursing by the newborn infant as is the integration of tongue and lip reflexes for the complex activity of sucking.

Gag Reflexes

A prolonged stimulation of the inside of the mouth with a glass rod, which probably included the back of the tongue and perhaps the pharynx as well, was followed by a rapidly executed gag reflex at 18.5 weeks (Fig. 8C). The action included closure of the mouth on the stimulator, its reopening, an inspiratory gasp with contraction of the diaphragm, and a second partial mouth closure (Humphrey, 1968a, 1969c). The gag reflex is almost always present in premature infants (Peiper, 1963) even if the infant is unable either to suck or to swallow.

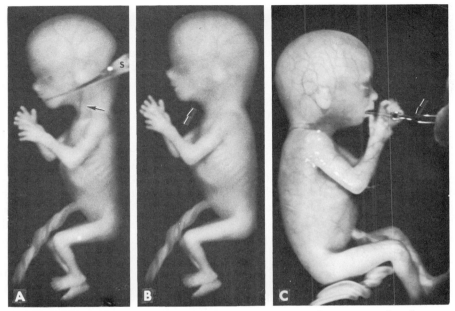

Fig. 8. A and B are photographs illustrating a swallowing reflex at 13 weeks of menstrual age (75.0 mm CR, No. 45). C shows a gag reflex at 18.5 weeks (144.5 mm CR, No. 111).

A. The area of the lower lip stroked by the stimulator (s) and the sharp outline of the sternocleidomastoid muscle (at *arrow*) are illustrated. B. The mouth has opened and the head extended slightly as the larynx moved upward, thus rounding the contour beneath the chin (at *arrow*) and obscuring the border of the sterno-cleidomastoid muscle. No movements of the extremities or of the trunk accompanied this reflex. The photographs are about 0.8 natural size.

C. The fullness in the floor of the mouth and one phase in the facial expression accompanying a gag reflex which was elicited by inserting a glass rod (at *arrow*) far into the mouth so that it stimulated the back of the tongue and possibly the posterior wall of the pharynx. No trunk or extremity movements accompanied the reflex. Almost 3 seconds elapsed after the glass rod was inserted before the rapid action began. The photograph is slightly less than half the size of the fetus.

However, it seems unlikely that gag reflexes would ever occur in utero under normal conditions.

Lip Movements and Sucking

Before 13.5 to 14 weeks (Hooker, 1952) the reflex opening and closing of the mouth has been due to lowering and lifting of the mandible and not to movements of the lips. At 14 weeks (Figs. 7A and B), however, there is clear evidence of upper lip movement of quite a different sort. The stimulus producing the reflex was an upward stroke of the stimulator from the angle of the jaw across the eyelids. The upper lip was raised ipsilaterally near the corner of the mouth and, in one reflex, the ala of the nose elevated also. In addition, the face rotated away from the side stimulated. With one of these reflexes extremity movements occurred also, but not with the other. An oral reflex of this type involves the muscles of facial expression about the mouth. These muscles develop later than those that depress the mandible but have attained a degree of differentiation that enables them to act at this age (Gasser, 1967).

In response to stimulation of the lower lip (Fig. 9A) this lip alone may be depressed as early as 15.5 weeks (Humphrey, 1968a). Stimulation of the upper lip may give rise to its protrusion at 17 weeks (Hooker, 1952; Humphrey, 1964a). Stimulation of the lower lip may result in its protrusion by 20 weeks (Figs. 9B and C) and in puckering the upper lip also. Puckering the lower lip has been seen at 22 weeks, when both lips may both pucker and protrude (Hooker, 1952; Humphrey, 1964a). According to Golubewa et al. (1959) sucking reflexes have been observed at 24 weeks. Sucking sufficiently strong to be audible was reported by Hooker (1958) at 29 weeks for one of the viable premature infants studied.

Popular publications, like those of Nilsson (1965) and Nilsson et al. (1966), refer to fetal thumb sucking in utero as early as 18 weeks. Their photographs show the thumb between the lips but without the lip puckering that is an essential

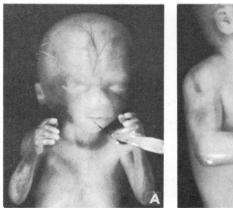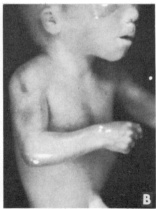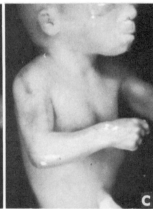

Fig. 9. A. Depression of the lower lip of a fetus of 15.5 weeks (No. 53, 110.5 mm CR, Graph 1) following stimulation of the vermilion border from the lateral side toward the middle. The tongue shows between the parted lips. No other action took place. The photograph is reproduced at about 0.7 the size of the fetus.

B and C. Puckering of the upper lip (shown by *vertical lines*) and protrusion of the lower lip following stimulation of the lower lip of a fetus of 20 weeks (No. 55, 166.0 mm CR, Graph 1). The tongue elevated and was thrust forward since it fills the space between the lips in C where the borders of the mentalis muscle are accentuated by its contraction. Before the movement began, in B, the open mouth was held with the upper lip elevated near the corner. The photographs are at about 0.4 of the size of the fetus. The lip action, both in the reflex in A and in that in B and C, is produced by the muscles of facial expression.

part of sucking. As just mentioned, both lips have not been shown to protrude and pucker simultaneously before 22 weeks, and sucking reflexes, even weak ones, have not been reported in scientific papers before 24 weeks. However, at 8.5 weeks of menstrual age (Figs. 2A and 3A) and later the hands are often close to the face after the fetus is removed from the amnion. Within the confined space of the amniotic sac, the hands often touch the face as shown in the photographs of Nilsson et al. (1966). Because the mouth often remains open, or partly so, from 14 weeks onward when the fetus is not moving (Figs. 7A, 9B, 10A, 10C, 11D), the thumb probably enters it earlier than true sucking is possible. Definite blisters on the thumb and other parts of the hands and lower forearms at birth have been interpreted by Murphy and Langley (1963) as the result of sucking these areas before birth. Inasmuch as sucking is often too weak in small premature infants to be adequate for nursing (Lundeen and Kunstadter, 1958), strong sucking must take place only during the last part of gestation. However, the close positional relationship of the hands and the face in utero provides ample opportunity for self-stimulation of the face during a large part of prenatal life.

Respiratory Reflexes

Windle et al. (1938) reported respiratory movements for a fetus of 62.0 mm CR (12 weeks menstrual age), and isolated respiratory chest contractions were mentioned by Hooker (1958) as early as 13 weeks menstrual age. At 14 weeks (Figs. 7C and D), drawing the stimulator upward along the back of the fetus resulted in a complex series of movements resembling the postnatal reaction to tickling. This reflex included an inspiratory gasp with flattening of the abdominal wall as well (Humphrey, 1968a, 1969c). At 18.5 weeks (Hooker, 1958) weak chest contractions have been seen both spontaneously and in response to chest stimulation, and at 22 weeks diaphragmatic contractions have been noted. It is at this age also that fetal hiccups, which are due to spasmodic contractions of the diaphragm, were first recorded by Norman (1942). When fetuses are artificially resuscitated at 23.5 weeks (Hooker, 1958), and possibly earlier, deep respiratory movements occur for a time with contraction of the diaphragm and of the abdominal and chest muscles. In the series of premature infants observed by Hooker, however, effective respiration could not be maintained until 27 weeks of menstrual age, although it could be artificially established much earlier on a temporary basis.

There is considerable evidence that respiratory movements may occur in utero (Windle et al., 1938; Davis and Potter, 1946; Windle, 1940, 1944; and others). It has been suggested that these movements are a normal part of intrauterine development that bring amniotic fluid into the developing lungs and so aid in the expansion of the alveolar spaces (Snyder and Rosenfeld, 1937; Bonar et al., 1938). However, the experimental evidence now available on subprimates demonstrates that the fluid present in the fetal respiratory passages is secreted by the lungs of the fetus, possibly some by the alveoli (Adams and Fujiwara, 1963). After being expelled into the amniotic cavity it is swallowed with the amniotic fluid or, to a lesser degree, passes directly into the pharynx and is swallowed. Only under conditions of fetal stress have respiratory movements been demonstrated to take place in utero. The evidence for this conclusion and the current views on its significance are discussed in the papers of Adams (1966) and Adams et al. (1967a, b).

Crying

According to Peiper (1963) premature infants weighing only 650 g cry audibly. This is approximately the size of the nonviable premature of 23.5 weeks for which the tonic neck reflex is illustrated (Figs. 11D and E). Audible crying with the wide open mouth and tongue movements typical of a crying infant were photographed for this fetus. The preliminary puckering up to cry is shown in Figure 11E. Scowling and tight contraction of the eyelid muscles accompany crying at this time, although the eyelids remain fused ordinarily until the seventh month (Patten, 1953; Arey, 1965). A single cry was reported by Golubewa et al. (1959) before 22 weeks and a series of cries by 22 weeks. Minkowski (1922) found crying at a comparable age (21 weeks).

On different occasions obstetricians have heard infants cry before delivery but after the membranes have ruptured (Ryder, 1943; Carmichael, 1954; Russell, 1957) so that air probably entered the uterus. Since the emission of sound, and so crying, depends on the expulsion of air as well as on the development of adequately maintained diaphragmatic and chest contractions, it will not take place in utero under normal circumstances. On the delivery of a premature infant with a sufficiently developed respiratory system to enable breathing to be established even temporarily, crying should be expected.

Reflexes Associated with the Eyes

As mentioned earlier, contraction of the orbicularis oculi muscle when it first occurs (10 to 10.5 weeks) on stimulation of the upper eyelid is not accompanied by other movements (Hooker, 1952, 1958). The corrugator supercilii reflex is also independent of other movements when it begins at 11 weeks. A week later the two reflexes (squint and scowl in type) may be seen together. These reflexes were not observed in conjunction with neck and trunk movements (Figs. 7A and B) until 13 to 14 weeks (Humphrey, 1964a). Still later (15.5 weeks) a quick mouth opening with the tongue behind the lips has been seen along with the squintlike reflex (Figs. 10A and B). A slight brief mouth closure may accompany the combination of squint and scowl type reflexes by 16 weeks (Figs. 10C and D).

Reflexes have not been secured from stimulating the ophthalmic fibers before the fibers touch the basement membrane, whereas they have been elicited from stimulating the maxillomandibular fibers when these fibers are as much as 13 μ from the epithelium. The ophthalmic nerve fibers do not make contact with the basement membrane of the upper eyelid epithelium until 10 weeks (37 mm CR), about a week later (9 to 9.5 weeks, 32 mm CR) than the maxillomandibular

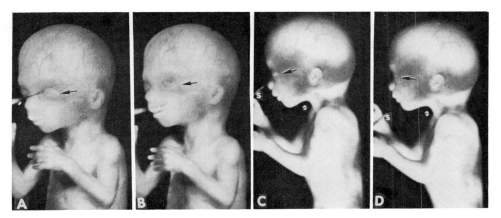

Fig. 10. Photographs illustrating reflex contraction of the orbicularis oculi muscle (squintlike reflex) in two different combinations with other reflex activity. A and B are photographs of a fetus of 15.5 weeks (No. 135, 107.5 mm CR). C and D show a different reflex combination from a fetus of 16 weeks (No. 27, 114.0 mm CR). Fertilization age as given by Patten (1953) and menstrual age based on the data of Mall (1910) may be checked against those above by consulting Graph 1.

A and B. The stimulator is touching the upper eyelid near the inner canthus in A, where the action has not yet begun, and is being lifted away from the face in the upper lip area in B. The contraction of the eyelid muscle is shown by the disappearance of the fusion line (at *arrow* on A) between the eyelids in B (at *arrow*) and by the flattening of the eyeball. In combination with this reflex there is a slight separation of the lips so that the tongue shows immediately behind them. The head extended slightly, and the fingers on the ipsilateral hand extended at the interphalangeal joints and flexed slightly at the metacarpophalangeal joints, but there was no other muscle activity. The photographs are reproduced at about 0.7 the size of the fetus.

C and D. The stimulator (s) that elicited this reflex was drawn down over the eyebrows on the left as well as along the inner canthus of the eye. As in the reflex shown in A and B, the lips were slightly parted before action began, but in this case they came together a little rather than parting more. In this reflex, both the orbicularis oculi and the corrugator supercilii contracted so that not only a squintlike reflex but also a scowllike reflex appeared. As in the reflex in A and B, the fusion line between the eyelids almost disappeared and the eyeball flattened (compare line at *arrow* in C with that in D). The slight movement caused by contraction of the corrugator is demonstrated only by the decrease in the size of the highlight in the eyebrow area in the two photographs, reproduced here at about half the size of the fetus.

fibers reach the same level of the cutaneous epithelium of the lips, and 1.5 weeks later (8.5 weeks, 27.1 mm CR) than they touch this membrane of the oral mucosa (Humphrey, 1966). In the spinal tract of the trigeminal nerve, likewise, the ophthalmic fibers arrive at their adult caudal level about a week later than the maxillomandibular fibers reach it (Humphrey, 1954). These differences in growth centrally and peripherally may account in part for the fact that the orbicularis oculi and corrugator reflexes are local in character when they appear, and the head and trunk movements accompany them only later.

Downward movements of both eyes were reported by Hooker (1952) following eyelid stimulation of two fetuses at 12.5 weeks, although at this age the eyelids are fused (Patten, 1953). Conjugate lateral movements of the eyes were noted first at 25 weeks with the eyelids open, and such movements were seen thereafter also. Eye movements undoubtedly occur during prenatal life in response to changes in position (Carmichael, 1954), but proof that this occurs is lacking. The neurons of the vestibular nuclei that mediate such reflexes are sufficiently differentiated at 13.5 weeks to function (Humphrey, 1965). Inasmuch as the other parts of the essential reflex arcs mature early, eye movement reflexes of vestibular origin may begin relatively early in development.

Reflexes from Stimulation of the Genital and Anal Regions

Reflexes have been elicited from stimulation of the genital area of fetuses as early in development as 10.5 and 11 weeks and have been seen also at 17 and 18.5 weeks (Humphrey and Hooker, 1961a, b; Humphrey, 1964a). The region of the genitofemoral sulcus as well as the phallus reacted to stimulation of the youngest fetus mentioned. The older fetuses reacted to stimuli over the penis and scrotum as well as to stroking the genitofemoral sulcus. By 32 weeks, stimulating the inside of the thigh may elicit the cremasteric reflex (Hooker, 1958), but Robinson (1966) found it present more often after that age for infants of normal weight as compared with those low in weight for their age.

Thus far the reflexes reported from genital stimulation have been lower trunk and lower extremity movements. Motion picture records were secured for only one of the fetuses listed above (18.5 weeks), so details of the reactions of the other fetuses were not secured. However, bilateral flexion of the thighs on the pelvis was seen for the youngest fetus (10.5 weeks) as well as for all of the older ones. Stimulation of the genitofemoral sulcus, or sometimes of the genital area (laterally), elicited an ipsilateral flexion of the thigh on the pelvis that, at 18.5 weeks, included flexion at the knee joint as well. At this age the bilateral reflex may include flexion at the hips, extension at the knees, dorsiflexion of the feet and toes with toe fanning, as well as ventral flexion of the lower back, and rotation of the pelvis to one side. Although action of the upper extremities and head has not been recognized with these reflexes, they are general body and extremity reflexes, not local reactions. Undoubtedly head and upper extremity movements will be found also when additional data are studied. The cremasteric reflex is the first local reflex, and the only one, that has been reported from genital stimulation as yet.

Fewer reactions have been seen from anal stimulation than from stimulation of the genital areas (Humphrey, 1964a). At 10.5 weeks, flexion of the pelvis on the trunk was noted. Later (17 weeks) with the fetus prone rather than supine, the reflex included flexion at the hips and knees as well as flexion of the pelvis on the trunk. For these reflexes stroking the anal surface with the esthesiometer was the effective stimulus. Introducing a glass rod into the anal canal was a less adequate stimulus.

Tonic Neck Reflexes

In the symmetric tonic neck reflex the upper and lower extremities are extended on the side toward which the face is turned and flexed on the side toward the occiput when the infant is in the supine position (Fig. 11D). Asymmetric tonic neck reflexes like that illustrated in Figure 11E are more common for nonviable premature infants, at least. Gesell and Amatruda (1947) indicate that the tonic neck reflex is present in the newborn infant and consider it a characteristic feature at 4 postnatal weeks. Some observers believe that the symmetric form of this reflex occurs only rarely (Illingworth, 1966; André-Thomas et al., 1960) and has little significance, whereas the asymmetric reaction is often seen. Others (Prechtl and Beintema, 1964) state that it may be present or absent at birth.

The Origin and Early Developmental History of Extremity Reflexes

Extremity reflexes, like active mouth opening reflexes, first appear in development as part of the total pattern lateral flexion reflexes. The backward movement of the arms at the shoulders (beginning arm extension, 25 mm) appears before there is any evidence that the lower extremities move as part of these contralateral reflexes. Almost at once, however, the separation of the soles of the feet (normally facing each other and in contact when the fetus is in the rest position) demonstrates a primitive sort of abduction at the hip joints. This movement has begun at 26.0 mm (Fig. 2), but the separation of the soles of the feet is slight, brief, and part of the reflex only when the action is forceful. As early as 27.1 mm, the two upper extremities may no longer move in exactly the same way, and by 34.3 mm a considerable difference between the arm movements on the two sides has been seen. During this period when the extremity movements are an integral part of the contralateral flexion reflexes following perioral stimulation (Fig. 3), the digits of both the hands and the feet appear to spread apart (Humphrey, 1968a, 1969c).

When the total pattern type of contralateral (and ipsilateral) flexion reflexes disappears, beginning at 10 to 10.5 weeks, the lower extremity movements commence to drop out of the reactions to perioral stimulation, whereas the upper extremity movements are still present (Humphrey, 1968a). The arm on the side ipsilateral to the stimulus may react to the facial stimulus after both upper extremities no longer participate (p. 782). Obviously both upper and lower extremity movements begin in response to perioral stimulation. Likewise they are suppressed as part of these reflexes after the extremities themselves (palms and soles) become sensitive.

Reflexes from Stimulating the Upper Extremity

AREAS SENSITIVE TO STIMULATION

The palm of the hand (Table 3) is both the most sensitive area of the upper extremity for eliciting reflexes, and the one that responds to stimulation earliest (Hooker, 1952, 1958). It is only rarely that stimulation over the shoulder areas has resulted in extension of the upper arm or brachium at 10.5 weeks (Hooker, 1958) or caused abduction by 11.5 weeks (Hooker, 1958). The reflexes elicited from palmar stimulation often involve only the fingers, but sometimes the hand, forearm, and upper arm are involved, and occasionally an oral area reflex is elicited as well (Fig. 6C) (Humphrey, 1969c, d).

REFLEXES ELICITED

Partial finger closure is the earlier reflex elicited by palmar stimulation. At about 10.5 weeks, "and possibly a little before" (Hooker, 1958), stimulation of the palm of the hand occasionally elicits quick, partial finger closure, without flexion of the thumb. By 11 weeks, the partial finger closure is quite consistently evoked by palmar stimulation (Figs. 11 A, B, and C), It is usually accompanied by participation of the hand, sometimes forearm flexion, and less commonly pronation of the forearm and rotation of the upper arm medialward. Finger closure becomes more complete by 13 weeks, and the thumb may come into apposition with the fingers, but only rarely. Finger closure is also more variable with the third to fifth digits shut more tightly and the index finger remaining extended (Humphrey, 1969d). By 13.5 to 14 weeks finger closure may be complete (Fig. 6C). Finger closure is maintained for a longer time by 15 to 15.5 weeks, and by 18.5 weeks Hooker (1958) found the fingers grasped a rod. The grasp of nonviable premature infants has become stronger by 23.5 weeks and is more variable (Figs. 11D and E). The thumb is sometimes folded inside the fingers (Fig. 11E) but lies along the side of the index finger more often (Fig. 11D). For a fetus of 27 weeks that proved viable, the grasp of one hand was apparently sufficiently strong to support most of the weight of the body, when it was lifted almost entirely away from the surface of the bed. The preceding account is based on the 1938, 1952, and 1958 papers of Hooker. The illustrations of Hooker showing the development of finger movements and grasping and photographs of finger movements are included in other papers (Humphrey, 1964a, 1969d).

HAND AND MOUTH INTERRELATIONSHIPS

When the total pattern types of flexion reflexes are suppressed by the development of inhibitory connections from higher centers (Humphrey, 1969d), arm and hand movements ipsilateral to the side of the face stimulated are seen after

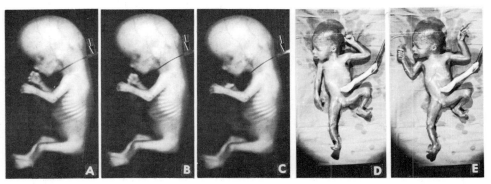

Fig. 11. A, B, and C. Photographs of a fetus of 11 weeks of menstrual age (No. 26, 48.5 mm CR length, Graph 1) illustrating the position of the fingers when the stimulator (at *arrows*) touched the palm in A, the partial closure of the fingers in B, and the flexion of the hand and arm movement with the added finger flexion in C. No other action accompanied this reflex. The photographs are at approximately 0.8 actual size.

D and E. Photographs of a fetus of 23.5 weeks of menstrual age (No. 56, 205.0 mm CR length, Graph 1) that was resuscitated with a respirator but was unable to maintain respiration adequately. In D, the characteristic position for the symmetric tonic neck reflex is demonstrated with the face turned toward the side where the extremities are extended. Although not crying, the mouth is open. The digits of the hand of the extended arm are extended also, whereas the fingers of the flexed arm are tightly closed with the thumb outside. In E, both upper extremities are in the flexion position, although the face is turned toward the side of the extended lower extremity in one of the asymmetric tonic neck reflex patterns. The fingers of the hand near the face are flexed with the thumb inside of the index finger. All of the digits of the other hand are extended, and the hand itself is adducted. The fetus is beginning to cry as indicated by the wider separation of the lips, the tightening of the eyelids, and the increased depth of the nasolabial fold. The disappearance of the border of the sternomastoid muscle is due to laryngeal movement upward, and the depression of the xiphoid process often occurs with the intake of air at this age. The photographs show this fetus at only about 0.1 of its size.

bilateral upper extremity movements following such stimuli have disappeared. Conversely, stimulation of one hand may be followed not only by some ipsilateral hand and finger action, but also by turning the face ipsilaterally as well, and by oral activity such as mouth opening, mouth closure, and tongue movements. This linkage of upper extremity and ipsilateral head movements (Figs. 6B and C) has been seen at 12.5 weeks and at 14 weeks (Humphrey, 1968a, 1969c). It has been demonstrated after 13.5 to 14 weeks by the fetal double simultaneous stimulation tests of face and ipsilateral hand. Before this age, when both face and palm are stimulated simultaneously the hand reflex tends to be suppressed. After this age the reflexes from both palmar and facial stimuli are more often elicited when the two stimuli are simultaneous (Hooker, 1954; Humphrey and Hooker, 1959).

At 14 weeks the close hand-mouth association has been seen following palmar stimulation. In one instance, a quite prolonged mouth opening with tongue pro-

trusion and retraction occurred, as well as tongue elevation, all combined with turning of the face toward the hand stimulated (Fig. 6C). This reflex has been suggested as the fetal forerunner of the Babkin reflex (Humphrey, 1969d) which is
elicited more frequently from premature than from newborn infants (Babkin,
1960; Peiper, 1963; Parmelee, 1963b). The intimate relationship between the
hand and the mouth is seen postnatally in the close association between grasp and
sucking (Prechtl, 1953; Peiper, 1963; Humphrey, 1969d). Another fetus of 14
weeks (No. 13, 88.5 mm CR) reacted to palmar stimulation by turning the head
toward the midline, elevating the ipsilateral upper lip near the corner and pulling
the corner laterally, contracting the eyelid muscles in the squintlike reaction, and
elevating the lower lip slightly. This reflex appears to be the fetal forerunner of
the palmomental reflex (Humphrey, 1969d) that was described by Marinesco
and Radovici (1920) for premature and term infants (Parmelee, 1963a) and is
seen occasionally in normal adults (Blake and Kunkle, 1951) as well as fairly
often in young children (Peiper, 1963).

Reflexes from Stimulating the Lower Extremity

AREAS SENSITIVE TO STIMULATION

The sole of the foot becomes sensitive to stimulation by 10.5 to 11 weeks, very
shortly after reflexes are elicitable from the palm of the hand (Hooker, 1952).
Although there is very little difference in their time of onset if the age group
is considered (Table 3), the palmar response for any single fetus is well established
when the plantar reaction is first secured. The retention of reflex finger closure
after anoxia suppresses the plantar reflex also demonstrates that the palmar reflex
develops earlier (Table 1), for the longer established reflexes function later than
newly matured reflex arcs under such conditions. The cutaneous areas of the leg
and thigh do not become sensitive until later than does the sole of the foot. At
17 weeks, stroking the surface of the buttock elicits a reflex (Humphrey, 1964a).
Probably other surfaces, such as the dorsum of the foot, also become sensitive,
but adequate testing has not been done. By 32 weeks the medial surface of the
thigh is also sensitive. However, the sole of the foot not only is the first lower
extremity surface to become sensitive, but also remains reflexogenous throughout
both fetal and postnatal life.

REFLEXES ELICITED

The initial response to plantar stimulation was found by Hooker (1958) to be
plantar flexion of all the toes (Figs. 12A and B), as originally reported by Minkowski (1923). Dorsiflexion of the great toe and toe fanning were elicited by
11.5 to 12 weeks by Hooker (1958). At 12.5 weeks, however, plantar stimulation may elicit either reflex, that is, plantar flexion of the toes or dorsiflexion of

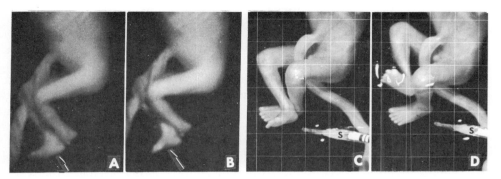

Fig. 12. Reflexes in response to stimulation of the sole of the foot at 13 weeks (No. 45, 75.0 mm CR length) in A and B and at 16.5 weeks (No. 43, 121.0 mm CR length) in C and D.

A shows the position of the foot before this planter flexion reflex began. In B, both the toes and the adjacent part of the foot are plantar flexed. The *arrow* points to the area of stimulation in A, and region of change in position in B. With this reflex, no other action took place, even for the lower extremities. The photographs are a little less than natural size.

C and D illustrate a Babinski reflex. On stroking the sole of the right foot with a 2-g stimulator (s), a rapid dorsiflexion of all toes took place accompanied by dorsiflexion of the foot, and flexion at the knee and at the hip joints. In D, however, neither dorsiflexion of the great toe nor toe fanning are complete, but both occurred a little later. There was no movement of the other lower extremity and no action elsewhere. The photographs are at about half the size of the fetus. The grid in these two photographs was used in an attempt to demonstrate the action more effectively.

the great toe with toe fanning (Figs. 12C and D). Either reflex may be accompanied by flexion at the ankle, knee, and hip and sometimes by rotation and abduction of the thigh (Hooker, 1952, 1958). The tabulations of reflexes by Hooker from the motion picture records show that plantar flexion continues to be elicited occasionally even as late as 18.5 to 20 weeks, although it occurs less frequently (see Humphrey, 1969d). However, dorsiflexion of the great toe with fanning of the other toes becomes more common during this period. The essential parts of the Babinski reflex, according to DeJong (1967), are dorsiflexion of the toes, and particularly the great toe, with spreading (or fanning) of the other digits. The Babinski reflex, therefore, develops in fetal life after plantar flexion has appeared. The plantar toe flexion reflex is comparable to the finger closure elicited by palmar stimulation. It has been suggested that it is the equivalent of the foot-grasp reflex present phylogenetically (Humphrey, 1964a). Perinatally, and especially with premature infants, plantar flexion is elicited more often on scratching the lateral aspect of the sole of the foot than is dorsiflexion of the great toe and toe fanning. However, plantar flexion is also elicited during this period by pressure on the ball of the foot, and the two reflexes are frequently confused in the literature (see Humphrey, 1969d).

The Sequence of Development of Sensitivity to Light Touch

In human development the areas about the mouth are the first ones to become sensitive to stimulation by stroking the surface lightly with a hair. For small fetuses that are not influenced by narcotics and/or anesthetics, like those in Figures 2 and 3, 25- or 50-mg stimulators are adequate to elicit reflexes before the oxygen supply is sufficiently depleted to suppress all reactions. As the amount of oxygen diminishes, stronger stimuli are necessary. In older fetuses that have a thicker surface epithelium, stronger stimuli are needed also. Although these stimulators exert very little pressure, even a 10-mg stimulator is easily felt when drawn across the palm of the hand. Because the growing nerve tips do not yet touch the basement membrane of the thin epithelium when sensitivity is first demonstrable, even the light stroking stimulus is thought to deform the nerve tips enough by displacement of the surrounding tissues to cause their excitation (Hogg, 1941).

The nerves functioning when the lips and adjacent perioral areas become sensitive to stimulation at 7.5 weeks (20 to 21 mm) are the maxillary and mandibular divisions of the trigeminal or fifth cranial nerve. Table 3 gives the chronologic order in which the surfaces of the body and oral cavity become sensitive to stimulation, as far as it has been possible to determine from the data available at the present time. Hooker (1952, 1958) found some indication that the maxillary fibers responded earlier than the mandibular fibers. There has been little difference shown between the distance of the nerve tips from the epithelium in the upper and lower lips, however, when they become sensitive (13 μ to 14 μ in rima oris region) at 7.5 weeks (Humphrey, 1966). The sensitive area widens out to cover the more peripheral perioral zones, including the alae of the nose and the chin by 9.5 weeks and the lower eyelids, the bridge of the nose, and the region below the lower eyelid by 10.5 weeks. None of the areas supplied by the ophthalmic division of the trigeminal nerve become sensitive until 10 to 10.5 weeks, when the upper eyelids are responsive to stimulation (Hooker, 1958). The superciliary ridges (eyebrow areas) and the forehead are added a little later (11 weeks) (Hooker, 1958), but the forehead rarely responds to stimulation. No reflexes have been reported from stroking the surface areas of the scalp which are supplied by ophthalmic fibers or from the other areas of the scalp that are supplied by cervical nerves.

It might be expected that surface sensitivity would spread regularly from the perioral facial areas peripheralward over the body and extremities. Such a regular sequence has not been demonstrated, however (Table 3). The palms of the hands, the genital areas, and the areas supplied by the ophthalmic fibers apparently become responsive to stimuli at approximately the same time. Touching the genital areas produces reflex action before stimulation of the back, the chest, or the abdominal wall becomes effective. Also the palms of the hands react to stimulation earlier than do the more centrally located shoulder, upper arm, and forearm areas. Likewise, the soles of the feet have been found to be sensitive earlier than either the thighs or legs.

These functional sequences do not necessarily mean that nerve fibers have not arrived as close to the surface of these intermediate regions as to the finger tips, for example. There are far fewer nerves terminating in these intermediate areas (Hogg, 1941). Consequently, there is little summation and so evidence of their functional capacity is difficult to secure. Reflexes elicited by cutaneous stimulation perinatally and postnatally likewise are mainly from the palms and soles, not from either the shoulder to wrist areas or buttock to ankle regions.

Although the ages given in Table 3 are subject to change as more data are accumulated, certain trends are clear. One is that the anterior end (oral area) and the posterior end (genital region) of the fetus become sensitive to external stimulation before the intervening regions. Likewise, the palmar and plantar surfaces or distal portions of the extremities become sensitive earlier than the proximal ones. From the morphologic viewpoint, it is evident at once that these areas—lips, genitalia, palms, and soles—are the cutaneous areas of the adult that contain both the greatest concentration of sensory nerve endings and the most highly specialized varieties of sensory receptors (Humphrey, 1964a).

Other Types of General Sensation

For the other types of sensory stimuli relatively little is known concerning function during fetal life. The literature on function of premature and full-term infants is discussed by Carmichael (1954) and Peiper (1963) and cannot be included here. Stretch reflexes like the localized reactions elicited by Windle (1944) by rapidly lifting and releasing a limb undoubtedly develop early, even though Cuajunco (1940) found the receptors (muscle spindles) only beginning development by 11 weeks of menstrual age in the biceps brachii. Whether these reflexes precede those elicited by light stroking of the skin remains an unsettled question. Two points, at least, favor the earlier functioning of the cutaneous reflexes: 1, They do not require specialized receptors, only naked end bulbs, even in the adult. 2, Until muscle contracts, there can be no stretch stimuli, and for higher mammals skeletal muscle does not contract before the reflex arcs function, although in birds, for example, spontaneous movements appear before reflexes can be elicited (Hamburger, 1963).

Sensations interpreted postnatally as painful have relatively little effect (Carmichael, 1954; Peiper, 1963). However, as soon as the fetus responds to perioral stimulation positively (turning toward) as well as negatively (turning away or avoiding), distinction is made on a reflex level. This occurs at 22.6 to 26.0 mm (Fig. 2). Whether this difference is due to the strength of stimulation (strong stimuli being nociceptive), as some believe, or is on some other basis it is not possible to say. Whether the area stimulated is peripherally or centrally situated may be a factor also.

Newborn infants and probably prematures also react more vigorously to stimuli colder than the body than to those warmer (Carmichael, 1954). In the observations of Hooker (1939, 1944, 1952, 1954, 1958) on fetuses, the temperature of the fluid bath was kept as near normal body temperature as possible. A stream of hot saline directed against the body of the fetus was tried a few times, but no definite information was secured. Cold saline was not tried. If the saline bath became overheated by 3 or 4°, reflexes were not obtained. However, reflexes have been elicited from fetuses of 11 weeks of menstrual age and older with the usual hair esthesiometers when the temperature has been as low as 80°F (Humphrey and Hooker, 1961b). This may indicate that sensitivity to temperatures colder than the body is greater than that to warmth in fetal life also. There is some evidence to indicate that temperature from the face is mediated through the rostral part of the spinal trigeminal nuclear complex (see Humphrey, 1969b). If so, then temperature sensitivity may be developing at the time that this region starts differentiation at 11 weeks (Brown, 1962), the age mentioned above.

So far as the other general sensory modalities mentioned are concerned, it is only possible to say that if they are related in any way to the development of the special receptors, such as Meissner's corpuscles and pacinian corpuscles, they may make their appearance in fetal life when these receptors begin to differentiate. This would probably be as the age of viability is approached, or attained, for cholinesterase activity has been demonstrated for pacinian corpuscles at 24 weeks and for Meissner's corpuscles at 28 weeks (Beckett et al., 1956).

The Special Senses During Intrauterine Life

Space does not allow more than brief comments on the questions of vestibular, gustatory, auditory, olfactory, and visual function in prenatal life. The reflex circuits that act at brain stem levels—vestibular, gustatory, and auditory reflex arcs—will mature earliest since differentiation proceeds from cervical levels cephalad as well as caudad (Kingsbury, 1924). For the spinal trigeminal nuclear complex (Brown, 1956, 1958, 1962) this order of maturation has been shown for human fetuses. It is indicated also for some reflex arcs (Humphrey, 1954, 1969d). The vestibular ganglion cells mature early, and the neurons of the lateral (Minkowski, 1922, 1928) and inferior vestibular nuclei are sufficiently mature to function at 9.5 weeks of menstrual age (Humphrey, 1965). Both Minkowski (1928) and Hooker (1942) have suggested that some movements observed by them might be due to vestibular stimulation. Abundant vestibular stimuli are certainly present in utero. Minkowski (1928) suggested that the almost weightless status of the fetus in utero provided a particularly advantageous medium for vestibular reflexes.

Concerning taste, Bradley and Stern (1967) conclude that taste buds are mature enough to function during the 13.5- to 15-week age period (apparently fertilization age). This age is later than the time that tongue movement has been demonstrated in our investigations. Swallowing begins at about the same age level as tongue movement, and undoubtedly amniotic fluid enters the mouth as it opens completely (9.5 weeks menstrual age). The addition of saccharine to amniotic fluid has been shown to result in increased swallowing by fetuses near term with hydramnios, but it is possible that other taste stimuli, such as bitter, or saccharine, for that matter, may be effective in eliciting reflexes much earlier. The literature on taste sensitivity of premature and newborn infants is controversial (see Peiper, 1963), but at least two types of reactions occur: grimacing and rejection as with quinine, for example, and swallowing and sucking movements as with sugar.

Fetal reactions to auditory stimuli have been demonstrated both by an increase in reflex activity and by an increase in fetal heart rate. The increase in heart rate has been shown at "about the beginning of the twenty-ninth week" (Sontag and Wallace, 1936) to "30 postconception weeks" (Murphy and Smyth, 1962) and is present until birth (Sontag and Wallace, 1936). Sontag and Wallace (1934) also report that both the mother's emotion (such as anger or fear) and fatigue increase the fetal heart rate. Increased movements in response to sound were first observed a little later than the change in heart rate, i.e., at the "beginning of the thirty-first week of intrauterine life" (Sontag and Wallace, 1935). Other literature on this subject is discussed by Carmichael (1954), Pratt (1954), and Peiper (1963).

As succinctly stated by Windle (1940), there can be no visual stimulation during intrauterine life. The information is controversial about the light reflexes of premature infants (Carmichael, 1954), but it is probably safe to say that the elicitation of this reflex is the first evidence of retinal function.

Because the olfactory portions of the telencephalon are relatively large in lower vertebrates, the assumption is sometimes made that olfactory sensitivity develops early embryologically. There is no evidence to support the view. Differentiation of the nervous system takes place from cervical levels cephalad, and the efferent pathways must reach the brain stem for reflexes to take place. Even if the necessary maturation occurs relatively early and there were an adequate stimulus, until the nasal plugs of epithelium in the external nares have resolved and disappeared, which may not be until four to six months (Schaeffer, 1910), no currents of fluid pass across the nasal epithelium. Therefore, until the infant is born there is little likelihood that there is any olfactory function taking place. The literature concerning the olfactory capacities of premature and full-term infants is extensive and controversial (Carmichael, 1954; Peiper, 1963), in part due to the use of irritants that stimulate the trigeminal endings in the nose rather than stimulate only the olfactory cells. However, it appears justifiable to conclude that when olfactory function begins, the reflex activity will indicate that the odor is either an agreeable or a disagreeable one.

Closing Comments

The development of nervous system function is an orderly process that is integrated from the beginning of the first reflex. Each added function is incorporated with the existing ones when it makes its appearance. Regardless of whether one reflex is suppressed and another performed, or whether two or more reflexes are combined, the reactions are integrated when they occur.

In response to cutaneous stimulation, at least, behavior begins with a reaction of the embryo as a whole. At first the reflex is limited, because only the earliest matured portions of the neuromuscular system have attained the capacity to respond. When additional regions are mature enough, the whole fetus reacts to the same stimulus—the head and trunk, the four extremities, including the hands and the digits, and even the mandible to open the mouth—all in response to a perioral stimulation (Fig. 3). Such reflexes meet all of the qualifications for the total pattern reflexes of Coghill. They constitute the only reflexes that have been recognized from known cutaneous stimuli of human fetuses until 10 to 10.5 weeks of menstrual age.

As cutaneous surfaces other than the perioral areas become sensitive to stimulation, inhibitory reactions develop. Local reflexes then begin to appear and increase in frequency. At the same time, the total pattern reflexes begin to disappear. The suppression of the total pattern reflexes elicited by facial stimulation takes place in a definite order. The lower extremity, lower trunk, and pelvic activity drop out of the responses first, and the bilaterality of arm movements becomes an ipsilateral arm reaction. The reflex activity that most often remains is ipsilateral head movement, usually in combination with oral reflexes. Other head movements form functional combinations of reflexes such as the head extension and ventral flexion that accompany mouth opening, mouth closure, tongue movements, and raising and lowering the larynx in swallowing (Humphrey, 1968a, 1969c, d).

In the total pattern lateral flexion reflexes, the activity is stereotyped and varies only in vigor and extent. Each extremity moves as a part of the general body and extremity reflex, not separately, although there may be action at all major joints—shoulder, elbow, and wrist, for example. Movement of some part of an extremity alone makes its appearance only when some surface area of that extremity becomes responsive to stimulation. This sequence is true for both the upper and lower extremities.

It is of some interest that mouth opening reflexes, although secured earliest by stimulation in the perioral region, may be elicited (usually combined with other activity) by stroking widely spread surfaces of the body, including the sole of the foot, the back, the forearm, the palm of the hand, and the external auditory canal. However, oral reflexes during later development usually are limited to stimulation of maxillomandibular zones of the face, although stimulation of the palm of the hand may be effective. Also active mouth opening reflexes by lowering the jaw are linked initially with contralateral flexion reflexes (avoiding reactions). Later they are associated with the reflexes related to feeding. The mouth opening reflexes elicited from areas distal to the mouth (and hand) are avoiding in type and some of them appear comparable to snapping and biting. Like mouth opening accompanying the total pattern lateral flexion reflexes, they disappear almost entirely, whereas the positive responses, such as turning toward the stimulus (and the actions associated with it), remain and increase in strength, in number, and in the variety of combinations that develop.

Throughout the preceding discussion, specific correlations have been made between the functional changes that take place during development and known morphologic changes in related areas of the nervous system. For the most part, however, it is only possible to speculate concerning what levels of the central nervous system are responsible for the activity described. On the one hand, both nuclear groups and fiber tracts in the telencephalon, for example, are identifiable long before there is any evidence that they become functional. On the other hand, in the development of the reflex arc mediating the first reflex that develops (Fig. 1), there appears to be an almost immediate onset of function (Humphrey, 1952,

1954). The author's speculations are that the reflex activities which have been demonstrated prior to 20 weeks of menstrual age are executed through the mesencephalon, the lower brain stem, and the spinal cord (Fig. 5) and do not involve diencephalic and telencephalic centers. After approximately 20 weeks, neural circuits through the diencephalon and striatal complex (or basal ganglia) become functional to an increasingly greater degree. In premature infants the lack of adequate temperature regulation indicates incomplete functional development of the hypothalamus. In both premature and newborn infants, the activity of the extremities is typically striatal in type. Electroencephalographic studies demonstrate that there is cortical activity in the brain during the perinatal period, but there is no indication that cortical function results in movements until the eyes of the postnatal infant are able to fix on a moving object and follow it at 4 weeks according to Gesell and Amatruda (1947). Function of additional extrapyramidal areas of the cortex probably begins when the infant endeavors to reach for the object on which the eyes are fixed. Much later, when fine finger movements make it possible to pick up a small pellet, undoubtedly the hand area of the motor cortex (area 4) is active.

Some mention should be made of the fact that activity sequences seen in fetal life are repeated perinatally and/or postnatally when higher levels of the nervous system, such as the striatal region, control activity. Likewise, when regulation is taken over by the cerebral cortex and becomes voluntary, the same general sequences may be repeated again, but with greater variability and complexity in detail. The development of fetal hand movements provides one example. Other instances are discussed by the author elsewhere (1969d) and explanations proposed as to the neuroembryologic background for this repetition.

ACKNOWLEDGMENTS

This investigation was supported by a Public Health Service research career program award, NB-K6-16716, from the National Institute of Neurological Diseases and Blindness and was aided by grant HD-00230, National Institute of Child Health and Human Development, National Institutes of Health. This paper is publication No. 54 in a series of physiologic and morphologic studies on human prenatal development begun in 1932 under the direction of Dr. Davenport Hooker. The data on which this paper is based were collected during periods of support in the past by grants from The Penrose Fund of the American Philosophical Society, The Carnegie Corporation of New York, The University of Pittsburgh, The Sarah Mellon Scaife Foundation of Pittsburgh, and Grant B-394 from the National Institute of Neurological Diseases and Blindness, National Institutes of Health to Davenport Hooker and/or to the author.

REFERENCES

Adams, F. H.   1966.   Functional development of the fetal lung. J. Pediat., 68:794-801.
———— and T. Fujiwara.   1963.   Surfactant in fetal lamb tracheal fluid. J. Pediat., 63:537-542.

——— D. T. Desilets, and B. Towers. 1967a. Control of flow of fetal lung fluid at the laryngeal outlet. Resp. Physiol., 2:302-309.

——— D. T. Desilets, and B. Towers. 1967b. Physiology of the fetal larynx and lung. Ann. Otol., 76:735-743.

André-Thomas, Y. C., and S. Saint-Anne Dargassies. 1960. The Neurologic Examination of the Infant. London, Wm. Heinemann Medical Books, Ltd.

Angulo y Gonzales, A. W. 1932. The prenatal development of behavior in the albino rat. J. Comp. Neurol., 55:395-442.

Anokhin, P. K. 1964. Systemogenesis as a general regulator of brain development. Progr. Brain Res., 9:54-86 (Discussion, 99-102).

Arey, L. B. 1965. Developmental Anatomy, 7th ed. Philadelphia and London, W. B. Saunders Company.

Arshavsky, I. A. 1959. Mechanisms of the development of nutritional functions during the intrauterine period and following birth. J. Gen. Biol., 20:104-114. (transl. from Russian).

Babkin, P. S. 1960. The establishment of reflex activity in early postnatal life. *In* Central Nervous System and Behavior. Translations from Fiziol. Zhi (Kiev), 44:922-927. Bethesda, Md., Scientific Translation Program, National Institutes of Health.

Barcroft, J., and D. H. Barron. 1939. Movement in the mammalian foetus. Ergebn. Physiol., 42:107-152.

Beckett, E. B., G. H. Bourne, and W. Montagna. 1956. Histology and cytochemistry of human skin: The distribution of cholinesterase in the finger of the embryo and the adult. J. Physiol. (London), 134:202-206.

Blake, J. R., and E. C. Kunkle. 1951. The palmomental reflex: A physiological and clinical analysis. Arch. Neurol. (Chicago), 65:337-345.

Bonar, B. E., C. M. Blumenfeld, and C. Fenning. 1938. Studies of fetal respiratory movements. I. Historical and present day observations. Amer. J. Dis. Child., 55:1-11.

Bradley, R. M., and I. B. Stern. 1967. The development of the human taste bud during the foetal period. J. Anat., 101:743-752.

Brown, J. W. 1956. The development of the nucleus of the spinal tract of V in human fetuses of 14 to 21 weeks of menstrual age. J. Comp. Neurol., 106:393-424.

——— 1958. The development of subnucleus caudalis of the nucleus of the spinal tract of V. J. Comp. Neurol., 110:105-134.

——— 1962. Differentiation of the human subnucleus interpolaris and subnucleus rostralis of the nucleus of the spinal tract of the trigeminal nerve. J. Comp. Neurol., 119:55-75.

Carmichael, L. 1954. The onset and early development of behavior. *In* Carmichael, L., ed. Manual of Child Psychology. New York, John Wiley & Sons, Inc., pp. 60-185.

Coghill, G. E. 1916. Correlated anatomical and physiological studies of the growth of the nervous system of Amphibia. II. The afferent system of the head of Amblystoma. J. Comp. Neurol., 26:247-340.

——— 1929. Anatomy and the Problem of Behaviour. Cambridge, England, Cambridge University Press. Reprinted, 1964, New York, Hafner Publishing Co.

Cuajunco, F. 1940. Development of the neuromuscular spindle in human fetuses. Carnegie Institution of Washington, Contrib. Embryol., 28:95-128.

Davis, M. E., and E. L. Potter. 1946. Intrauterine respiration of the human fetus. J.A.M.A., 131:1194-1201.

DeJong, R. N. 1967. The Neurologic Examination, 3d ed. New York, Hoeber Medical Division, Harper and Row, Publishers.

Fitzgerald, J. E., and W. F. Windle. 1942. Some observations on early human fetal movements. J. Comp. Neurol., 76:159-167.

Gasser, R. F. 1967. The development of the facial muscles in man. Amer. J. Anat., 120:357-376.

Gesell, A., and C. S. Amatruda. 1947. Development Diagnosis: Normal and Abnormal Child Development, 2nd ed. New York, Hoeber Medical Division, Harper and Row, Publishers.

Golubewa, E. L., K. V. Shulejkina, and I. I. Vainstein. 1959. The development of reflex and spontaneous activity of the human fetus during embryogenesis. Obstet. Gynec. (U.S.S.R.), 3:59-62.

Hamburger, V. 1963. Some aspects of the embryology of behavior. Quart. Rev. Biol., 38:342-365.

Heard, J. D., G. G. Burkley, and C. R. Schaefer. 1936. Electrocardiograms derived from eleven fetuses through the medium of direct leads. Amer. Heart J., 11:41-48. (Also Trans. Ass. Amer. Physicians, 50:335-341, 1935.)

Hogg, I. D. 1941. Sensory nerves and associated structures in the skin of human fetuses of 8 to 14 weeks of menstrual age correlated with functional capability. J. Comp. Neurol., 75:371-410.

Hooker, D. 1938. The origin of the grasping movement in man. Proc. Amer. Philosoph. Soc., 79:597-606.

———— 1939. A preliminary atlas of early human fetal activity. Published by the author.

———— 1942. Fetal reflexes and instinctual processes. Psychosom. Med., 4:199-205.

———— 1944. The Origin of Overt Behavior. Ann Arbor, University of Michigan Press.

———— 1952. The Prenatal Origin of Behavior. 18th Porter Lecture. Lawrence, University of Kansas Press. Reprinted, 1969, New York, Hafner Publishing Co.

———— 1954. Early human fetal behavior, with a preliminary note on double simultaneous fetal stimulation. Res. Publ. Ass. Res. Nerv. Ment. Dis., 33:98-113.

———— 1958. Evidence of Prenatal Function of the Central Nervous System in Man. James Arthur Lecture on The Evolution of the Human Brain for 1957. New York, American Museum of Natural History.

———— 1960. Developmental reaction to environment. Yale J. Biol. Med., 32: 431-440.

———— and T. Humphrey. 1954. Some results and deductions from a study of the development of human fetal behavior. Gaz. Med. Port., 7:189-197.

Humphrey, T. 1952. The spinal tract of the trigeminal nerve in human embryos between $7\frac{1}{2}$ and $8\frac{1}{2}$ weeks of menstrual age and its relation to early fetal behavior. J. Comp. Neurol., 97:143-209.

———— 1953. The relation of oxygen deprivation to fetal reflex arcs and the development of fetal behavior. J. Psychol., 35:3-43.

———— 1954. The trigeminal nerve in relation to early human fetal activity. Res. Publ. Ass. Res. Nerv. Ment. Dis., 33:127-154.

———— 1955. Pattern formed at upper cervical spinal cord levels by sensory fibers of spinal and cranial nerves. Arch. Neurol. (Chicago), 73:36-46.

———— 1964a. Some correlations between the appearance of human fetal reflexes and the development of the nervous system. Progr. Brain Res., 4:93-135.

————— 1964b. Embryology of the central nervous system: With some correlations with functional development. Alabama J. Med. Sci., 1:60-64.

————— 1965. The embryologic differentiation of the vestibular nuclei in man correlated with functional development. International Symposium on Vestibular and Ocular Problems, Tokyo, Japan, Society of Vestibular Research, University of Tokyo, pp. 51-56.

————— 1966. The development of trigeminal nerve fibers to the oral mucosa, compared with their development to cutaneous surfaces. J. Comp. Neurol., 126:91-108.

————— 1968a. The development of mouth opening and related reflexes involving the oral area of human fetuses. Alabama J. Med. Sci., 5:126-157.

————— 1968b. The dynamic mechanism of palatal shelf elevation in human fetuses. Anat. Rec., 160:369.

————— 1969a. The relation between human fetal mouth opening reflexes and closure of the palate. Amer. J. Anat., 125:317-344.

————— 1969b. The central relations of the trigeminal nerve. In Kahn, E. A., E. C. Crosby, R. C. Schneider, and J. A. Taren. Correlative Neurosurgery, 2nd ed. Springfield, Ill., Charles C Thomas, Publisher, pp. 477-492, 501-508.

————— 1969c. Reflex activity in the oral and facial area of human fetuses. In Bosma, J. F., ed. Second Symposium on Oral Sensation and Perception. Springfield, Ill., Charles C Thomas, Publisher.

————— 1969d. Postnatal repetition of human prenatal activity sequences with some suggestions on their neuroanatomical basis. In R. J. Robinson, ed. Brain and Early Behaviour: Development in the fetus and Infant. New York, Academic Press, Inc., pp. 43-84.

————— and D. Hooker. 1959. Double simultaneous stimulation of human fetuses and the anatomical patterns underlying the reflexes elicited. J. Comp. Neurol., 112: 75-102.

————— and D. Hooker. 1961a. Reflexes elicited by stimulating perineal and adjacent areas of human fetuses. Trans. Amer. Neurol. Ass., 86:147-152.

————— and D. Hooker. 1961b. Human fetal reflexes elicited by genital stimulation. In Transactions of the 7th International Neurological Congress, Rome, Italy, Vol. 2, pp. 587-590.

Illingworth, R. S. 1966. The Development of the Infant and Young Child, Normal and Abnormal, 3rd ed. Baltimore, The Williams & Wilkins Co.

Jacobs, M. J. 1970. The development of the human motor trigeminal complex and accessory facial nucleus and their topographic relations with the facial and abducens nuclei, J. Comp. Neurol, 138:161-194.

Jordan, H. E., and J. E. Kindred. 1942. Textbook of Embryology, 4th ed. New York, Appleton-Century-Crofts.

Kappers, C. U. Ariëns, G. C. Huber, and E. C. Crosby. 1936. The Comparative Anatomy of the Nervous System of Vertebrates, Including Man. New York, The Macmillan Company. (Reproduced without revision by Hafner Publishing Co., New York, 1960.)

Kingsbury, B. F. 1924. The significance of the so-called law of cephalocaudal differential growth. Anat. Rec., 27:305-321.

Kuo, Z.-Y. 1967. The Dynamics of Behavior Development: An Epigenetic View. New York, Random House, Inc.

Lundeen, E. C., and R. H. Kunstadter. 1958. Care of the Premature Infant. Philadelphia, J. B. Lippincott Co.

Mall, F. P. 1910. Determination of the age of human embryos and fetuses. In Keibel,

F., and F. P. Mall, eds. Manual of Human Embryology. Philadelphia, J. B. Lippincott Co., Vol. 1, pp. 180-201.

Marinesco, G., and A. Radovici. 1920. Sur un réflexe cutané nouveau à réflexe palmo-mentonnier. Rev. Neurol. (Paris), 27:237-240.

Minkowski, M. 1922. Über frühzeitige Bewegungen Reflexe und muskuläre Reaktionen beim menschlichen Fötus, und ihre Beziehungen zum fötalen Nerven- und Muskelsystem. Schweiz. Med. Wschr., 52:721-724; 751-755.

———— 1923. Zur Entwicklungsgeschichte, Lokalisation und Klinik des Fussohlenreflexes. Schweiz. Arch. Neurol. Psychiat., 13:475-514.

———— 1928. Neurobiologische Studien am menschlichen Foetus. In Abderhalden, E., ed. Handbuch der Biologischen Arbeitsmethoden. Abt. V, Teil 5B, Heft 5, Lief 253:511-618.

Moyers, R. E. 1950. An electromyographic analysis of certain muscles involved in temporomandibular movement. Amer. J. Orthodont., 36:481-515.

Murphy, K. P., and C. N. Smyth. 1962. Response of foetus to auditory stimulation. Lancet, 1:972-973.

Murphy, W. F., and A. L. Langley. 1963. Common bullous lesions—presumably self-inflicted—occurring in utero in the newborn infant. Pediatrics, 32:1099-1101.

Nilsson, L. 1965. Drama of life before birth. Life, 58:54-69.

———— A. Ingelman-Sundberg, and C. Wirsen. 1966. A Child Is Born: The Drama of Life before Birth. New York, Delacorte Press.

Norman, H. N. 1942. Fetal hiccups. J. Comp. Psychol., 34:65-73.

Parmelee, A. H., Jr. 1963a. The palmomental reflex in premature infants. Develop. Med. Child Neurol., 5:381-387.

———— 1963b. The hand-mouth reflex of Babkin in premature infants. Pediatrics, 31:734-740.

Patten, B. M. 1953. Human Embryology, 2nd ed. New York, The Blakiston Division, McGraw-Hill Book Company.

Peiper, A. 1963. Cerebral Function in Infancy and Childhood. New York, Consultants Bureau. Translation in Wortis, J. ed. Die Eigenart der kindlichen Hirntätigkeit, 3rd ed., 1961. Leipzig, Thieme Verlag.

Pratt, K. C. 1954. The neonate. In Carmichael, L., ed. Manual of Child Psychology, 2nd ed. New York and London, John Wiley & Sons, Inc., pp. 215-291.

Prechtl, H. F. R. 1953. Ueber die Koppelung von Saugen und Greifreflex beim Säugling. Naturwissenschaften, 12:347-348.

———— 1958. The directed head turning response and allied movements of the human baby. Behaviour, 13:212-242.

———— and D. Beintema. 1964. The Neurological Examination of the Full Term Newborn Infant, London, Wm. Heinemann Medical Books, Ltd.

Preyer, W. 1885. Specielle Physiologie des Embryo. Leipzig, Th. Grieben's Verlag.

Pritchard, J. A. 1965. Deglutition by normal and anencephalic fetuses. Amer. J. Obstet. Gynec., 25:289-297.

Robinson, R. J. 1966. Assessment of gestational age by neurological examination. Arch. Dis. Child., 41:437-447.

Root, R. W. 1946. The mechanics of the temporomandibular joint: Illustrated by two cases. Amer. J. Orthodont., 32:113-119.

Russell, P. M. G. 1957. Vagitus uterinus: Crying in utero. Lancet, 272:137-138.

Ryder, G. H. 1943. Vagitus uterinus. Amer. J. Obstet. Gynec., 46:867-872.

Schaeffer, J. P. 1910. The lateral wall of the cavum nasi in man, with especial reference to the various developmental stages. J. Morph., 21:613-707.

Snyder, F. F., and M. Rosenfeld. 1937. Direct observation of intrauterine respiratory movements of the fetus and the role of carbon dioxide and oxygen in their regulation. Amer. J. Physiol., 119:153-166.

Sontag, L. W., and R. F. Wallace. 1934. Preliminary report of the Fels Fund: Study of fetal activity. Amer. J. Dis. Child., 48:1050-1057.

———— 1935. The movement response of the human fetus to sound stimuli. Child Develop., 6:253-258.

———— 1936. Changes in the rate of the human fetal heart in response to vibratory stimuli. Amer. J. Dis. Child., 51:583-589.

Streeter, G. L. 1920. Weight, sitting height, head size, foot length, and menstrual age of the human embryo. Carnegie Institution of Washington, Contrib. Embryol., 11: 143-170.

Windle, W. F. 1940. Physiology of the Fetus. Origin and Extent of Function in Prenatal Life. Philadelphia, W. B. Saunders Company.

———— 1944. Genesis of somatic motor function in mammalian embryos: A synthesizing article. Physiol. Zool., 27:247-260.

———— 1950. Reflexes of mammalian embryos and fetuses. *In* Weiss, P., ed. Genetic Neurology. Chicago, University of Chicago Press, pp. 214-222.

———— and R. F. Becker. 1940. Relation of anoxemia to early activity in the fetal nervous system. Arch. Neurol. (Chicago), 43:90-101.

———— C. A. Dragstedt, D. E. Murray, and R. R. Greene. 1938. A note on the respiration-like movements of the human fetus. Surg. Gynec. Obstet., 66:987-988.

25

Neonatal Brain Mechanisms and the Development of Motor Behavior

F. J. SCHULTE ● **Department of Pediatrics, University of Göttingen, Germany**

Introduction

In the adult mammal, including the human, motor control has its representation at different levels of the central nervous system. A short review of motor control in the mature organism will precede each section dealing with the various brain mechanisms of neonatal motor behavior. Since Sherrington's (1898) basic experiments, a great wealth of data on spinal functions has been accumulated, thus allowing a detailed description of motor control at the spinal level. For neonatal studies, this is particularly advantageous, since the motor behavior of the newborn seems to be mainly under the control of the spinal cord and the medulla. On the other hand, our sparse knowledge of the neurophysiologic mechanisms of higher motor control, even in the adult, may well account for a tremendous overestimation of the significance of the spinal cord in neonatal motoricity.

Spinal Cord and Peripheral Nerves

The segmental efferent innervation of skeletal muscle (Fig. 1) is furnished by motoneurones with different axonal calibres of the A α type. The larger neurones prefer a more phasic, the smaller ones a more tonic discharge pattern (Granit et al., 1956; Eccles et al., 1957; Henatsch et al., 1959). The smallest motoneurones, with axons belonging to the A γ group, are not directly engaged in muscle contraction and limb movement. Activating the intrafusal muscle fibers inside the muscle spindle stretch receptors, the γ or fusimotoneurones increase the afferent discharge frequency of the receptors and their sensitivity to stretch (Leksell, 1945; Kuffler et al., 1951; Hunt and Paintal, 1958). The fusimotoneurones can be subdivided by means of different endings into γ-plate and γ-trail fibers, the former producing static, the latter producing dynamic changes in the afferent discharge pattern (Barker, 1962, 1966; ten Bruggencate et al., 1965).

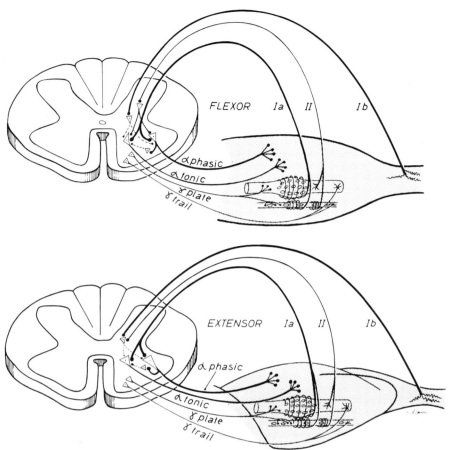

Fig. 1. Diagram of important pathways in the spinal motor system for flexor muscles (above) and for extensor mucles (below). Solid lines, excitatory connections; dashed lines, inhibitory connections. *a* phasic, phasic *a*-motoneurones which activate skeletal muscles and generally cause fast movements by means of short bursts of action potentials. *a* tonic, tonic *a*-motoneurones which activate skeletal muscles for longer periods of contraction by means of a series of repetitive action potentials. While still within the gray matter, axon collaterals of the *a*-motoneurones activate Renshaw cells which act as inhibitors of *a*-motoneurones. γ-plate and γ-trail, fusi-motoneurones innervating muscle fibers within the muscle spindles (intrafusal muscle fibers). Ia, II, Ib, Sensory afferent nerve fibers of muscle receptors activated by stretch. (From Schulte. 1968. *In* Bushe, K. A., and P. Glees, eds. Die Elektromyographie. Courtesy of Hippokrates Verl., Stuttgart.)

Two different types of intrafusal muscle fibers act on the sensory end-organ from the inside of the receptor: the nuclear bag and the nuclear chain muscle fibers (Boyd, 1962). Spiral or semispiral endings of the group Ia and group II fiber afferents are twisted around both. Group Ia fiber afferents produce monosynaptic excitation of the homonymous *a*-motoneurones while inhibiting motoneurones of antagonistic muscles, thus forming the proprioceptive reflex arc (Matthews, 1933;

Lloyd, 1944; Lloyd and Chang, 1948; Hunt, 1954; Eccles, 1964; Matthews, 1964). The group II fiber afferents, however, are monosynaptically connected only with flexor motoneurones, whereas even homonymous extensor motoneurones are inhibited via interneurones (Eccles and Lundberg, 1959; Laporte and Bessou, 1959). The Golgi tendon organ or group Ib afferents are connected with homonymous α-motoneurones via inhibitory interneurones, thus producing what is called "autogenetic inhibition" (Granit, 1950).

The α-motoneurones, before leaving the gray matter of the spinal cord, branch out into collaterals, activating inhibitory interneurones called "Renshaw cells" (Renshaw, 1941, 1946; Eccles et al., 1954). Both Renshaw cells and Golgi tendon organs comprise the main parts of two negative feedback systems, limiting the discharge frequency and the recruitment of spinal motoneurones (see p. 812).

IMMATURE ALPHA-MOTONEURONES

The differences between immature and mature motoneurones become evident in the two bioelectric properties of nerve cells: 1, the computational process of synaptic excitation or inhibition and 2, the conduction of impulses along myelinated axons.

SYNAPTIC TRANSMISSION

No direct information on the biochemical or electrophysiologic processes of intracentral impulse transmission in human infants is available. Eccles and Willis (1962) have shown that in kittens the postsynaptic potentials of immature motoneurones are greater than in adult cats. Thus, with an afferent volley produced by an electric stimulus to certain dorsal root fibers, a pool of motoneurones can easily be activated. In adult cats, however, an even greater number of ventral horn cells, although reached by the afferent volley, is not activated, since the depolarization does not reach the threshold. These motoneurones in the subliminal fringe can easily be coactivated either by additional, excitatory impulses after a slight delay, i.e., temporal summation, or by other afferent sources, i.e., spatial summation. The subliminal fringe of preactivated motoneurones is considerably smaller in newborn kittens compared with adult cats (Eccles and Willis, 1962). If this holds true for human infants as well, the recruitment of motoneurones, i.e., the increasing strength of muscle contraction, would occur stepwise rather than smoothly.

IMPULSE CONDUCTION

If the motoneurone membrane is depolarized to a certain degree by a sufficient amount of excitatory, postsynaptic potentials, a spike potential or all or none action potential is generated at the axon hillock of the nerve cell. This spike potential progresses along the myelinated axon by means of saltatory conduction, the action potential being regenerated at each Ranvier node (Tasaki, 1953; von Muralt, 1958).

The conduction velocity is dependent upon the thickness of the myelin sheath (Erlanger and Gasser, 1924; Hursh, 1939) which probably is positively related to the distance between the Ranvier nodes. Since myelination increases with age from conception (Carpenter and Bergland, 1957; Skoglund, 1960b; Ekholm, 1967), measuring the impulse conduction speed in peripheral nerves of human infants is a rather simple method of determining the menstrual age (Schulte et al., 1968c; Blom and Finnström, 1968; Ruppert and Johnson, 1968; Dubowitz et al., 1968) (Fig. 2). Nerve conduction velocity, in contrast to many other parameters, seems to be almost independent of abnormal influences (Schulte et al., 1969). Infants of either diabetic or toxemic mothers, dysmature and small-for-date, or hydropic babies and infants with moderate to severe but nonfatal degrees of intranatal hypoxia have a conduction velocity normal for conception age (Charts 1 and 2; Fig. 3). The slow conduction rate of the immature nerve has not much bearing upon the functional incapacity of the newborn infant (Schulte, 1968). The interneurone and the neuromuscular distances are shorter, thus, even more than compensating for the low speed (Fig. 4). However, other characteristics of the nerve, like maximum spike frequency, afterpotentials, oscillation of the membrane potential and excitability, vary also with myelination (Lloyd and Chang, 1948; Hunt, 1954). We have, as yet, no information about the significance of these parameters in the course of development toward a greater complexity of nervous functions.

NEUROMUSCULAR TRANSMISSION

The nerve action potential is transmitted to the muscle at the neuromuscular synapses by means of a chemical transmitter, acetylcholine (Dale et al., 1936).

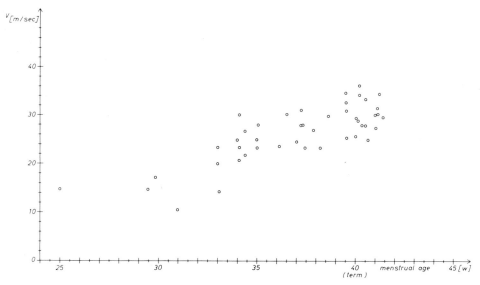

Fig. 2. Ulnar motor nerve conduction velocity in relation to menstrual age. Nerve conduction velocity increases with age. (From Schulte. 1968. *Fortschritte der Paedologie.* Courtesy of Springer-Verlag.)

N. ulnaris

	n	menstrual age [weeks]	weight (g)	conduction velocity β [m/sec] (p=0,05)
term	19	40,6 ± 0,61	3345 ± 349	* 30,4 ± 3,40 (31,87 / 28,82)
small for dates	16	40,3 ± 1,58	2068 ± 183	▲ 32,4 ± 7,25 (35,95 / 28,85)
preterm	17	35,8 ± 1,64	2129 ± 243	*▲ 25,9 ± 4,08 (27,87 / 24,0)

* $t = 4,520$ $p < 0,001$
▲ $t = 3,360$ $p < 0,005$

N. tibialis

	n	menstrual age [weeks]	weight (g)	conduction velocity β [m/sec] (p=0,05)
term	15	40,5 ± 0,20	3355 ± 316	* 25,8 ± 2,0 (26,85 / 24,82)
small for dates	24	40,7 ± 1,78	2139 ± 231	▲ 23,68 ± 4,02 (25,29 / 22,07)
preterm	20	36,3 ± 1,56	2224 ± 219	*▲ 18,6 ± 3,71 (20,26 / 17,0)

* $t = 5,934$ $p < 0,001$
▲ $t = 6,516$ $p < 0,001$

Chart 1. Statistic analysis (t test) of nerve conduction velocity in normal; full-term; preterm; and full-term, small-for-date infants. In each group the mean values and first standard deviations are given for conceptional ages and body weights at the time of examination and for both ulnar and tibial nerve conduction velocities. In addition, the confidence interval for the mean value of the conduction velocities is indicated under β when the probability is 95 percent (p=0.05). Statistically significant differences in ulnar or tibial nerve conduction velocities among the three groups of infants are indicated by * and + with the corresponding t values and the level of probability (p). (From Schulte et al. 1968c. *Pediatrics*, 42:17-26.)

	N	menstrual age [w] range ∣ mean		b_{yx}	r	p <	$\bar{y}_i$ [m/sec]
normal infants	38	25 - 42	37,5	1,08	0,78	0,001	29,6 ± 3,4
abnormal infants	43	34 - 47	39,5	1,07	0,63	0,001	30,9 ± 3,9

N   =   number of infants
b_{yx} =   regression coefficient
r   =   correlation coefficient (PEARSON)
$\bar{y}_i$ =   conduction velocity extrapolated at 40 weeks
              (mean and 1. standard deviation)

$$y_i = y - b_{yx}(x - x_i)$$

└──→ 40 weeks
└────→ actual menstrual age
└────→ regression coefficient
└────→ actual conduction velocity
└────→ conduction velocity, extrapolated at 40 w menstrual age

Chart 2. Regression and correlation coefficient for the ulnar nerve conduction velocity in
relation to menstrual age, as well as the conduction velocity, extrapolated to 40 weeks
of menstrual age, are strikingly similar in normal, newborn infants and in those
under various abnormal influences during pregnancy, birth, and the postnatal period.
(From Schulte et al. 1969. *Deutsch. Med. Wschr.*, 94:599-601.)

Whereas the maximum spike frequency electrically imposable on the neuronal
axon is about several hundreds per second, being limited only by the refractory
period in the order of 1 msec, the neuromuscular transmission, including its recovery

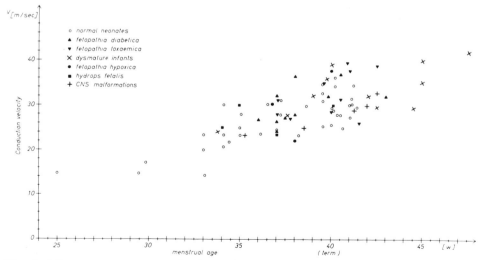

Fig. 3. Ulnar motor nerve conduction velocity in relation to menstrual age in normal
infants and in infants with various abnormalities. No differences in nerve conduction
velocity could be detected in infants with various pathologic conditions. (From
Schulte et al. 1969. *Deutsch. Med. Wschr.*, 94:599-601. Courtesy of Thieme-
Verlag.)

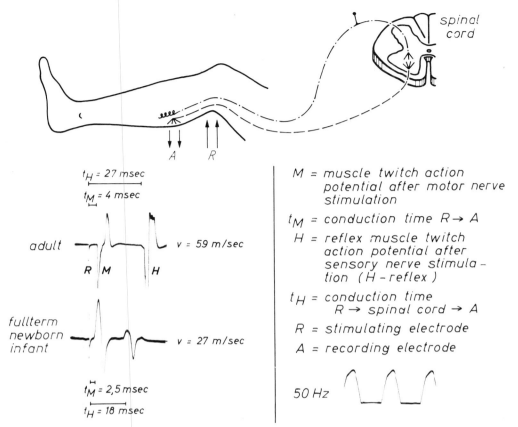

Fig. 4. The motor nerve conduction velocities and reflex times of an adult human subject compared with those of a normal, full-term newborn infant. Although motor nerve conduction velocity is significantly lower in the newborn infant, reflex times are shorter than in the adult because of the smaller distances. (From Schulte. 1968. *Fortschritte der Paedologie.* Courtesy of Springer-Verlag.)

cycle, is a more time-consuming process with a tendency to fatigue, the latter being more marked in newborn infants than in adults (Churchill-Davidson and Wise, 1963; Schulte and Michaelis, 1965). Neuronal spike frequencies of 50/sec are not transmitted to the muscle without decay (Harvey and Masland, 1941; Castillo and Katz, 1954). The higher the frequency, the more motor end-plates become refractory, and the resulting compound muscle action potential decreases (Fig. 5). It is still debatable whether the more limited neuromuscular transmission in the newborn infant is due to the immaturity of the enzyme systems of acetylcholine metabolism or whether it is due merely to differences in the distribution of electrolytes on both sides of the membrane. Both hypocalcemia and hyperpotassemia, i.e., a decreased potassium gradient from intracellular to extracellular fluid, are able to impair the neuromuscular transmission of impulses (Fatt and Katz, 1951; Castillo and Stark, 1952; Castillo and Katz, 1954; Takeuchi, 1963).

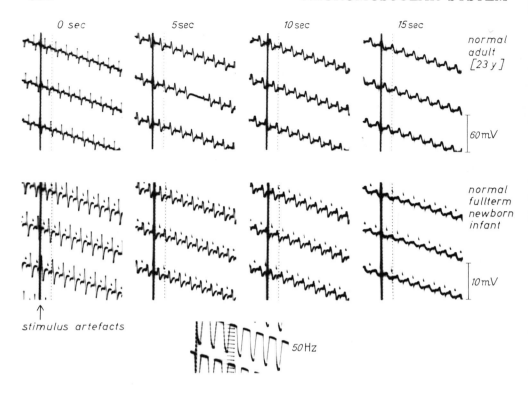

stimulus artefacts

50 Hz

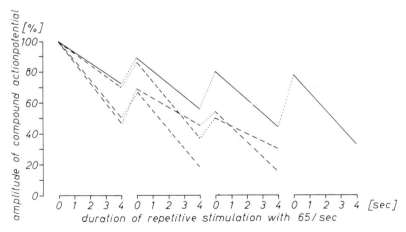

Fig. 5. Top and bottom. Muscle action potentials elicited by repetitive motor nerve stimulation. With repetitive motor nerve stimulation, the amplitude of the action potential decreases; this effect is more marked in newborn infants than in adults. (From Schulte and Michaelis. 1965. *Klin. Wschr.*, 43:295-300. Courtesy of Springer-Verlag.)

In preterm newborn infants the neuromuscular transmission capacity is unknown, and, particularly in very immature infants, it may be too limited to allow maximum muscle contraction over a longer period of time. However, in full-term newborn infants, neuromusclar transmission is not an important factor limiting muscle power.

GAMMA-MOTONEURONES AND MUSCLE SPINDLES
OF THE NEONATE

INTRAFUSAL INNERVATION

As shown in Figure 1 the intrafusal muscle fibers of the spindle stretch receptors are activated by γ-motoneurones. No information is available about γ-motoneurone and intrafusal activity in human infants, the data being extremely sparse even for adult humans. In kittens, the intrafusal activity, maintained by γ-motoneurone innervation, seems to be less tonic than that in adult cats (Skoglund, 1960c). This would imply decreased, afferent muscle spindle activity, the depolarization pressure, i.e., the excitatory drive on motoneurones, being diminished (Skoglund, 1960a).

The lack of γ-motoneurone support might be responsible for the absence of tonic, myotatic reflexes in preterm infants of less than 34 weeks of menstrual age (see p. 808) (Saint Anne-Dargassies, 1955, 1966; Amiel-Tison, 1968; Schulte et al., 1968a).

GROUP I MUSCLE SPINDLE AFFERENT FIBERS

Sensory nerve fibers with the highest conduction velocity, originating from spiral structures winding around intrafusal muscle cells, form the afferent pathway of the proprioceptive feedback circuit illustrated in Figure 1. The peripheral endings of these fibers, being the transducer membrane of the receptor, are depolarized by stretching of the muscle. This generator potential is transformed quantitatively by means of frequency modulation into spike potentials at the first Ranvier node. Maximum muscle spindle discharge frequency and its maintenance over a long period of time are severely restricted in the newborn kitten compared with the adult animal (Skoglund, 1960c). Both the absence of the tonic γ-motoneurone activity described above and particular membrane properties of the immature, receptive end-organ may account for the lack of tonicity in the afferent muscle spindle discharge pattern which, in turn, implies low γ-motoneurone activity and skeletal muscle hypotonia.

PROPRIOCEPTIVE REFLEXES OF NEWBORN INFANTS

PHASIC T AND H REFLEXES

A brisk tap on the tendon stretches the muscle, thereby exciting muscle spindles which, in turn, activate spinal α-motoneurones which give rise to a quick muscle twitch, called T (tendon) reflex. The receptors responsible for this reflex are located in the muscle rather than in the tendon (Hoffmann, 1922, 1934). The same reflex can be elicited by an electric stimulus to the afferent nerve, and it is then called H (Hoffmann) reflex. Both types of phasic, proprioceptive reflexes can already be obtained in the newborn infant, provided the infant is not asleep and particularly not in active or rapid eye movement (REM) sleep (see p. 830). In both animal and human, adult as well as newborn, muscle stretch reflexes are diminished or even abolished during active sleep (Hodes and Gribetz, 1962; Hodes and Dement, 1964; Giaquinto et al., 1964a, b; Prechtl et al., 1967). This fact has lead to considerable confusion in pediatric textbook literature about stretch reflexes. Since the examination of the newborn infant is sometimes accidentally carried out while the subject is asleep, many authors have erroneously assumed that some neonates do not have certain stretch reflexes. Even in the youngest preterm infant which we were able to study (25 weeks of menstrual age) proprioceptive reflexes in the quadriceps could be elicited by tendon tap (Schulte et al., 1968b). The reflex response, however, consisted of a burst of desynchronized impulses (Fig. 6) rather than of a single compound muscle action potential, as is usually seen in newborn infants above 30 weeks of menstrual age (Fig. 7).

TONIC MYOTATIC REFLEXES

In the normal adult human, a slow, gradual muscle stretch does not lead to an increased resistance against passive movement. In this case, the afferent drive from the muscle stretch receptors remains subthreshold, and motoneurones are not activated to a substantial degree. Contrarily, in healthy, full-term newborn infants, tonic myotatic reflexes, i.e., an increasing resistance against gradual stretch, can be

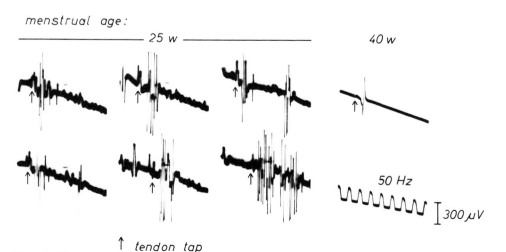

Fig. 6. The monosynaptic stretch reflex elicited by a tendon tap in a preterm infant (25 weeks of menstrual age) consists of a burst of impulses rather than of one compound muscle action potential. (From Schulte et al. 1969. *In* Robinson, R. J., ed. Brain and Early Behaviour. Courtesy of Academic Press, Inc., London.)

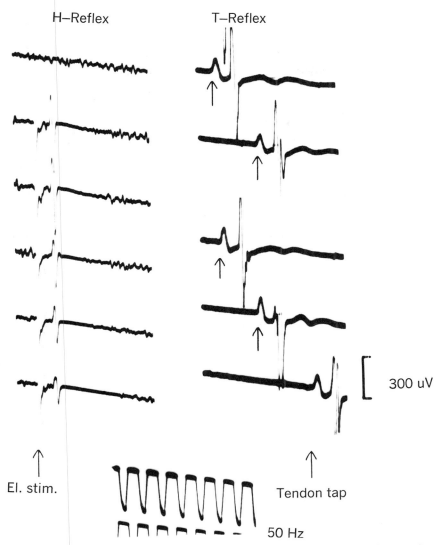

Fig. 7. Monosynaptic reflex of m. gastrocnemius in a one-day-old neonate. Left, H reflex (Hoffmann), elicited by electric stimulation of sensory nerve fibers of the n. tibialis. Right, T reflex (tendon) elicited by tendon tap. (From Schulte and Schwenzel, 1965. *Biol. Neonat.*, 8:198-215. Courtesy of S. Karger.)

elicited in almost all flexor and many extensor muscles (André-Thomas and Ajuriaguerra, 1949; André-Thomas and Saint Anne-Dargassies, 1952; André-Thomas et al., 1954; Peiper, 1963). A great number of the so-called primitive reflexes depend upon the tonic, myotatic reflex activity of the newborn—in the awake, full-term infant an extension of the lower arms is followed by a rather quick recoil into the flexed position (Fig. 8). If an infant, lying on his back, is pulled by his hands into the sitting position, the arms remain flexed (Fig. 9, bottom). The

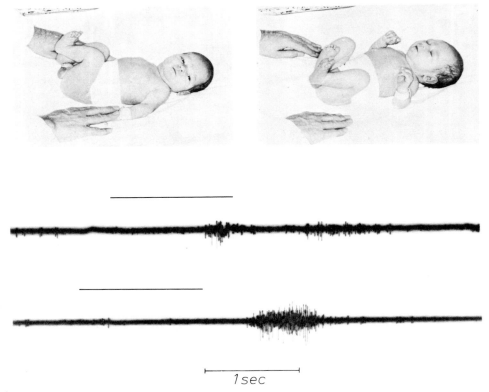

Fig. 8. Stretch and release of the forearms is followed by a quick recoil due to biceps
    muscle activity. Stretching of the elbows is indicated by a bar; the biceps electro-
    myogram of two recoils is given below.

palmar grasp can be reinforced by gradually extending the baby's fingers (p. 809).
A newborn infant standing on his legs usually activates hip and knee extensors if
the body weight is allowed to act on these muscles (p. 814). The motoneurone
activity demonstrated electromyographically during the recoil maneuver provides
clear evidence that this phenomenon is a spinal reflex rather than being caused by
mere elastic properties of muscles and ligaments.

Tonic, myotatic reflexes are more easily obtained in flexor than in extensor
muscles. They can hardly be demonstrated in infants of less than 34 weeks of
menstrual age and are normally present at 36 weeks (Saint Anne-Dargassies, 1955,
1966; Amiel-Tison, 1968; Michaelis et al., 1969).

CUTANEOUS AFFERENTS AND EXTEROCEPTIVE REFLEXES
OF THE NEWBORN INFANT

Stimulation of cutaneous receptors leads to a more or less stereotyped activation
of spinal motoneurones via many interneurones—exteroceptive polysynaptic reflexes.

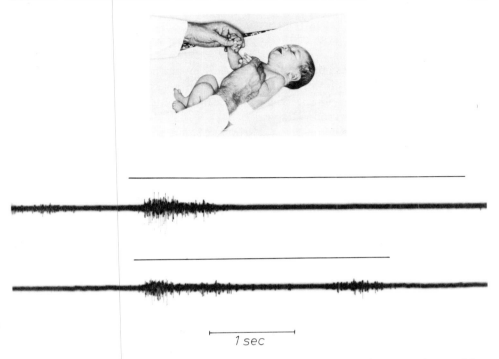

Fig. 9. Top, the elbows remain flexed while the infant is pulled to a sitting position. Bottom, the electromyogram of biceps muscle activity during two traction responses (traction indicated by a bar).

Reactions of this type are numerous, and they are an essential part of the neurologic examination of infants as well as of adults. In general, for all exteroceptive reflexes, the tendency to irradiate is greater in more immature subjects (Bergström et al., 1962; Hopf et al., 1964).

In the newborn there seems to be a principal difference in the behavior of proprioceptive and exteroceptive reflexes during sleep. Whereas proprioceptive reflexes are diminished in active, i.e., rapid eye movement (REM) sleep, exteroceptive reflexes are either diminished in quiet sleep (nonREM) or equally strong during wakefulness and both sleep states (Prechtl et al., 1967; Lenard et al., 1968). Particularly, motor responses to nociceptive stimuli, namely the abdominal skin, and the Babinski reflex were found to be surprisingly independent of the infant's behavioral state (Lenard et al., 1968).

The palmar and plantar *grasp reflexes* were first described by Robinson (1891) and van Woerkom (1912), respectively, and were more extensively investigated by Peiper (1963). The response can already be elicited in the fetus (see Ch. 24) and is present in every healthy newborn infant, both preterm and full-term (Stirnimann and Stirnimann, 1940; Dietrich, 1957; Pollack, 1960). The afferent stimulus consists of a light touch on the palmar or plantar surface of the infant's hands and feet achieved with the examiner's finger or with a pencil (Poeck, 1968). The infant closes his fingers in the following order: 3, 4, 5, 1, 2 (Prechtl, 1953). This exteroceptive reflex can easily be reinforced by an additional proprioceptive stimulus, stretching of the flexor muscles of the fingers. The grasp is stronger during sucking (Prechtl, 1953).

The *withdrawal reflex* is elicitable in every healthy newborn infant, both preterm and full-term, from any point of the skin. However, a semiquantitative assessment of the response strength and speed is most easily obtained when the stimulus is applied to the sole of the foot (Babinski, 1922). The leg is held in the flexed position as long as the stimulus lasts (Peiper, 1963). In newborn infants born in breech presentation the flexion response is hardly visible, and, paradoxically, a vigorous extension occurs (Prechtl and Knol, 1958).

The *Babinski reflex,* already present in the preterm newborn infant, is part of the withdrawal reflex. Richards and Irwin (1935) described seven different response patterns ranging from flexion to extension of one to five toes. Stimulating the skin of the foot only at the lateral and posterior part of the sole or at the instep avoids the grasp response and usually leads to the well-known extension of the big toe while the other toes are spread. In the newborn infant, however, this response might have a significance which is different from that in older children and adults. Wartenberg (1952) suggested that the spread of four toes is part of a climbing pattern, and, according to Schoch (1948, 1949), the extension of the first toe is the release part of a grasp reflex. This author still is inclined to believe that the true Babinski reflex pattern in the newborn infant, as well as in abnormal adults, is due to the lack of certain supraspinal influences mediated via the pyramidal tract, although Peiper (1963) disagreed with this hypothesis.

The *magnet response* is elicited by light pressure on the sole of the foot while the leg is flexed. The response consists of a continuous slow extension as long as the examiner maintains contact with the infant's foot (Balduzzi, 1932). Peiper (1963) states that the magnet response can be elicited in only 20 percent of newborn infants, and Lenard et al. (1968) also found a positive response in the awake and quiet, healthy, full-term infant only occasionally.

The *palmomental reflex* was first described by Marinesco and Radovici (1920). Scratching of the infant's hypothenar with the fingernail sometimes leads to a muscle contraction with lifting of the chin.

The *Babkin reflex* (Babkin, 1955; Lippmann, 1958) is present with particular strength in preterm infants (Parmelee, 1963). While the examiner applies firm pressure to the infant's palms, the neonate opens his mouth and occasionally lifts or turns his head.

The *lip tap reflex* was first described by Escherich (1888). Some authors believed this reflex to be abnormal, occurring only with hypocalcemia (Thiemich, 1900). Many authors, however, confirmed the original observation, noting that this reflex occurs in almost every healthy, full-term newborn infant (Thompson, 1903; Gamper and Untersteiner, 1924; Ingram, 1960). A sharp tap on the upper or lower lip is followed by a protrusion of the lips. Prechtl et al. (1967) have shown electromyographically that the lip tap response consists of two components with different latencies and durations. The first quick component is probably proprioceptive in origin, whereas the following long-lasting contraction of the orbicularis oris is supposed to be an exteroceptive reflex.

The *rooting reflex,* apparently first described by Pepsy (1933) as well as by Gentry and Aldrich (1948), was later studied by many authors (literature in Peiper, 1963). Tickling of the skin at the corner of the infant's mouth is followed by a rotation of the head to the side of the stimulus. The same stimulus applied to the upper lip leads to mouth opening and retroflection of the head; applied to the lower lip, it leads to mouth opening and jaw dropping. This response is particularly strong when the infant is hungry (Prechtl and Scheidt, 1950, 1951). If the stimulus is painful, the infant turns his head in the opposite direction (André-Thomas et al., 1954). The lip tap reflex and the rooting response are incorporated in the mechanism of food uptake. The main parts of this complex behavior, sucking and swallowing, are described in Chapter 24.

The *glabella reflex* is elicitable in newborn infants of more than 32 to 34 weeks of menstrual age through a sharp tap on the glabella (Robinson, 1966). The stimulus response is a blink with a short lasting, tight closure of the eyelids (Kugelberg, 1952; Rushworth, 1962; Gandiglio et al., 1965; Fra and Gandiglio, 1966). Like the lip tap, this response probably consists of two components; the short blink is a monosynaptically mediated proprioceptive reflex of the m. orbicularis occuli, and the following tonic contraction is maintained by polysynaptic activation of the same motoneurones.

A similar type of *blink reflex* can be elicited by tactile stimulation of the eyelashes and the cornea, as well as with sound and with bright light (Prechtl and Beintema, 1964). A tonically sustained contraction of the eyelids can easily be obtained through strong and unpleasant stimuli to the taste buds (Peiper, 1963).

The *pupil reaction to light,* an exteroceptive reflex in a broader sense, appears between 29 and 31 weeks of menstrual age (Bolaffio and Artom, 1924; Robinson, 1966). The dilatation of the pupils after painful skin stimuli was found invariably by Bartels (1904) and Bach (1908) in full-term and occasionally in preterm newborn infants (Peiper, 1926).

The *abdominal skin reflexes,* contrary to the assertions of several authors, are always present in full-term newborn infants, providing the subjects are not crying heavily with vigorous contraction of the abdominal muscles (Harlem and Lönnum, 1957; Lenard et al., 1968).

The *Galant reflex* (Galant, 1917), or incurvation of the trunk, first described by Bertolotti (1904), is present in all normal full-term and most preterm infants (Isbert and Peiper, 1927). A skin stimulus along a line parallel to the spine is followed by an extension of the lower trunk and an incurvation toward the side of the stimulus. Concomitantly, the contralateral hip and knee joints are extended.

The *cremaster reflex* is present in all full-term, and most preterm, newborn boys (Peiper, 1963) and is apparently not different from the same response in adults.

The *anal retraction response* is an important test for infants with spina bifida.

Vlach (1966, 1968) was able to demonstrate some principal rules for the occurrence of numerous exteroceptive reflexes in the newborn infant. Skin stimuli above flexors usually activate the motoneurones of the underlying muscles. The corresponding extensor activation from the skin is hardly visible or at least weak. The same results were obtained in newborn cats (Ekholm, 1967). For the trunk and the proximal part of the extremities, the sensitive area is located over the muscle bulk. For the distal part of the extremities, the exteroceptive reflexes are usually elicitable from skin areas over the tendons.

SPINAL INHIBITION

"No excitation without inhibition"; this basic rule of central nervous activity holds for neonatal, spinal motoricity as well. The monosynaptic, compound reflex action potential, as well as any synchronous burst of motoneurone activity, is followed by a short period of more or less complete inhibition, indicated by a silent period in the background activity called "Innervations-stille" (Hoffmann, 1922, 1934). In newborn infants, the duration of the silent period is dependent upon the amount of background activity, i.e., the depolarization pressure on spinal motoneurones (Schulte and Schwenzel, 1965). The duration of the silent period decreases with increasing background activity (Fig. 10), indicating that spinal

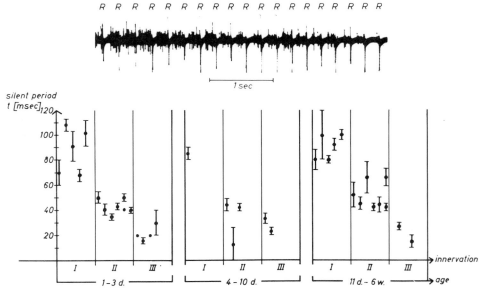

Fig. 10. Each quadriceps muscle reflex action potential evoked by tendon tap is followed by a silent period, the duration of which decreases with increasing background activity. The amount of background activity is indicated by I to III. I (weak), sparse activity, only single action potentials. II (moderate), background activity with one action potential immediately followed, sometimes even superimposed by another; III (strong), maximum activity with action potentials superimposing each other. The silent period is measured from the end of the reflex action potential to the recurrence of the background activity. Changes in the duration of the silent period which are possibly dependent on age were not statistically evaluated for the time after term-birth.

inhibitory mechanisms can in part be outweighed by supraspinal, excitatory drive (Paillard, 1954).

The duration of the silent period, i.e., the amount of inhibitory influences on spinal motoneurones subsequent to the monosynaptic stretch reflex, increases with menstrual age (Fig. 11). However, the minimum duration of the silent period after the monosynaptic reflex is almost equal for all ages during very strong supraspinal motoneurone excitation (Schulte et al., 1968b). This observation is consistent with the hypothesis that a minimum of postexcitatory inhibition, possibly due to basic membrane phenomena, is well developed in preterm infants of 30 weeks of menstrual age. However, surplus inhibition, due to more complex, computational synaptic mechanisms in the spinal cord, proceeds with menstrual age. In full-term newborn infants, the duration of the silent period is only slightly if at all, shorter than in older children and adults (Fig. 10).

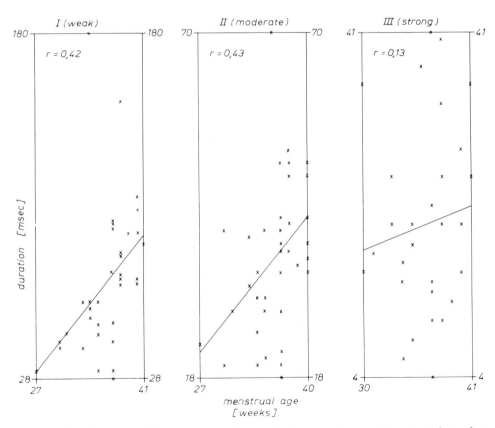

Fig. 11. The duration of the postreflex silent period (muscular quadriceps) is dependent upon background muscle activity (weak, moderate, strong), and it increases slightly with conceptional age. The Pearson correlation coefficient r is 0.42 during weak and 0.43 during moderate background activity. However, the duration of the silent period, subsequent to a monosynaptic reflex and elicited during strong muscle contraction, shows only little variation with age.

Spinal motoneurone inhibition is guaranteed by several mechanisms (see Fig. 1):

1. Each spike potential is followed by membrane hyperpolarization due to a postexcitatory increase of potassium membrane permeability. This membrane potential shift is called "positive afterpotential" (Henatsch, 1962; Patton, 1965).

2. Each motoneurone action potential, before leaving the gray matter of the spinal cord, activates interneurones called "Renshaw cells" which inhibit the surrounding motoneurones. This pathway represents an intraspinal, inhibitory feedback mechanism and is already active in newborn kittens (Naka, 1964).

3. The reflex muscle twitch activates Golgi tendon organs, the afferent impulses of which inhibit spinal motoneurones via interneurones. This pathway represents a musculospinal inhibitory feedback mechanism (see p. 799).

4. Muscle spindle afferents are silenced by the reflex shortening of the muscle; thus part of the continuous afferent drive of spinal motoneurones from peripheral sources is eliminated for the short period of time while the muscle is contracting.

5. Afferent fibers from both supraspinal and peripheral sources, before reaching spinal motoneurones, branch into collaterals with end-organs located at presynaptic excitatory nerve fibers. Action potentials reaching these presynaptic end-organs depolarize the underlying nerve fibers, thus diminishing the amplitude of the action potentials traveling along these fibers and thereby also the amount of transmitter secreted at the axodendritic motoneurone synapses. This mechanism is called "presynaptic inhibition" (Eccles et al., 1961, 1962a, b, c; Eccles and Willis, 1962). Thus, synaptic excitation of spinal motoneurones simultaneously produces presynaptic inhibition of the surrounding ventral horn cells.

COMPLEX MOTOR PHENOMENA OF THE NEWBORN INFANT

PLACING AND STANDING RESPONSE

If an infant is lifted while its insteps are touching the edge of a table, the feet are lifted and placed on the table (Saint Anne-Dargassies, 1954). When after this placing response, the trunk of the infant is lowered, a proprioceptive, tonic myotatic stretch reflex is produced and the leg extensors become activated. This standing response is variable but usually present in healthy, full-term newborn infants (Michaelis et al., 1969).

WALKING

If the infant is held in an upright position, and the soles of the feet are allowed to touch the surface of the table, stepping movements occur. The steps usually cross each other (Peiper, 1928; Stirnimann, 1938). The same movements can be elicited in any position of the body, horizontal or vertical, head up or head down, or even without the soles of the feet touching the table (André-Thomas and Saint Anne-Dargassies, 1952; Peiper, 1963).

CRAWLING

If the infant is awake and lying on its abdomen, crawling movements occur which can be reinforced by a light push on the sole of the feet (Blanton, 1917; Bauer, 1926; Stirnimann, 1938).

THE ASYMMETRIC TONIC NECK REFLEX

This reflex, first described in animals by Magnus (1924), can sometimes be demonstrated in newborn infants (Landau, 1923, 1925; Schaltenbrand, 1925; Isbert and Peiper, 1927; Byers, 1938; Gesell, 1938). If the infant's head is turned to the right and left after a few seconds the extremities become extended on the side to which the face is turned, whereas the contralateral arm and leg remain flexed. In many normal newborn infants, this response can hardly be seen because of interfering spontaneous movements. But, electromyographically, an ipsilateral increase of extensor muscle activity can always be demonstrated while the face is turned to one side (Fig. 12). The receptors of this reflex are very likely to be located in the muscles and joints of the neck.

THE RIGHTING RESPONSE

If the head of a healthy, full-term newborn infant is turned to one side, the trunk follows (Robinson, 1966). Again, the afferent sources of the righting reflex are located in the muscles and joints of the neck.

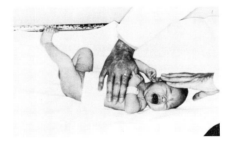

1 sec

Fig. 12. Asymmetric tonic neck reflex. If the infant's head is turned to one side, the corresponding extremities are stretched. Even if this reflex cannot be detected visually, an increase of extensor muscle activity can usually be recorded electromyographically as depicted below. The head turning is indicated by a bar.

THE MORO RESPONSE

The Moro reflex is a well-known phenomenon in newborn human infants. The motor pattern was first observed by Magnus and Kleijn (1912) during dorsal flexion of the infant's head. Moro (1918) elicited the reaction with a blow to the infant's mattress. At present, a brief head drop is most commonly used to elicit the Moro response (Prechtl and Beintema, 1964). It is still a matter of controversy whether under normal conditions the main afferent pathway of the reflex originates in the neck muscle (Freudenberg, 1931; André-Thomas and Hanon, 1947; André-Thomas and St. Anne-Dargassies, 1952; Parmelee, 1964) or in the labyrinthine receptors (Peiper, 1963; Prechtl and Lenard, 1968).

The characteristics of the observed Moro response pattern are dependent upon the infant's gestational age (Saint Anne-Dargassies, 1955, 1966; Babson and McKinnon, 1965; Brett, 1966; Schulte et al., 1968a). In preterm infants of less than 35 weeks of menstrual age, the reaction consists of a brisk extension and abduction of the upper extremities. The subsequent flexion and adduction component is missing or incomplete (Fig. 13). After 35 weeks of menstrual age the infant develops the characteristic flexion posture of the full-term neonate. Concomitantly, in the Moro response extension and abduction decrease, whereas flexion and adduction become increasingly prominent.

In spite of the high variability of the Moro response pattern, a statistically

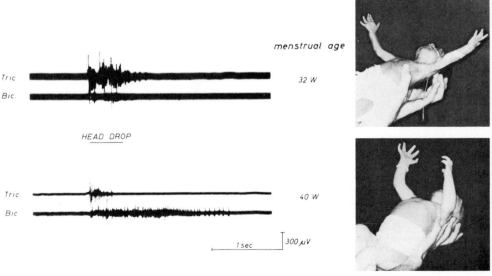

Fig. 13. At 32 weeks menstrual age, the Moro response consists of the extension and abduction of the upper extremities. With increasing maturity, both extension and abduction decrease, while adduction and flexion become more prominent. EMG activity, subsequent to the head drop, starts in the triceps muscle and is outlasted by the biceps in full-term newborn infants. (From Schulte et al. 1968a. *Develop. Psychobiol.*, 1:41-47. Courtesy of John Wiley and Sons, Inc.)

significant decrease with age of the triceps/biceps activity ratio can be demonstrated (Chart 3). Electromyographic analysis indicates that flexor predominance, which is dependent upon age, is due to an increase of flexor rather than a decrease of extensor activity (Fig. 14). The more tonic, i.e., long-lasting, discharge pattern of flexor motoneurones in term versus preterm infants may be explained by the following mechanisms: myogenic, intra- or supraspinal, and proprioceptive:

Myogenic mechanisms: Electromyographic data have shown that flexor preponderance with increasing age is not due to triceps/biceps muscle weight ratio which is dependent upon age because a true increase of spinal flexor motoneurone activity was observed. However, it cannot be ruled out that increasing flexor muscle power plays an additional role, although older studies on the weight of extensor and flexor muscles in newborn infants do not support such a theory (Theile, 1884; Ritter, 1924).

Spinal or supraspinal mechanisms: The early, immature Moro response consists of an immediate and strong activation of extensor motoneurones of the upper extremities. This reaction is already present in a preterm newborn infant of 25 weeks of menstrual age and remains almost constant through all ages. As we know from animal experiments a strong activation of extensor motoneurones very often implies a concomitant inhibition of flexors and vice versa (Sherrington, 1898; Ruch, 1965). At the very beginning of the Moro extensor response, sometimes a brief inhibition of flexor motoneurones can be detected (Schulte and Schwenzel, 1965). It is reasonable to assume that for flexor motoneurones in preterm infants the depolarization pressure, i.e., the excitatory afferent inflow from central and peripheral sources, is too weak to overcome the hyperpolarization pressure which is raised in the inhibitory interneurones of the spinal cord by strong synchronous bursts of extensor motoneurone activity. This hypothesis is supported by the finding that in preterm, more often than in full-term, newborn infants, the flexor Moro response starts only when the extensor activity has already ceased—Moro response with delayed biceps activity (Fig. 15). The increasing flexor Moro response with menstrual age can be due to an increase of intraspinal or supraspinal excitatory influences on flexor motoneurones in the course of the Moro reflex. At the moment, this hypothesis can neither be proven nor dismissed.

Proprioceptive mechanisms: Quite contrary to the purely hypothetic assumption of an increase of intra- or supraspinal flexor excitation, there is good evidence from animal experiments which would lead us to assume that proprioceptive influences enhance the Moro flexor reaction with increasing age. During the primary Moro extension response, flexor muscle spindles are stretched, thus eliciting phasic and/or tonic myotatic reflex activity in spinal flexor motoneurones. In kittens, the ability to sustain muscle spindle activity develops in the first weeks after birth, and in the immature animal only phasic and no tonic myotatic reflexes can be elicited (Skoglund, 1960a, c). It is likely that the same developmental sequence occurs in the human fetus and newborn infant. Thus, the brisk Moro extension creates a tonically sustained increase in flexor muscle spindle discharges and thereby tonic myotatic reflex activity in spinal flexor motoneurones of only the more mature infants. In the immature, preterm infant, the spindle discharge frequency rapidly accommodates. Thus the proprioceptive depolarization pressure on the flexor moto-

	menstrual age [w]	weight [g]	MORO-REFLEX duration of activity μ σ	β p=0,05	TRICEPS/BICEPS amount of activity μ σ	β p=0,05
term N = 18	40,17 ± 0,79	3344,74 ±348,94	*0,89 ± 0,66	1,20 0,58	*1,16 ± 0,94	1,59 0,72
preterm N = 21	36,19 ± 1,63	2194,76 ±250,09	*1,93 ± 1,99	2,78 1,08	*2,21 ± 1,76	2,97 1,46
			*t = 6,14; p < 0,001		*t = 4,18; p < 0,001	

Chart 3. Mean duration and amount of the Moro reflex expressed as a triceps/biceps activity ratio. (From Schulte et al. 1968a. *Develop. Psychobiol.* 1:41-47. Courtesy of John Wiley and Sons, Inc.)

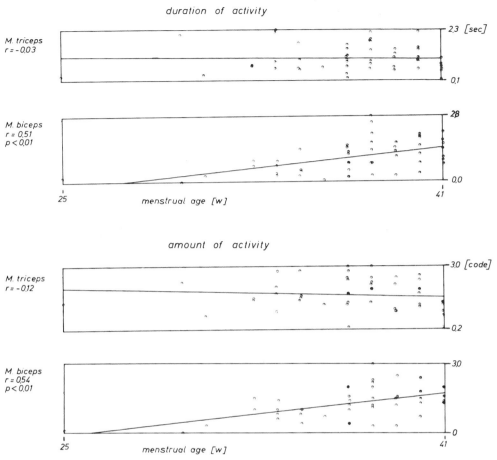

Fig. 14. Moro reflex. Regression lines for the amount and duration of biceps activity rise with increasing menstrual age; the product-moment correlation is significant. Triceps activity shows no significant alteration with age. (From Schulte et al. 1968a. *Develop. Psychobiol.*, 1:41-47. Courtesy of John Wiley and Sons, Inc.)

neurones definitely increases with maturation and is probably less in preterm than in full-term newborn infants.

RHYTHMIC MOTONEURONE ACTIVITY

In some infants part of the Moro reaction pattern consists of rhythmic, instead of tonic, motoneurone activity (Fig. 16). Frequently, similar rhythms occur spontaneously, particularly when the infant is crying. It is not absolutely clear whether all these rhythmic motoneurone activities have an identical neurophysiologic background. Most of our own experiments are based on rhythmic activities occurring with the Moro reflex and subsequent to muscle stretch. These rhythms show all

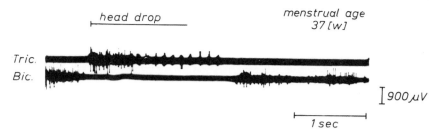

	N	infants with delayed biceps activity
preterm 25 – 33 w menstrual age	9	4 (44,5%)
preterm 34 – 38 w menstrual age	27	4 (14,8%)
term 39 – 41 w menstrual age	37	4 (10,8%)

Fig. 15. In the course of the Moro reflex biceps muscle activity starts after triceps muscle activity has ceased. This phenomenon occurs only in some newborns, particularly in prematures. (From Schulte et al. 1968a. *Develop. Psychobiol.*, 1:41-47. Courtesy of John Wiley and Sons, Inc.)

the characteristics of a clonus rather than a tremor (Schulte and Schwenzel, 1965). In preterm infants of less than 34 weeks of menstrual age the rhythmic activity in the arm and leg muscles is quite irregular, whereas interval histograms show increasing regularity, i.e., predominating discharge frequencies in more mature infants (Fig. 17). Under abnormal conditions both the amount and the regularity of rhythmic activity increase. Particularly in hypotonic and hyperexcitable infants, rhythmic motoneurone activity predominates. The clonus frequency is higher in the jaw compared with arm and leg muscles (Schulte, 1964). This might have something to do with the length of the reflex arc. On the other hand, the spontaneous discharge frequency of single motoneurones is higher in cranial than in spinal motor nuclei (Schaefer, 1965).

The Rhombencephalic Reticular Formation

The reticular formation as defined by anatomists (Brodal, 1957) consists of more or less diffuse aggregations of nerve cells and a great wealth of fibers. The reticular formation extends rostrally into the thalamic nuclei forming part of the midbrain and hypothalamic gray matter. Caudally, the reticular substance ends below the medullary pyramids, the interneurone network of the spinal cord usually not being referred to as reticular formation. As to function, the reticular neurones

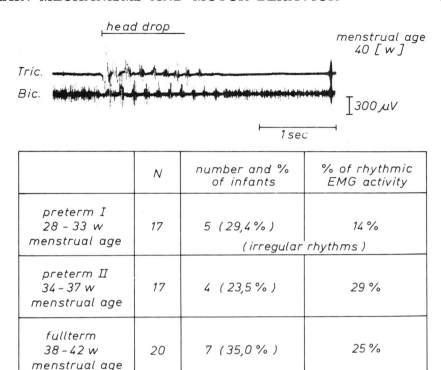

	N	number and % of infants	% of rhythmic EMG activity
preterm I 28 – 33 w menstrual age	17	5 (29,4 %)	14 %
		(irregular rhythms)	
preterm II 34 – 37 w menstrual age	17	4 (23,5 %)	29 %
fullterm 38 – 42 w menstrual age	20	7 (35,0 %)	25 %

Fig. 16. In some newborn infants, particularly in hyperexcitable babies, the Moro response consists of rhythmic, rather than tonic, motoneurone discharges.

influence 1, the behavioral state in the sleep/wakefulness cycle (Moruzzi and Magoun, 1949; Magoun, 1954; Moruzzi, 1960, 1964); 2, spinal motoneurone activity, i.e., muscle tone and contraction (Magoun and Rhines, 1946; Rhines and Magoun, 1946; Sprague and Chambers, 1954); 3, sensory perception (von Baumgarten et al., 1954; Scherer and Hernández-Péon, 1955; von Baumgarten, 1956; Duensing and Schaefer, 1957).

In this chapter we are dealing only with the influence of reticular formation on muscle tone and contraction.

Comparatively large neurones of the ventromedial and caudal parts of the rhombencephalic reticular formation give rise to descending, inhibitory pathways to spinal extensor motoneurones, while at the same time facilitating flexor motoneurones. Laterally, a more extensive part of the reticular formation, reaching from the subthalamus to the rhombencephalon, consists of smaller neurones with excitatory influence on spinal extensor and inhibitory influence on flexor motoneurones (Sprague and Chambers, 1954; Gernandt and Thulin, 1955). The reticulospinal tract is very likely to act via chains of interneurones, predominantly on γ- but probably on α-motoneurones as well (Granit and Kaada, 1952).

The reticular formation receives afferent impulses from almost all structures of the nervous system both central and peripheral. Descending from the cortex and

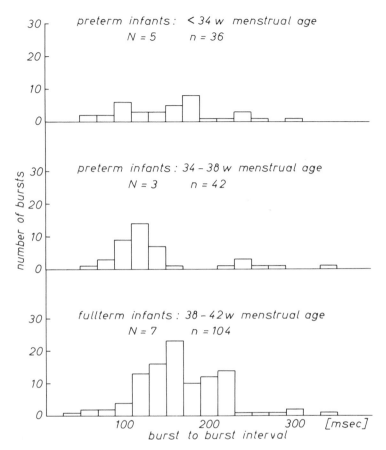

Fig. 17. Interval histograms of motoneurone bursts. The rhythmic motoneurone discharges in the course of a Moro reflex are more regular in full-term than in very immature preterm infants.

the basal ganglia, as well as from the cerebellum, and ascending from cutaneous, as well as from proprioceptive receptors, axon collaterals feed into the rhomben-cephalic reticular formation. A main source of excitatory afferents for the reticular activating system is provided by the chemoreceptors, their influence on rhomben-cephalic respiratory neurones being only one part of their alerting influence on the reticular formation (Schulte et al., 1959a; Hugelin et al., 1959). Baroreceptor afferents, on the other hand, inhibiting the reticular activating system or facilitating the deactivating system, decrease γ-motoneurone activity and muscle tone (Koch, 1932; Schweitzer and Wright, 1937; Schulte et al., 1959b).

Little is known about the development of dendrites in the brain stem reticular formation, particularly in structures responsible for respiration and muscle tone. Although the myelination of reticular axons is not complete for 10 years after birth, the influence of supraspinal structures on muscle tone is already quite obvious in the newborn period. Traumatic or hemorrhagic transection of the spinal cord immediately causes skeletal muscle hypotonia which is followed by spasticity after some days or weeks.

The Vestibular System and The Nucleus Ruber

Spinal and cranial nerve motoneurone activity is heavily influenced by afferents arising in the vestibular organ, which act via the vestibulospinal and the rubrospinal tract and produce both acceleratory and righting reflexes. In the adult human, these reflexes are partly masked by voluntarily controlled movements, but they are easily elicitable in newborn infants and in animals.

ACCELERATORY REFLEXES

Linear acceleration and gravity activate the macula receptors of the otolith organs mainly in the utricle (Camis, 1930). The corresponding receptors in the saccule are currently believed to be involved in the perception of slow vibration (McNalley and Stuart, 1942). If the animal is suddenly lowered, the legs become extended and the toes spread. Toward the end of the movement the legs become flexed. If the animal, standing on its legs, is lifted upward, the legs become flexed and later extended. These reflexes are particularly marked in the forelegs if the animal is in the vertical position, head pointed downward and upward, respectively.

Rotatory acceleration of the body on a vertical, a horizontal, or a sagittal axis activates receptors of the christa ampullaris, located in the ampulla of the semicircular canals (Camis, 1930). The reflex responses are identical in adults and newborn infants. If the infant is held in the upright position and spun around facing the examiner, the head and finally the trunk turn in the direction opposite to that of rotation, and nystagmus is induced with its quick or refixation component in the same direction as the rotation. The vestibular organ responds only to a change in the rate of movement rather than to a steady movement itself. When the rotation is suddenly discontinued, the same motorphenomena occur once again but in the opposite direction (Bartels, 1910; Alexander, 1911; Bárány, 1918; Schur, 1922; Duensing and Schaefer, 1957). Corresponding head and eye movements can be obtained while turning the infant around each one of the three axes. These are sensitive tests for both eye muscle and vestibular functions, but the responses are negative when the infant is asleep (Lawrence and Feind, 1953).

Thornval (1920-21), Schur (1922), and Berberich and Wiechers (1924) found eye muscle responses similar to those in adults following caloric stimulation of the auditory canal.

If the head is turned slowly to one side or upward and downward, the eyes move in the opposite direction (Doll's eye test) (Bartels, 1910; Esente, 1958). As for the afferent source of the Moro reflex, it is still debatable as to whether neck muscle or vestibular receptors are responsible for the Doll's eye reflex phenomenon. If the head is turned more rapidly, particularly in hyperexcitable infants, clonic eye muscle activity occurs (Schulte et al., 1965).

RIGHTING REFLEXES

The head always tends to turn back into the normal or resting position; this righting reflex is guaranteed by certain afferent impulse patterns from the macula receptors, probably in the utricle. If a cat is dropped with its legs upward, the head is immediately rotated and is followed by the upper and in turn by the lower body (Magnus, 1924; Rademaker, 1931; Rademaker and Ter Braak, 1936). These latter, neck righting reflexes are guaranteed by the activity of neck and trunk muscle proprioreceptors.

The Cerebellum

The archicerebellum (nodulus and flocculus) is connected to the vestibular nuclei by both afferent and efferent fibers (Fulton, 1952). Lesions in these structures lead to ataxia of the trunk, even in the sitting position (Dow and Moruzzi, 1958).

The paleocerebellum or lobus anterior, comprised of the lingula, the lobulus centralis, and the culmen, receives afferent inflow from muscle, joint, and skin receptors via the spino- and bulbocerebellar tract (Dow, 1942; Snider and Stowell, 1944; Hampson, 1949). Most of the efferent fibers originating in the Purkinje cells are interrupted at the cerebellar nuclei, such as the nucleus emboliformis, the nuclei globosi, and mainly the larger cells of the dentate nucleus (Brookhardt, 1961). Their efferents, in turn, project to the nucleus ruber and the reticular formation. Electric stimulation of the anterior lobe decreases muscle tone and decerebrate rigidity while its destruction leads to increased proprioceptive reflexes, opisthotonus, and tremor (Pollock and Davis, 1927; Connor, 1941).

The neocerebellum or posterior lobe receives afferent fibers from the contralateral motor cortex as well as from sensory areas of the parietal and occipital cortex. The different parts of the body are topically represented at the cerebellar cortex (Rossi, 1912; Hampson, 1949; Hassler, 1953a). The efferent Purkinje cell fibers in turn project back to the area 4 motor cortex with synaptic relays both at the smaller neurones of the dentate nucleus and at the ventral nucleus of the thalamus (Moruzzi, 1950; Hassler, 1950). The neocerebellum is part of the voluntary motor control system. Its destruction is followed by adiadochokinesis, hypotonia, dysmetria, ataxia, and intention tremor (Holmes, 1922, 1939; Dow and Moruzzi, 1958).

The cerebellum as a whole has no direct connection with the spinal motoneurones. Its influence, therefore, is only a regulating and stabilizing rather than an executing one. Complete absence of the organ might be asymptomatic, but its destruction usually implies dysregulation of muscle tone and posture, and walking and an inability to perform voluntary, skilled movements. As far as one can judge from the literature, the cerebellum is of little significance for neonatal motor behavior. Complete absence of the cerebellum, not easy to detect even later in life, can be asymptomatic in the newborn period.

The Basal Ganglia

According to anatomic classification the subcortical nuclei of the forebrain, the caudate nucleus, the putamen, and the pallidum are called "basal ganglia." Modern physiologic concepts of a reconsidered, extrapyramidal motor system include such structures as the subthalamic nucleus (corpus Luys), certain parts of the thalamus, the substantia nigra, the nucleus ruber, the cerebellar dentate nucleus, the brain stem reticular formation, and parts of the prefrontal cortical motor area. Hassler (1956) has shown that this system works by means of several feedback circuits, modifying and adding to the voluntary corticospinal output (Jung and Hassler, 1960). The main circuit seems to be formed by connecting fibers from the motor cortex to the putamen (Glees, 1944), from the putamen to the external and to the internal pallidum, from the pallidum to the nucleus ventralis oralis of the thalamus, and from the thalamus to the cortical motor area 6. This positive feedback circuit represents an activating system for corticospinal influences. In addition, there are other direct connections from the motor cortex to the putamen, to the external pallidum, as well as to the rostral nuclei of the thalamus, forming, at least in part, inhibitory shortcircuits.

The efferent fibers of the basal ganglia to the spinal motoneurones can be considered as two main tracts, from the putamen and the caudate nucleus, the nucleus niger is reached by inhibitory afferents influencing the nigrospinal and reticulospinal activity (Vogt, 1903; Jung and Hassler, 1960). Lesions in this strionigroreticulospinal system lead to rigidity, akinesis (poverty of movement), and resting tremor.

A second descending system, originating in the external pallidum, discharges to the subthalamic nucleus (corpus Luys), the nucleus ruber, and the reticular formation influencing rubrospinal activity. Lesions in this striopallidorubroreticulospinal system imply athetosis, chorea, and other forms of hyperkinesis. From each of these brain stem structures, the nucleus ruber, the corpus Luys, and the substantia nigra, reafferent connections feed back into the pallidum (Glees, 1944; Carpenter et al., 1960).

The functional significance of single parts of the extrapyramidal system is still obscure, perhaps mainly because this system works by means of circuits rather than centers. In birds the basal ganglia, together with the spinal cord, form a motor system capable of producing flying. Highly skilled movements can be obtained from striatal animals (cortex removed) (Wang and Akert, 1962; Ruch, 1965), and stimulation of the caudate nucleus can produce both stereotyped movements and an immediate arrest of cortically induced movements which is called "holding response" (Mettler et al., 1939; Laursen, 1962b).

Ever since 1913, when Foerster coined the word "Pallidumwesen," neonatal motor behavior has been supposed to be under the mere influence of the pallidal neurones. Flexor posture, climbing movements, grasp and palmomental reflex, recurring in adults with cortical and striatal lesions, probably represent the pallidal influences on spinal motoneurones. It is widely assumed that these motor phenomena disappear when the pallidum comes under striatal control (Peiper, 1963). Orthner and Roeder (1968) suggested a fascinating comparison of infantile motor development with extrapyramidal motor disturbances before and after stereotactic operations. These authors hypothesize that the choreaathetotic kicking-about of the newborn infant is a pallidum pattern which is replaced some weeks later by more ballistic movements under the influence of the corpus Luys. Interestingly enough, the nucleus niger, although myelination already occurs at two to three months after birth at term, becomes pigmented only when the extrapyramidal motor skill is almost fully developed at about three to four years of age. According to Hassler (1964) the nucleus niger has a direct regulating and desynchronizing effect on spinal motoneurones.

The Cerebral Motor Cortex

THE PRIMARY MOTOR AREA

In the precentral gyrus (area 4), the nerve cells of the central motoneurones are arranged in a relationship to each other which is similar to that of the muscles which can be activated by them. This somatotopic organization was postulated by Jackson in 1870 (see Taylor, 1956) and has been proved by several authors (Campbell, 1905; Brodmann, 1909; Vogt and Vogt, 1919; von Bonin and Bailey, 1947; Penfield and Jasper, 1954). It is mainly the pyramidal shaped Betz cells that give rise to descending fibers which activate single spinal motoneurones and, thereby, muscles in a volitional act of movement.

SUPPLEMENTARY CORTICAL MOTOR AREAS

Muscle contraction and movement can be obtained by electric stimulation of areas other than the precentral gyrus. In fact, movement can be elicited from almost the entire surface of the cerebral cortex (Lilly, 1958). Gross movements can be elicited particularly from areas 6 and 8 of the frontal lobe. However, motor nerve cells with pyramidal tract efferents become sparse in passing forward from the central fissure. Area 6 and 8 neurones are part of the extrapyramidal motor system (cortical extrapyramidal system: COEPS) with both efferent and afferent connections to the basal ganglia, the thalamus, and the cerebellum.

THE PYRAMIDAL TRACT

Thirty-one percent of its fibers belong to area 4 motoneurones and only 3 percent to Betz cells (Lassek, 1942; Mettler, 1944). The cellular origin of 29 percent lies in the sixth area, and of 40 percent in the postcentral fifth and seventh areas. The majority of the pyramidal tract fibers reach lower motoneurones via interneurones in the segmental level of the spinal cord.

EVIDENCES OF CORTICAL MOTOR CONTROL IN THE NEWBORN INFANT

Peiper (1963) thought that neonatal motor behavior was entirely subcortical, but he was constantly searching for cortical nerve cell activity.

EEG and evoked response studies have shown that bioelectric brain activity changes with certain behavioral states and reactions to stimuli, thus indicating that the cortex at least takes part in these states and response patterns.

Dendritic arborization of Betz cells, although occurring mainly postnatally, has already started before birth, particularly in the motor area of the trunk (Rabinowicz, 1964). The myelination of pyramidal tract fibers has started before birth, and we were able to elicit isolated movements of the toes and fingers by electric stimulation of unclassified cortical brain tissue in newborn infants with exencephaly.

Cortical lesions, due to pre- or perinatal pathology and later confirmed by radiographic studies, sometimes present themselves already in the newborn period when the infant is carefully examined.

Finally, in neonatal convulsions, cortical convulsive potentials occur synchronously with peripheral massive muscle contractions.

Admittedly, all these factors are not convincing evidence of cortical influence on normal neonatal motor behavior. However, in view of our present knowledge that behavioral mechanisms are the result of all computational processes in a countless number of neuronal feedback circuits, it is illogical to assume that well-documented cortical activity should have no influence on the infant's behavior.

Clinical Applications

MILESTONES OF MOTOR DEVELOPMENT AND THE ASSESSMENT OF GESTATIONAL AGE

During the past decade a number of neurophysiologic studies of the newborn, although aiming at diagnostic clues, have revealed the great variability of neonatal motor behavior with menstrual age. Both reflexes and complex motor phenomena appear or change at a certain time of the gestational period. A summary of these relations between menstrual age and behavior is given in Chart 4 and relies mainly on the work of Saint Anne-Dargassies (1955, 1966), Robinson (1966), Babson and McKinnon (1965), Amiel-Tison (1968), and Michaelis et al. (1969).

THE DEVELOPMENTAL PROFILE OF PRETERM AND FULL-TERM NEWBORN INFANTS

The relation between menstrual age and behavior was so striking that several authors suggested the assessment of menstrual age by means of a neurologic exami-

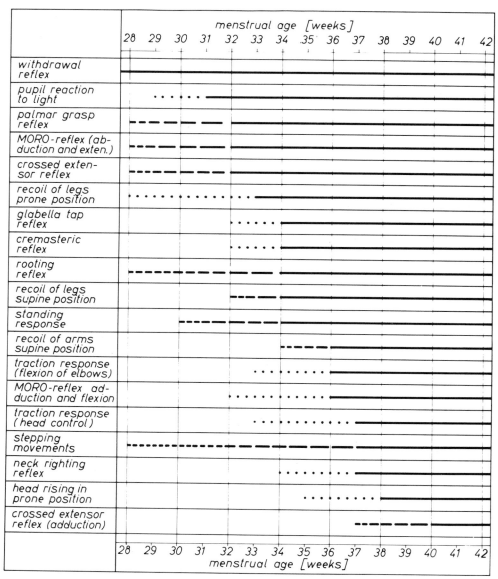

Chart 4. The developmental sequence of various reflexes and motor automatisms. (Data compiled by R. Michaelis according to Amiel-Tison, Babson and McKinnon, Michaelis, Robinson and Saint Anne-Dargassies.)

nation. However, neurophysiologic parameters, being dependent on menstrual age as well as on pathology, seem to be unreliable for both a neurologic diagnosis and an age estimate, if one of these factors is not known. According to our own experience the problem is even greater, since abnormal motor phenomena frequently mimic immature behavior. An infant supposed to be 32 weeks of menstrual age and having no pupil reactions to light is either younger or abnormal. Thus, every neurologic examination becomes an equation with two unknown factors. As shown in Graph 3, the triceps/biceps ratio of the Moro response decreases with menstrual age, since the flexor component gets stronger when the infant matures. Flexor motoneurone activity, however, is diminished or even abolished under many abnormal influences, thus the resulting triceps/biceps Moro response activity ratio increases and may become identical with the ratio of preterm infants. The same problem, although different in degree, arises with almost all parameters of motor behavior (Michaelis and Schulte, 1969).

Neurophysiologic data obtained from preterm and full-term newborn infants can be classified on a scale, the location on which indicates the sensitivity to abnormal influences as well as the dependency upon menstrual age (Fig. 18). Neurophysiologic mechanisms on the left side of the scale are mainly dependent upon structural maturation. These phenomena are rather independent of abnormal, environmental factors and are therefore suitable for an estimation of menstrual age. According to our experience, primarily two phenomena belong to this group—nerve conduction velocity as an indicator of myelination and basic EEG patterns, probably as an indicator of dendritic arborization and the subsequent formation of intracortical

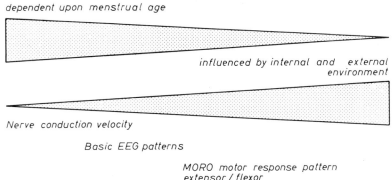

Fig. 18. Menstrual age, low birth-weight, and low activity. Brain mechanisms are dependent upon both structural maturation and environmental influences. Complex synaptic functions, like behavioral state homeostasis, are more easily altered by abnormal conditions and less suitable for an age estimate than are comparatively simple neuronal activities, such as impulse conduction.

synaptic connections (Parmelee et al., 1968; Nolte et al., 1969). The EEG patterns, however, may already be influenced by certain abnormal circumstances, particularly when they are of severe degree.

Neurophysiologic mechanisms on the right side of the scale show great variability, depending on the infant's external and internal environment. These phenomena seem to be most promising for detecting neurologic abnormalities, but they are less suitable for an age estimate, particularly under abnormal conditions. Complex nervous activity belongs in this group, the Moro response pattern being one example. Another example, probably even more revealing because it is more sensitive, is the behavioral state stability. Basic EEG patterns merely indicating the presence, the amount, and the sequence of bioelectric activity generators are dependent on age, but their circadian distribution and their coincidence with other parameters of respiration, heart rate, muscle activity, and so on are heavily influenced by environmental factors (Monod et al., 1967; Prechtl, 1968). All the phenomena on the right side of the scale also show various characteristics which are dependent upon menstrual age. This relationship, however, is immediately masked when abnormal conditions like hypoxia, hypoglycemia, electrolyte changes, polycythemia, hyperbilirubinemia, and many other unknown factors influence nervous activity.

For the future, a neurophysiologic evaluation of the newborn infant seems to be most promising when the results of different parameters in the form of a maturational age estimate are entered into a developmental profile. Smaller or larger discrepancies in neurophysiologic and behavioral maturity will probably indicate different kinds or degrees of abnormality. At present, however, for clinical purposes we still rely on a motor behavior oriented neurologic examination, the principles of which have been worked out mainly for the full-term newborn infant.

GENERAL PRINCIPLES FOR THE NEUROLOGIC EXAMINATION OF THE NEWBORN INFANT

It is not the purpose of this chapter to provide the reader with another scheme for the neurologic examination; such schemes have already been published by several authors (Prechtl and Beintema, 1964; Joppich and Schulte, 1968). All of the above described reflex and motor phenomena can be used in a routine or scientific study.

During the examination the infant should be in a certain behavioral state in order to make the results comparable from one infant to another. Preferably the infant should be awake but quiet. The examiner should be familiar with the characteristics of different behavioral states worked out by Wolff (1959) and Prechtl and Beintema (1964):

1. Eyes closed, regular respiration, no movements—quiet sleep (nonREM sleep).
2. Eyes closed, irregular respiration, many small movements—active sleep (REM sleep).
3. Eyes open, no gross movements—awake but quiet.
4. Eyes open, gross movements, no crying—awake and active.

5. Eyes open or closed, crying.

6. Other states which have to be described.

It is particularly important to know that during active sleep (REM) proprioceptive reflexes and during quiet sleep (nonREM) some exteroceptive reflexes are diminished or even abolished. During the examination the infant should be kept under a neutral temperature, i.e., 32°C.

The stimuli and the reflex responses should be quantified as much as possible and controlled by interscorer reliability studies.

Beintema (1968) has given a detailed description of slight physiologic changes in the motor behavior of the full-term newborn infant during the first days after birth. There is ample evidence now that during the first three days of life many behavioral parameters are less stable than thereafter. Thus a routine neurophysiologic examination should be done between four and eight days after birth, provided the infant is not severely ill and urgently in need of neurologic evaluation. Gross abnormalities are obvious at any time.

The results of all single tests can be summarized in order to classify the infant's motor behavior as normal, hyperexcitable, apathetic, hypertonic, hypotonic, hemilateral or focal, convulsive, or comatous. This classification is far from being a diagnosis. However, some of these groupings, although not specific, are typical for certain perinatal complications (Schulte et al., 1965). Infants of diabetic mothers are usually hyperexcitable; dysmature, small-for-date infants are frequently hypertonic; and infants with traumatic or inflammatory encephalopathies are usually found to have hemilateral, focal, and convulsive abnormalities.

The neurophysiologic classification of the newborn infant, by means of a quantitative assessment of each reflex response, gives little information about the nature of the underlying disease but indicates the degree and sometimes the localization of the functional disturbance.

Perspectives

The historic development of research on the nervous system of newborn infants, both normal and abnormal, is marked by three milestones, and for contemporary researchers the direction of the fourth step seems already to have been outlined.

The first effort was an anatomic approach linked with the names of Flechsig, Yllpö, and Schwartz. Second were the behavioral motor observations culminating in the work of Peiper and André-Thomas. Their work was carried further by a number of eminent authors who determined the third step which is characterized by a great wealth of quantitative data obtained through behavioral observations as well as electrophysiologic methods and which were subjected to statistic analysis. This approach can be called "brain engineering" (Prechtl). Undoubtedly, the fourth phase will be dominated by biochemical results which will have to be combined with structural, behavioral, and electrophysiologic findings as a true correlative study of the neonatal nervous system.

REFERENCES

Alexander, G. 1911. Die Reflexerregbarkeit des Ohrlabyrinthes am menschlichen Neugeborenen. Z. Sinnesphysiol., Abt. 2, 45:153-196.

Amiel-Tison, C. 1968. Neurological evaluation of the maturity of newborn infants. Arch. Dis. Child., 43:89-93.

André-Thomas, Y. C., and F. Hanon. 1947. Les premiers automatismes. Rev. Neurol. (Paris), 79:641.

———— and J. Ajuriaguerra. 1949. Etude Sémiologique du Tonus Musculaire. Paris, Flammarion.

———— and S. St. Anne-Dargassies. 1952. Etudes Neurologiques sur le Nouveau-né et le Jeune Nourrisson. Paris, Masson et Cie.

———— S. Autgaerden. 1959. Psycho-affectivité des Premiers Mois. Paris, Univ. Press, pp. 23 and 96.

———— Y. Chesni, and S. Autgaerden. 1954. A propos de quelques points de sémiology nerveuse du nouveau-né et du jeune nourrisson. Exploration de quelques afférences. Reactions aux excitations digitales et palmaires. Rythme; inhibitions de reflexes. Aptitude statique et locomotrice des membres superieurs. Affect et affectivité. Presse Med., 62:41-44.

Babinski, J. 1922. Réflexes de defense. Rev. Neurol. (Paris), 28:1049-1081.

Babkin, P. S. 1955. Jaw-rotating reflex of the head in infants. Zh. Nevropat. Psikhiat. Korsakova, 53:692-696.

Babson, S. G., and C. M. McKinnon. 1965. A preliminary report on the neuromuscular milestones in premature infant development. 13th Annual Meeting of the Western Society for Pediatric Research, Portland, Oregon.

Bach, L. 1908. Pupillenlehre. Anatomie, Physiologie und Pathologie. Methodik der Untersuchung. Berlin, S. Karger, p. 72.

Balduzzi, O. 1932. Die Stützreaktionen beim Menschen in physiologischen und pathologischen Zuständen. Z. Neurol., 141:1-29.

Bárány, R. 1918. Über einige Augen- und Halsmuskelreflexe bei Neugeborenen. Acta Otolaryng. (Stockholm), 1:97-102.

Barker, D. 1962. The structure and distribution of muscle receptors. Symposium on Muscle Receptors. Hong Kong, University of Hong Kong Press.

———— 1966. The motor innervation of the mammalian muscle spindle. Proceedings of the First Nobel Sympos. Stockholm, Almquist & Wiksell, p. 51.

Bartels, M. 1904. Pupillenverhältnisse bei Neugeborenen. Z. Augenheilk., 12:638-644.

———— 1910. Das Puppenaugenphänomen. Graefes Arch. Ophthal. 76:1-8.

Bauer, J. 1926. Das Kriechphänomen des Neugeborenen. Klin. Wschr., 4:1468.

von Baumgarten, R. 1956. Koordinationsformen einzelner Ganglienzellen der rhombencephalen Atemzentren. Pflueger. Arch. Ges. Physiol., 262:573-594.

———— A. Mollica, and G. Moruzzi. 1954. Modulierung der Entladungsfrequenz einzelner Zellen der substantia reticularis durch corticofugale und cerebelläre Impulse. Pflueger. Arch. Ges. Physiol., 259:56-78.

Beintema, D. J. 1968. A neurological study of newborn infants. Spastics Internat. Med. Publ. No. 28. London, W. Heinemann Medical Books, Ltd.

Berberich, J., and A. Wiechers. 1924. Symptomatologie des Geburtstraumas. Z. Kinderheilk., 38:59-102.

Bergström, R. M., P. E. Hellström, and D. Stenberg. 1962. Über die Entwicklung der elektrischen Aktivität im Großhirn des intrauterinen Meerschweinchen-Fetus. Ann. Chir. Gynaec. Fenn., 51:460.

Bertolotti, M. 1904. Étude sur la diffusion de la zone réflexogène chez les enfants; quelques remarques sur la loi à l'orientation des reflexes cutanés à l'état normal et à l'état pathologique. Rev. Neurol. (Paris), 12:1160-1166.

Blanton, M. G. 1917. The behaviour of the human infant during the first thirty days of life. Psychol. Rev., 24:456-483.

Blom, S., and O. Finnström. 1968. Motor conduction velocities in newborn infants of various gestational ages. Acta Paediat. Scand., 57:377-384.

Bolaffio, M., and G. Artom. 1924. Richerche sulla fisiologia del sistema nervosa del feto umano. Arch. Sci. Biol. (Bologna), 5:457-487.

von Bonin, G., and P. Bailey. 1947. The Neocortex of Macaca mulatta. Urbana, Illinois, University of Illinois Press.

Boyd, J. A. 1962. The nuclear-bag fibre and nuclear-chain fibre systems in the muscle spindles of the cat. In Granit, R., ed. Symposium on Muscle Receptors. Hong Kong, University of Hong Kong Press.

Brett, E. A. 1966. The estimation of foetal maturity by the neurological examination of the neonate. In Dawkins, M., and B. Mac Gregor, eds. Clinics in Developmental Medicine, No. 19. Publication of the Spastics Society for Medical Education. London, W. Heinemann Medical Books, Ltd., pp. 105-117.

Brett, E. M. 1966. Measurement of cerebrospinal fluid pressure in infants without puncture. Develop. Med. Child. Neurol., 8:207-210.

Brodal, A. 1957. The Reticular Formation of the Brain Stem. Anatomical Aspects and Functional Correlations. London, Oliver and Boyd.

Brodmann, K. 1909. Vergleichende Lokalisationslehre der Großhirnrinde in Prinzipien dargestellt auf Grund des Zellenbaues. Leipzig, J. A. Barth.

Brookhardt, J. M. 1961. The cerebellum. In Field, J., ed. Handbook of Physiology. Washington, D.C., American Physiological Society, Sect. I., ch. 51.

ten Bruggencate, H. G., H. D. Henatsch, and H. Bossmann. 1964. Reduction of dynamic sensitivity of primary muscle spindle endings in experimental tremor. Experientia, 20:554.

Byers, R. K. 1938. Tonic neck reflexes in children considered from prognostic standpoint. Amer. J. Dis. Child., 55:696-742.

Cajal, S., and Y. Ramon. 1949. Histologie du Système Nerveuse de l'Homme et des Vertêbrés. Paris, Univ. Press, p. 949.

Camis, M. 1930. The Physiology of the Vestibular Apparatus. Creed, R. S., trans. London, Oxford University Press.

Campbell, A. W. 1905. Histological Studies on the Localisation of Cerebral Function. Cambridge, Cambridge University Press.

Carpenter, F. G., and R. M. Bergland. 1957. Excitation and conduction in immature nerve fibres of the developing chick. Amer. J. Physiol., 190:371-376.

Carpenter, M. B., J. W. Correl, and A. Hinman. 1960. Spinal tracts mediating sulthalamic hyperkinesia: Physiological effects of selective partial cordotomies upon physikinesia in rhesus monkey. J. Neurophysiol., 23:288-304.

Castillo, J. Del., and L. Stark. 1952. The effect of calcium ions on the motor end-plate potential. J. Physiol. (London), 116:507-515.

——— and B. Katz. 1954. The effect of magnesium on the activity of motor nerve endings. J. Physiol. (London), 124:553-559.

Churchill-Davidson, H. C., and R. P. Wise. 1963. Neuromuscular transmission in the newborn infant. Anesthesiology, 24:271-278.

Connor, G. J. 1941. Functional localization within anterior cerebellum. Proc. Soc. Exp. Biol. Med., 47:205-207.

Dale, H. H., W. Feldberg, and M. Vogt. 1936. Release of acetylcholine at voluntary motor nerve endings. J. Physiol. (London), 86:353-380.

Dietrich, H. F. 1957. A longitudinal study of the Babinski and plantar grasp reflexes in infancy. Amer. J. Dis. Child., 94:265-271.

Dow, R. S. 1942. Cerebellar action potentials in response to stimulation of cerebral cortex in monkeys and cats. J. Neurophysiol., 5:121-136.

———— and G. Moruzzi. 1958. The Physiology and Pathology of the Cerebellum. Minneapolis, University of Minnesota Press.

Dubowitz, V., Ö. F. Whittacker, B. H. Brown, and A. Robinson. 1968. Nerve conduction velocity. Develop. Med. Child Neurol., 10:741-749.

Duensing, F., and K. P. Schaefer. 1957. Die Neuronenaktivität in der Formatio reticularis des Rhombencephalon beim vestibulären Nystagmus. Arch. Psychiat. Nervenkr., 196:265-290.

Eccles, J. C. 1964. The Physiology of Synapses. Berlin, Göttingen, Heidelberg, Springer-Verlag.

———— P. Fatt, and K. Koketsu. 1954. Cholinergic and inhibitory synapses in a pathway from motor-axon collaterals to motoneurones. J. Physiol. (London), 126: 524-562.

———— R. M. Eccles, and A. Lundberg. 1957. The convergence of monosynaptic excitatory afferents on the many different species of alpha motoneurones. J. Physiol. (London), 137:22-50.

———— R. M. Eccles, and F. Magni. 1961. Ventral inhibitory action attributable to presynaptic depolarisation produced by muscle afferent volleys. J. Physiol. (London), 159:147-166.

———— P. G. Kostyuk, and R. F. Schmidt. 1962a. Presynaptic inhibition of the central actions of flexor reflex afferents. J. Physiol. (London), 161:258-281.

———— F. Magni, and W. D. Willis. 1962b. Depolarisation of central terminals of Group I afferent fibres from muscle. J. Physiol. (London), 160:62-93.

———— R. F. Schmidt, and W. D. Willis. 1962c. Presynaptic inhibition of the spinal monosynaptic reflex pathway. J. Physiol. (London), 161:282-297.

Eccles, R. M., and A. Lundberg. 1959. Synaptic actions in motoneurones by afferents which may evoke the flexion reflex. Arch. Ital. Biol., 97: 199-221.

———— and W. D. Willis. 1962. Presynaptic inhibition of the monosynaptic reflex pathway in kittens. J. Physiol. (London), 165: 403-420.

Ekholm, J. 1967. Postnatal changes in cutaneous reflexes and in the discharge pattern of cutaneous and articular sense organs: A morphological and physiological study in the cat. Acta Physiol. Scand., (Suppl. 297):1.

Erlanger, J., and H. S. Gasser. 1924. Compound nature of action current of nerve as disclosed by cathode-ray oscilloscope. Amer. J. Physiol., 70:624-666.

Escherich, T. 1888. Über die Saugbewegungen beim Neugeborenen. München Med. Wschr., 1:687-689.

Esente, L. 1958. Physiologie de la Vision chez le Prématuré et le Nourrisson Normal. Paris, Univ. Press, p. 22.

Fatt, P., and B. Katz. 1951. An analysis of the end-plate potential recorded with an intra-cellular electrode. J. Physiol. (London), 115:320-370.

Foerster, O. 1913. Das phylogenetische Moment in der spastischen Lähmung. Klin. Wschr., 1:1217, 1255.

Fra, L., and G. Gandiglio. 1966. Risposte faciali reflessi da percussione dei distretti mimici. Studio EMG. Boll. Soc. Ital. Biol. Sper., 42:978-980.

Freudenberg, E. 1931. In Pfaundler-Schloßmanns Handbuch der Kinderheilkunde. Berlin, Springer-Verlag, 4 Aufl., Vol. 1, p. 785.

Fulton, J. 1952. Physiologie des Nervensystems. Stuttgart, G. Thieme, p. 483.

Galant, S. 1917. Der Rückgratreflex. Dissertation, Basel.

Gamper, E., and T. R. Untersteiner. 1924. Über eine komplex gebaute postencephalitische Hyperkinese und ihre möglichen Beziehungen zu dem oralen Einstellautomatismus des Säuglings. Arch. Psychiat. Nervenkr., 71:282-303.

Gandiglio, G., L. Fra, and B. Bergamasco. 1965. Risposte faciali reflessi da stimolazione elettrica delle tre branche terminali del trigemino. Studio EMG Boll. Soc. Ital. Biol. Sper., 42:385-388.

Gentry, E. F., and C. A. Aldrich. 1948. Rooting reflex in the newborn infant. Incidence and effect on it of sleep. Amer. J. Dis. Child., 75:528-539.

Gernandt, B. E., and C. A. Thulin. 1955. Reciprocal effects upon spinal motoneurones from stimulation of bulbar reticular formation. J. Neurophysiol., 18:113-129.

Gesell, A. 1938. Tonic neck reflex in human infant, morphogenetic and clinical significance. J. Pediat., 13:455-464.

Giaquinto, S., O. Pompejano, and J. Somogyi. 1964a. Supraspinal modulation of heteronymous monosynaptic and of polysynaptic reflexes during natural sleep and wakefulness. Arch. Ital. Biol., 102:245-281.

———— O. Pompejano, and J. Somogyi. 1964b. Descending inhibitory influences on spinal reflexes during natural sleep. Arch. Ital. Biol., 102:282-307.

Glees, P. 1944. Anatomical basis of cortico-striate connexions. J. Anat., 78:47-51.

Granit, R. 1950. Reflex self-regulation of muscle contraction and autogenetic inhibition. J. Neurophysiol., 13:351-372.

———— and B. Kaada. 1952. Influence of stimulation of central nervous structures on muscle spindles in cat. Acta Physiol. Scand., 27:130-160.

———— H.-D. Henatsch, and G. Steg. 1956. Tonic and phasic ventral horn cells, differentiated by post-tetanic potentiation in cat extensors. Acta Physiol. Scand., 37:114-126.

Hampson, J. L. 1949. Relationships between cat cerebral and cerebellar cortices. J. Neurophysiol., 12:37-50.

Harlem, O. K., and A. Lönnum. 1957. A clinical study of the abdominal skin reflexes in newborn infants. Arch. Dis. Child., 32:127-130.

Harvey, A. M., and R. L. Masland. 1941. A method for the study of neuromuscular transmission in human subjects. Bull. Hopkins Hosp., 68:81-93.

Hassler, R. 1950. Über Kleinhirnprojektionen zum Mittelhirn und Thalamus beim Menschen. Deutsch. Z. Nervenheilk., 163:629-671.

———— 1953a. Erkankungen des Kleinhirns. In Schwiegk, H., ed. Handbuch der Inneren Medizin. Berlin, Springer-Verlag, 4 Aufl., pp. 620-668.

———— 1953b. Extrapyramidalmotorische Syndrome und Erkrankungen. Handbuch der Inneren Medizin. Berlin, Göttingen, Heidelberg, Springer-Verlag, 4th ed., pp. 676-904.

———— 1956. Die extrapyramidalen Rindensysteme und die zentrale Regelung der Motorik. Deutsch. Z. Nervenheilk., 175:233-258.

———— 1964. Pathologische Grundlagen der Klinik und Behandlung extrapyramidaler Erkankungen. Klin. Wschr., 42:404.

Henatsch, H.-D. 1962. Allgemeine Elektrophysiologie erregbarer Strukturen. *In* Landau-Rosemann, H. V. ed. Lehrbuch der Physiologie des Menschen. München, Urban & Schwarzenberg, 28 Aufl. Bd. 2.

———— F. J. Schulte, and G. Busch. 1959. Wandelbarkeit des tonischen und phasischen Reaktionstyps einzelner Extensor-Motoneurone bei Variation ihrer Antriebe. Pflueger. Arch. Ges. Physiol., 270:161-173.

Hodes, R., and J. Gribetz. 1962. H-reflex in normal human infants; depression of these electrically induced reflexes in sleep. Proc. Soc. Exp. Biol. Med., 110: 577-580.

———— and W. C. Dement. 1964. Depression of electrically induced reflexes in man during low voltage EEG sleep. Electroenceph. Clin. Neurophysiol., 17:617-629.

Hoffmann, P. 1922. Untersuchungen über Eigenreflexe (Sehnenreflexe) menschlicher Muskeln. Berlin, Springer-Verlag.

———— 1934. Die physiologischen Eigenschaften der Eigenreflexe. Ergebn. Physiol., 36:15-108.

Holmes, G. 1922. Clinical symptoms of cerebellar disease and their interpretation. Lancet, 1:1177-1182, 1231-1237. 2:59-65, 111-115.

———— 1939. Cerebellum of man. Hughlins Jackson Memorial Lecture. Brain, 62: 1-30.

Hopf, H. C., H. J. Hufschmidt, and J. Ströder. 1964. Über die "Ausbreitungsreaktion" nach Trigeminusreifung beim Säugling. Ann. Paediat. (Basel), 203:89-100.

Hugelin, A., M. Bonvalet, and P. Dell. 1959. Activation réticulaire et corticale d'origine chimoreceptie au cours de l'hypoxie. Electroenceph. Clin. Neurophysiol., 11:325-340.

Hunt, C. C. 1954. Relation of function to diameter in afferent fibres of muscle nerves. J. Gen. Physiol., 38:117-131.

———— and A. S. Paintal. 1958. Spinal reflex regulation of fusimotor neurones. J. Physiol. (London), 143:195-212.

Hursh, J. B. 1939. The properties of growing nerve fibres. Amer. J. Physiol., 127: 140-153.

Ingram, T. T. S. 1960. Little Club Summer Meeting, Groningen.

Isbert, H., and A. Peiper. 1927. Über die Körperstellung des Säuglings. Jb. Kinderheilk., 115:142-176.

Joppich, G., and F. J. Schulte. 1968. Neurologie des Neugeborenen. Berlin, Springer-Verlag.

Jung, R., and R. Hassler. 1960. The extrapyramidal motor system. *In* Field, J., ed. Handbook of Physiology. Washington, D.C., American Physiological Society, Sect. I, Vol. 2, pp. 863-927.

Koch, E. 1932. Die Irradiation der pressoreceptorischen Kreislaufreflexe. Klin. Wschr., 11:225-227.

Kuffler, S. W., C. C. Hunt, and J. P. Quilliam. 1951. Function of medullated small-nerve fibres in mammalian ventral roots: Efferent muscle spindle innervation. J. Neurophysiol., 14:29-54.

Kugelberg, E. 1952. Facial reflexes. Brain, 75:385-396.

Landau, A. 1923. Über einen tonischen Lagereflex beim älteren Säugling. Klin. Wschr., 2:1253-1255.

———— 1925. Über motorische Besonderheiten des zweiten Lebenshalbjahres. Mschr. Kinderheilk., 29:555-558.

Laporte, Y., and P. Bessou. 1959. Modification d'excitabilité de motoneurones homonymes provoqués par l'activation physiologique de fibres afférentes d'origine musculaire du groupe II. J. Physiol. (Paris), 51:897-908.

Lassek, A. M. 1942. Human pyramidal tract; study of mature myelinated fibres of pyramid. J. Comp. Neurol., 76:217-225.

Laursen, A. M. 1962a. Movements evoked from the region of the caudate nucleus in cats. Acta Physiol. Scand., 54:175-184.

———— 1962b. Inhibition evoked from the region of the caudate nucleus in cats. Acta Physiol. Scand., 54:185-190.

Lawrence, M. M., and C. R. Feind. 1953. Vestibular responses to rotation in newborn infants. Pediatrics, 12:300-305.

Leksell, L. 1945. The action potential and excitatory effects of the small ventral root fibres to skeletal muscle. Acta Physiol. Scand., 10 (Suppl. 3): 1-84.

Lenard, H. G., H. von Bernuth, and H. F. R. Prechtl. 1968. Reflexes and their relationship to behavioural state in the newborn. Acta Paediat. Scand., 57:177.

Lilly, J. C. 1958. In Harlow, H. F., and C. N. Woolsey, eds. Biological and Biochemical Bases of Behavior. Madison, University of Wisconsin Press.

Lippmann, C. 1958. Über den Babkin'schen Reflex. Dissertation, Leipzig, 1958. Arch. Kinderheilk., 157:234.

Lloyd, D. P. C. 1944. Functional organization of the spinal cord. Physiol. Rev., 24:1-17.

———— and H. T. Chang. 1948. Afferent fibres in the muscle nerves. J. Neurophysiol., 11:199-207.

Magnus, R. 1924. Körperstellung. Berlin, Fischer Verlag.

———— and A. de Kleijn. 1912. Die Abhängigkeit des Tonus der Extremitätenmuskulatur von der Kopfstellung. Pflueger. Arch. Ges. Physiol., 145:455-548.

Magoun, H. W. 1954. The Waking Brain. Springfield, Ill., Charles C Thomas, Publisher.

———— and R. Rhines. 1946. Inhibitory mechanism in the bulbar reticular formation. J. Neurophysiol., 9:165-171.

Marinesco, G., and A. Radovici. 1920. Sur une réflexe cutané nouveau réflexe palmo-mentonier. Rev. Neurol. (Paris), 27:237-240.

Matthews, B. H. C. 1933. Nerve endings in mammalian muscles. J. Physiol. (London), 78:1-53.

Matthews, P. B. C. 1964. Muscle spindles and their motor control. Physiol. Rev., 44:219-288.

McNalley, W. J., and E. A. Stuart. 1942. Physiology of labyrinth reviewed in relation to seasickness and other forms of motion sickness. War Med. (Chicago), 2:683-771.

Mettler, F. A. 1944. An origin of fibres in pyramid of primate brain. Proc. Soc. Exp. Biol. Med., 57:111-113.

———— H. W. Ades, E. Lipman, and A. A. Culler. 1939. Extrapyramidal system; experimental demonstration of function. Arch. Neurol. (Chicago), 41:984-995.

Michaelis, R., and F. J. Schulte. 1969. Neurological examination and estimation of postmenstrual age in abnormal newborn infants. In preparation.

———— F. J. Schulte, and R. Nolte. 1970. Motor behavior of small for gestational age newborn infants. J. Pediat., 76:208-213.

Monod, N., J. Eliet-Flescher, and C. Dreyfus-Brisac. 1967. The sleep of the full-term newborn and premature infant. Biol. Neonat., 11:216-247.

Moro, E. 1918. Das erste Trimenon. München. Med. Wschr., 65:1147-1150.

Moruzzi, G. 1950. Problems in Cerebellar Physiology. Springfield, Ill. Charles C Thomas, Publisher.

———— 1960. Synchronizing influences of the brain stem and the inhibitory mechanisms underlying the production of sleep by sensory stimulation. *In* Jasper, H. H., and G. D. Smirnow, eds. Moscow Collokquium, 1958. Electroenceph. Clin. Neurophysiol., 12 (Suppl. 13) : 231.

———— 1964. Reticular influences on the EEG. Electroenceph. Clin. Neurophysiol., 16: 2-17.

———— and H. W. Magoun. 1949. Brain stem reticular formation and activation of the EEG. Electroenceph. Clin. Neurophysiol., 1:455-473.

von Muralt, A. 1958. Neue Ergebnisse der Nervenphysiologie. Berlin, Springer-Verlag.

Naka, K. J. 1964. Electrophysiology of the fetal spinal cord. II. Interaction among peripheral and recurrent inhibition. J. Gen. Physiol., 47:1023-1038.

Nolte, R., et al. 1969. Bioelectric brain maturation in small-for-dates infants. Develop. Med. Child Neurol., 11:83-93.

Orthner, H., and F. Roeder. 1969. Die Entwicklung der Motorik beim Menschen. In preparation.

Paillard, J. 1954. Eléments d'une étude psychophysiologique du "Tonus musculaire." Bull. Psycho. (Paris), 12:653.

Parmelee, A. H. 1963. The palmomental reflex in premature infants. Develop. Med. Child Neurol., 5:381-387.

———— 1964. A critical evaluation of the Moro reflex. Pediatrics, 33:773-788.

———— et al. 1968. Maturation of EEG activity during sleep in premature infants. Electroenceph. Clin. Neurophysiol., 24:319-329.

Patton, H. D. 1965. Special properties of nerve trunks and tracts. *In* Ruch, T. C., and H. D. Patton, eds. Physiology and Biophysics. Philadelphia, W. B. Saunders Company, pp. 73-94.

Peiper, A. 1926. Über das Pupillenspiel des Säuglings. Jb. Kinderheilk., 112:179-183.

———— 1928. Die Hirntätigkeit des Säuglings. Berlin, Fischer Verlag.

———— 1963. Die Eigenart der kindlichen Hirntätigkeit. Leipzig, VEB Thieme.

Penfield, W., and H. Jasper. 1954. Epilepsy and the Functional Anatomy of the Human Brain. Boston, Little, Brown and Company.

Pepsy, S. 1933. *Cited in* K. C. Pratt, Murchison's Handbook of Psychology, 2nd ed. Worcester, Mass., Clark University Press.

Poeck, K. 1968. Die Bedeutung der Reizqualität für die Greifreflexe beim menschlichen Neugeborenen und Säugling. Deutsch. Z. Nervenheilk., 192:317-327.

Pollack, S. L. 1960. The grasp response in the neonate: Its characteristics and interaction with the tonic neck reflex. Arch. Neurol. (Chicago), 3:574-581.

Pollock, L. J., and L. Davis. 1927. Influence of cerebellum upon reflex activities of decerebrate animal. Brain, 50:277-312.

Prechtl, H. F. R. 1953. Über die Kopplung von Saugen und Greifreflex beim Säugling. Naturwissenschaften, 40:347.

———— 1968. Polygraphic studies of the fullterm newborn. II. Computer analysis of recorded data. *In* Bax, M., and R. C. McKeith, eds. Studies in Infancy. London, S. J. M. P. Heinemann.

———— and W. M. Scheidt. 1950. Auslösende und steuernde Mechanismen des Säuglings. I. Z. Vgl. Physiol., 32:257-262.

———— and W. M. Scheidt. 1951. Auslösende und steuernde Mechanismen des Saugaktes. II. Z. Vgl. Physiol., 33:53-62.

———— and A. R. Knol. 1958. Der Einfluß der Beckenendlage auf die Fußsohlenreflexe beim neugeborenen Kind. Arch. Psychiat. Nervenkr., 196:542.

———— and D. Beintema. 1964. The Neurological Examination of the Newborn. London, William Heinemann Medical Books, Ltd.

———— and H. G. Lenard. 1968. Verhaltensphysiologie des Neugeborenen. *In* Linneweh, F., ed. Fortschritte der Paedologie. Berlin, Springer-Verlag.

———— V. Vlach, H. G. Lenard, and P. K. Grant. 1967. Exteroceptive and tendon reflexes in various behavioural states in the newborn infant. Biol. Neonat., 11:159-175.

Rabinowicz, T. 1964. The cerebral cortex of the premature infant of the 8th month. Prog. Brain Res., 4:39-86.

Rademaker, G. G. J. 1931. Das Stehen. Berlin, Springer-Verlag.

———— and J. W. G. Ter Braak. 1936. Das Umdrehen der fallenden Katze in der Luft. Acta Otolaryng. (Stockholm), 23:313-343.

Renshaw, B. 1941. Influence of discharge of motoneurons upon excitation of neighboring motoneurons. J. Neurophysiol., 4:167-183.

———— 1946. Central effects of centripedale impulses in axons of spinal ventral roots. J. Neurophysiol., 9:190-204.

Rhines, R., and H. W. Magoun. 1946. Brain stem facilitation of cortical motor response. J. Neurophysiol., 9:219-229.

Richards, T. W., and O. C. Irwin. 1935. Iowa Studies in Child Welfare. Iowa, Vol. 11, No. 1.

Ritter, C. 1924. Über das Verhältnis von Extremitätenbeugern zu Streckern beim Neugeborenen unter Berücksichtigung seiner Haltung. Jb. Kinderheilk., 104:293-300.

Robinson, L. 1891. *In* Darwinismus in the nursery. Nineteenth Century, 30:831.

Robinson, R. J. 1966. Assessment of gestational age by neurological examination. Arch. Dis. Child., 41:437-447.

Rossi, G. 1912. Singli effetti conseguenti alla stimolazione contemporanea della corteccia cerebrale e di quella cerebellare. Arch. Fisiol., 10:389-399.

Ruch, T. C. 1965. Physiology and Biophysics. Philadelphia, W. B. Saunders Company.

Ruppert, E. S., and E. W. Johnson. 1968. Motor nerve conduction velocities in low birth weight infants. Pediatrics, 42:255-260.

Rushworth, G. 1962. Observations on blink reflexes. J. Neurophysiol., 25:93-108.

Saint Anne-Dargassies, S. 1954. Méthode d'examin neurologique sur la nouveau-né. Étud. Neonat. 3:101.

———— 1955. La maturation neurologique du prémature. Rev. Neurol. (Paris), 93:331-340.

———— 1966. Neurological maturation of the premature infant of 28-42 weeks gestational age. *In* Faulkner, F., ed. Human Development. Philadelphia, W. B. Saunders Company.

Schaefer, K. P. 1965. Die Erregungsmuster einzelner Neurone des Abducens-Kernes beim Kaninchen. Pflueger. Arch. Ges. Physiol., 284:31-52.

Schaltenbrand, G. 1925. Normale Bewegungs- und Lagereaktionen bei Kindern. Deutsch. Z. Nervenheilk., 87:23-59.

Scherer, H., and R. Hernández-Péon. 1955. Inhibitory influence of reticular formation upon synaptic transmission in facialis nucleus. Fed. Proc., 14:132.

Schoch, E. O. 1948. Über die stammesgeschichtliche Bedeutung und die biologische Zusammengehörigkeit der Fußsohlenreflexe. Grenzgeb. Med., 1:111-113.

———— 1949. Die Fußsohlenreflexe als phylogenetisch bedingte Greif- und Loslassreflexe. Homo 1,1 Bd., 148-149.

Schulte, F. J.   1964.   Reflex activation and inhibition of spinal motoneurones of the newborn. *In* Symposuim on Neurology of the Newborn, Rome, April, 1964.

———— 1968.   Gestation, Wachstum und Hirnentwicklung. *In* Linneweh, F., ed. Fortschritte der Paedologie, Vol. II. Berlin, Springer-Verlag, pp. 46-64.

———— and R. Michaelis.   1965.   Zur Physiologie und Pathophysiologie der neuromuskulären Erregungsübertragung beim Neugeborenen. Klin. Wschr., 43:295-300.

———— and W. Schwenzel.   1965.   Motor control and muscle tone in the newborn period. Electromyographic studies. Biol. Neonat., 8:198-215.

———— G. Albert, and R. Michaelis.   1969.   Gestationsalter und Nervenleitgeschwindigkeit bei normalen und abnormen Neugeborenen. Deutsch. Med. Wschr., 94: 599-601.

———— G. Busch, and H.-D. Henatsch.   1959a.   Antriebssteigerungen lumbaler Extensor-Motoneurone bei Aktivierung der Chemoreceptoren im Glomus caroticum. Pflueger. Arch. Ges. Physiol., 269:580-592.

———— H.-D. Henatsch, and G. Busch.   1959b.   Über den Einfluß der Carotissinus-Sensibilität auf die spinalmotorischen Systeme. Pflueger Arch. Ges. Physiol., 269: 248-263.

———— R. Michaelis, and E. Filipp.   1965.   Neurologie des Neugeborenen. I. Ursachen und klinische Symptomatologie von Funktionsstörungen des Nervensystems bei Neugeborenen. Z. Kinderheilk., 93:242-263.

———— J. Linke, R. Michaelis, and R. Nolte.   1968a.   Electromyographic analysis of the Moro-reflex in term, preterm and small-for-dates newborn infants. Develop. Psychobiol., 1:41-47.

———— J. Linke, R. Michaelis, and R. Nolte.   1968b.   Excitation, inhibition and impulse conduction in spinal motoneurones of preterm, term, and small-for-dates newborn infants. *In* Robinson R., ed. CIBA Foundation Study Group, London, February 12-16, 1968.

———— R. Michaelis, J. Linke, and R. Nolte.   1968c.   Motor nerve conduction velocity in term, preterm and small-for-dates newborn infants. Pediatrics, 42:17-26.

Schur, E.   1922.   Studien über das statische Organ normaler Säuglinge und Kinder. Z. Kinderheilk., 32:227-239.

Schweitzer, A., and S. Wright.   1937.   Effects on knee jerk of stimulation of the central end of the vagus and of various changes in the circulation and respiration. J. Physiol. (London), 88:459-475.

Sherrington, C. S.   1898.   Decerebrate rigidity and reflex coordination of movements. J. Physiol. (London), 22:319.

Skoglund, S.   1960a.   On the postnatal development of postural mechanisms as revealed by electromyography and myography in decerebrate kittens. Acta Physiol. Scand., 49:299-317.

———— 1960b.   The spinal transmission of proprioceptive reflexes and the postnatal development of conduction velocity in different hindlimb nerves in the kitten. Acta Physiol. Scand., 49:318-329.

———— 1960c.   The activity of muscle receptors in the kitten. Acta Physiol. Scand., 50:203-221.

Snider, R. S., and A. Stowell.   1944.   Receiving areas of tactile, auditory and visual systems in cerebellum. J. Neurophysiol., 7:331-357.

Sprague, J. M., and W. W. Chambers.   1954.   Control and posture by reticular formation and cerebellum in intact, anesthetized and unanesthetized, and in decerebrated cat. Amer. J. Physiol., 176:52-54.

Stirnimann, F. 1938. Das Kriech- und Schreitphänomen der Neugeborenen. Schweiz. Med. Wschr., 68:1374-1376.

———— and W. Stirnimann. 1940. Der Fußgreifreflex bei Neugeborenen und Säuglingen. Seine diagnostische Verwendbarkeit. Ann. Paediat. (Basel), 154:249-264.

Takeuchi, N. 1963. Effects of calcium on the conductance change of the end plate membrane during the action of transmitter. J. Physiol. (London), 167:141-155.

Tasaki, J. 1953. Nervous Transmission. Springfield, Ill. Charles C Thomas, Publisher.

Taylor, J., ed. 1956. Selected Writings of John Huglings Jackson. New York, Basic Books, Inc.

Theile, F. W. 1884. Nova Acta physiko-medica Acad. Leopold-Carol. (D.) 46, no. 3, p. 133. Cited by Peiper, A. 1963. Die Eigenart der kindlichen Hirntätigkeit. Leipzig.

Thiemich, M. 1900. Über Tetanie und tetanoide Zustände im ersten Kindesalter. Jb. Kinderheilk., 51:222.

Thomson, J. 1903. On the lip-reflex of newborn children. Rev. Neurol. Psychiat., 1: 145-148.

Thornval, A. 1920-21. L'épreuve laborique chez les nouveau-nés. Acta Otolaryng. (Stockholm), 2:451-454.

Vlach, V. 1966. Exteroceptive trunk reflexes in the newborn infant. Cs. Neurol., 29: 240-247.

———— 1968. Some exteroceptive skin reflexes in the limbs and trunk in newborn. Clinics in Developmental Medicine, 27. Spastics International Medical Publications. London, W. Heinemann Medical Books, Ltd.

Vogt, C., and O. Vogt. 1919. Allgemeine Ergebnisse unserer Hirnforschung. J. Psychol. Neurol. (Leipzig), 25:279-461.

Vogt, O. 1903. Zur anatomischen Gliederung des Cortex cerebri. J. Psychol. Neurol. (Leipzig), 2:160-180.

Wang, G. H., and K. Akert. 1962. Behaviour and reflexes of chronic striadal cats. Arch. Ital. Biol., 100:48-85.

Wartenberg, R. 1952. Die Untersuchung der Reflexe. Cited by Peiper, A. 1963. Die Eigenart der kindlichen Hirntätigkeit. Leipzig.

von Woerkom, W. 1912. Sur la signification physiologique des réflexes cutanés des membres inférieurs; quelques considerations à propos de l'article de Marie et Foix. Rev. Neurol. (Paris), 20:285-291.

Wolff, P. H. 1959. Observations on newborn infants. Psychosom. Med., 21:110-118.

26

Biochemistry of Muscle Development

JEAN CLAUDE DREYFUS and FANNY SCHAPIRA •
Institut de Pathologie Moléculaire, Paris, France

Myogenesis

The striated musculature of vertebrates is from mesodermal origin. Boyd (1960) named the first stage of embryonic muscle cell "premyoblast." This cell cannot be distinguished from the associated fibroblasts.

The next stage of development following the premyoblast is the myoblast which is elongated but does not exhibit transverse striation. Then the cells become multinucleated with the nuclei still centrally situated, and at that stage the striation appears forming the myotube. Progressively the pale axial cytoplasmic core of the myotube disappears, while the nuclei migrate under the sarcoplasmic membrane. The mature muscular fiber is characterized by the transverse striation and peripheral nuclei.

Fenichel (1966) and Karpati and Engel (1968) have performed extensive histochemical studies on the development of the human skeletal muscle. From the fifth through the eighth weeks of gestation the muscle shows a syncytium of premyoblasts without mitotic figures. Multiple nuclei are located in the central region, and mitochondria are concentrated beneath the sarcolemma. Mitochondrial enzyme activity and glycogen are intense in regions of myofibrillar formation. From the tenth to the twentieth weeks of gestation the number of myotubes increases. At 20 weeks of gestation the myocytes become mature. There are differences among species regarding the fiber differentiation at birth. Dubowitz and Pearse (1960, 1961) have shown the existence of two distinct types of fibers (see below, p. 846). In newborn infants, in guinea pigs, and in rabbits the fibers are fully differentiated at birth; but in the rat the differentiation into two types of fibers occurs between the seventh and tenth postnatal days (Dubowitz, 1963).

During the later stages of embryonic development and during fetal life, the number of muscle fibers increases considerably. Couteaux (1941) has shown that this increase is due to the differentiation of fibroblastlike cells which surround the muscle fibers.

Konigsberg (1963) has studied myogenesis in the chick embryo in tissue cultures.

Multinucleated myotubes seem to be formed through a process of successive cell fusion which is the predominant, or even the sole, mechanism to form multinuclearity. Recently, Mintz and Baker (1967) showed that in skeletal muscle of allophenic mice, which consists of a mosaic of cells, a hybrid isoenzyme form of isocitrate dehydrogenase occurred, and they demonstrated that in each muscle cell nuclei of diverse origin are at work. They have consequently confirmed the origin of the syncytium by myoblast fusion. Proliferation of muscle cells does not affect their capacity to differentiate; but it is true that the myofibril formation begins not earlier than after proliferation is completed (Konigsberg, 1963).

Muscle Proteins

The soluble sarcoplasmic fraction of muscle protein is relatively greater in fetuses than in adults. In skeletal muscle of 16-day-old rabbit fetuses, the sarcoplasmic nitrogen concentration was found to be higher than myofibrillar nitrogen (Perry and Hartshorne, 1963). During gestation the percentage of the sarcoplasmic nitrogen fraction decreases while the myofibrillar fraction increases.

MYOFIBRILLAR PROTEINS

Striated myofibrils may be detected very early; however, a contractile reaction to direct electric stimulation cannot be demonstrated before the sixteenth day in the rabbit fetus. At the end of gestation the relative amount of myofibrillar proteins suddenly increases. Csapo and Herrmann (1951) have initiated these studies (see also Herrmann, 1952). By measuring the decrease in viscosity the authors found a sharp increase in the actomyosin content beginning on the twelfth day of gestation, but some myosin was already present before the ninth day. Actin appears later than myosin, but its rate of increase is faster than that of myosin. The formation of other extractable proteins seemed to be slower.

In the chick embryo traces of myosin have been detected as early as 16 hours after the beginning of incubation by an immunologic technique, and actin and myosin in skeletal muscle were found after 3 days of incubation.

Perry and Hartshorne (1963) have prepared myosin from fetal rabbit muscle. The electrophoretic pattern and pH activity curve were similar in the fetus and adult, but adenosine triphosphatase (ATP-ase) activity was low in fetal myosin; it was only 10 percent on the sixteenth day and 60 percent on the thirtieth day compared to the ATP-ase activity of adult muscle.

Barany et al. (1965a) have measured the nucleoside triphosphatase activity of myosin in newborn rabbits, and they found a low activity. However, the combination with actin is of the same extent as measured for adult myosin. Muscles of newborn mammals are physiologically slow in reactivity; Barany et al. (1965b) assigned this property to the low nucleoside triphosphatase activity and compared it to the slow muscles of adults.

Crepax (1952) has shown that fetal actomyosin migrates faster electrophoretically than that of adult muscles. The different content of nucleic acids could explain the different speed of migration. In this context it might be important that fetal actin forms a complex with nucleic acids (Ravikovitch and Kasavina, 1952). Villafranca (1956) suggested that an inactive myosin exists in fetal muscle before the appearance of myosin with ATP-ase activity.

Marcaud-Raeber (1959a, b, c) discovered a new component in myofibrils, the "metamyosin," which is especially abundant in fetal muscle and which disappears almost completely before birth. This protein does not combine with actin, has no ATP-ase activity, and is very viscous. Marcaud-Raeber separated two types of metamyosin; in fetal muscle the electrophoretically slow type predominates. These observations raise the question as to whether a similar precursor of metamyosin exists also for other proteins. The metamyosin from fetal pig and sheep muscles contains salt-soluble collagen (Needham and Williams, 1963). Furthermore, it might be interesting to note that Engel et al. (1964) have compared protein of rods found in nemaline myopathy to the metamyosin.

Recently, Trayer et al. (1968) described a difference in the amino acid composition of fetal and adult myosin; in some peptides of adult myosin histidine is replaced by 3-methyl-histidine; however, methyl-histidine is present in actin of adult and fetal animals.

MYOGLOBIN

Myoglobin is much less abundant in fetal than in adult muscle as was demonstrated in man by Kagen and Christian (1966). However, the very conflicting problem remains as to whether a specific fetal form exists.

In 1952, Jonxis and Wadman prepared a purified solution of myoglobin from heart muscle of a full-term bovine fetus. Its alkali denaturation and solubility revealed that it is different from adult myoglobin. However, improved purification techniques showed discrepant results. Rossi-Fannelli et al. (1959) were able to obtain a crystalline myoglobin from human and bovine fetal heart. They separated three components by electrophoresis and chromatography. The amino acid composition and physicochemical properties were revealed to be the same in fetal and in adult myoglobins. Nevertheless, Singer et al. (1955) found different absorption spectrums and electrophoretic mobilities in fetal and adult human myoglobins.

Perkoff (1966) studied 34 fetal human muscles and isolated the muscle heme proteins. From chromatographic, electrophoretic, and spectralanalytic studies he concluded that a fetal form of myoglobin does actually exist. He (1964) compared it to abnormal myoglobin as described in some cases of muscular dystrophy and as recently analyzed by Miyoshi et al. (1968). Wolfson et al. (1967) investigated fetal myoglobin that has been prepared by two different techniques; they were able to show that the electrophoretically fast moving component of fetal heme protein is similar to fetal hemoglobin. More recent immunologic studies confirmed the identity of this fraction with fetal hemoglobin; the other fractions are identical with adult myoglobin. Perkoff (1968) has now recognized that there is no evidence for the existence of a specific heme protein in fetal muscle.

SARCOPLASMIC PROTEINS

The soluble proteins are more acidic in fetal than in adult muscle. On the sixteenth day of gestation the basic fraction accounts for about 16 percent in fetal rabbit muscle. It increases to 30 percent at birth and reaches 80 percent not earlier than several months after birth. Hartshorne and Perry (1962) have shown that starch gel electrophoresis reveals more cathodic bands in adult than in fetal rabbit muscle. Chromatography on diethylamino-ethyl cellulose revealed that fetal sarcoplasmic proteins are more similar in composition to heart proteins than to skeletal muscle proteins of adults. Further studies have confirmed these facts and, moreover, have shown that some analogies exist between red (slow) adult muscles and fetal muscles; however, the latter contain little myoglobin.

Enzymes

The enzymatic development in muscle was studied mainly by histochemical techniques.

Dubowitz (1966) has shown that in mammalian and avian muscles a reciprocal relationship exists between phosphorylase (representative for glycogenolysis) and oxidative enzymes (of which succinate dehydrogenase has been mainly studied). The same author described two types of fibers in human muscle: The group of larger fibers has high phosphorylase activity and low activities of oxidative enzymes, and the group of smaller fibers has low phosphorylase and high oxidative enzyme activities. Engel (1962) has found that ATP-ase activity is correlated with phosphorylase activity. According to Pearse (1961) the larger fibers are rich in glycerol-3-phosphate dehydrogenase.

The onset of differentiation into the two types of fibers varies in different species. Cosmos (1966) and Cosmos and Butler (1967) have studied the ontogenic differentiation in chicken muscle. In chick embryo the development of red fibers (slow contraction) precedes that of white fibers (fast contraction). Phosphorylase activity is low in the embryo, and phosphorylase a is almost absent. Phosphorylase activity increases rapidly in white fibers after hatching and reaches the adult value at 6 weeks of age. In embryonic breast muscle glycerol-3-phosphate dehydrogenase and lactate dehydrogenase activities are low, while succinate dehydrogenase is high. After hatching, succinate dehydrogenase decreases at the time when red fibers disappear, while the other enzymes increase. Fenichel (1966) has studied the muscle development in human fetuses. From 5 to 8 weeks of gestation the majority of cells form a syncytium of premyoblasts. From 8 to 10 weeks myotubes predominate, and they have central nuclei and a positive ATP-ase reaction (type II fibers); mitochondrial enzyme activity is intense but type I fibers are still small. From 10 to 20 weeks the nuclei are migrating, and at 20 weeks the two fiber types become equal in number; the type I fibers are growing larger than the type II ones. Fenichel (1966) compares this evolution to the development of the same fibers in fetal mice, as studied by Wirsen and Larsson (1964). Dubowitz (1966) has studied this enzymatic ontogeny more extensively by histochemical methods. Before the eighteenth week of gestation the pattern does not show fiber differentiation; some skeletal muscles display a certain enzyme pattern, other muscles another one, but this does not occur systematically. From 20 to 26 weeks a differentiation occurs between the two types of fibers of which the majority belongs to the phosphorylase-rich type. At the end of gestation the distribution of the two types is approximately equal, and the pattern resembles that of the adult.

Experimental cross-innervation of slow and fast muscles showed not only an interconvertibility of muscle types but also consequent enzyme changes. Yellin (1967) and Guth and Watson (1967) performed these experiments in adult rats and demonstrated the important role of innervation in physiologic and biochemical differentiation. Dubowitz (1967) has performed cross-innervation experiments in newborn animals; fast or mixed muscles show a transformation to a pattern resembling the m. soleus pattern; but in the m. soleus of newborns the changes were less extensive.

Cholinesterase is found in myoneural junctions, and it plays a fundamental role in the transmission of nervous stimulation to the muscle fiber; histochemically this was detected by Couteaux (1955). Mavrenskaya (1963) has shown that cholinesterase appears first along the nerve fibers (at six weeks of gestation) and then in the neuromuscular junction; in the beginning it shows a pattern, and later it becomes more localized. The appearance of cholinesterase activity coincides with the first movements.

Creatine kinase is very specific for muscle, and its ontogeny is of great interest. In a tissue culture of chick embryo, Konigsberg (1963) detected no creatine kinase activity before the seventh day; its later increase correlates well with the initiation of contraction. Stave (1964) found that the activity is much lower in rabbit fetuses at the end of gestation and in newborn than in adult muscles (see Fig. 3, p. 849). In skeletal muscle of chick embryo, Eppenberger et al. (1962-63) showed that the development of creatine kinase activity is similar in comparison to actomyosin appearance; the author defined four stages of development: 1, Creatine kinase synthesis begins in the myoblast, but phosphocreatine (substrate) is very low, and consequently it seems that the enzyme cannot function. 2, Cross-striation and contractile proteins appear, but phosphocreatine remains low. 3, On the thirteenth day true myofibrils appear. Actomyosin and creatine kinase concentrations increase sharply, and soon phosphocreatine becomes abundant. 4, After hatching, the concentration of specific proteins and enzymes increases.

Eppenberger et al. (1964) also studied other cytoplasmic enzymes, and they concluded from their work on chick embryos that in the first days glycolysis is the only source of energy in most tissues, including muscle. However, their data do not indicate that glucose is the only source of substrates for glycolysis. It seems that amino acids are another important source for yielding metabolic fuel.

Bocek and Beatty (1967) found that glycogenolysis is especially high in muscles from monkey fetuses near term (on the one hundred and fiftieth day of gestation), and this finding may explain, partially, the increased resistance of the fetus to anoxia.

The possible role of exercise to induce the biosynthesis of several enzymes in newborn animals has been emphasized by Kendrick-Jones and Perry (1967).

These authors studied and compared the diaphragm and leg muscles of rat and rabbit; the activities of creatine kinase, AMP deaminase, and adenylate kinase reach adult values at birth in the diaphragm and considerably later in leg muscle. In other species which are more mature at birth, as, for example, chick and guinea pig, a relatively high level of these enzymes appears in skeletal muscle during fetal life.

The pentose phosphate cycle is more active in fetal than in adult muscle; this has been shown for several species, especially the monkey (Beatty et al., 1965) and the rabbit (Ilyin, 1965-66). Glucose-6-phosphate dehydrogenase and 6-phosphogluconate dehydrogenase are high in fetal muscle while these activities are very low in adult muscle, particularly in white fibers.

Little is known about the postnatal development of muscle enzymes in *man*. Hooft et al. (1966) have studied 14 muscle biopsies from children between birth and the age of 14 years. The activities of sarcoplasmic enzymes, such as creatine kinase, aldolase, and lactate dehydrogenase, increase with age. However, the mitochondrial malate dehydrogenase seems to decrease postnatally.

The perinatal changes of glycolytic and Krebs cycle enzyme activities have been studied by biochemical methods in m. psoas major of the rabbit (Stave, 1964). Figures 1 and 2 demonstrate the low specific activity of five glycolytic enzyme activities in the perinatal period. Hexokinase, however, was found to be up to 27 times higher immediately after birth than in adults. Thereafter it decreases rapidly. This observation might explain the very active prenatal glycogen deposition in skeletal muscles, since the blood glucose is channeled into the muscle cells by this

Fig. 1. Enzyme activities of perinatal rabbit muscle (m. psoas major), calculated in units per extracted protein and expressed in percent of adult values. HK, hexokinase (EC 2.7.1.1); G A P D H, glyceraldehydephosphate dehydrogenase (EC 1.2.1.9); GDH, glycerol-3-phosphate dehydrogenase (EC 1.1.1.8); LDH, lactate dehydrogenase (EC 1.1.1.27). (Data from Stave, 1964. Revised and supplemented, courtesy of Dr. Stave.)

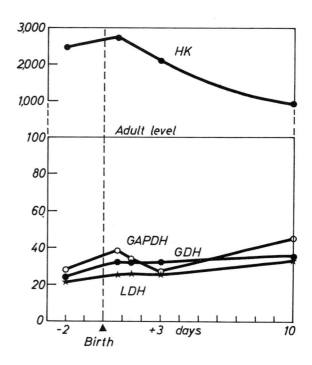

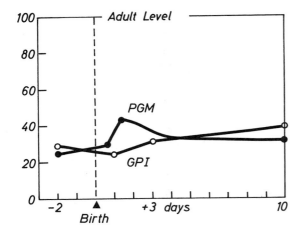

Fig. 2. Enzyme activities of perinatal rabbit muscle; same presentation as in Figure 1. PGM, phosphoglucomutase (EC 2.7.5.1); PGI, glucose-phosphate isomerase (EC 5.3.1.9). (Data from Stave, 1964. Revised and supplemented, courtesy of Dr. Stave.)

phosphorylation process. In Figure 3 some enzyme activities of the Krebs cycle and related reactions are shown for the perinatal period. All of those increase in the immediate perinatal period, and all are several times higher in fetal and newborn than in adult muscle. From this observation, the simultaneous low glycolytic enzyme activities, and the exceptionally high concentrations of amino acids (see below),

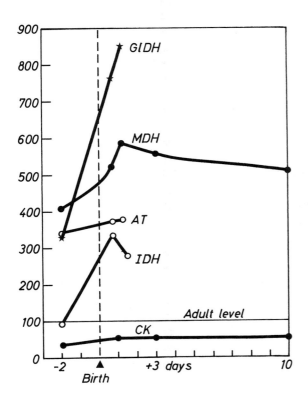

Fig. 3. Enzyme activities of perinatal rabbit muscle; same presentation as in Figure 1. GlDH, glutamate dehydrogenase (EC 1.4.1.2); MDH, malate dehydrogenase (EC 1.1.1.37); AT, aspartate aminotransferase (EC 2.6.1.1); IDH, isocitrate dehydrogenase (EC 1.1.1.42); CK, creatine kinase (EC 2.7.3.2). (Data from Stave, 1964. Revised and supplemented, courtesy of Dr. Stave.)

one might speculate that the perinatal skeletal muscle utilizes amino acids for energy production in preference to glucose.

ISOENZYMES

The study of enzymatic ontogeny has been stimulated by the discovery of multiple molecular forms of enzymes (isoenzymes). Pfleiderer and Wachsmuth (1961) showed first that the isoenzyme pattern of lactate dehydrogenase (LDH) changes during ontogeny in human tissues; animal tissues have been analyzed by Markert and Møller (1959), Appella and Markert (1961), Markert and Ursprung (1962), and Cahn et al. (1962). Two basic types of LDH subunits exist, the muscle type (M) and the heart type (H). Each LDH isoenzyme is composed of four of these subunits, and the random combination leads to the formation of five different isoenzymes of the same molecular weight, but they are of different charge. The five LDH isoenzymes can be separated by electrophoresis (on starch gel, agar, cellulose acetate, and so on). At alkaline pH, the most anodic isoenzyme (1) is a pure tetramer of H-subunits; the most cathodic isoenzyme (5) is a pure tetramer of M-subunits. The intermediary isoenzymes are hybrids. Several other methods (Dreyfus and Schapira, 1967) have also been used to separate these isoenzymes, but the different methods are in good agreement. A distinct ontogenetic evolution can be observed in muscles of some species, especially man: Of the LDH isoenzyme subunits the type M is predominant in adult muscle, while the type H predominates in fetuses. This fact was first noted by Dreyfus et al. (1962) for man. Chicken embryo and rabbit fetal muscle show an analogous development (Kaplan and Cahn, 1962; Fine et al., 1963). In beef and sheep the same evolutionary change from H type toward the M type occurs (Masters, 1964). This is in contrast to rat and mouse muscle (Schapira and Dreyfus, 1965), where no specific LDH isoenzyme pattern changes occur, and the fetal and the adult muscle contain only type M. Goodfriend et al. (1966) have shown that oxygen represses the biosynthesis of M-subunits; however, it remains difficult to explain the differences in the ontogenic evolution of isoenzymes among species.

The histochemical difference between the two types of muscle fibers applies also to the isoenzyme pattern. The rabbit m. soleus, which is a red muscle with slow contraction, has a predominant H type pattern (similar to the heart) while white muscles, as, for example, the m. gastrocnemius or the breast muscles of chicken, both with fast contraction, show a predominant type M pattern. The isoenzyme pattern of red muscles is similar to the isoenzyme pattern of fetal white muscles.

In long-term tissue cultures, Vesell et al. (1962) have shown that various tissues tend to assume a similar LDH isoenzyme pattern—the sequential alteration is the same for fetal muscles of different species, and it always develops in a predominantly M type form (effect of aging in culture and/or lack of oxygen).

Takasu and Hughes (1966) have emphasized that the isoenzyme pattern varies considerably in the various muscles of human adults. This is in contrast to young fetuses which have a more uniform pattern; at term the pattern is already less different from adults.

The isoenzymes of several other enzymes show also an ontogenic development. Creatine kinase, for example, has been shown to be a dimer and was especially studied (Eppenberger et al., 1964; Dawson et al., 1965; Dance and Watts, 1962). Each subunit may be of muscle type (M) or brain type (B); electrophoretically separated at an alkaline pH, type B is the most anodic. The hybrid MB has an intermediate position. In embryonic chicken Eppenberger et al. (1964) found only the isoenzyme BB (pure brain type); later the isoenzyme BB disappeared slowly, and the hybrid BM type appeared. Finally at hatching only the pure muscle type MM was found.

In rats the ontogenic evolution is similar but much slower. In fetuses of gestational age of 11 days, only the brain type BB exists. In 90-day-old rats the isoenzyme BB is replaced by the BM type, and in very old rats the hybrid disappears and only the MM type remains.

Schapira et al. (1968) have studied the ontogenic evolution of creatine kinase in some other species. In the rabbit, the developmental changes are slow; on the twenty-fifth day of life the muscle isoenzymes of creatine kinase are still of brain type. However, in mice no difference was found between the adult and fetal isoenzyme pattern. In man the ontogenic evolution occurs very early; isoenzyme BB was found only in the first trimester of gestation.

Aldolase isoenzymes have also been studied (Schapira, 1965; 1967; Herskovitz et al., 1967; Masters, 1968). In fetal rabbit muscle an aldolase isoenzyme was separated that revealed kinetic and electrophoretic characteristics similar to brain type aldolase (aldolase C), and furthermore, the embryonic chicken muscle also contains primarily this aldolase isoenzyme C; during late gestation, before hatching, the isoenzymes A-C appear.

Among other muscle enzymes with multiple molecular forms the ontogenic evolution of the intracellular distribution of two forms of malate dehydrogenase (Wiggert and Villee, 1964) and of carboxyl and aryl esterases (Holmes and Masters, 1967) might be mentioned.

It is remarkable that in muscle diseases either of myopathic or neurogenic origin, a shift toward the fetal pattern was observed for LDH (Dreyfus et al., 1962), creatine kinase, and aldolase isoenzymes (Schapira, 1965, 1968).

Peptides and Amino Acids

The typical muscle dipeptides anserine and carnosine are of low concentration in fetal skeletal muscle of rabbits. The postnatal increase is much more pronounced for anserine than for carnosine. The glutathion content is about the same shortly before and after birth, but the adult muscle contains less glutathion than that of the newborn rabbits (Stave and Armstrong, 1968). Glutathion might have a specific function in protecting SH groups of several enzymes, and it also might function as an enzyme activator (Stave, 1965). The perinatal changes of free amino acids in rabbit skeletal muscle (m. psoas major) are shown in Table 1. Compared with

TABLE 1. Developmental Changes of Muscle Free Amino Acids[a]
Average in μmoles per g wet weight

Amino acids	Fetuses (−1 day) n = 13/3[b]	Newborns 3 hours n = 6	Newborns 3rd day n = 6	Adults n = 7
Taurine	5.09	7.14	8.13	0.276
Aspartic acid	0.614	0.602	0.588	0.211
Threonine	0.261	0.444	0.426	0.221
Serine	1.425	1.032	0.933	0.399
Glutamine	6.131	4.70	3.10	0.928
Asparagine[c]	0.462			
Proline	0.822	0.488	0.503	0.313
Glutamic acid	5.791	2.91	2.72	0.526
Glycine	2.965	3.49	2.42	1.72
Alanine	2.955	3.10	1.77	1.258
Valine	0.112	0.220	0.374	0.265
Cystine[c]	0.03			
Methionine	0.042	0.102	0.101	0.088
Isoleucine	0.088	0.166	0.108	0.079
Leucine	0.116	0.167	0.231	0.159
Tyrosine	0.116	0.202	0.181	0.132
Phenylalanine	0.124	0.105	0.073	0.083
Ornithine	0.740	0.699	0.469	0.031
Lysine	1.23	1.52	0.371	0.090
1-methyl-histidine	0.081	0.114	0.028	0.029
Histidine	0.306	0.256	0.183	0.122
Arginine	1.03	0.630	0.170	0.064
Total amino acids:	30.53	28.08	22.88	6.99
Peptides:				
Carnosine	3.11	6.05	4.53	5.88
Anserine	0.430	0.445	0.532	30.02
Glutathione	1.056	1.072	1.339	0.864

[a]Data from Stave and Armstrong, 1968.
[b]First number indicates the total number of animals used, the second number indicates the reduced number of values because of pooling samples.
[c]In all but fetal muscle, ASN was not separated from GLN, and also CYS from VAL.

adult muscle, the several times higher concentrations in perinatal muscle are of special significance.

Glycogen

Glycogen concentration in muscle as well as in liver of various mammals increases rapidly during the later period of gestation (Shelley, 1960; see also Ch. 13). The carbohydrate reserve is three to four times higher at birth than in the adult. Bocek and Beatty (1967) have followed the glycogen content of muscle in the perinatal period; in the rhesus monkey it rises from 0.8 g/100 g fresh tissue at 20 days of gestational age to 2.8 g/100 g at 160 days. After birth, values decreased rapidly toward the adult level, averaging 0.68 g/100 g muscle. The glycogen level in the skeletal muscle is not significantly decreased during hypoxia, while the liver becomes depleted of glycogen (see Ch. 35).

Syrovy and Gutman (1967) found a reciprocal relationship between the muscle glycogen concentration and the RNA concentration. In mammals, the fast muscles are richer in glycogen than the slow muscles, but the turnover is higher in the latter ones.

Conclusions

The biochemical composition of muscle varies considerably during pre- and postnatal development. The general trend is toward a more differentiated pattern that develops mainly after birth. The factors governing the biosynthesis of constituents which are specific for the adult muscle remain to be defined; however, the onset of a purposeful use of muscles and the respective nervous stimulation after birth seem to accelerate the maturation of the skeletal muscle, directly or indirectly, to a great extent.

Acknowledgments

This work was supported by l'Institut National de la Santé et de la Recherche Médicale, le Centre National de la Recherche Scientifique, and the Muscular Dystrophy Associations of America.

REFERENCES

Appella, E., and C. L. Markert. 1961. Dissociation of lactate dehydrogenase into subunits with guanidine hydrochloride. Biochem. Biophys. Res. Commun., 6:171.

Barany, M., E. Gaetjens, K. Barany, and E. Karp. 1964. Comparative studies of rabbit cardiac and skeletal myosins. Arch. Biochem., 106:280.

———— K. Barany, T. Reckard, and A. Volpe. 1965a. Myosin of fast and slow muscles of the rabbit. Arch. Biochem., 109:185.

———— et al., 1965b. Myosin of new born rabbits. Arch. Biochem., 111:727.

Beatty, C. H., G. M. Basinger, and R. M. Bocek. 1965. Pentose cycle activity in muscle from fetal, neonatal and infant rhesus monkeys. Arch. Biochem., 117:275.

Bocek, R. M., and C. H. Beatty. 1967. Glycogen metabolism in fetal neonatal and infant muscle of the rhesus monkey. Pediatrics, 40:412.

Boyd, J. O. 1960. Development of striated muscle. In Bourne, G. H., ed. The Structure and Function of Muscle. New York, Academic Press, Inc., Vol. I, p. 63.

Cahn, R. D., N. O. Kaplan, L. Levine, and E. Zwilling. 1962. Nature and development of lactic dehydrogenase. Science, 136:962.

Cosmos, E. 1966. Enzymatic activity of differentiating muscle fibers. Develop. Biol., 13:163.

———— and J. Butler. 1967. Differentiation of fiber types in muscle of normal and dystrophic chickens. In Milhorat, A. T., ed. Exploratory Concepts in Muscular Dystrophy. New York, Excerpta Medica Foundation, p. 197.

Couteaux, R. 1941. Recherches sur l'histogénèse du muscle strié des mammifères et la formation des plaques motrices. Bull. Biol. France Belg., 75:101.

———— 1955. Localization of cholinesterases at neuromuscular junctions. Int. Rev. Cytol., 4:604.

———— 1958. Sur le mode de terminaison des myofibrilles et leurs connections avec la membrane sarcoplasmique au niveau de la jonction musculo-tendineuse. C.R. Acad. Sci. [D] (Paris), 246:307.

Crepax, P. 1952. Étude électrophorétique d'extraits de muscles doués de différentes propriétés morphologiques et fonctionnelles. Biochim. Biophys. Acta, 9:385.

Csapo, A., and H. Herrmann. 1951. Quantitative changes in contractile proteins of chick skeletal muscle during and after embryonic development. Amer. J. Physiol., 165:701.

Dance, N., and D. C. Watts. 1962. Comparison of creatine phosphotransferase from rabbit and brown-hare muscle. Biochem. J., 84:114.

Dawson, D. M., M. Eppenberger, and N. O. Kaplan. 1965. Creatine kinase: Evidence for a dimeric structure. Biochem. Biophys. Res. Commun., 21:346.

Dreyfus, J. C., and F. Schapira. 1967. Lactic dehydrogenase isozymes. In Bajusz, C., ed. Methods Achievements in Experimental Pathology. Cambridge, Mass., Harvard University Press.

———— F. Schapira, G. Schapira, and J. Demos. 1962. La lactico-déshydrogénase musculaire chez le myopathe: Persistance apparente du type foetal. C. R. Acad. Sci. [D] (Paris), 254:4384.

Dubowitz, V. 1963. Enzymic maturation of skeletal muscle. Nature (London), 197: 1215.

———— 1966. Enzyme histochemistry of developing human muscle. Nature (London), 211: p. 884.

———— 1967. Cross innervation of fast and slow muscle: Histochemical, physiological and biochemical studies. In Milhorat, A. T., ed. Exploratory Concepts in Muscular Dystrophy. New York, Excerpta Medica Foundation, p. 164.

———— and A. G. E. Pearse. 1960. Reciprocal relationship of phosphorylase and oxidative enzymes in skeletal muscle. Nature (London), 185:701.

———— and A. G. E. Pearse. 1961. Enzymic activity of normal and dystrophic human muscle: A histochemical study. J. Path. Bact., 81:365.

Engel, W. K. 1962. The essentiality of histo- and cytochemical studies of skeletal muscle in the investigation of neuromuscular diseases. Neurology (Minneap.), 12:778.

———— T. Wanko, and G. Fenichel. 1964. Nemaline myopathy. Arch. Neurol. (Chicago), 11:22.

Eppenberger, H. M., K. von Fellenberg, R. Richterich, and H. Aebi. 1962-63. Die Ontogenese von zytoplasmatischen Enzymen beim Hühner Embryo. Enzym. Biol. Clin. (Basel), 2:139.

———— M. Eppenberger, R. Richterich, and H. Aebi. 1964. The ontogeny of creatine kinase isozymes. Develop. Biol., 10:1.

Fenichel, G. M. 1966. A histochemical study of developing human skeletal muscle. Neurology (Minneap.), 16:741.

Fine, I. H., N. O. Kaplan, and D. Kuftinec. 1963. Developmental changes of mammalian lactic dehydrogenases. Biochemistry, 2:116.

Goodfriend, T. L., D. Sokol, and N. O. Kaplan. 1966. Control of synthesis of lactic acid dehydrogenases. J. Molec. Biol., 15:18.

Guth, L., and P. K. Watson. 1967. The influence of innervation on the soluble proteins of slow and fast muscles of the rat. Exp. Neurol., 17:107.

Hartshorne, D. J., and S. V. Perry. 1962. A chromatographic and electrophoretic study of sarcoplasm from adult and fetal rabbit muscles. Biochem. J., 85:171.

Herrmann, H. 1952. Studies of muscle development. Ann. N.Y. Acad. Sci., 55:99.

Herskovitz, J., C. J. Masters, P. M. Wassarman, and N. O. Kaplan. 1967. On the tissue specificity and biological significance of aldolase C in the chicken. Biochem. Biophys. Res. Commun., 26:24.

Holmes, R. S., and C. J. Masters. 1967. The developmental multiplicity and isoenzyme status of rat esterases. Biochim. Biophys. Acta, 146:138.

Hooft, C., P. de Caey, and Y. Lambert. 1966. Etude comparative de l'activité enzymatique du tissu musculaire de l'enfant normal et d'enfants atteints de dystrophie musculaire progressive aux différents stades de la maladie. Rev. Franç. Etud. Clin. Biol., 11:510.

Ilyin, V. 1965-66. Central regulation of enzyme activity and synthesis in embryonal and adult mammalian tissues. Biol. Neonat., 9:215.

Jonxis, J. H. P., and S. K. Wadman. 1952. A fetal form of myoglobin. Nature (London), 169:884.

Kagen, L. J., and C. L. Christian. 1966. Immunologic measurement of myoglobin in human adult and fetal skeletal muscle. Amer. J. Physiol., 211:655.

Kaplan, N. O., and R. D. Cahn. 1962. Lactic dehydrogenases and muscular dystrophy in the chicken. Proc. Nat. Acad. Sci. U.S.A., 48:2123.

Karpati, G., and W. K. Engel. 1968. Correlative histochemical study of skeletal muscle. Neurology (Minneap.), 18:681.

Kendrick-Jones, J., and S. V. Perry. 1967. Protein synthesis and enzyme response to contractile activity in skeletal muscle. Nature (London), 213:406.

Konigsberg, J. R. 1963. Clonal analysis of myogenesis. Science, 140:1273.

Marcaud-Raeber, L. 1958. Contribution à l'étude d'une nouvelle protéine myofibrillaire chez l'animal adulte et chez le foetus (lapin, mouton): La métamyosine. These Doct. es-Sci, Paris, p. 61.

——— 1959a. Sur une nouvelle protéine myofibrillaire: La métamyosine. Observation et isolement. Bull. Soc. Chim. Biol. (Paris), 41:283.

——— 1959b. Hétérogénéité de la métamyosine. Bull. Soc. Chim. Biol. (Paris), 41:297.

——— 1959c. Comparaison de la métamyosine avec les autres protéines myofibrillaires. Bull. Soc. Chim. Biol. (Paris), 41:315.

Markert, C. L., and F. Møller. 1959. Multiple forms of enzymes: Tissue, ontogenetic, and species specific patterns. Proc. Nat. Acad. Sci. U.S.A., 45:753.

——— and H. Ursprung. 1962. The ontogeny of isozyme patterns of lactate dehydrogenase in the mouse. Develop. Biol., 5:363.

Masters, C. J. 1964. The developmental progression of ruminant lactate dehydrogenase. Biochim. Biophys. Acta, 89:1.

——— 1968. The ontogeny of mammalian fructose-1-6-diphosphate aldolase. Biochim. Biophys. Acta, 167:161.

Mavrenskaya, I. F. 1963. Histochemical study of cholinesterase during development of somatic musculature in the human fetus. Fed. Proc. (Transl. Suppl.), 22:T597.

Mintz, B., and W. B. Baker. 1967. Normal mammalian muscle differentiation and gene control of isocitrate dehydrogenase synthesis. Proc. Nat. Acad. Sci. U.S.A., 58:592.

Miyoshi, K., et al. 1968. Myoglobin subfractions: Abnormality in Duchenne type of muscular dystrophy. Science, 159:736.

Needham, D. M., and J. M. Williams. 1963. Salt soluble collagen in extracts of uterus muscle and in fetal metamyosin. Biochem. J., 89:546.

Pearse, A. G. E. 1961. Direct relationship of phosphorylase and mitochondrial α-glycerophosphate dehydrogenase activity in skeletal muscle. Nature (London), 191:504.

Perkoff, G. T. 1964. Studies of human myoglobin in several diseases of muscle. New Eng. J. Med., 270:263.

——— 1966. Evidence for a specific human fetal muscle heme protein. J. Lab. Clin. Med., 67:685.

——— 1968. Further consideration of fetal muscle heme protein. J. Lab. Clin. Med., 71:610.

Perry, S. V., and D. J. Hartshorne. 1963. The proteins of developing muscle. In Gutman, E., and P. Hnik, eds. The Effect of Use and Disuse on Neuromuscular Function. Prague, Publishing House of the Czechoslovak Academy of Sciences, p. 491.

Pfleiderer, G., and E. D. Wachsmuth. 1961. Alters und funktionsabhängige Differenzierung der Lactatdehydrogenase menschlicher Organe. Biochem. Z., 334:185.

Ravikovitch, C. M., and B. S. Kasavina. 1952. Acad. Sci. U.S.S.R., 82:115. Cited by Marcaud-Raeber, L. 1958.

Rossi-Fanelli, A., E. Antonini, C. de Marco, and S. Benerecitti. 1959. Studies on foetal myoglobin. In Wolstenholme G. E. W., and C. M. O'Connor, eds. Biochemistry of Human Genetics. London, Churchill Ltd., p. 144.

Schapira, F. 1965. Modification de spécificité de l'aldolase musculaire au cours de l'atrophie expérimentale. C. R. Soc. Biol. (Paris), 159:2189.

——— 1966. Modification des isozymes de la créatine kinase musculaire au cours de l'atrophie. C. R. Acad. Sci. [D] (Paris), 262:2291.

——— 1967. Type embryonnaire de l'aldolase musculaire chez le poulet myopathe. C. R. Acad. Sci. [D] (Paris), 264:2654.

——— 1968. Ontogenetic evolution and pathogenic modifications of multiple forms of lactate dehydrogenase, creatine kinase and aldolase. In Thoai, U. V., and J. Roche, eds. Homologous Enzymes and Biochemical Evolution. New York, Gordon and Breach.

——— and J. C. Dreyfus. 1965. Différences de comportement au cours de l'atrophie des isozymes de la lactico-deshydrogenase musculaire selon l'espèce animale. Bull. Soc. Chim. Biol. (Paris), 47:2261.

——— J. C. Dreyfus, and G. Schapira. 1965. Fetal-like patterns of lactic dehydrogenase and aldolase isozymes in some pathological conditions. Enzym. Biol. Clin. (Basel), 7:98.

——— J. C. Dreyfus, and D. Allard. 1968. Les isozymes de la créatine kinase et de l'aldolase du muscle foetal et pathologique. Clin. Chim. Acta, 20:439.

Shelley, H. J. 1960. Blood sugars and tissue carbohydrate in fetal and infant lambs and rhesus monkeys. J. Physiol. (London), 153:527.

Singer, K., B. Angelopoulos, and B. Ramot. 1955. Studies on human myoglobin. Blood, 10:987.

Stave, U. 1964. Age dependent changes of metabolism. Biol. Neonat., 6:128.

——— 1965. Age dependent changes of metabolism: Influence of hypoxia on tissue enzyme patterns of newborn and adult rabbits. Biol. Neonat., 8:114.

————— 1967a. Age dependent changes of metabolism: The effect of prolonged hypoxia upon tissue enzyme activities of newborn and adult rabbits. Biol. Neonat., 11:310.

————— 1967b. Importance of proper substrate concentration for enzyme assays in tissue homogenates for developmental studies. Enzym. Biol. Clin. (Basel), 8:21.

—————and M. D. Armstrong. 1968. Developmental changes of free amino acids in liver, kidney, skeletal muscle, and plasma in rabbits. Memoirs XIIth Internat. Congr. Pediatrics, Mexico City, Vol. 3, pp. 13-14.

Syrovy, J., and E. Gutman. 1967. Metabolic differentiation of the anterior and posterior latissimus dorsi of the chick during development. Nature (London), 213:937.

Takasu, T., and B. P. Hughes. 1966. Lactate dehydrogenase isoenzymes in developing human muscle. Nature (London), 212:609.

Trayer, J. P., C. J. Harris, and S. V. Perry. 1968. 3-methyl histidine and adult and fetal forms of skeletal muscle myosin. Nature (London), 217:452.

Vesell, E. S., J. Philip, and A. G. Bearn. 1962. Comparative studies of the isozymes of lactic dehydrogenase in rabbit and man. J. Exp. Med., 116:797.

de Villafranca, G. W. 1956. A study on the nature of the A band of cross striated muscle. Arch. Biochem., 61:378.

Wiggert, C., and C. A. Villee. 1964. Multiple molecular forms of malic and lactic dehydrogenase during development. J. Biol. Chem., 239:444.

Wirsen, C., and K. S. Larsson. 1964. Histochemical differentiation of skeletal muscle in fetal and newborn mice. J. Embryol. Exp. Morph., 12:759.

Wolfson, R., Y. Yakulis, R. D. Coleman, and P. Heller. 1967. Studies on fetal myoglobin. J. Lab. Clin. Med., 69:728.

Yellin, H. 1967. Neural regulation of enzymes in muscle fibers of red and white muscle. Exp. Neurol., 19:92.

27

The Autonomic Nervous System

ALFRED STEINSCHNEIDER and JULIUS B. RICHMOND ●
Department of Pediatrics, State University of New York, Upstate
Medical Center, Syracuse, New York

Introduction

It must be recognized at the outset that the autonomic nervous system is, for the most part, a conceptual system and not a system functioning independently of the remainder of the nervous system or of other bodily systems. To postulate independent action not only would lead to erroneous conclusions but would seriously limit our understanding of the complex functioning of the human organism. By referring to the autonomic nervous system we are attempting to isolate a specific set of functions and controls, those dealing with the neurogenic influences on glandular and smooth and cardiac musculature.

In general the autonomic nervous system consists of both central as well as peripheral structures. However, studies on the intact organism are severely limited to an elaboration of the effects of controlled inputs on readily measurable outputs. Consequently, much of what we know of the functioning of central mechanisms is deduced either from these latter types of studies or from investigations of organisms other than man.

Our understanding of the autonomic nervous system in fetal and neonatal life is made even more difficult by the fact that developmental changes are also taking place in the autonomic end-organs as well. Thus changes in response to a constant physiologic alteration may be a reflection of maturational alterations in neural control, in the end-organ, or both.

The discussion to follow will be limited almost entirely to studies performed on the human fetus and neonate. This is done in the recognition that a significant body of knowledge has developed from the study of nonhuman subjects. The decision to concern ourselves with human studies was motivated not only by the appreciation of species differences but also by the desire to identify more readily the weaknesses as well as the strengths in our understanding of autonomic nervous system function in the human fetus and neonate.

Initial Value and Reactivity

In a relatively recent report, Wilder (1967) reviewed extensively the literature regarding the significance of organ function prior to stimulation on the subsequent response to a standard stimulus. On the basis of such a consideration, Wilder has argued not only that the initial value is a significant determiner of the response to stimulation but that there is, in general, a directional aspect to this effect. This relationship has been called the "law of initial value."

Given a standard stimulus and a standard period of time, the extent and direction of response of a physiological function at rest depends to a large measure on its initial (pre-experimental) level. The relations are as follows: the higher the initial value, the smaller the response to function-raising, the larger the response to function-depressing stimuli. Beyond a certain medium range of initial values, there is a tendency to paradoxic (reversed) responses, increasing with the extremeness of initial values. (Wilder, 1967).

It must be clear that this law is proposed as an empiric relationship and does not imply anything about causal factors.

Several studies have demonstrated that applicability of the law of initial value to the autonomic nervous system functions in full-term newborn infants. These investigations have employed, for the most part, the cardiac rate response to external stimulation.

In general, external stimulation results in an initial cardiac rate increase followed by a subsequent decline to near prestimulation levels. Figure 1 contains the maximal initial change in heart rate as a function of the prestimulus heart rate. These data were obtained from a single neonate repeatedly stimulated by a standard five-second duration jet of air delivered to an area of skin cephalad to the umbilicus. Comparable data have been obtained for other infants and stimulus conditions. It is apparent from an examination of this figure that greater increments in cardiac rate occur to a standard stimulus presented at a time when the heart rate is low. It can also be seen that at high prestimulus heart rates the initial response to the same stimulus is one of deceleration. A detailed examination of the cardiac rate response curve to stimulation has revealed that the initial value is of importance when considering the magnitude aspects of the response but does not appear to relate to the temporal aspects (Lipton et al., 1961). Similar observations have been made for the respiratory response to stimulation (Lipton et al., 1965).

The initial value is also of importance in determining the response to stimulation of premature newborn infants. Unfortunately, no data are available on the effect of gestational age on the relative importance of the initial value. Significant for this discussion is the additional observation by Lipton et al. (1966) that the slope of the line describing the relationship between the response magnitude and the initial value increases during the first five months of postnatal life. This is most apparent for the return portion of the cardiac rate response. Thus a constant change in the initial heart rate has less of an effect on the responsiveness of newborn infants

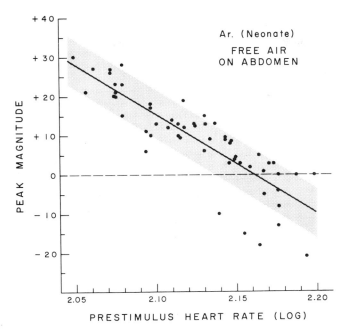

Fig. 1. The maximal heart rate response (peak magnitude) as a function of the prestimulation level as obtained from a single neonate. The best fit regression line is
represented by the solid line and the shaded area indicates $\pm S_{yx}$. (From Lipton et al.,
1965. *Pediatrics*, Suppl., 35:521-567.)

than on that of infants five months of age. Comparable data are needed relative to
the influence of gestational age.

Visceral Stimulation and Physiologic Processes

The autonomic nervous system of neonates is an extremely labile system, one that
demonstrates frequent spontaneous changes as well as responses to clearly identifiable sensory stimuli. Examination of the spontaneous changes occasionally reveals
them to be associated with definable physiologic processes and respiratory activity.

General or tonic changes in the level of autonomic activity are related to overall
level of arousal or the sleep-wake continuum. This has been demonstrated from an
examination of a number of different end-organs. Thus, in the full-term newborn
a decrease in arousal or the state of sleep is associated with a decrease in heart rate
(Bridger et al., 1965), an increase in skin resistance (Wenger and Irwin, 1936),
a decrease in skin potential (Stechler et al., 1966), a decrease in diastolic and
systolic pressure (Moss et al., 1963), and an increasing regularity of respiratory
activity. In a sense, the changes associated with sleep can be viewed as a shift in
the parasympathetic-sympathetic axis toward the parasympathetic side.

In addition to these tonic shifts, phasic responses have been observed to occur in conjunction with a wide variety of physiologic processes and complex stimulus situations. Although sinus arrhythmia had been considered an infrequent observation in the newborn, it is becoming increasingly apparent that this phenomenon does occur in most, if not all, premature and full-term newborns (Lipton et al., 1964; Morgan et al., 1965; Morgan and Guntheroth, 1965).

Vallbona et al. (1963) observed an immediate and transient bradycardia associated with a sneeze in newborns. Straining on defecation and hiccups were also noted to result in sudden brief bradycardia (Lipton et al., 1964). The bradycardia of defecation has been found to occur in premature infants as well (Phillips et al., 1964). Lipton et al. (1964) observed a total of 59 spontaneous yawns in 24 newborn infants and noted the gradual development of bradycardia. The lowest heart rate usually occurred between two and five seconds following the behavioral onset of the yawn. In a most interesting study, Cotton and O'Meara (1964) were able to demonstrate that the sudden increase in negative intrapleural pressure (a sigh) resulted in both a cardiac slowing (an average decrease of about 40 beats per minute) and a decrease in systolic blood pressure. This latter study was performed on infants less than 12 hours of age. Gavage feeding of premature infants has been found to result in a significant bradycardia (a drop in rate of 35 beats per minute or greater) in 53 percent of babies. The very passage of a nasogastric tube has been observed to produce abrupt and marked bradycardia in premature infants (Lipton et al., 1964).

A number of investigators have noted cardiac rate changes in association with nutritive as well as nonnutritive sucking. These observations have been made on full-term and premature infants. Some authors have observed cardiac rate acceleration (Halverson, 1941; Greenberg et al., 1963; Gottlieb and Simner, 1966) whereas others emphasize cardiac rate deceleration (Phillips et al., 1964; Winter et al., 1966) as a concomitant of sucking. This discrepancy can be understood on the basis of the results obtained by Boschan and Steinschneider (1968). These latter investigators observed that, in general, the onset of a sucking burst is associated with an increase in heart rate whereas the cessation of sucking results in an average decrease in rate. Of significance is the additional observation that the magnitude of the cardiac rate increase with sucking was negatively correlated with the heart rate prior to sucking. Thus, increasing presucking heart rate resulted in a decrease in the magnitude of the heart rate increase. Furthermore, at high presucking heart rates, the cardiac response to sucking was one of deceleration. These results, once again, point to the significance of the initial value as a possible determiner of the subsequent response to stimulation.

External Stimulation

Studies performed on both full-term and premature newborns clearly demonstrate that discrete external stimulation is capable of eliciting autonomic nervous system responses. Sontag and his colleagues (Bernard and Sontag, 1947; Sontag and Wallace, 1936; Sontag et al., 1969) as well as Murphy and Smyth (1962) have presented data suggesting that the fetal heart rate as well is influenced by stimuli presented to the mother. The presentation of a sound stimulus to the mother was found to result in a transient tachycardia in fetuses of 28 to 30 weeks' gestation. Whether the fetal tachycardia is in response to stimulation of fetal sensory systems or somehow mediated via maternal responses is at present unclear.

Available data do not permit any firm conclusions regarding the effect of gestational age on the characteristics of the autonomic response to sensory stimulation.

Relatively well-controlled studies have demonstrated that the characteristics of the phasic response are related to the properties of the stimulating conditions. Thus the response has been shown to vary as a function of the intensity and duration of the stimulus as well as of the area of tactile stimulation.

Employing sound stimulation in full-term newborns, Bartoshuk (1964) and Steinschneider et al. (1966) observed a progressive increase in the magnitude of the cardiac rate acceleration with increasing intensity. In addition, the more intense sounds resulted in a decrease in the cardiac response latency and an increase in the duration of the accelerative phase of the overall response. Respiratory reactivity also is sensitive to the intensity variable. Stubbs (1934) found a greater frequency of respiratory responses, and Suzuki et al. (1964) found a greater tendency for a sudden deep inspiration to occur to the more intense sound. Analyzing the phasic change in respiratory period in a manner similar to that employed for cardiac rate, Steinschneider (1968) observed that the more intense sounds produced a greater magnitude of respiratory response simultaneous with a decrease in the time the maximum response occurred.

Stimulus duration also appears to influence both the magnitude as well as the temporal characteristics of the cardiac response to stimulation. Keen et al. (1965), using a sound stimulus, and Steinschneider et al. (1965), employing a tactile stimulus, found the magnitude of cardiac rate increase to be positively correlated with stimulus duration. The latter investigators also noted that increased stimulus duration resulted in an increase in the duration of the initial portion of the cardiac response and an increase in the latency of the return portion.

The data from a number of studies are suggestive that the autonomic response of newborns is conditioned by the location of tactile stimulation. Stimulation of the mucous membranes of the lips produced greater cardiac rate increases when compared with comparable stimulation of the abdomen (Lipton et al., 1958). Furthermore, the cardiac rate increase to abdominal stimulation was greater than that for anal stimulation. The latter type of stimulation frequently produced cardiac rate deceleration (Richmond and Lipton, 1959).

Grossman and Greenberg (1957) recorded the cardiac rate and skin temperature (forehead, abdomen, toe) responses to tactile stimulation applied to a variety of sites. The largest increase in toe temperature was noted following stimulation of the genitalia. This contrasts with the abdominal skin temperature which was observed to show greatest change in association with tactile stimulation of the abdomen.

Studies in adults have demonstrated that repetitive presentation of a stimulus results in a progressive decrement in the magnitude and frequency of occurrence of the autonomic response. This has been referred to as *habituation*. Several investigators have obtained evidence of habituation in full-term newborns while studying the cardiac rate response to an auditory stimulus (Bartoshuk, 1962a, b; Bridger, 1961, 1962). It would appear from these studies that the development of habituation can be facilitated by utilizing long-duration stimuli and brief interstimulus intervals. Habituation cannot be attributed simply to fatigue, for slight shifts in the stimulating condition will result in a recurrence of the earlier response magnitude. Furthermore, in one study, habituation was noted to persist for at least 24 hours (Keen et al., 1965). An exciting alternative to the fatigue hypothesis concerns the possibility that habituation is a form of learning.

Employing a variety of approaches, investigators have observed significant individual differences in reactivity to a standard stimulus. Bridger and Reiser (1959) obtained the cardiac rate response to an air stream stimulus in a group of full-term infants on two successive days. A number of intraindividual response measures were obtained on each of the days, and correlation coefficients were then determined across days. Statistically significant coefficients were obtained for almost all the response measures employed. Another approach utilized in the identification of individual differences has been to test the same neonates under a variety of experimental conditions and to determine whether an individual maintained his same degree of relative reactivity across experimental conditions. In studies employing varying degrees of motor restraint (Lipton et al., 1965), different intensities of white noise (Steinschneider et al., 1966), and three durations of a tactile stimulus (Steinschneider et al., 1965), subjects tended to respond in a consistent fashion. These data, however, do not allow for any conclusions regarding the basis for these differences between subjects, that is, whether they are a reflection of differences in genetic composition, intrauterine experiences, unique characteristics of the labor and delivery, or subtle unidentified testing variables.

By simultaneously recording responses from a number of different end-organs, it has been possible to inquire into the extent to which the relative degree of intra-individual reactivity is comparable across response systems. Several studies have failed to find consistency across response systems (Grossman and Greenberg, 1957; Schachter et al., 1966; Steinschneider, 1968).

Labor

Further evidence of autonomic nervous system activity derives from the study of cardiac rate control during the process of labor and delivery. To a large extent these investigations were initiated in the hopes of better identifying fetal distress. The development of electronic instrumentation allowing for constant monitoring has resulted in a considerable increase in our knowledge of the qualitative and quantitative changes in cardiac rate occurring during labor. There also has evolved a greater understanding of the probable mechanisms responsible for the changes in fetal heart rate.

The heart rate of fetuses near term is marked by considerable moment-to-moment variation (Swarthwout et al., 1961). As a means of better understanding the mechanisms as well as the significance of the observed variations, several classification schemes have been developed. For the purpose of this discussion we will employ the notation used by Caldeyro-Barcia et al. (1966).

Superimposed on what might be called the "basal heart rate" are "rapid fluctuations" consisting of slight fluctuations (1 to 8 beats per minute) with a frequency ranging from 3 to 10 cycles per second. In addition to the rapid fluctuations there are "transient increases" (less than 30 seconds in duration), "spikes" (rapid and brief bradycardia), and "dips" (transient bradycardia associated with uterine contractions). Two types of dips have been differentiated primarily on the basis of the time interval between the peak increase of intrauterine pressure and the maximal development of the bradycardia. It has been proposed that the lag time for the type I dips be less than 18 seconds whereas dips with longer lag times be labeled as of the type II variety. In addition to the longer lag times, the type II dips are of a longer duration.

Of considerable interest to this discussion are the observations on the effect of atropine on fetal heart rate and the transient changes noted during labor. Stern et al. (1961) injected atropine into the umbilical veins of fetuses weighing between 100 and 525 g. These six fetuses were made available while performing cesarean sections for the purpose of a legal abortion. Atropine was found to have little or no effect on the configuration of the ECG or the cardiac rate. In this same study compression of the umbilical cord failed to elicit any consistent change in cardiac rate. These observations were interpreted as support for the hypothesis that vagal influence of cardiac function does not develop until late in the life of the fetus. Consistent with this formulation is the additional observation that atropine administered either directly or indirectly to the fetus at or near term had a considerable influence not only on the basal heart rate but on a number of changes observed during labor (Hellman et al., 1961; Hon, 1963; Hon, et al., 1961; Mendez-Bauer et al., 1963). In brief, atropine resulted in an increase in the basal cardiac rate and in a total disappearance of all the above discussed patterned changes except the type II dips. It thus appears that the near term fetal heart rate is under constant vagal tone and demonstrates changes reflecting phasic modifications in tone. The type II dips continued to occur even under the influence of atropine, although the degree of bradycardia was markedly decreased.

Investigators have suggested that the reflex bradycardia associated with increased intrauterine pressure results from umbilical cord compression and/or increased intracranial pressure (secondary to compression of the fetal brain). These hypotheses would be consistent with experimental data demonstrating that compression of the fetal brain and compression of the umbilical cord will produce a marked and sudden reflex bradycardia (Kelly, 1963; Lee and Hon, 1963).

Vasomotor Control

PERIPHERAL VASCULATURE

Peripheral vasomotor control in neonates has been studied primarily by determining the effect of applied temperature changes on bloodflow. These temperature modifications have taken the form of either general ambient temperature changes or the local application of temperature stimuli.

Laupus et al. (1963) applied a cold stimulus to a group of full-term newborn infants on the first day of life and failed to observe significant digital vasoconstriction. These investigators also followed several newborns during the first week of life. They concluded that the vasoconstrictor response to the local application of cold gradually matures postnatally. In contrast, Brück (1961) observed vasoconstriction to low ambient temperatures in full-term and premature infants from the first day of life. Brück also obtained reflex vasoconstriction when the face was cooled by a current of cool air. These latter observations, however, must be evaluated in the light of Brück's additional observation (see Ch. 16) that peripheral vasoconstriction may occur as a result of the mechanical stimulation of facial cutaneous receptors.

Bower (1954) studied the effect of local application of heat (upper extremity) on the reflex skin temperature response of the foot. The youngest baby examined was 2 days of age. Comparison with adult responses indicated that the reflex response in infants was slower and failed to achieve as high a skin temperature level. Furthermore, adult type reflex vasodilatation was observed in all children over 3 months of age. To some extent these results agree with those obtained by Young (1962). Young also noted developmental changes in vasomotor responsiveness. Body warming during the first 3 days of age frequently failed to elicit vasodilatation (as measured by skin temperature) and, when noted, the response was delayed. However, the response in infants older than 3 days was comparable to that observed in adults. The observations by Richmond and Lustman (1955) are consistent with the above results. In addition, these latter investigators demonstrated marked subject differences in reflex vasodilatation. Of 31 infants studied between the ages of 3 and 4 days, 10 failed to demonstrate any change in the temperature response of the left toe following immersion of the right foot in warm water. The maximal temperature response ranged from 0.1°F to 6.0°F in the remaining neonates.

A considerable increase in peripheral blood flow in response to an increase in ambient temperature was observed by Brück (1961) in premature and full-term infants. This applied to all but those in the first day of life. An ambient temperature between 32° and 34°C did not invariably produce an increase in peripheral blood flow within the first 24 hours. In an important follow-up study, peripheral blood flow was measured as a function of both rectal temperature and age (up to 14 days). Clearly, vasodilatation (increase in blood flow) could be induced at all ages (even during the first few hours of life). However, in the younger newborns higher rectal temperatures were required before an increase in blood flow became apparent.

Wilkes et al. (1966) employed a very different approach in assessing vasomotor control. The development of reflex vasodilatation in response to varying dosages of intradermal histamine was determined in adults and full-term infants less than 48 hours old. Although reflex vasodilatation was observed in the newborn, higher concentrations of histamine were required (relative to the adults) before vasodilatation first occurred. Two alternative hypotheses were suggested to explain these results. The first suggested a lessened responsiveness of the vascular smooth muscle. The second hypothesis considered the possibility of greater vasoconstrictor tone in the newborn as compared with adults. No data are available to allow for a reasonable choice of these alternative hypotheses.

In summary, there is sufficient evidence to conclude that the newborn, full-term as well as premature, is born with a considerable degree of peripheral vasomotor responsiveness. This responsiveness, however, differs quantitatively from that of the adult. It is still unclear whether these differences are a reflection of developmental features (local or central), environmental differences, the birth process, or a combination of all.

PULMONARY VASCULATURE

A good deal of research has demonstrated considerable lability of the pulmonary circulation of the fetal and newborn lung. Sufficient evidence is now available to demonstrate that the pulmonary arterial pressure in the fetus is significantly greater than that in the normal breathing newborn. Furthermore, the pulmonary vascular resistance and pulmonary arterial pressure decrease, and pulmonary blood flow increases with the advent of pulmonary ventilation, the decrease in Po_2, and the increase in Pco_2.

The influence of neural factors has been studied in animals in an effort to elucidate the mechanisms by which pulmonary ventilation and changes in serum Po_2 and Pco_2 alter the tone of the pulmonary vasculature. One such investigation was that performed by Lauer et al. (1965). These researchers studied lambs near term delivered by cesarean section while the umbilical circulation was maintained intact. Changes in pulmonary vascular resistance in response to ventilation with 10 percent CO_2 and 90 percent O_2 were measured before and after bilateral vagotomy. The decrease in vascular resistance to this gas mixture was not influenced by the surgical procedure. In still another small group of fetal lambs the vascular response to ventilation with 100 percent O_2 was studied before and after the administration of atropine and ismeline. Neither blocking agent was found to influence the vasodilatation resulting from ventilation.

Confirmatory observations have been made by Colebatch et al. (1965), also studying fetal lambs. Bilateral vagotomy and thoracic sympathectomy failed to alter the vascular response to positive pressure ventilation or acute asphyxia.

The above studies should not be interpreted as a demonstration of a lack of autonomic nervous system influence on the pulmonary vasculature. Rather, these studies reveal that the effect of pulmonary ventilation and changes in blood gases and pH is not mediated primarily by the autonomic nervous system. Neural control of the pulmonary vasculature has been observed by Colebatch et al. (1965) and Campbell et al. (1966). Both investigations were performed on lambs. Electric stimulation of the cervical vagus resulted in an increase in pulmonary blood flow secondary to vasodilatation which was blocked by the administration of atropine. In contrast, comparable stimulation of the thoracic sympathetic produced pulmonary vasoconstriction and a decrease in pulmonary blood flow.

The data obtained by Campbell et al. (1966), although reported in brief, also suggest that neural influences become more manifest in later fetal life. These investigators employed the technique of cross-circulation between twins as a means of maintaining the relative constancy of blood gases. Compression of the umbilical cord in lambs of 91 to 92 days' gestation had no influence on the pulmonary vasculature, providing the arterial blood supply from the twin donor was maintained intact. A comparable procedure performed on lambs of 98 to 143 days' gestation was associated with a small pulmonary vasoconstriction. Significantly, this latter effect was abolished following surgical interruption of the left sympathetic supply to the left lung.

Blood Pressure

Several investigators have documented the changes in blood pressure taking place during the first few hours and weeks of life. This subsection will not be concerned with these studies nor with those dealing with problems of obtaining blood pressure. Rather we will consider the changes in blood pressure in response to a variety of stimuli and the extent to which baroreceptor mechanisms are effective in maintaining a stable pressure.

Young and Holland (1958) found little, if any, differences in systolic blood pressure between the quiet and the crying newborn of less than 3 days of age. At subsequent ages crying was associated with a significant elevation in systolic pressure. These results are at variance with those obtained by Moss et al. (1963). In their study of premature and full-term infants of 77 hours of age or less, both systolic and diastolic pressures were higher during periods of crying. The discrepancy between these two studies might be attributable to differences in blood pressure recording. Young and Holland (1958) obtained blood pressures by palpation, an exceedingly difficult procedure, especially in crying infants, whereas Moss et al. (1963) recorded pressure from the descending aorta by means of an indwelling catheter. However, in a still more recent study, Gupta and Scopes (1965), using an indirect as well as a direct method of recording blood pressure, observed increases in blood pressure during crying even during the first 24 hours of life.

Blood pressure changes have been noted to occur during bottle feeding. Both Hakulinen et al. (1962) and Gupta and Scopes (1965) reported higher systolic pressures during sucking.

Moss et al. (1963) also studied the effect of immersing the foot in ice water (4° to 5°C for one minute) in both full-term and premature infants. In the vast majority of newborns studied (77 hours of age or less) there was an increase in heart rate and systolic and diastolic pressures.

Attempts to assess the ability of the newborn to adjust to changes in position have led to contradictory results. Employing indirect methods of blood pressure recording, Young and Holland (1958) and Hakulinen et al. (1962) failed to find changes in pressure in association with alteration in body position (i.e., supine to upright position) during the first three days of life. In older neonates higher systolic pressures were recorded when the infant was placed upright. It should be clear that the recording procedures were such that the posttilt pressure was obtained at a point in time comparable to the recovery period in the adult (that is, at the time when the adult blood pressure would have returned to normal following an initial fall). Of additional interest, Young and Holland (1958) observed cardiac rate acceleration to tilting upright during the first day of life. Observations of direct arterial pressures have failed to yield consistent results. In their initial study employing premature and full-term newborns, Moss et al. (1963) reported an immediate increase in systolic pressure to upright tilt followed by a drop and then a return to pretilt values. The initial small pressure increase was attributed to the impact of blood on the catheter. The upright tilt also produced an increase in heart rate. These results are interpreted as an indication that premature and newborn infants respond in a manner comparable to that of the adult. A subsequent study by Moss et al. (1968) essentially confirmed their earlier observations. Contradictory results were obtained by Gupta and Scopes (1965) who observed an increase in *both* systolic and diastolic pressures which persisted for at least two minutes following an upright tilt. The results obtained by Young and Cottom (1966) tend to agree with those of Gupta and Scopes (1965). It should be noted that Young and Cottom (1966) found considerable response variability; in 13 infants there was a slight increase in systolic and diastolic pressure, in 4 there was no change, and in 8 infants there was a slight decrease (no greater than 3 mm Hg). Young and Cottom (1966) also observed a good deal of variability in the cardiac rate response, although this appeared to be less than that observed for pressures. Of the 25 babies studied, 18 demonstrated a tachycardia averaging 7 beats per minute.

In view of the unresolved differences between investigators regarding the actual blood pressure response to changes in position, it is difficult to know to what extent, if any, the baroreceptor mechanism of infants differs from that of adults. It would be surprising, in view of the previous discussion on vasomotor control, if differences were not obtained. This should not be interpreted as indicating a deficiency of baroreceptor activity. Failure to elicit a blood pressure response in infants comparable to that seen in adults could represent a difference in vasomotor reactivity. This possibility is supported by the observation that the cardiac rate response to position change is similar in direction for adults and neonates. Young and Cottom (1966) also commented on the difference in responsiveness of the cardiac and peripheral vascular systems in their discussion of the effects of blood withdrawal. Bleeding in neonates was found to be associated with an increase in cardiac rate but a reduction in mean pressure.

Conclusions

It should be apparent that our knowledge of autonomic nervous system functioning in the human neonate is extremely fragmentary. This conclusion applies with even greater force to the human fetus.

Recognizing the severe limitations imposed by the available data, it is still reasonable to conclude that the autonomic nervous system exerts a progressively increasing influence on the functioning of the developing organism. Clearly, autonomic activity is modified by a wide variety of internal as well as external conditions. Furthermore, it is sufficiently developed at birth to respond quantitatively to variations in the stimulus input.

It seems appropriate to conclude that the autonomic nervous system does not respond in an all-or-none fashion; that is, all end-organs innervated by the autonomic nervous system do not react to the same degree. Thus it is possible that efferent discharges from central autonomic structures either do not cause a response in all autonomically innervated end-organs or if they do, under certain circumstances, the response is not of the same relative magnitude.

The development of autonomic functioning is far from complete in the full-term neonate. A considerable degree of additional modifications can be anticipated for some time subsequent to delivery. The point in time at which autonomic control becomes apparent in fetal life is far from clear and probably varies considerably depending upon the specific functional system under study.

The influence exercised by the autonomic nervous system has also been implicated, to varying degrees, in the development of a variety of abnormal states. Thus, Morgan et al. (1965) consider immaturity of the sympathetic and parasympathetic cardiac regulatory mechanisms of possible significance in the development of cardiac arrhythmias in prematures. The autonomic innervation of the pulmonary vasculature could exert an influence in the pulmonary vasoconstriction considered, by some, of vital importance in the etiology of the respiratory distress syndrome (Strang, 1966). It has also been suggested that some of the sudden unexplained deaths in infancy are due to a hyperactive vagal response resulting in the development of fatal cardiac arrhythmias and/or laryngospasm (Valdes-Dapena, 1967).

It would be in error to view the developing role of autonomic nervous system control solely in terms of maturity or immaturity. Rather, more is to be gained by studying the extent, both quantitative as well as qualitative, to which it influences various end-organs and assists in maintaining organismic integrity. Furthermore, it is essential that this influence be viewed within the framework of a developing nervous system and its interaction with an almost constantly changing organism and environment, both internal and external.

REFERENCES

Bartoshuk, A. K. 1962a. Human neonatal cardiac acceleration to sound: Habituation and dishabituation. Percept. Motor Skills, 15:15-27.

———— 1962b. Response decrement with repeated elicitation of human neonatal cardiac acceleration to sound. J. Comp. Physiol. Psychol., 55:9-13.

———— 1964. Human neonatal cardiac responses to sound: A power function. Psychon. Sci., 1:151-152.

Bernard, J., and L. W. Sontag. 1947. Fetal reactivity to tonal stimulation: A preliminary report. J. Genet. Psychol., 70:205-210.

Boschan, P. J., and A. Steinschneider. 1968. Cardiac rate and bottle feeding in the neonate. Presented at the annual meeting of the American Psychosomatic Society, Boston, Mass., March 29, 1968. Unpublished data.

Bower, B. D. 1954. Pink disease: The autonomic disorder and its treatment with ganglion-blocking agents. Quart. J. Med., 23:215-230.

Bridger, W. H. 1961. Sensory habituation and discrimination in the human neonate. Amer. J. Psychiat., 117:991-996.

———— 1962. Sensory discrimination and autonomic function in the newborn. J. Amer. Acad. Child Psychiat., 1:67-82.

———— and M. F. Reiser. 1959. Psychophysiologic studies of the neonate: An approach toward the methodological and theoretical problems involved. Psychosom. Med., 21:265-276.

———— B. M. Birns, and M. Blank. 1965. A comparison of behavioral ratings and heart rate measurements in human neonates. Psychosom. Med., 27:123-134.

Brück, K. 1961. Temperature regulation in the newborn infant. Biol. Neonat., 3:65-119.

Caldeyro-Barcia, R., et al. 1966. Control of human fetal heart rate during labor. In Cassels, D. E., ed. The Heart and Circulation in the Newborn and Infant. New York, Grune & Stratton, Inc. pp. 7-36.

Campbell, G. M., F. Cockburn, G. S. Dawes, and J. E. Milligan. 1966. Pulmonary blood flow and cross-circulation between twin foetal lambs. J. Physiol. (London), 186:96P-97P.

Colebatch, H. J. H., G. S. Dawes, J. W. Goodwin, and R. A. Nadeau. 1965. The nervous control of the circulation in the foetal and newly expanded lungs of the lamb. J. Physiol. (London), 178:544-562.

Cotton, E. K., and O. P. O'Meara. 1964. Cardiovascular response to sighing in newborn infants. Presented at the annual meeting of the American Pediatric Society, June 16-18, 1964. Unpublished data.

Gottlieb, G., and M. L. Simner. 1966. Relationship between cardiac rate and nonnutritive sucking in human infants. J. Comp. Physiol. Psychol., 61:128-131.

Greenberg, N. H., P. R. Cekan, and J. G. Loesch. 1963. Some cardiac rate and behavioral characteristics of sucking in the neonate. Presented at the annual meeting of the American Psychosomatic Society, Atlantic City, N.J., April 27-28, 1963.

Grossman, H. J., and N. H. Greenberg. 1957. Psychosomatic differentiation in infancy. I. Autonomic activity in the newborn. Psychosom. Med., 19:293-306.

Gupta, J. M., and J. W. Scopes. 1965. Observations on blood pressure in newborn infants. Arch. Dis. Child., 40:637-644.

Hakulinen, A., L. Hirvonen, and T. Peltonen. 1962. Response of blood pressure to sucking and tilting in the newborn infant. Ann. Paediat. Fenn., 8:56-61.

Halverson, H. M. 1941. Variation in pulse and respiration during different phases of infant behavior. J. Genet. Psychol., 59:259-330.

Hellman, L. M., H. L. Johnson, W. E. Tolles, and E. H. Jones. 1961. Some factors affecting the fetal heart rate. Amer. J. Obstet. Gynec., 82:1055-1063.

Hon, E. H. 1963. The foetal heart rate. In Carey, H. M., ed. Modern Trends in Human Reproductive Physiology. Washington D.C., Butterworth & Co., Inc. pp. 245-256.

———— A. H. Bradfield, and O. W. Hess. 1961. The electronic evaluation of the fetal heart rate. V. The vagal factor in fetal bradycardia. Amer. J. Obstet. Gynec., 82:291-300.

Keen, R. E., H. H. Chase, and F. K. Graham. 1965. Twenty-four hour retention by neonates of an habituated heart rate response. Psychon. Sci., 2:265-266.

Kelly, J. V. 1963. Compression of the fetal brain. Amer. J. Obstet. Gynec., 85:687-694.

Lauer, R. M., J. A. Evans, H. Aoki, and C. F. Kittle. 1965. Factors controlling pulmonary vascular resistance in fetal lambs. J. Pediat., 67:568-577.

Laupus, W. E., Z. Bilsel, L. W. Collins, and J. T. Stubbs, Jr. 1963. Vasoconstrictor responses in the young infant. Circulation, 28:755.

Lee, S. T., and E. H. Hon. 1963. Fetal hemodynamic response to umbilical cord compression. Obstet. Gynec., 22:553-562.

Lipton, E. L., A. Steinschneider, and J. B. Richmond. 1961. Autonomic function in the neonate. IV. Individual differences in cardiac reactivity. Psychosom. Med., 23:472-484.

———— A. Steinschneider, and J. B. Richmond. 1964. Autonomic function in the neonate. VIII. Cardiopulmonary observations. Pediatrics, 33:212-215.

———— A. Steinschneider, and J. B. Richmond. 1965. Swaddling, a child care practice: Historical, cultural and experimental observations. Pediatrics (Suppl.), 35:521-567.

———— A. Steinschneider, and J. B. Richmond. 1966. Autonomic function in the neonate. VII. Maturational changes in cardiac control. Child Develop., 37:1-16.

———— J. B. Richmond, H. Weinberger, and L. Hersher. 1958. An approach to the evaluation of neonate autonomic responses. Presented at annual meeting of the American Psychosomatic Society, Cincinnati, O., March 31, 1958.

Mendex-Bauer, C. et al. 1963. Effects of atropine on the heart rate of the human fetus during labor. Amer. J. Obstet. Gynec., 85:1033-1053.

Morgan, B. C., and W. G. Guntheroth. 1965. Cardiac arrhythmias in normal newborn infants. J. Pediat., 67:1199-1202.

———— R. S. Bloom, and W. G. Guntheroth. 1965. Cardiac arrhythmias in premature infants. Pediatrics, 35:658-661.

Moss, A. J., E. R. Duffie, and G. Emmanouilides. 1963. Blood pressure and vasomotor reflexes in the newborn infant. Pediatrics, 32:175-179.

———— G. C. Emmanouilides, M. Monset-Couchard, and B. Marcano. 1968. Vascular responses to postural changes in normal, newborn infants. Pediatrics, 42:250-254.

Murphy, K. P., and C. N. Smyth. 1962. Letters to the editor. Lancet, 1:972-973.

Phillips, S. J., F. J. Agate, Jr., W. A. Silverman, and P. Steiner. 1964. Autonomic cardiac reactivity in premature infants. Biol. Neonat., 6:225-249.

Richmond, J. B., and S. L. Lustman. 1955. Autonomic function in the neonate. I. Implications for psychosomatic theory. Psychosom. Med., 17:269-275.

———— and E. L. Lipton. 1959. Some aspects of the neurophysiology of the newborn and their implications for child development. In Jessner, L., and E. Pavenstedt, eds. Dynamic Psychopathology in Childhood. New York, Grune & Stratton, Inc., pp. 78-105.

Schachter, J., et al. 1966. Behavioral and physiologic reactivity in human neonates. Ment. Hyg., 50:516-521.

Sontag, L. W., and R. F. Wallace. 1936. Changes in the rate of the human fetal heart in response to vibratory stimuli. Amer. J. Dis. Child., 51:583-589.

———— W. G. Steele, and M. Lewis. 1969. The fetal and maternal cardiac response to environmental stress. Hum. Develop., 12:1-9.

Stechler, G., S. Bradford, and H. Levy. 1966. Attention in the newborn: Effect on motility and skin potential. Science, 151:1246-1248.

Steinschneider, A. 1968. Sound intensity and respiratory responses in the neonate: Comparison with cardiac rate responsiveness. Psychosom. Med., 30:534-541.

———— E. L. Lipton, and J. B. Richmond. 1965. Stimulus duration and cardiac responsivity in the neonate. Presented at the biennial meeting of the Society for Research in Child Development, Minneapolis, Minn., March 24-27, 1965. Unpublished data.

———— E. L. Lipton, and J. B. Richmond. 1966. Auditory sensitivity in the infant: Effect of intensity on cardiac and motor responsivity. Child Develop., 37:233-252.

Stern, L., J. Lind, and B. Kaplan. 1961. Direct human foetal electrocardiography (with studies of the effects of adrenalin, atropine, clamping of the umbilical cord, and placental separation of the foetal ECG). Biol. Neonat., 3:49-62.

Strang, L. B. 1966. The pulmonary circulation in the respiratory distress syndrome. Pediat. Clin. N. Amer., 13:693-701.

Stubbs, E. M. 1934. The effect of the factors of duration, intensity, and pitch of sound stimuli on the responses of newborn infants. Univ. Iowa Stud. Child Welf., 9:75-135.

Suzuki, T., Y. Kamijo, and S. Kiuchi. 1964. Auditory test of newborn infants. Ann. Otol., 73:914-923.

Swarthwout, J. R., W. E. Campbell, Jr., and L. G. Williams. 1961. Observations of the fetal heart rate. Amer. J. Obstet. Gynec., 82:301-303.

Valdes-Dapena, M. A. 1967. Sudden and unexpected death in infancy: A review of the world literature. Pediatrics, 39:123-138.

Vallbona, C., et al. 1963. Cardiodynamic studies in the newborn. II. Regulation of the heart rate. Biol. Neonat., 5:159-199.

Wenger, M. A., and O. C. Irwin. 1936. Fluctuations in skin resistance of infants and adults and their relation to muscular processes. Univ. Iowa Stud. Child Welf., 12:143-179.

Wilder, J. 1967. Stimulus and Response: The Law of Initial Value. Bristol, John Wright and Sons, Ltd.

Wilkes, T., R. I. Friedman, J. Hodgman, and N. E. Levan. 1966. The sensitivity of the axon reflex in term and premature infants. J. Invest. Derm., 47:491-492.

Winter, S. T., et al. 1966. Neonatal cardiac deceleration on suckle feeding. Amer. J. Dis. Child., 112:11-20.

Young, I. M. 1962. Vasomotor tone in the skin blood vessels of the newborn infant. Clin. Sci., 22:325-332.

———— and W. W. Holland. 1958. Some physiological responses of neonatal arterial blood pressure and pulse rate. Brit. Med. J., 2:276-278.

———— and D. Cottom. 1966. Arterial and venous blood pressure responses during a reduction in blood volume and hypoxia and hypercapnia in infants during the first two days of life. Pediatrics, 37:733-742.

28

The Visual System

DAVID S. WALTON ● Massachusetts Eye and Ear
Infirmary, Boston, Massachusetts

Introduction

Visual behavior patterns dominate early neonatal development. From birth the wakefulness of the neonate is closely correlated with visual activity (Gesell, 1949). At birth he is sensitive to light, possesses reactive pupils, demonstrates conjugate eye movements, and opens his lids as if to see.

Within hours of birth the neonate may be observed to fixate on a near object. This stare, which is often uniocular, may be associated with slowing of body movement, raising of the eyelids, and cessation of crying. If moved, the visual stimulus may be pursued, a chase characterized by coarse conjugate refixation movements.

The month following delivery is characterized by rapid visual development. Periods of visual activity become longer, fixation and following become refined, binocularity becomes the rule, and the range of visual interest expands outward. In the weeks that follow, visual activity accelerates, mirrored by expressions of interest, curiosity, and joy.

It is the purpose of this chapter to describe the functional development of the visual system of the newborn, and to present in an integrated fashion selected data from the literature supporting these various levels of development.

Visual Function

VISUAL ACUITY

The clinical concept of visual acuity is the qualitative measurement of visual performance based on the recognition or interpretation of distant target forms. As a physiologic parameter, it is employed as an expression of overall ocular function and may be influenced by many factors, such as target contrast and illumination, pupillary size, clarity of ocular media, and refractive error, as well as by retinal factors, which include retinal sensitivity and histologic development. The ability of the retina to distinguish separate points or components of a target is the most common and useful test of visual acuity and is dependent upon the number of photoreceptors per unit area in the retina. Visual acuity is the most useful expression of visual achievement.

Measurement of visual acuity in the newborn period has required the use of an objective technique, and for this, optokinetic nystagmus has been utilized, varying the size of the targets. By correlating the onset of nystagmus in the infant with the separation of a series of moving targets, the visual acuity of premature and term infants has been estimated. This technique has shown good correlation with Snellen visual acuity values when tested with older subjects (Wolin and Dillman, 1964; Reinecke and Cogan, 1958). The Snellen system is based on a resolution of one minute of arc designated as 20/20.

Gorman et al. (1957) found 93 of 100 newborns responsive to a pattern equivalent to 20/670. Dayton et al. (1964b) concluded from results with 18 full-term infants that the expected visual acuity in this age group is at least 20/150. Kiff and Lepard (1966), in examining premature infants, estimated a visual acuity of 20/820 for such infants, with the earliest such response occurring in an infant weighing 1,418 g.

Application of this same optokinetic nystagmus technique to rhesus monkeys has demonstrated the development of visual acuity in the first postnatal months in eight neonates from approximately 20/400 after birth to 20/80 at age one month (Ordy et al., 1965).

FIXATION

Fixation is the visual reflex act, which functions to maintain the image of the object of regard on the retinal foveal area of maximum visual acuity. Successful following of an object, such as the optokinetic nystagmus test objects or an examiner's light, depends on the integrity of this fundamental ocular mechanism. The infant who does not soon locate and fixate his mother and nearby attractive objects becomes suspect of blindness.

Examination of full-term newborn infants of less than 10 days of age has demonstrated the presence of an intact fixation reflex in 17 out of 30 subjects alert enough for testing (Dayton et al., 1964a). A qualitative evaluation of the fixation reflex in 163 normal infants from birth to 6 months of age has described its refinement through this period (Dayton and Jones, 1964). The amplitude of readjustment movements during periods of successful following of a moving object was found to decrease markedly during the first 10 days of life, followed by a more gradual decrease in the frequency of such movements over the first 6 months of life.

Haith (1968) has demonstrated preferential fixation in the newborn for certain types of objects. A vertical edge induced many fixations, while a horizontal edge induced essentially none. When presented with an acute angle, fixations were seen to be concentrated at its apex. Such studies suggest that fixation in the newborn infant is not only present but in addition has become complex and refined.

RETINAL DEVELOPMENT

In the sixteenth century the retina was established as the light-sensitive element of the eye. The true optical function of the crystalline lens was later described by Dioptrics in 1610. In the centuries that have followed, investigators have studied the retina in search of answers to many questions, including those related to estimating and explaining the visual capacity of the newborn.

The retina is an appendage of the central nervous system. Impulses initiated in its photosensitive cells (rods and cones) are relayed by axons of the ganglion cell layer to an intracranial relay center. The histologic development of the human neonatal retina has reached a level of maturation approximating that of an adult; however, the visually important foveal region at its center is the least developed of its parts. Its relative underdevelopment, and subsequent rapid differentiation during the first four postnatal months, has historically provided support for the belief that neonates should have little visual capacity (Duke-Elder, 1963a). More recent studies lend support to the quite advanced degree of human neonatal visual function already described.

Morphology

Light microscopy of the retina of the newborn human and rhesus monkey demonstrates fully structured rods and cones, pigment epithelium, and inner adult retinal layers. Thinning of the retina with peripheral spread of the ganglion cells away from the central foveal depression has already begun. Refinement occurs in the postnatal period. Foveal cones increase in number concomitant with elongation and thinning of their outer segments. The fovea's high density of cones, already present at birth and increased postnatally, is the anatomic basis for its selective high visual acuity. These changes are completed by the fifth postnatal month (Duke-Elder, 1963a). The neonatal retinal architecture of the human (Duke-Elder, 1963a) and the rhesus monkey (Ordy et al., 1965) is similar and markedly more advanced at birth than that of the dog and rat, whose retinas at birth correspond to the level achieved by the human fetus during the fifth gestational month. The subsequent retinal development in these animals is rapid, with a level equivalent to the human neonate reached by the end of the first postpartum month.

Electron Microscopy

Electron microscopy of the important cone outer segments in the foveal region of the newborn rhesus monkey shows well-developed bimembraneous lamellar plates closely resembling those seen in the adult (Ordy et al., 1965). Wiedman and Kuwabara (1968) have used the electron microscope to illustrate the development stages of the rat retina. This important work, describing retinal development paralleling human prenatal development, demonstrates the rapid early formation of the outer segments (rods and cones) of the photoreceptors concomitant with the development of the retinal cellular layers and their synaptic unions in the outer plexiform layer. The electroretinographic quiet present at this stage is shown to end with the development of inner synapses with the ganglion cell layer. Only further cellular differentiation is still required to reach a stage equivalent to the human neonatal retina.

Electrophysiology

The electroretinogram is a recording of the change in corneoretinal potential evoked by a light stimulus and occurring secondary to retinal synaptic electric activity. The ERG is influenced by the wavelength of the light, the state of light adaptation of the eye, the intensity of light reaching the retina, and the maturation of the retina. Since 1951 electroretinography has been applied to the interpretation of the visual performance of the newborn (Letterstrom, 1951). Suspected absence of an ERG response in term and premature newborns, followed by progressive development during the first six months of life, was felt consistent with the suspected low level of visual function in the neonate (Letterstrom, 1951, 1952).

In 1960, Horsten and Winkelman reported the appearance of the ERG in developing dog retina at a stage comparable to the human during the seventh fetal month. The appearance of the response was found at considerably higher intensity than was required for a mature retina, and it was also favorably affected by prolongation of dark adaptation. Examination of newborn rhesus monkeys revealed discernible ERG potentials on the day of birth, followed by rapid maturation to adult responses during the first two months of life (Ordy et al., 1965). Reexamination of term and premature infants followed, employing higher intensity stimuli. It was shown that the ERG is present in the newborn and that it does not differ in form from that of the adult (Horsten and Winkelman, 1962). Action potentials were increased by dark adaptation and reached adult size over the first three months (Letterstrom, 1951). The presence in the newborn ERG of a demonstrable negative A wave, as well as a positive B wave, gives support to the presence of an active photopic (cone) retinal visual system. Electroretinographic evidence of fusion of repeated light flashes at adult frequencies (Horsten and Winkelman, 1962), and more recently, the finding of the photopic X wave in newborn ERG when stimulated with long wavelength light, also indicate that cone vision is functional in the neonate (Barnet et al., 1965).

LOWER AND CENTRAL VISUAL PATHWAYS

The lower visual pathway is formed by the axons of retinal ganglion cells directed to central thalamic and tegmental centers. This pathway is recognized grossly by its three anatomic divisions: the optic nerves, chiasm, and optic tracts. The central visual pathway is formed by the paired lateral geniculate subcenters in the thalami, their projections in the cerebral cortex, and the association tracts arising in the occipital lobes.

Morphology

By the end of the first fetal trimester the lower visual pathway is well developed with recognizable nerve fibers extending posteriorly to the chiasm where partial decussation occurs, followed by extension to the embryologic thalami. During the middle trimester, septal vessels grow into the optic nerve, and the dural, arachnoid, and pial sheaths are completed. The final trimester is characterized by cellular differentiation and myelin formation. Myelination is initiated and then proceeds distally from the geniculate bodies, becoming evident in the optic tracts in the sixth month, in the optic nerves in the seventh month, and reaching the eye during the ninth gestational month (Duke-Elder, 1963b). This process has been found to be completed in the optic tract of term newborns, but present only in the axial fibers of the optic nerve (Nakayama, 1968). The macular fibers are those first myelinated in the optic nerve (Bembridge, 1956). There appeared to be no acceleration of myelination in premature infants compared with term newborns of a similar gestational age (Nakayama, 1968).

It might be well to recall that nerve function is thought to be poorly correlated with myelination; pupillary responsiveness to light has been seen at six months in premature infants long before the completion of myelination (Magitot, 1909).

Development of the upper visual pathways and primary and association neuronal centers in the occipital lobe may be the limiting link in the visual system of the newborn. Myelination in these pathways is first seen at about the time of birth, occurring first in the cortical projection system, which carries the primary visual stimulus from the geniculate bodies to area 17 in the occipital lobe. Myelination proceeds forward centrifugally from the occipital centers and is later seen in the association tracts. Not until the fourth postnatal month is myelination of all the main visual fiber tracts completed (Duke-Elder, 1963c).

Functional correlation with this histologic evidence of early visual tract development is provided by the presence in the newborn of the optokinetic reflex, location and fixation of an object, following of an object, pupillary reactivity, and other signs of visual responsiveness. The behavior of the normal seeing newborn is in marked contrast to that of the blind infant (Knox, 1964).

Electrophysiology

Light-evoked cortical potentials have been examined in the newborn. In a group of 120 human newborns, including 58 prematures, responses were obtained from the occipital regions following light stimulus in all except 3 of the prematures (Hrbek and Mares, 1964). Responses differed from those of older children and adults in the shape of the wave response, fatigability, and time lapse (latency) between the stimulus and initial positive wave response registered in the occipital region. The shape of evoked potentials in prematures resembled full-term responses. Absent response in one 1,700-g premature became present after 10 days. The latency period was greatest in the prematures and decreased progressively with age in all the newborn subjects. The fatigability of the responses at relatively low stimulus frequencies (3 per second) was suggested due to the slowness of the metabolic process in newborn nerve cells (Hrbek and Mares, 1964).

Similar examinations using newborn rhesus monkeys demonstrated progressive diminution of the latency period, reaching adult values by the third month of life (Ordy et al., 1965).

Hubel and Wiesel (1963) have studied single occipital cortical cell responses to patterned retinal stimuli in visually inexperienced and experienced newborn kittens and compared their receptive field organization, cellular binocular interaction, and functional architecture with results from similar studies using adult cats. The responses from kitten cortical cells were found to be strikingly similar to those of the adult cat, suggesting that highly complex neural connections are developed in the newborn and do not await the arrival of light stimulation or other visual experience (Hubel and Wiesel, 1963).

Ocular Motility

Each eye acquires motility within its respective facial socket by the action of six extraocular muscles. The higher the mammal is in the phylogenetic scale, the more highly developed are the extraocular muscles and eye movements (Cogan, 1956a). An increased range of movement allows for the preservation of a wide visual field, in spite of the developmental shift of the eyes from the side to the front of the head, associated with the climb up the phylogenetic scale.

From an early embryonic stage, the four rectus muscles are seen in the orbit in their adult arrangement, directed to the globe from their origin at the apex of the orbit. The medial rectus appears more fully developed than the lateral rectus muscle during embryologic development. The oblique muscles' development parallels that of the rectus muscles. During the course of fetal development the muscles lengthen and narrow until at term they resemble the mature state.

The extraocular muscles are voluntary and, within the family of striated muscles, they have unique pharmacologic, histologic, and physiologic characteristics which have been well described (Cogan, 1956b; Adler, 1959b). One of the unique features of these muscles is their constant state of electric activity, even when the eye is in the straight ahead position, which contrasts to the electric quiet of a relaxed skeletal muscle.

The position of an eye or its velocity is determined by the relative innervation received by opposing pairs of ocular muscles. Centers which control this innervation are the following: from the labyrinth in response to body position or acceleration, from the retina in response to light intensity, eccentric fixation, and disparateness of retinal images (i.e., not falling on corresponding retinal receptor areas), and from cerebral centers participating in voluntary and object-elicited eye movements, in movements in response to sound, and in following or pursuit eye movements. These centers work simultaneously to determine the momentary resultant ocular muscle equilibrium.

It has often been the custom, when describing the ocular movements of the newborn and their development, to speak of their sequential development (Kestenbaum, 1961). Vestibular movements were conceded to be present at birth, followed by the appearance of random movements followed at age two weeks by (object) optically elicited movements. Following movements were said then to occur at age four months, followed later by acoustically elicited eye movements and voluntary movements at age five months. The loss of oculomotor function in the reverse order in progressive deterioration of the central nervous system with the uncovering of the various stages of development may be indirect evidence to support this sequential pattern of development (Jampel and Quaglio, 1961). Recent studies have at least moved the timetable ahead by demonstrating a complex system of eye movements to be already present in the neonate. They are usefully described in the order applied above.

Forced conjugate deviation of the eyes in response to vestibular stimulation is perhaps the first and simplest eye movement in the developmental hierarchy. These movements are analogous to the residual doll's head movements seen with rotation of the head in the presence of acquired paralysis of the other sources of conjugate gaze. Forced deviation of the eyes appeared to be the only type of induced eye movement present in resting premature infants of 32 to 34 weeks of gestational age (Pendleton and Paine, 1961).

Following stimulation, premature infants first demonstrated the onset of post-rotatory vestibular nystagmus at 33 weeks of gestational age and at subsequent ages regularly demonstrated vestibular nystagmus similar to that seen in full-term infants when subjected to body rotation. Vestibular nystagmus consists of forced deviation secondary to the effect of rotation on the semicircular vestibular end-organs and of a reflex quick return component of uncertain origin but probably utilizing pathways related to voluntary gaze. Vestibular nystagmus, in response to rotation, is best seen as a postrotatory phenomenon and is a constant finding in the awake, full-term neonate. Its absence is a sensitive sign of a normal or pathologic variation in the state of consciousness. Vestibular nystagmus in response to caloric stimulation in the newborn has been variously reported as present or absent. Its presence should be expected in the alert neonate.

During the clinical examination, object-elicited movements are difficult to initiate in response to a hand light or other objective until about three weeks of age. Their association with head movements soon appears after this time. In contrast, following movements can usually be demonstrated to either side in the immediate postnatal period using simple targets by beginning the test in the center of the field.

Following movements have been shown to be well developed in the neonate (Dayton and Jones, 1964) and to possess a high degree of conjugation. The difference between the following movements of infants and those of older children is in the number and amplitude of necessary refixations required to correct the tendency of the following eye to fall behind the moving target. Refinement of these following movements occurs over the first year of life, with the amplitude of the refixations decreasing rapidly during the first two neonatal weeks. The angular velocity of the refixation movements is very rapid compared with the relatively slow following or pursuit movement. There is both anatomic and neurophysiologic support for the presence of independent rapid (saccadic) and slow (pursuit or following) oculomotor systems (Miller, 1968). Their integrated activity produces successful following movements.

It is interesting that normal voluntary eye movements are never slow eye movements but rather resemble the rapid saccadic refixations or the object-elicited type movement. It is a moot question when the neonate first shows voluntary eye movement. The presence of the rapid phase of vestibular nystagmus, and the saccadic refixation with following movements in the term and premature neonate, suggest that the initiation of voluntary gaze movements awaits only the development of an intellectual desire for them.

Convergence and divergence eye movements are first seen during the third month (Haith, 1968).

The Intraocular Pressure

An important characteristic of an eyeball is its internal pressure. Only arterial pressure is greater than the intraocular pressure among body organ systems. The chief function of intraocular pressure is to maintain the shape of the cornea. Variations out of the normal pressure range decrease corneal transparency. Increased pressure causes edema and clouding of the cornea, and decreased pressure allows corneal wrinkling to occur.

The eye may be considered a sphere of constant volume, with relatively little elasticity. The anterior chamber, behind the cornea, is shallow in the newborn and communicates with the posterior chamber through the pupil. These chambers are filled with an aqueous solution. Although affected momentarily by arterial pulsation and external pressure, intraocular pressure is chiefly determined by the balance between aqueous humor formation and rate of outflow. The aqueous humor is secreted from the ciliary processes of the ciliary body, exists in equilibrium with iris blood vessels, and is finally filtered out through the trabecular meshwork to reach the extraocular venous network. Alteration in aqueous formation and drainage occurs to produce normal and abnormal variations in the intraocular pressure.

The development of the anterior segment occurs after the fifth gestational month. The anterior chamber and posterior chamber become defined by the growth of iris mesoderm, and the angle structures form concomitant with the cleavage of mesoderm between the developing iris and cornea. At birth, the angle of the anterior chamber is well developed, and in the postnatal period its development continues with circumferential migration of its apex, with widening of the angle, and with the occurrence of pigmentation. These stages have been well illustrated (Duke-Elder, 1963d). Study of the embryologic and postnatal development of the corneoscleral angle has shown the intimate relationship of the ciliary body musculature and filtering trabecular meshwork (Kupfer, 1962).

Tonometeric pressure readings in the premature newborn were first reported by Brockhurst (1955), who examined 59 premature infants under topical anesthesia. Three infants, born nearly 3 months prematurely, demonstrated hypotony, while the others had an average pressure of 24 mm Hg (1948 Friedenwald Standard Tonometer Scale). Thirty-two tonometer readings in one-hour-old, full-term neonates revealed high normal pressures (Giles, 1959). Examination of 100 eyes in full-term newborns during the first week of life using topical anesthesia revealed an average pressure of 16 mm Hg, with values ranging between 11 and 24 mm Hg (1955 Friedenwald Scale) (Horven, 1961). In this study, lower pressure determination correlated with newborns of greater birth-weight. The intraocular pressure of 356 normal eyes of children from age 1 day to age 10 years has been measured under ether general anesthesia (Kornblueth et al., 1964). Ninety-six of these eyes, examined during the first year of life, had an average pressure of 21 mm Hg (1955 scale). Later childhood years correlated with a progressive diminution of the intraocular pressure.

The Pupil

The pupil is the round aperture seen in the center of the iris annulus. Functional iris components include a central sphincter muscle and a peripheral dilator muscle. The sphincter fibers appear in an early embryologic stage and give the pupil movement in response to light as early as the sixth gestational month. The dilator muscle does not make its appearance until the sixth month and is not fully formed and functional until after birth.

The pupil at birth is usually small and shows only moderate movement in response to light. Enlargement of the resting pupil may occur early in the postnatal period or may be delayed until one year of age. Its size then progresses to reach a maximum size during adolescence.

Lacrimal System

The function of the lacrimal system is the maintenance of a normal precorneal and conjunctival tear film. Tears act as a lubricant, possess antibacterial properties, and enhance the optical characteristics of the front of the cornea. To accomplish these functions and others, tears have a complex composition and organized layering (Mishima, 1965; Adler, 1959a).

The basic physiologic tear fluid seen under usual conditions is mostly the secretion of accessory lacrimal glands associated intimately with the conjunctival fornices. These glands are present at birth but have not completed their development. Excessive tear production, as seen secondary to corneal irritation or to psychic stimulation, is produced by the main lacrimal gland. This structure appears early in embryologic development and, though well formed at birth, does not reach full development until age three to four years (Kirchstein, 1894).

Obstruction of the lacrimal drainage passage is a common clinical problem in pediatric ophthalmology. The development of the nasolacrimal passages has been well described and illustrated (Cassidy, 1952; Sjogren, 1955). Canalization of the system begins early at its ocular end. The lacrimal puncta open on the lid margins during the seventh month; however, the lower end of the nasolacrimal duct, even at birth, is frequently separated from the nasal cavity. This block consists of a membrane formed by the opposed mucosal linings of the nasal fornix and lacrimal duct. An investigation of 15 full-term stillborn fetuses revealed this abnormality in 73 percent of their lacrimal ducts (Cassidy, 1952).

When basic tear production was examined in 65 noncrying, premature newborns using Schirmer litmus paper, secretion was found to be proportionate to body weight (Apt and Cullen, 1964). Only 14 percent of prematures of less than 1,500 g had normal tear production, while 63 percent of those weighing between 2,000 and 2,500 g had normal lacrimation. Tear secretion increases progressively during the first postnatal month following premature birth (Sjogren, 1955). Lacrimation in the premature newborn is increased with crying (Apt and Cullen, 1964).

Lacrimation in the full-term newborn is usually normal. Eighty-two percent of 140 eyes belonging to noncrying, one-day-old newborns demonstrated normal secretion using the adult Schirmer standard (Apt and Cullen, 1964). This percentage increased with the crying state or with retesting at one week of age.

Paper electrophoresis of tear samples from eight newborns demonstrated normal globulin, albumin, and lysozymal concentration when compared with adult tear fluid (Apt and Cullen, 1964). Assay for the presence of lysozymal antibacterial activity was also in an adult normal range (Apt and Cullen, 1964).

Psychic weeping is usually delayed until the third or fourth postnatal month.

Refractive State

Vision depends on the production of focused images on the retina. The anterior surface of the cornea is the principal refracting surface and is aided by the lens inside the eye. The lens can vary its power, and so can function as the fine focusing component. Refraction in the eye is a function of the corneal and lens curvatures (lens power), the distance between these lenses, and their distance from the retina.

Compared with the body, the eye grows little, increasing its volume only threefold from birth to maturity. Seventy percent of this increment, however, is attained by age four (Kaiser, 1926). The main growth occurs in the posterior segment.

The cornea of the newborn is proportionately larger than that of the mature eye and is geometrically similar to that of an adult (Mandell, 1967) (Fig. 1). The radius of curvature of its center is about 1 mm less than that of an adult cornea (Mandell, 1967). The flattening of the cornea with postnatal growth helps to mask the myopic effect of axial elongation.

The lens also flattens with continued postnatal growth and occupies proportionately less volume.

The total refractive error of full-term newborns is usually (in 80 percent of infants tested) hyperopic and between one and four diopters (Cook, 1951). Astigmatism is found more frequently in the hyperopic newborn than in the myopes (Cook, 1951). With postnatal growth, the eye becomes more hyperopic into early childhood, followed by a progressive myopic growth pattern (Slataper, 1950).

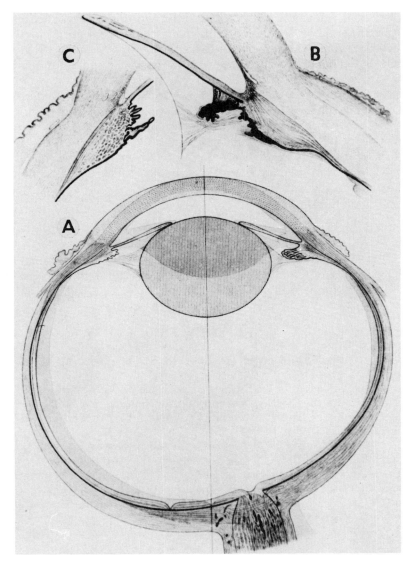

Fig. 1. The eye of the newborn. A. Horizontal sections of infant and adult eyes adjusted for size and superimposed. B. Adult corneoscleral angle. C. Newborn corneoscleral angle. Note position of Schlemn's canal and retention of mesodermal tissue, compared with Figure B. (Merkel and Orr. 1892, *Anat. Hefte,* 1:273-296.)

Examination of 150 premature infants found a predominance of emmetropia or myopia (Graham and Gray, 1963).

Conclusions

Visual behavior in the newborn is active and develops rapidly. The visual acuity of the newborn is about 20/200 and improves steadily. He can fixate immediately at birth. Retinal development is advanced at birth, awaiting only macular refinement in the neonatal period. Electroretinography indicates the presence of a well-developed visual cone system. Myelination of the optic pathways is completed after birth.

At birth, the eye moves well in response to vestibular stimuli and to moving objects.

Structures controlling aqueous humor dynamics are incompletely developed in the newborn. The intraocular pressure in the newborn may be slightly higher than in the normal adult when measured with a Schiotz tonometer.

The pupil is small and reactive in the newborn.

Basic tear production is qualitatively and quanitatively normal in the neonate.

The newborn refractive error is usually hyperopic. The eye is proportionately large at birth, compared with the body as a whole.

Acknowledgment

The author is indebted to Dr. Richard M. Robb, Children's Hospital Medical Center, Department of Ophthalmology, for his personal assistance, and to Miss Carol M. Turnbull for her editorial assistance.

REFERENCES

Adler, F. H. 1959a. Physiology of the Eye, 3rd ed. St. Louis, C. V. Mosby Co., pp. 33-42.
———— 1959b. Physiology of the Eye, 3rd ed. St. Louis, C. V. Mosby Co., pp. 356-386.
Apt, L., and B. F. Cullen. 1964. Newborns do secrete tears. J.A.M.A., 189:951-953.
Barnet, A. B., A. Lodge, and J. C. Armington. 1965. Electroretinogram in newborn human infants. Science, 148:651-654.
Becker, B. 1958. The decline in aqueous secretion and outflow facility with age. Amer. J. Ophthal., 46:731-736.
Bembridge, B. A. 1956. The problem of myelination of the central nervous system with special reference to the optic nerve. Trans. Ophthal. Soc. U.K., 76:311.
Brockhurst, R. J. 1955. The intraocular pressure of premature infants. Amer. J. Ophthal., 39:808-11.
Cassidy, J. V. 1952. Developmental anatomy of the nasolacrimal duct. Arch. Ophthal. (Chicago), 47:141-158.
Cogan, D. G. 1956a. Neurology of the Ocular Muscles. Springfield, Ill., Charles C Thomas, Publisher, p. 7.
———— 1956b. Neurology of the Ocular Muscles. Springfield, Ill., Charles C Thomas, Publisher, Ch. 3.
Cook, R. C. 1951. Refractive and ocular findings in the newborn. Amer. J. Ophthal., 34:1407.
Dayton, G., and M. Jones. 1964. Analysis of characteristics of fixation reflex in infants by use of direct current electrooculography. Neurology, 14:1152-1156.
———— M. Jones, B. Steele, M. Rose. 1964a. Developmental study of coordinated eye movements in the human infant. II. Fixation reflex. Arch. Ophthal. (Chicago), 71:871-875.
———— M. Jones, R. Rawson, B. Steele, and M. Rose. 1964b. Developmental study

of coordinated eye movements in the human infant. I. Visual acuity determined by electrooculography. Arch. Ophthal. (Chicago), 71:865-870.

Duke-Elder, W. S. 1963a. System of Ophthalmology. St. Louis, C. V. Mosby Co., Vol. 3, Part 1, pp. 96-99.

——— 1963b. System of Ophthalmology. St. Louis, C. V. Mosby Co., Vol. 3, Part 1, p. 119.

——— 1963c. System of Ophthalmology. St. Louis, C. V. Mosby Co., Vol. 3, Part 1, p. 125.

——— 1963d. System of Ophthalmology. St. Louis, C. V. Mosby Co., Vol, 3, Part 1, pp. 171-179.

——— 1963e. System of Ophthalmology. St. Louis, C. V. Mosby Co., Vol. 3, Part 1, pp. 241-246.

Gesell, A. 1949. Vision: Its Development in Infant and Child. New York, Paul B. Hoeber, Inc.

Giles, G. L. 1959. Tonometer tensions in the newborn. Arch. Ophthal. (Chicago), 61:517-519.

Gorman, J., et al. 1957. An apparatus for grading the visual acuity of infants on the basis of optokinetic nystagmus. Pediatrics, 19:1088-1092.

Graham, M. V., and O. Gray. 1963. Refraction of premature babies' eyes. Brit. Med. J., 1:1452-54.

Haith, M. 1968. Personal communication.

Horsten, G. P. M., and J. E. Winkelman. 1960. Development of the ERG in relation to histological differentiation of the retina in man and animals. Arch. Ophthal. (Chicago), 63:232-242.

——— and J. E. Winkelman. 1962. Electrical activity of the retina in relation to histological differentiation in infants born prematurely and at full-term. Vision Res., 2:269-276.

Horven, I. 1961. Tonometry in newborn infants. Acta Ophthal. (Kobenhavn), 39:911-918.

Hrbek, A., and P. Mares. 1964. Cortical evoked responses to visual stimulation in full-term and premature newborns. Electroenceph. Clin. Neurophysiol., 16:575-581.

Hubel, D. H., and T. Wiesel. 1963. Receptive fields of cells in striate cortex of very young, visually inexperienced kittens. J. Neurophysiol., 26:994-1002.

Jampel, R. S., and N. Quaglio. 1961. Eye movements in Tay-Sachs disease. Neurology, 11:1013-1019.

Kaiser. 1926. Graefe. Arch. Klin. Exp. Ophthal., 116:288.

Kestenbaum, A. 1961. Clinical Methods of Neuro-ophthalmologic Examinations. New York, Grune & Stratton, Inc.

Kiff, R., and C. Lepard. 1966. Visual response of premature infants. Arch. Ophthal. (Chicago), 75:631-633.

Kirchstein, F. 1894. Ueber die Tränendrüse der Neugeborenen. Dissertation. Berlin.

Knox, L. 1964. Cortically blind infants. Amer. J. Ophthal., 58:617-621.

Kornblueth, W. 1959. Influence of general anesthesia on intraocular pressure in man. Arch. Ophthal. (Chicago), 61:84-87.

——— et al. 1964. Intraocular pressure in children measured under general anesthesia. Arch. Ophthal. (Chicago), 72:489-490.

Kupfer, C. 1962. Relationship of ciliary body meridional muscle and corneoscleral trabecular meshwork. Arch. Ophthal. (Chicago), 68:818-822.

Letterstrom, B. 1951. The clinical electroretinogram. IV. The electroretinogram in children during the first year of life. Acta Ophthal. (Kobenhavn), 29:295-304.

——— 1952. The electroretinogram in prematurely born children. Acta Ophthal. (Kobenhavn), 30:405-408.

Magitot, A. 1909. L'Apparition précoce du réflexe photomoteur au cours du développement foetal. Ann. Oculist (Paris), 141:161.

Mandell, R. B. 1967. Corneal contour of the human infant. Arch. Ophthal. (Chicago), 77:345-348.

Merkel, F., and W. Orr. 1892. Das Auge des Neugeborenen an einem schematischen Durchschnitt erläutert. Anat. Hefte, 1:273-296.

Miller, D. 1968. Saccadic and pursuit systems: A review. J. Pediat. Ophthal., 5:39-43.

Mishima, S. 1965. Some physiological aspects of the precorneal tear film. Arch. Ophthal. (Chicago), 73:233-241.

Nakayama, K. 1968. Studies on the myelination of the human optic nerve. Jap. J. Ophthal., 11:132-140.

Ordy, J. M., et al. 1965. Postnatal development of vision in a subhuman primate. Arch. Ophthal. (Chicago), 73:674-686:

Pendleton, M. E., and R. Paine. 1961. Vestibular nystagmus in newborn infants. Neurology, 11:450-458.

Reinecke, R., and D. Cogan. 1958. Standardization of objective visual acuity measurements. Arch. Ophthal. (Chicago), 60:418-421.

Sjogren, H. 1955. Lacrimal secretion in newborn premature and fully developed children. Acta Ophthal. (Kobenhavn), 33:557-560.

Slataper, F. J. 1950. Age norms of refraction and vision. Arch. Ophthal. (Chicago), 43:466-481.

Wiedman, T. A., and T. Kuwabara. 1968. Postnatal development of the rat retina. Arch. Ophthal. (Chicago), 79:470-484.

Wolin, I., and A. Dillman. 1964. Objective measurement of visual acuity. Arch. Ophthal. (Chicago), 71:822-826.

29

Morphologic and Functional Development of the Skin

J. GLEISS • Kinderabteilung St. Josef-Hospital, Oberhausen-Sterkrade, Germany and G. STÜTTGEN • Hautklinik der Freien Universität, Berlin, Germany

Introduction

The skin of our body performs many functions: it is the outer covering, storage, regulator of body temperature, and a secreting organ as well as a sense-organ.

This biologically uniform organ is composed of the ectodermal epidermis and the mesodermal corium (cutis).

The skin of the newborn differs considerably from that of the adult. The epidermal layers are thinner, particularly the transitional and cornified layers. The sebaceous glands, which in the newborn are temporarily functioning under the influence of maternal androgenous hormones, are as yet insufficiently developed. However, the function of the eccrine sweat glands is established. Due to the incomplete development of immunobiologic resistance, the susceptibility to bacterial infections is high, particularly for certain types of diseases (hidradenitis suppurative). Because of its physical and biochemical qualities the skin of the newborn and of the young infant is very vulnerable to even the least irritation, easily forming blisters. The turgor of the skin and the lack of histamine make intercellular diffusion easy, and this accounts for the almost complete absence of urticarial eruptions.

Our present knowledge of the physiology of the newborn and of the infant skin in particular is by no means complete; especially fragmentary is the role of hormonal, nervous, and intermediary metabolic regulations.

Morphologic and physiologic proven data are therefore the basis of our paper on the physiology and pathophysiology of the skin in the perinatal period, and functional relationships are mentioned where appropriate. Genetic factors determine to a high degree physiologic and pathologic changes in the skin of the newborn. In numerous publications (Jadassohn, 1966) more than 150 anomalies of the skin have been reported due to different genes: autosomal dominant 105, autosomal recessive 31, and gonosomal x:8, y:1. The connection between mutation of genes and skin anomalies is in most cases unknown.

Since the knowledge of the physiology of the newborn's skin is relatively sparse, it seems desirable to supplement it with already existing data on animals of corresponding ages. Even though valuable information is obtained through test data, we cannot unconditionally transfer these from the animal to the human. Similarities have been surmised in the development of the epidermis of the chicken and the human, and these have for the most part been confirmed (Pasteels, 1936-37).

Fetal Skin

Examinations of 1-month-old fetuses of Yorkshire pigs show that the thickness of the epidermis ranges from 2 to 5 cell layers and that blood vessels, blood isles, and hair follicles are present around the snout. On days 50 to 53 the epidermal cells are enlarged, and the epidermis consists of 15 cell layers which include a stratum germinativum and a stratum spinosum, a two-layered dermis containing fat, and a prominent panniculus adiposus in the abdominal and axillary skin regions. At this stage the sinus hair can be distinguished from regular hair. Nonsecreting sebaceous glands, tubular sweat glands of the eyelid and of the dorsal region of the neck, as well as mammary anlagen are present. At the age of 72 to 74 days there is an increase in vascularization and innervation of the arrector pili muscles in the corium, and hairs in groups of three to five follicles are present. Sebaceous glands and hair ducts can be seen, and on day 95 the epitrichium covering the dorsal neck region is 2 to 3 layers thick. The skin now resembles that of an adult animal.

The collagen fractions of the pig embryo skin which are soluble in neutral salt solutions contain only traces of globular, loosely bound proteins and 2 to 4 percent polysaccharide-protein complexes (Tustanovsky et al., 1964).

The use of alkaline solvents recovers, in addition to residues insoluble in hydrochloric acid and citric salt solution, up to 65 percent of procollagen proteins of different stages of maturity which appear to be bound to the outer microphase of the collagen fiber.

Hydroxyproline is a component of collagen; it occurs in the nonsoluble tissue residue. The composition of this residue resembles pure preparations of almost completely mature colostromines. Colostromine belongs to the group of collagen precursors and contains polypeptides of varying degrees of polymerization and maturation.

There is general agreement that water- and salt-soluble collagen fractions diminish with age in different groups of animals and man. This process is correlated with the number and strength of bonds between the collagen macromolecules and with the extractability in different electrolyte solutions. The accumulation of noncollagenous proline during early stages of development, and its diminution with increasing age, further elucidates this process. In addition, distinct relationships exist between hydroxyproline and aging (Gonzales-Cadavid et al., 1963).

Skin of the Newborn

In contrast to the skin of the adult, that of the newborn mouse absorbs large amounts of proline and transforms it into hydroxyproline (McLennan and Karasek, 1966).

In the newborn rat the hexosamine:collagen ratio is higher than in older and mature rats. Cortisone causes a decrease of the collagen and hexosamine content of the skin in all age groups, and this cortisone effect is strongest in the newborn rat.

Eleven-day-old chicken skin cultures rapidly lose the ability to incorporate thymidine. This is coincidental with the loss of the columnar arrangement of the basal cells of the epidermis. However, addition of fresh epidermis cells to aged skin cultures reverses these changes. Apparently the cellular incorporation of thymidine depends upon special conditions in the epidermis, which in turn seem to depend upon specific mesenchymal influences upon the developing epidermis (Wessells, 1963).

Experiments with salamander skin (Hay, 1964) revealed that the epidermis is able to secrete certain substances which form the basal lamella together with fibro-blasts of the cutis. These experiments also demonstrate that the epidermis secretes a protein which participates in collagen formation.

The cell-specific functions of the epidermis appear to change in accordance with phenotypic variations. When 15-day-old mouse skin was converted into a suspension of single cells by trypsin and shaking (Moscona and Moscona, 1965) these single cells had the tendency to aggregate and to form cell complexes capable of depositing glycogen and keratohyalin granula; also, hair formation could be observed with the onset of keratin deposition. The same observation could be noted when these cell suspensions were placed on the chorioallantoic membrane of chicken embryos; a typical mouse skin with hair follicles developed within 6 days. This phenomenon of embryonal skin formation could be inhibited if the mouse epidermis cell suspension was first spread as a monocellular layer on a liquid culture medium for 24 hours and then washed off, resuspended, and allowed to aggregate. It is of particular interest that no development of feathers occurs when epidermis cell suspensions of the mouse and chicken are mixed. From these observations the conclusion may be reached that, in contrast to hair development, the formation of feathers depends upon dermal factors (Moscona and Moscona, 1965).

Phosphodiesterase is highly concentrated in the cells of the skin of newborn mice (Žaruba et al., 1968). This enzyme activity is present in all tissues in rather high concentrations. However, the skin and intestinal epithelium have much higher concentrations than the brain and muscles.

Treatment of the human skin with vitamin A increases the rate of mitosis as observed from enhanced DNA incorporation of tritiated thymidine (Christophers, 1968). The same observation can be made on cultured embryonic rat cells. In contrast, addition of vitamin A to cell cultures of embryonic chicken skin results in formation of glandular epithelium rather than in the growth of epidermal cells. This is accompanied by a change in sensitivity of the cell cultures to different viruses (influenza and vaccinia) (Huang and Bang, 1964). We have mentioned these examples to point out the possibility that cell differentiation can be altered through various manipulations. Addition of 14-day-old skin cells to a 6- to 8-day-old cultured chicken skin cell aggregate suppresses completely feather formation. Likewise, there are reciprocal influences between corium and epidermal growth rates (Garber, 1967).

Through modern immunoelectrophoresis, skin-specific antigens can be identified during the development of the skin or feathers following induction of appropriate antibodies (Ben-Or and Bell, 1965). Specific antigens are identified on day 6 (skin) and on day 13 (feathers) in the chicken. Two stage-specific antigens which are still missing on days 3, 4, and 5 can be demonstrated on the sixth day of incubation. Still another stage-specific antigen is apparent on day 11 or 12. The appearance of these new antigens on day 6 is related to feather induction which occurs between days 5 and 6. Chemical relationships have been identified between a specific antigen which appears first on day 13 and another antigen which is composed of stable polygonal complexes and which is already present at an earlier stage but not activated prior to day 13 (Ben-Or and Bell, 1965).

Morphology of the Embryonic and Neonatal Skin

This topic has been extensively studied by Becker (1954), Rhodin (1965), Töndury (1964), Breathnach and Wyllie (1965a, b), Riegel (1965), Koboyasi (1966), and by Hashimoto and his associates.

Epithelial cells regenerate from the stratum germinativum, which forms epidermal buds during the third month and which later differentiates into sebaceous and sweat glands. The absence of eccrine sweat glands in cases of congenital anhydrotic ectodermosis is due to lack of this differentiation. The dermal papilla of the hair is formed by mesenchymal cells around epidermal buds (follicle formation). Developmental disturbances at this stage lead to congenital atrichosis.

Following the fifth month of gestation the anuclear stratum corneum gradually replaces the periderm. A disturbance of this process results in abnormalities of keratinization. The vernix caseosa protects the newly formed stratum corneum during the last trimester. Angiogenesis commences during the second month. Concurrent with the proliferation of epithelial cells leading to formation of papillae and globuli in the deeper layers, eccrine and apocrine glands develop from vascular and ectodermal elements.

The components of the corium originate in the undifferentiated mesenchyme. Fibroblasts form delicate networks (positive silver staining) during the third month. These fibers increase in number and thickness, forming bundles of collagen like those in adults. Disturbances during this stage lead to the Ehlers-Danlos syndrome, among other diseases. Subcutaneous fetal fat can be detected during the third month, and it persists through the neonatal period. Chemical changes of the fetal fat may lead to subcutaneous fat necrosis and sclerema neonatorum. A peculiarity of this fat is its brown color. Cutis and epidermis remain a biologic unit and interact with each other. Inflammatory reaction of the cutis causes passive and active alterations of the epidermal layers, such as scaling and formation of blisters. The skin participates in disturbances of other organic systems through alterations of its own metabolism. Examples are increased secretion of sodium chloride through sweat glands in cases of cystic fibrosis, hyperpigmentation in Addison's disease, and disturbances of protein and amino acid metabolism, such as phenylketonuria. Neurofibromatosis, Albright's syndrome, tuberous sclerosis, and similar diseases are other examples which demonstrate the close relationship between the skin and systemic diseases.

Anatomy of the Skin

Epidermis and cutis are connected with each other through a basal membrane into which epidermal roots protrude. This basal membrane is a PAS-positive, continuous layer which is missing in certain skin diseases; therefore, it can be of diagnostic importance if it is undisturbed.

Melanocytes are imbedded in the stratum basale. Close to the middle layer of the stratum spinosum light cells can be observed. The origin and differentiation of those Langerhans cells has been mentioned above. The stratum spinosum has been named according to microscopically visible bridges among the cells. By electron microscopy these bridges were identified as desmosomes without syncytial connection to the cells. The number of desmosomes per cell was found to be between 2,000 and 3,000. The stratum spinosum is covered by the stratum granulosum which is characterized by flattening of the cells and the occurrence of cytoplasmic keratohyalin granula. The next layer is the stratum lucidum that, by light microscopy, can only be detected on the palms and soles. The top layer of the skin is the stratum corneum that consists of multiple lamellas and represents the final stage of keratinization. Half of the material forming the stratum corneum is keratin; the other half of the material originates from transformed cells into cornified lamellas.

PIGMENT CELLS

There is no doubt that pigment cells originate from the neural cord and probably also to a certain degree from the neural tube. This, at least, has been proven for amphibians and birds. Heteroplastic skin grafts of albino and pigmented newborn mice revealed that the hairs growing in the peripheral areas of the implant showed the color characteristics of the host while the hairs in the center of the implant demonstrated color characteristics of the donor, due to the fact that the skin already contained melanophores at the time of the experiment (Reed and Henderson, 1940). Hence, it is possible to combine the hairs of one genotype with the pigment cells of another genotype.

The formation of the neural cord and the migration of mesoderm occurs around the sixth week of gestation. The precursors of melanocytes are detectable around the tenth week. Melanoblasts of the Negro fetus are not distinguishable from mesenchymal cells up to the ninth week (Becker et al., 1952). Hence, there is a time interval of three to four weeks which has not been bridged in the human through direct observations. Observations in animals could close this gap. It has been found that the precursors of pigment cells migrate from the neural cord into the dermis and that these appear first in the head region. Melanoblasts migrate from the dermis toward the epidermis; the invasion occurs about the eleventh or twelfth week. Incorporation of pigment granula into epithelial cells through dendritic melanocytes has been observed around the fifth month. Finally the reservoir of melanocytes will be exhausted except for small residuals in various regions of the body (e.g., pigmented nevi).

Variations in location and migration of melanocytes are responsible for pigment anomalies. Examples are the blue nevus of Jadassohn, pigmented nevi, nevus Ota (in which melanin-carrying melanocytes are located in the corium), and nevus cell nevi as well as melanocytic nevi. Melanocytes possess numerous tiny branches which surround neighboring cells with a fine network of dendrites. They virtually inject these neighboring epidermal cells with their pigment. Melanocytes originate in the neural cord from which they migrate dorsoventrally along the craniocaudal axis into all regions of the embryo. They increase rapidly in number beginning between the twelfth and fourteenth weeks, and at the end of the thirteenth week their number exceeds $1{,}000/mm^3$. The genetic constitution of the melanocytes determines their differentiation. Melanin bodies are formed in each genotype and eventually are deposited in the epidermis. Exogenous factors are apparently influencing developmental potentials. The fetal skin is not pigmented during its development (Töndury, 1964), and the melanoblasts are distributed independently of the segmented regions of the body since there is no segmental division of the epidermis and cutis.

Melanogenesis of the epidermis of bush babies (*Galago senegalensis* and *Galago crassicaudatus*) commences during fetal life, reaches its peak at the time of birth, and disappears permanently during early postnatal life. The epidermis of the hair-growing skin is almost completely pigment-free except for the ears which remain pigmented throughout life. Dendritic melanocytes are present in the upper portions of fully mature hair follicles. These melanocytes are active only during the early stages, and then they become dormant until the next growth cycle (Yun and Montagna, 1965).

Electronmicroscopic examinations of melanocytes and Langerhans cells (the latter having been recently studied more extensively by Niebaur, 1968) in the skin of the 14-week-old human fetus revealed that epidermal melanocytes located in the basal and lower intermediate layers of the epidermis contain nonmelanized premelanosomes.

No melanocytes were discovered in the cutis. Melanoblastlike cells could not be classified because of lack of specific criteria for their identification. The few Langerhans cells of neonatal skin which are identical with those found in the adult contain no premelanosomes. Therefore, the Langerhans cells are "not the outworn remnant of a previously melanogenic melanocyte" (Breathnach and Wyllie, 1965).

SKIN SURFACE

A characteristic finding for skin of the various age groups is the relief formation of the skin surface. These are present in the newborn at the buttocks, axillas, and folds of the inner aspect of the thighs (adductor folds and horizontal folds at the level of the umbilicus). The folds of the joints as well as those of the plantar region of the foot and the palm of the hand are well formed in the newborn. Those of the foot are more varied in the newborn than in the adult because they are the point of insertion of the palmar and plantar aponeurosis.

Papillary lines are prominent on the fingers, palm, plantar regions of the foot, and toes of the newborn although they are flatter than in the adult. The width of these papillary lines in the volar aspect of the finger of the newborn varies between 0.18 and 0.22 mm versus 0.4 to 0.5 mm in the adult. Three systems of folds can be identified on fingers. One originates at the base of the finger, another around the nail bed, and the third at the tip of the finger. These extend in the distal, volar, and centrifugal aspects. Due to this distribution they form curves, loops, and whirls. The number of papillary lines depends upon the thickness of the epidermis, i.e., the thinner the epidermis the greater the surface of the tip of the finger and the larger the number of lines. The fine surface relief of the skin is covered with vernix caseosa in the newborn. This gray white or blue yellow matter is fatty and viscous and covers the face, ears, axillas, inguinal folds, and sacrum. The vernix is composed of desquamated cells of the stratum corneum and is rich in cholesterol, glycogen, and elcidin. The pH is almost neutral.

Following removal of the vernix caseosa the skin of the newborn has a pale cyanotic appearance which changes into a healthy red after the first few breaths. In premature infants the outer layers of the skin are remarkably transparent, and numerous blood vessels can be observed by the naked eye.

Desquamation of cornified cells starts a few days after birth, and with increasing strength of the stratum corneum the shedding of the remaining vernix is completed. A laminar separation and desquamation of portions of the stratum corneum is unphysiologic.

The thickness of the epidermis varies individually and at various areas of the body. The cornified layer of the newborn is very thin because of the small number of cell layers in the epidermis of the newborn, but the stratum corneum grows rapidly during the first few months. Becker (1954) applies the term "physiologic parakeratosis" to the first few days of life referring to keratinized cells with faintly staining nuclei. Becker (1954) measured the thickness of the stratum corneum in newborn autopsies and found the unfixed newborn skin to be 0.05 to 0.1 mm in thickness at the buttocks and abdomen. Following subtraction of loosely attached layers which desquamate postnatally, it measured only 0.01 to 0.05 mm with the exception of the plantar region of the foot and the palm of the hand. It varies from 0.1 to 0.9 mm in the adult.

DEVELOPMENT OF THE DIFFERENT EPIDERMIC LAYERS

The stratum germinativum of the newborn consists of only three to four cell layers. The basal cells are very irregular in outline, and no clear separation from the papillary projections is possible. The prickle cell layer is thin. Its cells are round or polygonal with relatively large, chromatin-poor nuclei and fibrillous, foamy cytoplasm. Intercellular bridges are difficult to identify except in the palm of the hand and the plantar region of the foot. The tonofibrils are less numerous than in the adult. The granular layer is incomplete, with the exception of the foot and hand, and consists of only one layer. This probably explains the transparency and pink color of the newborn skin, because, with the increase of keratohyalin granules, more light is reflected, and the skin appears white. The stratum lucidum is well developed only on the soles of the feet and palms of the hands. The collagenous fibers of the deep portions of the corium are thicker and more voluminous than are the fine collagen fibers around the papillary projections (stratum reticulare).

Electronmicroscopic examination of the ectoderm from the regio ulnaris of the palm of 25- to 60-mm human embryos reveals a special thickness and basal accumulation of cytoplasm of the embryonal ectoderm in those areas where surface growth was retarded. Shortly before birth the cell nuclei move into a more basal location and the basal cytoplasm zone disappears. Cells of the palm show an increased amount of mitochondria and osmophilic granula. The relation between cell nucleus and cell plasma shifts in favor of the cell nucleus in human embryos of 60-mm length. At the same time glycogen-rich areas of the cytoplasm disappear, and there, instead, an endoplasmic reticulum develops that is rich in ribosomes. Fibroblasts form intracytoplasmic filaments during the embryonal period, and these reach the extracellular space by transcellular permeation. These filaments are connected to collagen fibrils.

Elastic fibrils are presumably formed by similar filaments. The meshlike texture of the cutis is formed by filaments and fibers which run vertically through the outer surface of the corium. This structure strengthens the union between epidermis and dermis. A basal membrane can already be seen in 12-week-old human fetuses (Kobayasi, 1966).

The superficial layers of the fetal epidermal cells are rich in microvilli and cytoplasmic vacuoles (Breathnach and Wyllie, 1965b). This could imply that these cells are functionally active in the human embryo, performing secretory and absorptive functions. Electronmicroscopic examinations of 12- to 22-week-old human embryos showed the first anlagen of intraepidermal eccrine sweat glands in 12- to 13-week-old embryos and sweat gland ducts in 14- to 15-week-old embryos (Hashimoto et al., 1965). Glycogen was present in the intercellular spaces of eccrine sweat glands of 12- to 13-week-old embryos.

The cytoplasm of the stratum intermedium contained glycogen particles, and the amount of intracellular glycogen increased progressively in the upper layers of the epidermis.

Nail formation begins during the third month of gestation on the dorsal surface of the fingertips by an invagination of the epidermis. The nail originates in the nail bed. The matrix produces hard keratin, analogous to the development of the hair. Up to the fifth month the outer cell layer of the epidermis, the periderm, is composed of cuboidal cells. During the second month the periderm begins to flatten out and loses its ability to divide. The cytoplasm changes into a cornified substance which is resistant to proteolytic enzymes. Fortuyn (1927) demonstrated that the nail grows more in length than in width during the fifth through tenth months of gestation, but the individual variations are too great to use the nail for establishing the fetal age.

The first nail anlagen were observed in 16- to 18-week-old embryos in the form of a ventral and dorsal matrix (Hashimoto et al., 1966b). Proximal to the level of cornification (a fourth of the distance between matrix and cuticula) there is no keratinization of the cells. Some of these proximal matrix cells show even vacuoles.

At the border between the volar and dorsal epidermis of the finger axis a mushroomlike accumulation of vacuolized cells has been observed during the third week and has been thought to be the anlage of the distal matrix, while the real proximal nail matrix later develops dorsally. Distal to the vertical cornification layer, basal, ventral, and dorsal matrix cells mature into squamous cells. The tonofibrils and somewhat later granulated cells are enriched with keratohyalin granules, eventually changing into cornified cells (nail cells), densely packed with keratin which cannot be differentiated from keratin of the epidermis. While this process of maturation is in progress the basal, ventral, and dorsal matrix cells accumulate along the axis of the matrix. The matrix cells meet along the geometric midline of the primordial matrix at the most vertical point of keratinization.

Glycogen is being formed in the dorsal matrix, and melanocytes appear in the area of the cuticula. The thickness of the ventral matrix increases gradually and reaches a plateau beneath that layer of the cuticula where the ventral matrix is transformed into the nail bed. The ventral matrix produces later on only new cells for the nail plate.

During early keratinization SH groups can be detected histochemically in the nail plate, and PAS-positive mucopolysaccharides are formed. Electron microscopically, numerous granules can be seen in the nail bed which may contain mucopolysaccharides because of their histochemical characteristics.

Biochemical Development

Histochemical-enzymatic reactions of the embryonic skin have been investigated by Hashimoto et al. (1966). The activity of glucose-6-phosphate dehydrogenase (G-6-PDH) increases with the keratinization of the skin and also with the development of hair and sweat glands in the 10- to 18-week-old embryo. The hair canal shows G-6-PDH activity in very early stages and can be differentiated easily from surrounding epidermal cells. Hair papillae have the same property but lose it during further development.

The activity of cholinesterase in the embryonic rat skin is similar to that in the human adult skin. The enzyme reaction is often apparent at the time of the anlage of the organ. This is not so in sebaceous glands, epidermis, and musculi arrectores pilorum where the enzymatic activity appears about 10 days after formation of the anlage. Contrary to this finding, the activity of the enzyme in the subepidermal and perifollicular plexus of the skin reaches the maximal intensity on the fifth day.

From there on, there is a decrease in cholinesterase activity which correlates with the increase in skin mass. The intensity of monoaminooxidase in embryonic and adult rat skin increases with maturation and is most intense in the cutaneous nerve fibers. This mitochondrial enzyme is related to the amino acid metabolism of the cell, and it participates in the deamination of sympathomimetic amines in nerve fibers.

Alkaline phosphatase changes its histochemical distribution rapidly in the fetal skin. During early fetal life most cells of the skin, like most cells with a rapid rate of growth and differentiation, show a high alkaline phosphatase activity, including the endothelium of the dermal blood vessels which can therefore be easily traced. Only minimal quantities of alkaline phosphatase are present in hair follicles and sebaceous glands (Serri et al., 1963).

Phosphorylase activity has been demonstrated not only in all glycogen-forming cells, but also in those without demonstrable glycogen (Serri et al., 1962). From the beginning of differentiation the eccrine sweat glands are rich in phosphorylase, but the apocrine glands show little activity (Serri et al., 1962). Nails and hair are always rich in glycogen and phosphorylase. More than 80 percent of the energy required for the skin metabolism of the embryo is supplied by glycolysis.

The cells of the epidermis remain rich in glycogen until keratinization begins; thereafter glycogen is confined to the basal layer. However, glycogen can still be found in certain regions of the epidermis, such as in the palm of the hand and sole of the foot, even after the beginning of cornification. In the fetal dermis it can be demonstrated not only in cells but also in the intercellular substance, but it decreases with maturation of the fetus. The sebaceous glands are rich in glycogen and phosphorylase.

Hoyes (1967) demonstrated the presence of acid mucopolysaccharides on the surface of the periderm of the human fetal skin. It is possible that these mucopolysaccharides are formed by the cells of the periderm.

The content of histamine in the fetal skin increases with maturation. The number of mast cells is correlated to the amount of intracellular histamine (Zachariae, 1964).

Physiology of the Embryonic Skin

Cell desquamation in the newborn increases rapidly with advancing postmaturity, and it has been used as a measure for the length of gestation. However, this applies only to eutrophic children because desquamation is much more pronounced in sick children without delayed delivery. In dystrophic children increased desquamation is a characteristic sign of the placental insufficiency syndrome.

The average pH of the skin of the arm in 2- to 24-week-old infants is below 5, age and sex notwithstanding (Peck and Botwinick, 1964). Immediately after washing with soap solution with a pH of 10 the pH of the newborn skin increases by 2.55 in contrast to an increase of 0.97 after washing with a neutral solution. In 75 percent of the infants washed with a soapy solution more than 60 minutes are required for the skin to return to the initial pH value. These findings support the modern tendency to use neutral detergent solutions for washing infants.

SKIN FLORA

At the time of birth by cesarean section the skin of the infant is sterile, and that of the spontaneously born is usually contaminated with nonpathogenic staphylococci and diphtheroid bacilli (Sarkany and Gaylarde, 1967). Coliform bacteria and streptococci are found less frequently. The pattern of the skin flora is usually a reflection of routine manipulations, such as washing of the child or the use of forceps at the time of birth. Diphtheroid bacilli are found most often at the time of birth, and their number reaches a plateau after two days.

WATER CONTENT OF THE SKIN

Conduction measurements, i.e., measurements of the electric conductivity of the skin tissue in relation to its water content, showed that the initial postnatal reduction in weight up to the fourth day is related to the decrease in extracellular water contents and that this is almost twice as high in the newborn than in the adult (Bielecka-Winnicka, 1965a). In postterm babies less extracellular hydration of the subcutaneous tissue was found. In the first six days of life a constant increase in extracellular hydration of the subcutaneous tissue can be observed, and it reaches a normal value on the sixth day (Bielecka-Winnicka, 1965b). Dysmature newborns show a considerably higher extracellular hydration than healthy mature babies. Skin turgor is particularly dependent upon the water content. In human newborns examinations of skin turgor have not been done as yet. The amount of retraction is a measure for the presence of elastic forces, and the resistance to compression is related to the colloidal composition of the skin.

SKIN METABOLISM

Changes in skin potentials through sensual stimulation have been observed by Stechler et al. (1966). The newborn while stimulated by a visual object shows a decreased motility and increased reactivity of the skin potential, both of which are less in an awake but inattentive newborn. The facial skin of the newborn and adult alike is very important in regulating the temperature. The central temperature stimulates the metabolism less than the temperature of the skin when the body is exposed to cold (see Ch. 16).

Experiments with mice as well as with human fetuses have shown a cutaneous respiration when the animals are placed in incubators filled with liquids. The solution in the incubator and its oxygen tension do not influence the rate of survival in mice under normal atmospheric conditions. Human fetuses between 9 and 24 weeks of age have been placed in solutions at 35°C with an oxygen tension of 250 PSI (pounds per square inch) and have survived as long as 23 hours. This seems to demonstrate that cutaneous respiration can suffice to meet the demand for oxygen of an extrauterine fetus for a limited period of time.

The metabolic effect of warming and cooling of the face with infra-red rays in a fully wrapped premature infant at a room temperature of 20 to 22°C showed that a minimal oxygen consumption can be attained when the face is warmed; when the face was cooled an increase in oxygen consumption occurred accompanied by strong muscular activity (Mestyan et al., 1964a, b).

The precursor of fat cells is derived from mesenchymal cells of the wall of precapillary vessels. The labile condition of the fat tissues in the newborn permits hematopoiesis and storage of fat analogous to that in the bone marrow. The chemical characteristics of the skin fat in the newborn have not been thoroughly studied. The iodine index for the content of unsaturated fatty acids increases with age up to 12 months. The average content in the newborn is 43 and 62 in the 12-month-old child. Therefore, the fat of the newborn contains less oleic acid than that of the adult: its consistency is more solid and its melting point is higher.

Repeated efforts have been made to determine the maturity of a newborn by the thickness of its skin folds. The average thickness in 300 newborn babies (162 males and 138 females) of different gestational ages and less than 48 hours of age, was 0.6 mm more in girls than in boys (scapula, arms, chest, and abdominal wall) (Farr, 1966). Mature babies have thicker skin folds than premature ones. Those of postterm boys are thinner than those found in mature boys, and postterm girls have thicker skin folds than term born girls. The thickness of the skin folds in the mother is not significantly correlated to that of her newborn (Gampel, 1965). In general, the correlation between the thickness of skin folds and gestational age is not high enough for exact determinations of the maturity of a newborn.

PIGMENTATION

Pigmentation in the basal layer of the epidermis begins at birth. Therefore, the different skin pigmentation in human races begins postnatally. Pigmented nevi are considered to be an atavistic phenomenon which is promoted by interracial mixing. They are formed by cutaneous melanoblasts in the deeper layers of the corium. The linea fusca appears as a fine line of pigmentation in the midline of the abdomen, usually visible at the age of three to six months and less frequently during the second, or as late as in the eighth week of life. The hypothesis that this could be a response to maternal hormones has been questioned.

Development of the Vascular System

The vascular system of the mature newborn corresponds in number and arrangement to that of the adult. In embryos, regularly distributed vessels penetrate the skin diagonally, and it is not until the number of fibrillary elements increases and the sebaceous glands have matured further that they appear in their final horizontal position. The terminal loops of skin capillaries are well developed in the newborn and show a distinct differentiation of the arterial and venous portions. The appearance of the capillaries is not a good index for maturity. The intracapillary pressure increases during the first year of life from 90/23 to 95/30 mm Hg. The resistance of the skin capillaries decreases with age. This is interesting in view of the fact that the permeability of the capillary wall is increased for soluble and colloidal substances during the first trimenon and that the permeability and physical resistance of the vessels are not necessarily correlated. The variation in luminal diameter is considerable. For example, the lumen of a vessel in the subcutis of the calf is often wider than in one in the abdominal subcutis of the newborn. The number of vessels per unit of space decreases with age.

Skin Nerves

The terminal nerves of the newborn are immature. Meissner's bodies are preformed before birth, and they mature in the postnatal period. They are elliptic in shape and have numerous horizontal stripes. Their diameter averages 0.022 mm. Double contoured nerve fibers have an average thickness of 0.0027 mm. Free-ending intraepithelial terminal nerve fibers are comparatively numerous (Becker, 1954). Vater-Pacini bodies have been observed to appear in the fifth and sixth months of gestation and are similar in the newborn and adult but seem smaller in size in the newborn and have little or no fluid between the lamellae. Well-developed terminal nerves and free-ending nerve fibers are scarce in the external genitalia of the newborn. They are particularly numerous in the deeper layer of the suction pads.

Hair of the Newborn

The change of hair after birth is similar to the first hair anlagen in the embryo. The first hair appears between the second and fifth months of gestation. Hair growth begins on the head and extends from there over the rest of the body.

The fetal lanugo covers equally all hair-growing parts of the body. A differentiation into hair types can be observed only after the first change of hair has taken place shortly before or right after birth. The localization of hair on the body determines the different hair types, but what these determining factors are has not been established as yet. All possible hair types have been found in dermoid cysts. Apparently the determining factor resides in the skin itself since transplanted skin retains its characteristic hair. The presence of marrow in the hair of the head can be used as proof that the fetus or child was alive. Marrow in the cilias can be used as an index for fetal maturity. Examinations of twins demonstrated the heredity of development and distribution of hair.

DEVELOPMENT AND FORMATION

Basal cells with deeply staining nuclei develop in groups in the as yet undifferentiated epidermis. Through mitosis aggregates of cells appear which soon arrange into columns (hair bud), and fibroblasts containing alkaline phosphatase accumulate around the base. These cell groups form the papilla of the hair which then grows toward the dermis. While this columnar structure becomes longer, a coat of proliferating cells grows around the papilla, encircling it completely. At this time two new budlike structures appear. The upper one develops into a sebaceous gland, the lower into the terminal permanent portion of the hair follicle. Accordingly, the hair bulb, the hair matrix, and hair shaft differentiate within the cell column. The hair bulb is formed through widening of the caudal section of the column which surrounds the papilla and contains pigmented and trichohyalin-rich cells in its upper portion and nonpigmented cells in the lower part. The inner section of the hair shaft originates in the trichohyalin-containing cells of the upper portion of the hair bulb and is later transformed into a keratinizing cellular tube. At this time the original epithelial column consists of an outer cylinder, the outer shaft, and of an incomplete cylinder of the inner shaft in which the hair will grow. The hair keratin can be differentiated from that of the shaft. Meanwhile two layers of cells develop within the cluster surrounding the follicle; the lower develops into the glass membrane and the upper cell layer forms the musculus errector pili. After a certain time the hair changes into the catagen and telogen exactly as in postnatal life.

The anatomy of the human follicle and its hair follows a certain cycle. Three phases are distinguished in the human and animal: 1, the stage of growth (proliferation) or anlagen formation; 2, transitional or catagen stage; and 3, resting or telogen stage.

The first change of hair occurs during the eighth month of intrauterine life and lasts into childhood. The hair of the eyebrows, forehead, lips, crown of the head, trunk of the body, arms, legs, back of hands, and feet changes in this order with certain individual differences. The time for hair regeneration seems to vary considerably in different regions of the body. Differences in hair of various body areas are already discernible in the newborn. Lanugo hair is silky and contains little pigment. Throughout life it persists as body hair and is only partly replaced later in life by terminal hair. Lanugo hair consists of soft downs and coarse, woollike hair (wellus hair). Wellus hair appears on the head about six months after birth and remains until puberty. This type is also found in some of the eyelashes and brows. Up to the thirteenth year of life and sometimes even longer this woollike hair remains the predominant type; its anatomic structure is similar to that of the terminal hair.

The eyelashes are comparatively well developed at birth and are prominently pigmented in brunette children. The eyebrows have often already changed at the time of birth and appear in a prominent arclike pattern.

COLOR CHANGE

The color of lanugo hair at birth is not always the permanent color throughout life, i.e., children with dark hair at birth can become blond as the hair continues to grow (wellus and terminal hair) and vice versa. The change in hair color of a child corresponds to the hair change in animals in whom usually the lighter colored hair is exchanged for the terminal hair.

Conclusions

The skin of the mammalian newborn is morphologically and functionally different from adult skin. Fundamental changes occur in the newborn period, and many of those can be interpreted as an adaptation of the fetal skin to extrauterine life. In addition, skin function and morphology reflect metabolic changes of the organism in general and of single organ systems. Therefore, dysfunctions and anomalies of other tissues can be manifested on the skin. Thus, the clinical diagnosis of systemic diseases and metabolic disorders will benefit greatly from the knowledge and understanding of developing skin functions. For example, the electrolyte concentration in sweat is typically disturbed in cystic fibrosis (mucoviscidosis); abnormal pigmentation is found in adrenal dysfunctions or disorders of the amino acid or protein metabolism; histologic and histochemical examinations of skin biopsies can verify diseases of the lipid metabolism, connective tissue, and many others. Finger and foot prints as well as palm lines become increasingly important for detecting and differentiating chromosomal aberrations. The width of papillary ridges has disclosed marked differences between infants with chromosomal aberrations and healthy newborns. These examples may elucidate the important role that skin morphology and function play in clinical neonatology and in developmental physiology.

Desquamation of the newborn's skin occurs in close relation to gestational age; scaling increases more rapidly when the term-date has passed. Infants born one to two days after term already show a marked increase in skin desquamation. In conjunction with other symptoms the degree of desquamation can be used for evaluating the stage of maturity or postmaturity. Dystrophic newborns always suffer from extensive scaling which symptom thus becomes indicative of the placental insufficiency syndrome.

Our present knowledge about the functional development of the skin during the fetal and neonatal period consists of a great number of studies of varying topics. A comprehensive study is urgently needed for envisioning an intelligent meaning of this scattered information on perinatal skin physiology. Among the gaps to be filled, future investigations have to deal particularly with interactions between skin and body metabolism, and with problems of maturation and adaptation of cutaneous functions in the early postnatal period.

REFERENCES

Becker, J. 1954. Die Haut. *In* Brock, J., ed. Biologische Daten für den Kinderarzt, 2nd ed. Berlin, Springer-Verlag, pp. 1042-1081.

Becker, S. W., Jr., T. B. Fitzpatrick, and H. Montgomery. 1952. Human melanogenesis: Cytology and histology of pigment cells (melanodendrocytes). Arch. Derm. Syph. Chicago, 65:511-523.

———— and A. A. Zimmerman. 1955. Further studies on melanocytes and melanogenesis in the human fetus and newborn. J. Invest. Derm., 25:103-112.

Bekhor, I. J., Z. Mohseni, M. E. Nimni, and L. Bavetta. 1965. The biosynthesis of microsomal-bound collagen precursors in rabbit embryo skin in vitro. Proc. Nat. Acad. Sci. U.S.A., 54:615-622.

Ben-Or, S., and E. Bell. 1965. Skin antigens in the chick embryo in relation to other developmental events. Develop. Biol., 11:184-201.

Bielecka-Winnicka, A. 1965a. Conductometric investigations in subcutaneous and muscular tissues of postmature newborns with syndromes of skin dehydration. Biol. Neonat., 8:321-328.

———— 1965b. An attempt to determine hydration changes in subcutaneous and muscular tissues of a newborn by conductometric method. Ann. Paediat., 204:377-386.

Breathnach, A. S., and L. M. Wyllie. 1965a. Electron microscopy of melanocytes and Langerhans cells in human fetal epidermis at 14 weeks. J. Invest. Derm., 44:51-60.

———— and L. M. Wyllie. 1965b. Fine structures of cells forming the surface layer of the epidermis in human fetuses at fourteen and twelve weeks. J. Invest. Derm., 45:179-189.

Burke, R. C., T. H. Lee, and V. Buettner-Janusch. 1966. Free amino acids and water soluble peptides in stratum corneum and skin surface film in human beings. Yale J. Biol. Med., 38:355-373.

Christophers, E. 1968. Wachstumsdynamik von Epidermis und Papillarkörper nach lokaler Applikation von Vitamin A- Säure. Arch. Klin. Exp. Derm., 233:99-106.

Farr, V. 1966. Skinfold thickness as an indication of maturity of the newborn. Arch. Dis. Child., 41:301-308.

Fortuyn, A. B. D. 1927. A catalogue of the first 400 specimens of the human embryological collection in the department of anatomy of the Peking Union Medical College. Chin. Med. J., 41 (Suppl.):1-94.

Fowler, E. H., and M. L. Calhoun. 1964. The microscopic anatomy of developing fetal pig skin. Amer. J. Vet. Res., 25:156-164.

Gampel, B. 1965. The relation of skinfold thickness in the neonate to sex, length of gestation, size at birth and maternal skinfold. Hum. Biol., 37:29-37.

Garber, B. 1967. Aggregation in vivo of dissociated cells. II. Role of developmental age in tissue reconstruction. J. Exp. Zool., 164:339-349.

———— and A. A. Moscona. 1967. Suppression of feather morphogenesis in co-aggregates of skin cells from embryos of different ages. J. Exp. Zool., 164:351-361.

Gonzales-Cadavid, N., B. Denduchis, and R. E. Mancini. 1963. Soluble collagens in normal rat skin, from embryo to adulthood. Lab. Invest., 12:598-605.

Goodlin, R. C. 1963. Cutaneous respiration in a fetal incubator. Amer. J .Obstet. Gynec., 86:571-579.

Griffiths, A. D. 1966. Skin desquamation in the newborn. Biol. Neonat., 10:127-139.

Hashimoto, K., and W. F. Lever. 1966. Histochemical demonstration of glucose-6-phosphate dehydrogenase in the skin of human embryos. J. Invest. Derm., 47:421-425.

———— K. Ogawa, and W. F. Lever. 1963a. Histochemical studies of the skin. III. The activity of cholinesterases during the embryonic development of the skin in the rat. J. Invest. Derm., 40:15-26.

———— K. Ogawa, and W. F. Lever. 1963b. Histochemical studies of the skin. IV. The activity of monoamine oxidase during the embryonic development of the skin of the rat. J. Invest. Derm., 41:81-90.

———— B. G. Gross, and W. F. Lever. 1965. The ultrastructure of the skin of human embryos. I The intraepidermical eccrine sweat duct. J. Invest. Derm., 45:139-151.

———— B. G. Gross, R. J. Di Bella, and W. F. Lever. 1966a. The ultrastructure of the skin of human embryos. IV. The epidermis. J. Invest. Derm., 47:317-335.

———— B. G. Gross, R. Nelson, and W. F. Lever. 1966b. The ultrastructure of the skin of human embryos. III. The formation of the nail in 16-18 weeks old embryos. J. Invest. Derm., 47:205-217.

Hay, E. D. 1964. Secretion of a connective tissue protein by developing epidermis. In Montagna, W., and W. C. Lobitz, eds. The Epidermis. New York, Academic Press, Inc.

Hoyes, A. D. 1967. Acid mucopolysaccharide in fetal epidermis. J. Invest. Derm., 48: 598-601.

Huang, J. S., and F. B. Bang. 1964. The susceptibility of chick embryo skin organ cultures to influenza virus following excess vitamin A. J. Exp. Med., 120:129-148.

Jadassohn, J., ed. 1966. Handbuch Haut und Geschlechtskrankheiten. Erg. Werk, Vol. 7: Vererbung von Hautkrankheiten. Gottron, H. A., and U. W. Schnyder, eds. Berlin, Springer-Verlag.

Kobayasi, T. 1966. Development of fibrillar structures in human fetal skin, an electron microscope study. Acta Morph. Neerl. Scand., 6:257-269.

Kollar, E. J. 1966. An in vitro study of hair and vibrissae development in embryonic mouse skin. J. Invest. Derm., 46:254-262.

Kopsch, F. 1940. Lehrbuch und Atlas der Anatomie des Menschen. Leipzig, Thieme, Vol. 3, p. 478.

Larson, C. A. 1967. The skin: Problems of inheritance. Science, 155:488-489.

Malt, R. A., and K. A. Hartman, Jr. 1963. Infra-red spectra of embryonic chick feathers. Nature (London), 200:703-704.

McLennan, J., and M. Karasek. 1966. Incorporation of proline and conversion to hydroxyproline in newborn mouse skin. Biochim. Biophys. Acta, 117:184-192.

Mestýan, J., I. Járai, G. Bata, and M. Fekete. 1964a. Surface temperatures versus deep body temperature and the metabolic response to cold of hypothermic premature infants. Biol. Neonat., 7:230-242.

———— I. Iárai, G. Bata, and M. Fekete. 1964b. The significance of facial skin temperature in the chemical heat regulation of premature infants. Biol. Neonat., 7:243-254.

Mishima, Y., and S. Widlan. 1966. Embryonic development of melanocytes in human hair and epidermis: Their cellular differentiation and melanogenic activity. J. Invest. Derm., 46:263-277.

Moscona, A. A. 1964. Studies on stability of phenotypic traits in embryonic integumental tissues and cells. In Montagna, W., and W. C. Lobitz, eds. The Epidermis. New York, Academic Press, Inc.

Moscona, M. H., and A. A. Moscona. 1965. Control of differentation in aggregates of embryonic skin cells: Suppression of feather morphogenesis by cells from other tissues. Develop. Biol., 11:402-423.

Nelson, W. E., ed. 1966. Textbook of Pediatrics, 8th ed. Philadelphia, W. B. Saunders Company.

New, D. A. 1965. Effects of excess vitamin A on cultures of skin from the tail and pads of the embryonic rat, and from the trunk, tail and pads of the embryonic rabbit. Exp. Cell. Res., 39:178-183.

Niebauer, G. 1968. Dendritic Cells of Human Skin. Basel, S. Karger.

Pasteels, J. 1936-37. Etudes sur la gastrulation des vertébrés méroblastiques. III. Oiseux. IV. Conclusions générales. Arch. Biol., 48:381-488.

Peck, S. M., and I. S. Botwinick. 1964. The buffering capacity of infants skin against an alkaline soap and a neutral detergent. J. Mount Sinai Hosp. N. Y., 31:134-137.

Pullar, P., and C. Liadsky. 1965. Dehydrogenase systems of human foetal skin. Brit. J. Derm., 77:314-321.

Reed, S. C., and J. M. Henderson. 1940. Pigment cell migration in mouse epidermis. J. Exp. Zool., 85:409-418.

Rhodin, J. 1965. Ultrastructure of human skin. J. Pediat., 66:171-177.

Riegel, P. 1965. Die Frühentwicklung der Ultrastruktur in der Epidermis menschlicher Embryonen. Z. Morph. Anthrop., 56:195-205.

Sarkany, I., and C. C. Gaylarde. 1967. Skin flora of the newborn. Lancet, 1:589-590.

Serri, F., W. Montagna, and H. Mesconi. 1962. Studies of the skin of the fetus and the child. II. Glycogen and amylophosphorylase in the skin of the fetus. J. Invest. Derm., 39:199-217.

———— W. Montagna, and W. M. Huber. 1963. Studies of the skin of the fetus and the child. I. The distribution of alkaline phosphatase in the skin of the fetus. Arch. Derm., 87:234-245.

Smith, Q. T. 1964. Body weight, cutaneous collagen, and hexosamine of cortisone treated female rats of various ages. J. Invest. Derm., 42:353-357.

Stechler, G., S. Bradford, and H. Levy. 1966. Attention in the newborn: Effect on motility and skin potential. Science, 151:1246-1248.

Steigleder, G. K. 1964. Verhalten von Gefässen und Bindegeweben in der Haut des menschlichen Unterschenkels in verschiedenen Altersperioden. Zbl. Phlebol., 3:231-242.

Töndury, G. 1964. Embryologie und Hauttopographie. Arch. Klin. Exp. Derm., 219:12-24.

Tustanovsky, A. A., G. L. Myagkaya, and Z. I. Volkava. 1964. Comparative studies on the production of collagen. The collagen fractions of pig embryo skin. Gerontologia, 9:28-35.

Vukas, A. 1965. Embryogenetic aspects in dermatology. Dermatologica, 131:293-303.

Wessells, N. K. 1963. Effects of extra-epithelial factors on the incorporation of thymidine by embryonic epidermis. Exp. Cell. Res., 30:36-55.

Winter, V. 1968. Fluoreszenzmikroskopische Studien der menschlichen embryonalen Haut. I. Entwicklung des menschlichen Haares. Dermatologica, 136:29-34.

Yun, J. S., and W. Montagna. 1965. The skin of primates 25: Melanogenesis in the skin of the bushbabies. Amer. J. Phys. Anthrop., 23:143-148.

Zachariae, H. 1964. Histamine and mast cells in human fetal skin. Proc. Soc. Exp. Biol. Med., 117:63-65.

Zaruba, F., E. M. Karasek, and E. M. Farber. 1968. Isolation and properties of a phosphodiesterase from newborn mouse skin. J. Invest. Derm., 49:537-543.

Zelickson, A. S. 1963. Electron Microscopy of Skin and Mucous Membrane. Springfield, Ill., Charles C Thomas, Publisher.

Part VI

ENDOCRINE SYSTEM

30

Steroid Hormone Formation and Metabolism

EDUARDO ORTI ● Department of Pediatrics, State University of New York Downstate Medical Center, Brooklyn, New York

Introduction

The adrenal cortex is essential for life in mammals. The steroids secreted by the adrenal are well known to exert important regulatory actions on carbohydrate, lipid, and protein metabolism. The nature of their contribution to the physiologic phenomena that occur during intrauterine life remains to be established. The phylogenetic appearance of adrenal cortical glands is a much earlier phenomenon than placentation. Both the adrenal and the placenta are steroid secreting organs. It is, therefore, of considerable interest to understand how the biosynthetic function of the placenta has interdigitated itself with that of the adrenal. We have limited the review to the human species when available data are adequate and referred to research done in rodents when information is not available for the human fetus. There is always a considerable risk of error when applying to one species notions obtained in another. For the adrenal and placenta this general caution cannot be overemphasized. The adrenal biosynthetic pathways are well known to vary among mammals; the corticosteroids secreted into the blood are different in the rat from those in the guinea pig, rabbit, and man. As for the placenta it is probably the organ that has the greatest variability from species to species.

Embryologic Development of the Adrenal Cortex in Man

In man the adrenal cortical primordium appears toward the fourth week of gestation when the crown to rump (CR) length is about 6 to 8 mm. At this time its dimensions are $0.5 \times 0.3 \times 0.1$ mm (Velican, 1946-47), and it is composed mainly of large acidophilic cells. In the fifth week in the 12-mm CR embryo the adrenal has doubled in size ($0.8 \times 0.6 \times 0.4$ mm), and a smaller type of basophilic cell has appeared, presumably derived from the coelomic epithelium, as were the

909

earlier acidophilic cells (Keene and Hewer, 1927) over which the basophilic cells soon spread. These small cells give rise to the definitive cortex, while the initial migration becomes the distinctive fetal zone. According to this interpretation of Keene and Hewer, which is supported by the work of Uotila (1940), the cells of the fetal and definitive zones of the fetal cortex are cytologically different from the time of their earliest differentiation. The question of their separate origin by a succession of two separate migrations is not accepted by some recent workers (Gruenwald, 1946; Crowder, 1957). Whatever its embryologic origin, the definitive cortex appears on electron microscopic studies to be inactive, while the mitochondria of the fetal zone studied by Ross (1962) appear to be active in fetuses between the sixth and seventeenth weeks of gestation. In the 20-mm CR embryo (7 to 8 weeks) when the adrenal dimensions are $1.2 \times 1.0 \times 0.8$ mm the fetal zone accounts for 30 to 50 percent of the cross-sectional area of the cortex. Its relative prominence increases during pregnancy, particularly during the last trimester, at which point it constitutes about 80 percent of the cortex (Swineyard, 1943). During the first month of postnatal life the involution of the fetal zone is largely completed.

Onset of Functional Capability in the Fetal Adrenal

The functional capabilities for which the human fetal adrenal has been studied to date comprise its steroidogenic capability (spontaneous or with added precursors) by comparison with the known synthetic pathways of the adult cortex, and its enzymatic content as shown by histochemical studies. Studies on DNA, RNA, and protein synthesis of the fetal adrenals still remain to be done. The first studies on the biosynthetic capability of the fetal adrenal were made using in vitro incubation of surviving fetal glands. They aimed at ascertaining whether the sequence of synthetic reactions known to occur in the adult gland also took place in the fetal ones. In that sequence, as shown in Figure 1, cholesterol is synthesized from acetate. The side-chain of cholesterol is then broken down by a desmolase to pregnenolone. Pregnenolone, like cholesterol, has a hydroxyl in position 3 and is unsaturated in position 5-6. The next step involves the formation of progesterone and consists in the conversion of the 3 hydroxyl into a 3 ketone and the shift of the double bond from position 5-6 to position 4-5; the first step of dehydrogenation is done by an enzyme called "3β-hydroxysteroid dehydrogenase" (3β-HSD). The second step or shift (isomerization) of the double bond can take place spontaneously in vitro; in vivo it is believed to be performed by an isomerase. In this review we will refer to both of the actions jointly as mediated by 3β-HSD. When this enzyme acts on $\Delta 5$ pregnenolone, the product is progesterone. In the normal sequence of events in the adult adrenal cortex, progesterone is hydroxylated in position 17 by a 17 hydroxylase to produce 17 hydroxyprogesterone. 17 hydroxyprogesterone is then acted upon by 21 and 11 hydroxylases to yield, respectively, 17 hydroxycorticosterone and cortisol. It is against this sequence of biosynthetic steps known to occur in the adult cortex that the fetal cortex or its two individual zones have been compared.

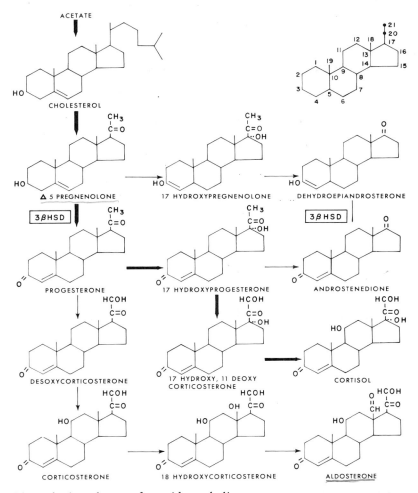

Fig. 1. Biosynthetic pathways of steroid metabolism.

In 1956, Davis and Plotz demonstrated for the first time that the adrenals from human fetuses in the third to fifth months could perform the first step of steroid biosynthesis in vitro, converting C14-labeled acetate to cholesterol.

Lanman and Silverman (1957) and Lanman et al. (1957) showed that the adrenals of fetuses obtained in abortions and those of premature infants had little spontaneous steroidogenic capability, but after the addition of progesterone to the medium they were able to recover cortisol, corticosterone, and 17 hydroxycortico-sterone, thereby demonstrating that at those stages of development the human adrenal cortex had the capacity to hydroxylate in positions 11, 17, and 21. They were the first to postulate that the 3β-HSD system was either deficient or inhibited in the fetus.

Solomon et al. (1958) using material from fetuses obtained in abortions between the tenth and twenty-second weeks of gestation dissected the fetal zone and the definitive type cortex and were able to show that both zones could convert progesterone to 17 hydroxyprogesterone and androstenedione. The latter C^{19} steroid is assumed to derive from 17 hydroxyprogesterone by cleavage of the $C^{20,21}$ side-chain. The in-vitro capacity of the adrenal cortex to perform the complete synthesis from acetate to cortisol was soon demonstrated (Bloch and Benirshke, 1959) for fetuses between 12 and 22 weeks. Products identified after addition of C^{14} acetate were dehydroepiandrosterone (DHA), pregnenolone, androstenedione, 11 hydroxyandrostenedione, and cortisol; sought but not found were progesterone, 17 hydroxyprogesterone, corticosterone, testosterone, and adrenosterone (Δ^4-androstene 3, 11-17 trione). These results showed that capability for complete adultlike synthesis of cortisol from acetate was present in the fetal adrenal cortex as a whole and brought into the picture the synthesis of DHA; also, they confirmed the presence of 11, 17, and 21 hydroxylases, and even though the study was qualitative in nature the authors believed their results pointed to a restricted activity of 3β-HSD. Villee et al. (1959), using human fetuses of 11 to 26 weeks of age, confirmed that adrenal cortices could transform progesterone to cortisol but were more efficient if 17 hydroxyprogesterone were the added precursor. They were unable to confirm that Porter Silber chromogens (which include cortisol) appeared after the addition of precursors more primitive than progesterone ($\Delta 5$ pregnenolone, cholesterol, and acetate). They again interpreted their findings to indicate either a deficiency or a lability of 3β-HSD activity in the whole fetal cortex. Studies on the secretory capability of the fetal zone were carried out after dissection of the fetal cortex by several authors. Solomon et al. (1958) showed that fetal zone tissue essentially free from definitive cortex had the capacity to convert C^{14} progesterone to 17 hydroxyprogesterone and androstenedione. These findings were confirmed and extended by Bloch and Benirshke (1959, 1962) who demonstrated the capability of the fetal zone tissue of embryos 12 weeks or older to synthesize DHA, androstenedione, and cortisol from C^{14} acetate. In these experiments the amount of androstenedione plus cortisol ($\Delta 4$ compounds) produced was only one fourth to one sixth the amount of DHA (the major $\Delta 5$ compound isolated). Thus, in early pregnancy the isolated fetal zone in the human fetus has full corticosteroidogenic capability, and its 3β-HSD activity is as limited as that of the adrenal as a whole.

Villee and Villee (1964) used incubations of homogenized adrenals in vitro to study the quantitative developmental changes in enzyme contribution to steroid synthesis. Adrenals of fetuses of less than 10 cm CR length produce in-vitro androstenedione, 11β-hydroxyandrostenedione, 16α-hydroxyprogesterone, 16α, 17 dihydroxyprogesterone, desoxycorticosterone, corticosterone, and cortisol from progesterone. Under their conditions androstenedione was a major metabolite of progesterone in the fetus of less than 10 cm CR length. Beyond this stage of fetal growth the adrenal homogenates produced much less if any androstenedione or 11β-hydroxyandrostenedione from the same precursor any increased quantities of corticosterone and cortisol. In the same preparation pregnenolone was converted largely to DHA, with small amounts of 17 hydroxypregnenolone, 16α-hydroxypregnenolone, and androstenedione. In summary, very early in fetal development the adrenal has complete capability for synthesis of cortisol from acetate. However, the step between Δ5 pregnenolone and progesterone mediated by 3β-HSD is very restricted in in-vitro studies. As a consequence of this block, progesterone must be supplied to the adrenal from an outside source if any significant corticosteroid synthesis is to take place. The major androgen produced in vitro from pregnenolone is DHA and that produced from progesterone is androstenedione.

ENZYME DEMONSTRATION IN FETAL ADRENAL BY HISTOCHEMICAL METHODS

Histochemical staining to reveal the presence of enzymes that are known to be implicated in steroid biosynthesis has given some information on the presence of those enzymes at different stages of fetal development. Goldman et al. (1964, 1966) reported 3β-HSD activities in the adrenals of fetuses larger than 15 cm CR. Cavallero and Magrini (1966) used DHA, pregnenolone, 17α-hydroxypregnenolone, and androstenediol as substrate for the demonstration of 3β-HSD. This enzyme could not be demonstrated by them in the fetal zone at any gestation age from the second month of intrauterine life to birth. The definitive cortex, on the other hand, showed no evidence of 3β-HSD activity in the first two to three months of intrauterine life, but a positive reaction was faintly visible at four to six months and increased to the point of being quite evident in the neocortex of the newborn. The best substrates were found to be DHA and androstenediol.

Steroid Metabolism in the Perfused Previable Fetus at Midterm

Further studies of the synthesis and metabolism of adrenal steroids have frequently been made by the perfusion of the previable fetus in cases in which elective legal abortion was performed. Most of the information yielded by this approach concerns the fetus at midpregnancy (15 to 20 weeks). The results obtained by perfusion of the previable fetus with steroid precursors, followed by isolation of the metabolites from blood and various tissues, are a considerable step forward in the study of the integrated metabolism of steroid hormone.

The work of Solomon in collaboration with the group of Diczfalusy has greatly helped to clarify many aspects of the metabolism of neutral steroids in the fetus and placenta. This work has been recently summarized by Solomon (1966), Solomon et al. (1967), and Solomon and Friesen (1968).

The previable fetus of 18 to 22 weeks' gestation age when perfused for 60 minutes can synthesize cholesterol from C^{14} acetate in its liver and adrenal. When the same preparation was perfused with tritium-labeled cholesterol and C^{14}-labeled acetate, only minute amounts of Δ5 pregnenolone or 17α-hydroxypregnenolone could be isolated from the adrenal with either label. Perfusion with cholesterol sulfate yielded no transformation products. Solomon et al. (1967) concluded from this experiment that the human fetus at midterm must use precursors reaching it from the placenta or the mother in order to synthesize neutral steroids.

Injection of Δ5 pregnenolone into the umbilical vein in a fetus at 13 weeks' gestation, with clamping of the veins 20 seconds after the injection, resulted in the isolation from the adrenal of 14.6 percent nonmetabolized Δ5 pregnenolone; 2.8 percent of the radioactivity in the adrenal appeared as DHA sulfate and 2.3 percent as 17α-hydroxypregnenolone sulfate. All tissues studied contained only unmetabolized Δ5 pregnenolone and 20α-dihydropregnenolone sulfate. After perfusion of the previable fetus with progesterone $^4C^{14}$, extensive metabolism of the precursor occurred, the major sites of which were the adrenal and the liver. Hydroxylated metabolites were recovered exclusively from the adrenal and included 16α-hydroxyprogesterone, 17α-hydroxyprogesterone, and cortisol. The perfusate contained 16α-hydroxyprogesterone and small amounts of corticosterone and 6β-hydroxyprogesterone. Reduced metabolites were recovered from the adrenal (20α-dihydroprogesterone), but most came from the liver (20α-dihydroprogesterone, 3α15β-pregnan 20 one, and pregnane 3α, 20αdiol). Lung, kidney, and intestine contained lesser amounts and number of reduced metabolites of progesterone. In all tissues Δ4-androstenedione was searched for but could not be detected. These experiments were repeated after fetal adrenalectomy in order to assess to what extent the hydroxylated and reduced metabolites found in the perfusate and nonadrenal tissues were of adrenal origin. It was concluded that a number of tissues of the fetaus can reduce progesterone to a variety of products but that the adrenals are the main site for the formation of the hydroxylated products isolated from the tissues of the intact perfused fetuses.

When 17α-hydroxyprogesterone $^4C^{14}$ was injected into the umbilical vein of a male fetus (19 weeks' gestation) and a female fetus (8 weeks' gestation), no labeled androstenedione or testosterone could be detected in the adrenal extract. Therefore, as far as this preparation is concerned, there is apparently no functioning 17, 20 desmolase in the fetal at midterm. Similar studies with 16α-hydroxyprogesterone, a major product of the perfusion with progesterone, supported the conclusion that the fetal adrenal at midterm does not further hydroxylate this steroid nor is it extensively metabolized in the fetal tissues.

Aldosterone secretion was considered to be absent at midpregnancy because of the nonsecretory aspect of the zona glomerulosa. Longchamp (1965) claimed that the 18 hydroxylase system required for the synthesis of aldosterone develops shortly before term. However, Pasqualini et al. (1966) were able to isolate aldosterone from the adrenal of fetuses at midterm, after perfusion with corticosterone.

Dell'Acqua et al. (1966) studied the metabolism of androgens in the perfused fetus. They perfused two male and two female fetuses at midpregnancy with C^{14}-labeled androstenedione and tritium-labeled testosterone. Very little interconversion of androstenedione to testosterone was found in any of the fetal tissues studied with the exception of the liver. In the fetal liver, complete interconversion of these two compounds was found. The resting tissues transform testosterone into androstenedione (Benagiano et al., 1967) and both androgens into several metabolites including etiocholanolone, etiocholanediol, dehydrotestosterone, and etiocholanedione. Androsterone was isolated only from the lung. Fetal aromatization of the two androgens also takes place only in the liver, while the fetal adrenals can produce 11β, 15α, and 16α hydroxylated derivatives.

The fetal circulation contains levels of estrogen about tenfold those of the maternal blood, estriol being in concentration 50 to 100 times higher than estrone or estradiol. Yet little, if any, of this estrogen circulating in the fetus originates in fetal tissues. The contribution of the fetal adrenal to estrogen metabolism consists probably in the synthesis of DHA (Fig. 2) which is a precursor for the placental synthesis of estrone and estradiol and 16α-OHDHA, which the placenta will cyclize to estriol. Estrogens reaching the fetus from the placenta are conjugated by most fetal tissues to their sulfate derivatives, and once in conjugated form are further transformed by hydroxylation (Ryan, 1965; Diczfalusy, 1965).

Placental Contribution to the Metabolism of Steroids

The placenta is a very efficient synthesizer within a very limited range of steroid biosynthesis. One might well say that it is a highly specialized organ if one takes as comparative standard the accepted steroidogenic sequence and scope of the adult human adrenal. Its capability appears to include total synthesis of progesterone from acetate. However, evidence from in-vitro perfusion experiments suggests that synthesis from acetate is quantitatively a very insignificant capability of the placenta (Levitz et al., 1960; Van Luesden and Villee, 1965).

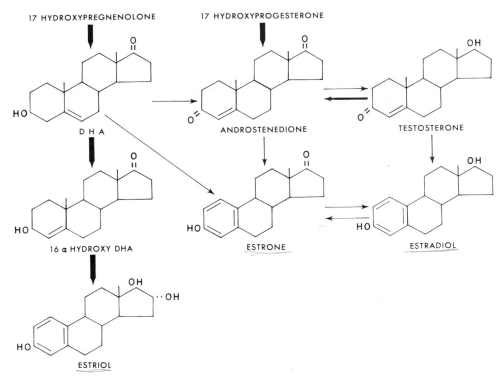

Fig. 2. Biosynthetic pathways of estrogen.

PARTIAL BIOSYNTHESIS OF PREGNENOLONE AND PROGESTERONE FROM CHOLESTEROL

The midterm placenta does have 3β-HSD and is capable of producing pro-gesterone from pregnenolone and 17 hydroxyprogesterone from 17 hydroxy-pregnenolone (Pion et al., 1965); most important, it can produce pregnenolone from cholesterol (Jaffe et al., 1966). When placental homogenates were incubated in vitro with adequate precursors, Jungmann and Schweppe (1967) also found evidence of 16α and 17α hydroxylases which have not been shown to be operational in in-situ perfusion. The placenta appears to be incapable of metabolizing or further hydroxylating progesterone to corticosteroid compounds. Therefore, it would seem as if its main precursor is cholesterol and its main products are pregnenolone and progesterone. From in vitro incubation studies of placental homogenates and mitochondria, Ryan et al. (1966) concluded that pregnenolone (from the fetus) was also a placental precursor of progesterone but quantitatively less important than cholesterol.

Histochemical studies by Cavallero and Magrini (1966) found 3β-HSD activity in the trophoblast amniotic epithelium and in chorion, using DHA and andro-stenediol as substrates.

The placenta can also resynthesize progesterone from reduced metabolites (20α-hydroxyprogesterone) of that steroid produced in the fetal liver and adrenal when they are recirculated into the placenta (Zander, 1962).

Arguments have recently been presented by Diczfalusy (1967) to support the notion that the main source of cholesterol for placental pregnenolone and proges-terone synthesis is maternal blood cholesterol and, to a lesser extent, fetal blood cholesterol. Davis and Plotz (1957) had previously shown that administration of tritiated cholesterol to pregnant women resulted in the production of tagged preg-nandiol excretion, which implied the synthesis of progesterone from cholesterol. They calculated that 70 percent of the progesterone elaborated in the placenta came from maternal blood cholesterol.

While the placenta does not have corticosteroid synthetic capability, it can dehydrogenate cortisol to cortisone (Sybulski and Venning, 1961). This conversion may be of considerable importance, for it has been found that cortisone rather than cortisol predominates in cord blood. This might explain the hyperfunction of the fetal pituitary, since only cortisol appears to have biologic activity in most target organs (Bush, 1962) and presumably also in inhibiting the pituitary.

PARTIAL BIOSYNTHESIS OF ESTROGEN BY THE PLACENTA

Estriol, the estrogen quantitatively most abundant in fetal and maternal circu-lation and urine during pregnancy, originates from 16α-hydroxydehydroepiandros-terone (16 OHDHA) and 16α-hydroxydehydroepiandrosterone sulfate (16 OHDHAS) which, in turn, has been formed from DHA and DHAS in the fetal liver. The placenta reduces the ring A of 16 OHDHA to produce estriol (Magen-dantz and Ryan, 1964) (Fig. 2).

If DHA is perfused through the placenta rather than the 16α hydroxylated relative, no estriol is formed; only estrone and estradiol appear, indicating that the placenta lacks 16 hydroxylating ability. Using a different technique, Siiteri and MacDonald (1966) have demonstrated that maternal DHAS can be a quantitatively important precursor of estradiol; they further showed that in the normal pregnant woman estriol may be formed by more than one mechanism. The most important is the one already described which uses 16α-OHDHAS derived from the fetus as a precursor. Estradiol may be further hydroxylated in position 16 by the fetus and thus make a minor contribution to estriol formation.

METABOLISM OF ANDROGENS BY THE PLACENTA

This aspect of placental synthetic function has been extensively studied by Diczfalusy et al. (1957). DHA and its sulfate are found in substantial amounts in cord blood (Colás et al., 1964). The placenta will cyclize and transform DHA and DHAS to estrone and estradiol (Boltè et al., 1964a, b, c) when they are injected into a uterine artery or perfused into the placenta in situ. Synthesis of androgens in the placenta using DHA as a precursor has also been suggested by the work of Lamb et al. (1967). They perfused with DHA the fetal side of the midterm placenta while it was attached to the uterus and isolated testosterone and androstenedione from the perfusate.

STEROID TRANSFER BY THE PLACENTA BETWEEN MOTHER AND FETUS

The placenta allows all steroids that have been studied to cross in both directions. However, the rate at which this happens varies greatly from steroid to steroid and depends on the form of conjugation with glucuronic and/or sulfuric acid in which the steroid is present in blood.

This problem has been extensively studied by Migeon et al. (1961, 1962) at midpregnancy and by Migeon et al. (1957) near term. Originally, using Nelson and Samuel's method for estimation of total 17 OH-corticosteroids in blood, they found the concentration of 17 OH-corticosteroids to be higher in maternal blood than in cord blood by a factor of 2:5, which allowed them to postulate that the latter was derived from the former (Migeon et al., 1956). In a series of subsequent studies (Migeon et al., 1961, 1962) they established unequivocally that cortisol transversed rapidly the placental barrier, and they confirmed for cortisol a mother-to-fetus gradient of the same order of magnitude as that previously shown by them to exist for 17 OH-corticosteroids as a group. These authors interpreted the observed gradient to be a consequence of the high concentration of transcortin in maternal blood during pregnancy rather than an active placental function. The findings at midpregnancy were similar to those at term. Other steroids studied included C^{14}-labeled corticosterone, progesterone, estrone, and 17β-estradiol. In all cases, there was a bidirectional transfer of the steroids, the specific rate of transfer for each steroid varying by a factor of more than 3, cortisol and estrone being the fastest and corticosterone, progesterone, and estriol being at a slower and approximately similar rate among themselves.

However, most of the steroids found in cord blood are in conjugated form, mainly as sulfates and also as glucosiduronides (Eberlein, 1965). The transference and/or previous deesterification of the steroid by the placenta is probably the most important factor in regulating the retention of steroids in the fetus or their transfer to the mother for ulterior elimination. Dancis et al. (1958) and Levitz et al. (1960) have extensively studied this problem. They have demonstrated for estrone and its glucosiduronide, estradiol and its sulfate, and estriol sulfate and glucosiduronide (Levitz, 1966), that the free forms of the hormone go through the placenta many times faster than do the conjugates. The sulfate is transferred at about three times the rate of the glucosiduronide, probably because the placenta has a powerful sulfatase activity which liberates the free steroid from its sulfated conjugate. The glucosiduronide is probably not split by the placenta in vivo even though β glucuronidase activity has been reported in the placenta in vitro (Fishman and Anlyan, 1947).

Integrated Steroid Synthesis and Metabolism in the Fetoplacental Unit

The results of the experiments on perfusion of fetus and placentas in situ and of in-vitro incubations led to the understanding that both the fetal adrenal and the placenta are incomplete endocrine organs. The synthetic and metabolic capabilities are complementary except in the synthesis of cholesterol in which both appear to be defective at midpregnancy. However, if cholesterol is supplied by the maternal and fetal livers the combined capabilities of both organs cannot only carry out all the synthetic steps of the adult human adrenal, but also are capable of performing several other synthetic reactions that do not exist in the adult organ. Diczfalusy et al. (1967) deserve the credit of having established firmly the notion of the fetoplacental unit as a functional whole.

The methodology of direct study of steroid metabolism in the fetoplacental unit is complicated by the fact that the precursors must be injected while the fetoplacental circulation is still intact, in cases of legal abortion produced by hysterotomy at midterm. The circulation is allowed to continue for some time before the cord is ligated, and the metabolites are extracted from blood, placenta, and fetal tissues and in some cases from maternal urine. Other important data have been obtained by steroid fractionation and identification in cord blood at term (Eberlein, 1965) or by the study of quantitative differences of steroid content in blood from the umbilical arteries and umbilical vein (Gardner and Walton, 1954).

NEUTRAL STEROIDS

Synthesis of cholesterol appears to take place in the maternal and fetal livers rather than in either placenta or fetal adrenal. Maternal blood contains a higher cholesterol level and is probably the major contributor (Schreier, 1964). The placenta can produce Δ5 pregnenolone and progesterone from the cholesterol (Fig. 3). These two precursors are secreted to the fetal and maternal circulation. The adrenal does not, at midpregnancy, transform Δ5 pregnenolone to progesterone because it has little or no 3β-HSD activity. Δ5 pregnenolone is sulfonated by the adrenal and is hydroxylated to 17 hydroxypregnenolone sulfate which serves as precursor within the adrenal to DHAS. In the fetal liver the same precursor may be either hydroxylated in position 16 to yield 16α-hydroxypregnenolone sulfate or reduced to 20α-hydroxypregnenolone. The latter steroid may, on returning to the placenta, be used to resynthesize progesterone.

Progesterone produced by the placenta may go into the maternal circulation to the liver, be transformed to pregnandiol, and be excreted by maternal urine. A large amount goes into the fetus. In the fetal adrenal progesterone may be hydroxylated in positions 17, 21, and 11 to yield corticosteroids-corticosterone sulfate, 11 desoxycorticosterone sulfate, 11 dehydrocorticosterone sulfate, hydrocortisone, and its sulfate. Hydrocortisone will be oxidized in the fetus to cortisone which is as

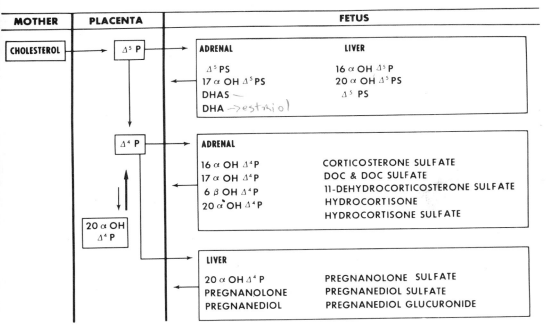

Fig. 3. A scheme for the metabolism of pregnenolone and progesterone in the human placenta and fetus at midpregnancy. Δ⁵ P, pregnenolone; Δ⁵ PS, pregnenolone sulfate; 17αOHΔ⁵ PS, 17α-hydroxypregnenolone sulfate; DHAS, dehydroisoandrosterone sulfate; DHA, dehydroisoandrosterone; 16αOHΔ⁵ P, 16α-hydroxypregnenolone; 20αOHΔ⁵ PS, 20α-dihydropregnenolone sulfate; 16αOHΔ⁴ P, 16α-hydroxyprogesterone; 17αOHΔ⁴ P, 17α-hydroxyprogesterone; 6βOHΔ⁴ P, 6β-hydroxyprogesterone; 20αOHΔ⁴ P, 20α-dihydroprogesterone; DOC, deoxycorticosterone. (From Solomon et al. 1967. Recent Progr. Hormone Res., 23:297-349.)

such probably devoid of biologic activity and incapable of repressing the pituitary release of ACTH. Other forms of hydroxylation of progesterone in the fetal adrenal that do not enter in the corticosteroid biosynthetic pathway are 16a and 6a-hydroxylation to 16a-hydroxyprogesterone and to 6a-hydroxyprogesterone, respectively.

In the fetal liver and other tissues progesterone may be transformed into pregnandiol and its sulfate or reduced to 20a-hydroxyprogesterone.

ANDROGENS AND ESTROGENS

DHAS secreted by the fetal (and maternal) adrenal may undergo, on returning to the placenta, two types of transformations: 1, cyclizing of ring A to yield estrone and/or estradiol or 2, by the action of placental 3β-HSD be transformed to androstenedione, which in turn may be transformed to testosterone by a 17 reductase. Both these androgens can be secreted to the maternal and fetal circulations or they can be cyclized within the placenta to estrone and estradiol. DHAS may also be hydroxylated by the fetus to 16a-hydroxydehydroisoandrosterone sulfate which, upon repassage through the placenta, will serve as the main precursor for estriol sulfate and estriol (Fig. 4), the quantitatively most important estrogen in pregnancy.

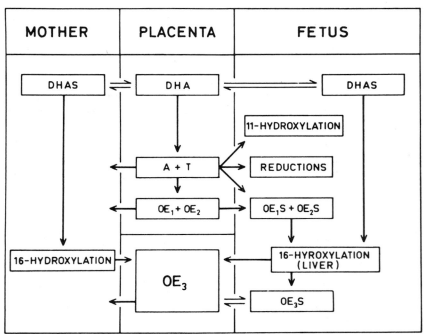

Fig. 4. Schematic representation of the metabolism of dehydroepiandrosterone sulfate by the fetoplacental unit at midpregnancy. DHAS, dehydroepiandrosterone sulfate; DHA, dehydroepiandrosterone; A, androstenedione; T, testosterone; OE$_1$, estrone; OE$_2$, 17β estradiol; OE$_3$, estriol; OE$_1$S, estrone sulfate; and OE$_2$S, 17β-estradiol 3-sulfate. (From Diczfalusy. 1967. *In Fetal Homeostasis*, Vol. 2. Courtesy of New York Academy of Sciences.)

Estriol is excreted in maternal urine, but it is also abundantly distributed in all fetal tissues where recent evidence (Gurpide et al., 1966) indicates it can be further hydroxylated to a tetrol derivative.

Eberlein (1965) made an important contribution to the knowledge of steroid content in pooled fetal blood retained in the placenta after vaginal delivery of full-term infants. He detected in this blood 23 steroids and 5 sterols. Twenty of these steroids appeared to exist in fetal blood as sulfoconjugates; only 17 hydroxy-progesterone was found in free state, and the only glucosiduronide detected was 5β-pregnane-3α, 20α diol. This author found 2 populations of steroids in fetal blood. One group was composed of Δ4 compounds, including progesterone and its metabolites. The second group included the majority of the steroids and all 5 sterols; they were found to be Δ5 3β hydroxysteroids. Eberlein believes these Δ5 hydroxysteroids originate in the fetal zone of the fetal adrenal cortex, which is markedly deficient in 3β-HSD at term as well as at midpregnancy.

CONJUGATION AND CONJUGATE HYDROLYSIS IN THE FETOPLACENTAL UNIT

Most fetal tissues, including the skin, have an intense steroidsulfokinase activity but scarce sulfatase activity. Therefore, steroid sulfates formed by the fetal tissues from circulating free steroids will remain as conjugates as long as they are in the fetal organism. On the other hand, the placenta has powerful aryl, a sterol sulfatase capable of hydrolyzing most steroid sulfates. (Goebelsmann et al., 1965, 1966). Glucuronide conjugation is quantitatively less important than sulfate conjugation. Out of 23 steroids isolated by Eberlein (1965) from cord blood, 20 were recovered by a transesterification method (Eberlein, 1965) which appears to be specific for sulfates, and only 1 (5β-pregnane-3α, 20α diol) was present as a glucosiduronate. Levitz (1966) has given figures for the relative amounts of 3 types of conjugates of estriol in cord blood: 67 percent is present as estriol sulfate, 20 percent as glucosiduronate, and about 10 percent each for the unconjugated or diconjugated estriols.

Control of Fetal Adrenal Secretion

The question of trophic control of the fetal adrenal has intrigued workers in this field for years. Factors suggesting a strong trophic stimulus were the large size of the fetal adrenal relative to body weight and the peculiar pattern of its development in intrauterine life followed by involution in the first three weeks after birth. This involution is mainly accounted for by the development followed by necrosis of the distinctive fetal zone. It appeared probable that this stimulus was due to a trophic hormone different from ACTH, since the anatomic pattern of the hypertrophy was peculiar and the hypertrophy was confined to the duration of pregnancy. It is not surprising that chorionic gonadotropin was considered for some time a likely candidate for the trophic role (Gardner, 1956; Gardner and

Walton, 1954). The fact that both the fetal zone and a luteinizing type of chorionic gonadotropin are peculiar to the human species and restricted to pregnancy made this speculation extremely attractive. However, attempts to stimulate the adrenal in vivo or in vitro with chorionic gonadotropins failed. Experimental evidence relevant to the problem of pituitary control was not easy to obtain in humans because the crucial experiments of fetal hypophysectomy could not be performed.

Anencephalic fetuses fail to produce a fetal zone in the second half of pregnancy, probably because of lack of pituitary stimulation. Lanman (1962) was able to produce adrenal hypertrophy equivalent in size to that of the normal fetus in these anencephalic fetuses by injection of zinc ACTH, while chorionic gonadotropin did not result in fetal zone stimulation.

Lanman (1961) reviewed the available evidence and concluded that in the human fetus the pituitary is responsible for the maintenance of the fetal zone. The pituitary control of the fetal adrenal is now widely accepted. However, the question of what makes the adrenal involute after birth has not been adequately answered. It would probably be necessary to postulate either hyperactivity of the fetal pituitary in the second half of pregnancy or a partial pituitary insufficiency or adrenal unresponsiveness after birth.

Jost (1966) and Jost et al. (1962) working with rats and rabbits have accumulated an impressive body of evidence in support of an active role of the pituitary in the hypertrophy, maintenance, and secretion of the adrenal in utero. Evidence has also been found in animals that a feedback mechanism exists between the fetal adrenal and the fetal pituitary, unilateral adrenalectomy being followed by enlargement of the remaining gland (Kitchell, 1950). This can be prevented by decapitating the fetus. In humans the evidence for a feedback is much less explicit. Babies born to mothers that have received large doses of prednisone during the later part of the pregnancy may show evidence of adrenal insufficiency after birth (von Hottinger, 1959), but this type of experience has been neither abundant nor conclusive, and larger series of pregnant women treated with prednisone make no reference to the occurrence of adrenal insufficiency in the neonate (Warrell and Taylor, 1968). The studies of steroid production and metabolism in the fetoplacental unit previously outlined suggest that a closed loop feedback control mechanism between the pituitary and the adrenal probably does not exist in the fetus. Because of the deficient 3β-HSD system in the fetal adrenal the earlier steps of steroid metabolism which are supposed to be the steps at which the stimulatory effect of ACTH is largely exerted do not result in the formation of corticosteroids. Rather, Δ5 pregnenolone is used in the pathway leading to the formation of DHA, 16αOH DHA, and estriol, none of which is efficient as far as we know in inhibiting the pituitary. Large amounts of progesterone of placental origin are continuously offered the adrenal. The adrenal has all the enzymatic equipment to transform this progesterone into cortisol, and cortisol can be isolated from the fetal adrenal after progesterone perfusion. But cortisol is probably dehydrogenated in the placenta to cortisone (Seely, 1964; Eberlein, 1965), and cortisone is presumably not capable of inhibiting the pituitary. The progesterone which is presumed to be the precursor of hydrocortisone is mainly of placental origin, and pituitary ACTH is not known to stimulate any of the biosynthetic steps leading to the synthesis of progesterone from cholesterol by the placenta. No known feedback exists between the placenta and the pituitary. The remaining possible source of cortisol would be the maternal circulation. This cortisol would presumably also be subject to the conversion to cortisone in the placenta, and in any case this exogenous cortisol could not explain how the regulatory loop including the fetal adrenal could be closed. In conclusion, there is little doubt that fetal pituitary ACTH is the trophic stimulus to the fetal adrenal.

The pituitary may be influenced by the level of circulating cortisol, and because this level is low, the pituitary tends to overstimulate the adrenal. A closed loop regulatory system with the fetal adrenal or one of its components may not be operational during fetal life.

Function of the Fetal Adrenal Cortex

There is scarce information on the function of the adrenal cortex of the human fetus. Forsham (1967) has recently discussed the biochemical phenomena in a physiologic perspective. Experimental evidence in rats indicates that adrenalectomy of mother and fetus on day 18.5 does not result in death of the fetus or interruption of pregnancy. In the anencephalic human fetus, in which the adrenals frequently fail to show the usual hypertrophy, mainly at the expense of the fetal zone, no correspondent failure in somatic development results; the fetus develops normally to term. A large number of experiments done by Jost et al. (1962) in rabbits and rats has established that in those species the fetal adrenal cortex is not required for fetal growth. The main function found by this author for the rat adrenal cortex is that it influences the deposition of glycogen in the fetal liver and fetal myocardium (Jacquot, 1959). The size of the fetal thymus is also influenced by adrenocortical secretions. Jost et al. (1962) have shown that intrauterine decapitation of the fetus at day 17.5 reduces by 90 percent the medullary activity of the enzyme phenyl-ethanolamine-N-methyl transferase, the enzyme that mediates the synthesis of adrenaline from noradrenaline. These works have been recently summarized by Jost (1966, 1967).

Present knowledge does not permit a physiologic interpretation of the many changes in corticosteroid and sex hormone production and metabolism that the biochemists have unveiled in the last decade. Indeed, thinking in terms of what little is known of the biologic activities of these steroids, the high circulating levels of androgens and estrogens in fetal blood would appear to be a liability rather than an asset. Nor is it in any way clear that the high levels of androgens and estrogens in the fetoplacental unit play a symbiotic role, the end-organ of which is in the maternal organism, with the possible exception of the maternal elevation of transcortin as a response to placental estrogen. Steroids as well as chorionic gonado-tropin or the placental lactogen have yet to be assigned a convincing role in the physiology of pregnancy. Yet it would be rash to conclude at the present stage of our knowledge that any of these hormones is superfluous. Our understanding of the biologic effect of the steroids at the cellular level is rudimentary. The determinating factors of tissue differentiation are almost completely unknown. The non-rejection of the placenta by the maternal organism, the successful competition of fetal tissues versus maternal tissues for available nutrients, and the factors that determine the initiation of labor are all problems that await elucidation.

Steroids may have a role in some of these mechanisms. The fetal adrenal does not appear to be necessary for fetal development in the rat as shown by Jost et al. (1962) nor in the human species as suggested by the normal development of the anencephalic fetus. As for the maternal adrenal, it is well known that Addison's disease in the mother is no impediment to a successful pregnancy (Davis and Plotz, 1956). One may, therefore, surmise that the adrenal plays a role in survival only in extrauterine life and that the gland is not necessary in utero. But unlike the other unused systems, such as the sensory organs, the adrenal is active, and that activity may not be pertinent or may be deleterious to fetal development. Hypercorticism of the mother is known to be detrimental to the fetus (Cope and Raker, 1955), and corticosteroid, progestin, and sex hormone treatments all have adverse side effects on the fetus at certain moments of its development. In this light the sequence of biosynthetic transformations described may represent a huge dumping operation by which the fetal organism is defended against the noxious steroids.

The lack of 3β-HSD could be understood as the essential block whereby production of corticosteroids is prevented and the superabundant precursors are shifted to the synthesis of more innocuous estriol. The inactivity of 3β-HSD itself may be due to a late developmental schedule for this enzyme, or it may be due, as Ville (1966) has suggested, to inhibition by its normal reaction product, progesterone, originated in the placenta. The reductive pathways of progesterone in the liver would serve a similar purpose by withdrawing progesterone from corticosteroid synthesis. The ubiquitous sulfokinase of fetal tissues would serve to impede the biologic action of estrogens, androgens, and progestins alike. Two additional mechanisms would defend the fetus against maternal cortisol—the increased transcortin in maternal blood and the rapid dehydrogenation of free cortisol to cortisone by placental cortisol dehydrogenase.

MATERNAL COMPARTMENT

The fetoplacental unit is in dynamic equilibrium with the larger continent of the maternal organism. Levels of steroids and their metabolites in the fetoplacental circulation depend, to a considerable extent, on mechanisms that operate in the mother. Maternal secretion, metabolism, and excretion of steroids regulate the composition of the milieu in which the fetoplacental unit extracts precursors and excretes metabolites. While a detailed exposition of steroid metabolism in the pregnant woman is outside the scope of this chapter, some of the pertinent facts will be summarized.

Plasma cortisol and corticosteroids have consistently been found to be elevated in maternal plasma during pregnancy (Assali et al., 1955; Bayliss et al., 1955; Birke et al., 1958; Cohen et al., 1958; reviewed by Jayle and Pasqualini, 1965). This is probably secondary to the increase in cortisol-binding globulin (CBG)

(Slaunwhite and Sandberg, 1959). The concentration of CBG is 29 to 30 mg/liter in nonpregnant plasma. It starts to rise in the second or third month of pregnancy and reaches a mean level of 70 mg/liter at term. This concentration is much higher than that of cord blood (Daughaday, 1958, 1967), which probably accounts for the lower corticosteroid level found in the fetal circulation. Bound cortisol is probably not biologically active, and pregnant women show no clinical manifestations of hypercorticism.

The half-life of cortisol in the plasma of pregnant women is greatly prolonged (Migeon et al., 1957), and its glucuronic conjugation in the liver is decreased. This, together with the increase of CBG, probably accounts for its increased concentration in blood in spite of the fact that cortisol production rates by the adrenal are decreased in pregnancy except at the time of labor (Migeon et al., 1968). Testosterone concentration in maternal blood is significantly increased independent of sex in the fetus (Rivarola et al., 1968). Androstenedione and dehydroepiandrosterone are also increased although only slightly. Pregnancy increases the protein binding of testosterone and DHA but does not affect binding of androstenedione.

Estriol concentration in maternal plasma increases an average of fivefold from the twenty-fifth to the fortieth weeks. Values given by various authors have varied considerably depending on the techniques used. Nachtigall et al. (1966) introduced a method in which synthetic conjugated estriol is used to correct for recovery losses. They found values ranging between 9.3 and 56 mg/100 ml of plasma with a mean of 27 mg/100 ml in normal late pregnancy. Most of it was in the form of a sulfoglucosiduronate diconjugate (Touchstone et al., 1963).

Adrenal Function in the Neonatal Period

During the first 3 to 4 weeks of life the adrenal is undergoing a dramatic structural reorganization. The fetal zone starts to involute shortly before term and by the end of the first month has completely regressed. The definitive cortex, on the contrary, develops to adopt the three zone structure of the adult gland. It is now believed that this structural change does not compromise the function of the neonate's adrenal. The adrenal appears to be competent to carry out its metabolic functions and electrolyte regulation, as well as to react to stress. It is presently felt by most authors that there is no transient adrenal insufficiency in the first weeks of life, a notion that was entertained by some a decade earlier. This physiologic competence does not mean that the quantitative and qualitative patterns of steroids in blood and urine are identical to those of the adult.

Several factors require special caution in interpreting results in the first 48 hours of life. They have been reviewed by Seely (1961, 1964) and Ulstrom et al. (1961). During the first 24 hours, concentrations of plasma and urine corticosteroids probably represent an unknown proportion of corticosteroids of maternal origin (Bertrand et al., 1965).

During delivery both maternal and fetal adrenals are responding to stress, resulting in elevated values. When the Porter-Silber reaction is used, bilirubin and ketone may interfere with the reaction. The large number of pregnane derivatives present in blood and urine during the first day may also contribute color in several steroid reactions used. The newborn has a circadian rhythm, and the time of day at which the sampling is done must be taken into consideration for the comparison of different sets of blood values.

17 hydroxycorticosteroids in plasma decrease from the high values found in cord blood (19 μg 100 ml, Bertrand et al., 1965) to somewhat subnormal values (9 μg 100 ml, Bertrand et al., 1965; 5.4 μg 100 ml, Seely, 1964) during the first three weeks of life and return to normal adult levels in the fourth week and there-after. During that period the proportion of blood conjugated versus free cortico-steroid is in a ratio of 1:1.

This decrease of blood corticosteroids is probably not due to a decreased ability of the adrenal to respond to ACTH (Lanman, 1953; Bertrand et al., 1965) or to a low cortisol production rate. The cortisol production rate in the neonatal period is not lower than that of the adult in terms of mg per unit of body surface (Migeon, 1959). The half-life of cortisol has consistently been found to be considerably increased (Bongiovanni et al., 1958; Cranny et al., 1960; Migeon, 1959).

On the other hand, the half-life of injected tetrahydrocortisol, the main excretion product of cortisol, is not increased (Bongiovanni et al., 1958; Grumbach et al., 1959). The deficiency is probably in the reduction of ring A in the liver to form the tetrahydro derivative from cortisol. There is ample evidence for a similar deficiency in glucuro conjugation. The proportion of free to conjugated corticoste-roids in plasma shows a disproportionate amount of free corticosteroids when compared with adult blood. ACTH produces an increase of the free corticosteroid fractions but no elevation of the conjugated fraction during the first three weeks of life (Bertrand et al., 1965).

Another peculiarity of the neonate consists in the inability of estrogen administra-tion to produce an elevation of blood corticosteroids, probably because the corticoste-roid-binding globulin fails to increase at this age. Seely (1964) and Eberlein (1965) found that corticosteroids in cord blood were mainly, if not exclusively, in the form of cortisone. The equilibrium of 11 ketones versus 11 hydroxy com-pounds is shifted in the direction of the 11 ketones. This peculiarity of cortisol metabolism in cord blood has been attributed to the presence of an 11 dehydrogenase in the placenta.

However, the effect persists for about three weeks postpartum. It is, therefore, probable that the liver in the neonatal period has the capability of transforming most of the secreted cortisol to cortisone, a reaction which takes place normally but to a lesser extent in adult life and which is an important regulatory factor of the half-life of cortisol. In urine there is a parallel excess of tetrahydro E over tetrahydro F. Thus, THF/THE equals 0.003 in the infant, while this ratio has a value of 2.0 for older children (Bertrand et al., 1965).

Another feature of adrenal cortical secretion in the neonatal period is the pre-dominance of corticosterone over cortisol (Exley and Norymberski, 1963). The physiologic significance of these differences of steroid metabolism in the neonate is poorly understood.

The levels of total blood 17 ketosteroids measured by the Zimmermann reaction rise during and immediately after delivery (Eberlein, 1965), remain elevated during the first week of life, and decline thereafter. Using simultaneously the Zimmermann reaction for total 17 ketosteroids and the Oertel-Eik-Nes (1959) reaction for Δ5 3β hydroxysteroids, Eberlein (1965) showed that during the first week of life blood levels of Δ5 3β hydroxysteroids are higher than those for total 17 ketosteroids, while the reverse is true after the first week.

Finally, 16α-hydroxylated C19 steroids have been detected in the infant's urine during the neonatal period (Cleary and Pion, 1968). They probably represent the persistence during this time of the same mechanisms that are responsible for the production of estriol precursors in the fetus. Infants born to mothers whose estriol excretion during pregnancy was reduced have decreased rates of excretion of the latter compounds.

Conclusion

Both the fetal adrenal and the placenta appear to be very active steroidogenic organs. The steroid spectrum secreted by the fetal adrenal is very different from that of the adult gland.

Some of the most important differences can be accounted for by postulating a deficiency of 3β-HSD, a contention which has considerable experimental support. Extensive 16 hydroxylation is also a distinctive capability of the fetal adrenal.

The placenta is a potent synthesizer of pregnenolone and progesterone from maternal and fetal blood circulating cholesterol. These two products are potential precursors for corticosteroid synthesis by the fetal adrenal and can be catabolized by different reductive reactions in the fetal liver and maternal liver; the catabolic reactions are probably of greater quantitative importance than those of adrenal corticosteroid synthesis. A second placental function is that of steroid transformation. Only some of those are known: 16 OHDHAS from the fetal adrenal is converted to estriol sulfate, the most abundant estrogen of the fetal circulation. DHA is converted to estrone and estradiol, and possibly to testosterone and androstenedione. Cortisol is dehydrogenated to cortisone. A third important function of the placenta is the transfer of corticosteroids from mother to fetus, and of estrogens and possibly androgens from fetus to mother.

Finally, the fetus conjugates most steroids in its circulation as steroid sulfates. The placenta can split these sulfates and efficiently transfer the steroid to the maternal circulation. It is probable that the estrogens are then responsible for the increase of CBG in the maternal circulation. All these combined activities of the fetal adrenal and placenta result in large amounts of circulating steroids, particularly androgens and estrogens in both circulations. Corticosteroids are elevated in the mother but not in the fetus. It is tempting to infer that these unusually high levels are of physiologic consequence to the fetal development, but evidence in this direction is conspicuous by its absence. The simplest explanation may be that the fetoplacental unit is functioning to inactivate biologically active steroids.

In the neonatal period most of the qualitative and quantitative peculiarities of steroid composition of the infant's blood seem to be due to a continuing activity of the fetal pathways during the first few days of life, to the excretion of the large amounts of metabolites accumulated in fetal tissues, and to the stress of labor.

REFERENCES

Assali, N. J., J. B. Garst, and J. Vosikan. 1955. Blood level of 17 hydroxycorticosteroids in normal and toxemic pregnancy. J. Lab. Clin. Med., 46:385-390.

Bayliss, R. S., J. M. Browne, B. P. Round, and A. W. Steinbeck. 1955. Plasma corticosteroids in pregnancy. Lancet, 1:62-64.

Benagiano, G., et al. 1967. Metabolism of C19 steroids in the fetoplacental unit. III. Metabolism of androstenedione and teststerone by previable fetuses at mid pregnancy. Acta Endocr. (Kobenhavn), 56:203-220.

Bertrand, J., B. Loras, J. M. Saez, and B. Cantenet. 1965. Hydroxycorticosteroid secretion and metabolism in neonates and infants up to the age of three months. *In* Jayle, M. F., ed. Hormonology of Human Pregnancy. Oxford, Pergamon Press, Inc., pp. 165-187.

Birke, G., C. A. Gemzell, L. O. Plautin, and H. Robbe. 1958. Plasma levels of 17 hydroxycorticosteroids and urinary excretion pattern of ketosteroids in normal pregnancy. Acta Endocr. (Kobenhavn), 27:389-402.

Bloch, E., and K. Benirschke. 1959. Synthesis in vitro of steroids by human fetal adrenal gland slices. J. Biol. Chem., 234:1085-1089.

——— and Benirschke, K. 1962. Steroidogenic capacity of fetal adrenal in vitro. *In* Currie, A. R., T. Symington, and J. K. Grant, eds. The Human Adrenal Cortex. Baltimore, The Williams & Wilkins Co., pp. 580-589.

Boltè, E., et al. 1964a. Studies on the aromatization of neutral steroids in pregnant women. I. Aromatization of C19 steroid by placentas perfused in situ. Acta Endocr. (Kobenhavn), 45:535-559.

——— et al. 1964b. Studies on the aromatization of neutral steroids in pregnant women. II. Aromatization of dehydroepiandrosterone and of its sulfate administered simultaneously into a uterine artery. Acta Endocr. (Kobenhavn), 45:560-575.

——— et al. 1964c. Studies on the aromatization of neutral steroids in pregnant women. III. Overall aromatization of dehydroepiandrosterone sulfate circulating in the fetal and maternal compartments. Acta Endocr. (Kobenhavn), 45:575-599.

Bongiovanni, A. M., W. R. Eberlein, M. Wetphal, and T. Boggs. 1958. Prolonged turnover rate of hydrocortisone in the newborn infant. J. Clin. Endocr., 18:1127-1130.

Boyd, E. M., and K. M. Wilson. 1935. Exchange of lipids in umbilical circulation at birth J. Clin. Invest., 14:7-15.

Bush, I. E. 1962. Chemical and biological factors in the action of steroid hormones. *In* Currie, A. R., T. Symington, and J. K. Grant, eds. The Human Adrenal Cortex. Baltimore, The Williams & Wilkins Co., pp. 138-171.

Cavallero, A., and U. Magrini. 1966. Histochemical studies on 3β hydroxysteroid dehydrogenase and other enzymes in the steroid secreting structures of human fetus. Int. Congr. on Hormonal Steroids. Amsterdam, Excerpta Medica Foundation ICS, 132:667-674.

Cleary, R. E., and J. Pion. 1968. Urinary excretion of 16α hydroxy dehydroepiandrostenedione and 16α keto androstenediol during early neonatal period. J. Clin. Endocr., 28:372-378.

Cohen, M., M. Steifel, W. J. Reddy, and J. C. Laidlaw. 1958. The secretion and disposition of cortisol during pregnancy. J. Clin. Endocr., 18:1076-1192.

Colás, A. L., W. Heinrichs, and H. Talum. 1964. Pettenkoffer chromogen in the maternal and fetal circulations. Steroids, 3:417-434.

Cope, C. L., and E. Black. 1959. The hydrocortisone production in late pregnancy. J. Obstet. Gynec. Brit. Emp., 66:404-408.

Cope, O., and J. W. Raker. 1955. Cushing's disease: The surgical experience of 46 cases. New Eng. J. Med., 253:119-127.

Cranny, R. L., J. F. K. Vink, and V. C. Kelley. 1960. The half life of hydrocortisone in normal newborn infants. Amer. J. Dis. Child., 99:437-443.

Crowder, R. E. 1957. The development of the adrenal gland in man with special reference to origin and ultimate location of cell types and evidence in favor of the cell migration theory. Carnegie Institute Contrib. Embryol., 36:195-210.

Dancis, J., W. L. Money, G. P. Condon, and M. Levitz. 1958. The relative transfer of estrogens and their glucuronides across the placenta in the guinea pig. J. Clin. Invest., 37:1373-1378.

Daughaday, W. H. 1958. Binding of corticosteroids by plasma proteins. V. Corticosteroids-binding globulin activity in normal human beings and in certain disease states. Arch. Intern. Med. (Chicago), 101:286-290.

———— 1967. The binding of corticosteroids by plasma protein. In Eisenstein, A. N., ed. The Adrenal Cortex. Boston, Little, Brown and Company, pp. 385-403.

Davis, M. E., and E. J. Plotz. 1956. Hormonal interrelationships between maternal adrenal, placenta and fetal adrenal function. Obstet. Gynec. Surv., 11:1-43.

———— and E. J. Plotz. 1957. The metabolism of progesterone and its clinical use in pregnancy. Recent Progr. Hormone Res., 13:347-388.

Dell'Acqua, S., et al. 1966. Androgen metabolism in the fetoplacental unit at midterm. In Proc. 2nd Int. Congr. on Hormonal Steroids. Amsterdam, Excerpta Medica Foundation ICS, 132:639-645.

Diczfalusy, E. 1965. In vivo biogenesis and metabolism of oestrogens in the fetoplacental unit. In Proc. 2nd Int. Congr. of Endocr. Amsterdam, Excerpta Medica Foundation ICS, 83:732-736.

———— 1967. Endocrinology of the fetoplacental unit. In Wynn, R. M., ed. Fetal Homeostasis. New York, New York Academy of Sciences, pp. 268-361.

———— G. Tellinger, and A. Westman. 1957. Studies on estrogen metabolism in newborn boys. I. Excretion of oestrone oestradiol-17β and estriol during the first few days of life. Acta Endocr. (Kobenhavn), 26:303-312.

Eberlein, W. R. 1963. Transesterification method for the measurement of plasma 17 ketosteroid sulfates. J. Clin. Endocr., 23:990-995.

———— 1965. Steroids and sterols in umbilical cord blood. J. Clin. Endocr., 25:1101-1118.

Exley, D., and J. K. Norymberski. 1964. Urinary excretion of 17-deoxy-corticosteroids by man. J. Endoc., 29:293-302.

Fishman, W. H., and A. J. Anlyan. 1947. β glucuronidase activity in human tissues: Some correlations with the process of malignant growth and with the physiology of reproduction. Cancer Res., 7:808-817.

Forsham, P. H. 1967. The adrenal cortex in pregnancy. *In* CIBA Foundation Study Group No. 27. The Human Adrenal Cortex: Its Function Throughout Life. Boston, Little, Brown and Company, pp. 48-59.

Gardner, L. I. 1956. Adrenocortical metabolism of the fetus, infant and child. Pediatrics, 17:897-924.

——— and R. L. Walton. 1954. Plasma 17 ketosteroids of the human fetus: Demonstration of concentration gradient between cord and maternal circulation. Helv. Paediat. Acta, 4:311-316.

Goebelsmann, U., G. Eriksson, N. Wiqvist, and E. Diczfalusy. 1965. Metabolism of oestriol-3-sulfate and oestriol-16 (17?)-glucosiduronate in pregnant women. Acta Endocr. (Kobenhavn), 50:273-288.

——— et al. 1966. Fate of intra-amniotically administered oestriol-15^{3}H-3 sulfate and oestriol-16-^{14}C-16-glucosiduronate in pregnant women at midterm. Acta Endocr. (Kobenhavn), 52:550-564.

Goldman, A. S., W. C. Takovac, and A. M. Bongiovanni. 1966. Development of activity of 3B hydroxysteroid dehydrogenase in human fetal tissue and in two anencephalic newborns. J. Clin. Endocr., 26:14.

——— A. M. Bongiovanni, W. C. Takovac, and A. Prader. 1964. Study on Δ5 3B hydroxysteroid dehydrogenase in normal, hyperplastic and neoplastic adrenal tissue. J. Clin. Endocr., 24:894-909.

Gruenwald, P. 1946. Embryonic and postnatal development of the adrenal cortex: Particularly the zona glomerulosa and accessory nodules. Anat. Rec., 95:391-422.

Grumbach, M. M., J. R. Ducharme, and A. Norishima. 1959. The metabolism of hydrocortisone and its metabolite in premature and newborn infants: Evidence for defective degradation and impaired laydrolysis of steroidesters. Amer. J. Dis. Child., 98:672-673.

Gurpide, E., et al. 1966. Fetal and maternal metabolism of estradiol in pregnancy. J. Clin. Endocr., 26:1355-1365.

von Hottinger, A. 1959. Vorübergehende, passive Nebennereninsuffizienz beim Neugeborenen. Schweiz. Med. Wschr., 11:419-472.

Jacquot, R. 1959. Recherches sur le controle endocrinien de l'accumulation de glycogene dans le foie chez le fetus de rat. J. Physiol. (Paris), 51:655-721.

Jaffe, R. B., G. Erikson, and E. Diczfalusy. 1966. In situ perfusion of the midterm human placenta with cholesterol. Excerpta Medica Foundation ICS, 99:182.

Jayle, M. F., and J. R. Pasqualini. 1965. Metabolism of adrenocortical hormones in the course of human pregnancy. *In* Jayle, M. F., ed. Hormonology of Human Pregnancy. Oxford, Pergamon Press, pp. 127-154.

Jost, A. 1966. Problems of fetal endocrinology: The adrenal glands. Recent Progr. Hormone Res., 22:541-574.

——— 1967. The function of the fetal adrenal cortex. *In* CIBA Foundation Study Group No. 27. The Human Adrenal Cortex: Its Function Throughout Life. Boston, Little, Brown and Company, pp. 11-28.

——— R. Jacquot, and A. Cohen. 1962. The pituitary control of the fetal adrenal cortex. *In* Currie, A. R., T. Symington, and J. K. Grant, eds. The Human Adrenal Cortex. Baltimore, The Williams & Wilkins Co., pp. 569-579.

Jungmann, R. A., and J. S. Schweppe. 1967. Biosynthesis and metabolism of neutral steroids by human midterm placenta and fetal liver. J. Clin. Endocr., 27:1151-1160.

Keene, M. F. L., and E. E. Hewer. 1927. Observations on the development of the human suprarenal gland. J. Anat., 61:302-324.

Kitchell, R. L. 1950. Compensatory hypertrophy of the intact adrenal of fetal rats subjected to unilateral adrenalectomy. Proc. Soc. Exp. Biol. Med., 75:824-827.

Lamb, E., et al. 1967. Studies on the metabolism of C19 steroids in the human facto-placental unit. Acta Endocr. (Kobenhavn), 55:263-277.

Lanman, J. T. 1953. Adrenal function in premature infants. II. ACTH treated infants and infants born of toxemia mothers. Pediatrics, 12:62-71.

———— 1960. An interpretation of human foetal adrenal structure and function. In Currie, A. R., T. Symington, and J. H. Grant, eds. The Human Adrenal Cortex. Baltimore, The Williams & Wilkins Co., pp. 547-558.

———— 1961. The adrenal gland in the human fetus: An interpretation of its physiology and unusual developmental patterns. Pediatrics, 27:140-158.

———— and L. M. Silverman. 1957. In vitro steroidogenesis in the human neonatal adrenal gland, including observations on the human adult and monkey adrenal glands. Endocrinology, 60:433-445.

———— S. Solomon, J. Lind, and S. Lieberman. 1957. In vitro biogenesis of steroids by the human fetal adrenal. Amer. J. Dis. Child., 94:504-505.

Levitz, M. 1966. Conjugation and transfer of fetal-placental steroid hormones. J. Clin. Endocr., 26:773-777.

———— G. P. Condon, W. L. Money, and J. Dancis. 1960. The relative transfer of estrogens and their sulfates across the guinea pig placenta: Sulfurylation of estrogens in the placenta. J. Biol. Chem., 235:973-977.

Longchamp, J. 1965. Biogénèse des steroids par les corticosurrénales foetales. In Jayle, M. F., ed. Hormonologie de la Grossesse Humaine. Paris, Gauthiers-Villars, pp. 205-218.

Magendantz, H. G., and K. G. Ryan. 1964. Isolation of an estriol precursor, 16α-hydroxyepiandrosterone, from human umbilical sera. J. Clin. Endocr., 24:1155-1162.

Migeon, C. J. 1959. Cortisol production and metabolism in the neonate. J. Pediat., 55:280-295.

———— J. Bertrand, and C. A. Gemzell. 1961. The transplacental passage of various steroid hormones in midpregnancy. Recent Progr. Hormone Res., 17:207-248.

———— J. Bertrand, and C. A. Gemzell. 1962. The transplacental passage of 4C14 cortisol in midpregnancy. In Currie, A. R., T. Symington, and J. K. Grant, eds. The Human Adrenal Cortex. Baltimore, The Williams & Wilkins Co., pp. 580-588.

———— J. Bertrand, and P. E. Wall. 1957. Physiological disposition of 4-C14 cortisol during late pregnancy. J. Clin. Invest., 36:1350-1362.

———— F. M. Kenny, and F. H. Taylor. 1968. Cortisol production rate. VIII. Pregnancy. J. Clin. Endocr., 28:961-968.

———— H. Prystowsky, M. M. Grumbach, and M. C. Byron. 1956. Placental passage of 17 hydroxycorticosteroids: Comparison of the levels in maternal and fetal plasma and effect of ACTH and hydrocortisone administration. J. Clin. Invest., 35:488-493.

Nachtigall, L., et al. 1966. A rapid method for the assay of plasma estriol in pregnancy. J. Clin. Endocr., 26:941-948.

Nelson, D. H., and L. T. Samuels. 1952. A method for the determination of 17-hydroxycorticosteroids in blood: 17-Hydroxycortisone in the peripheral circulation. J. Clin. Endocr., 12:519-526.

Oertel, G. W., and K. B. Eik-Nes. 1959. Determination of Δ5-3 beta-hydroxysteroids. Anal. Chem., 31:98-100.

Pasqualini, J. R., N. Wiquist, and E. Diczfalusy. 1966. Biosynthesis of aldosterone by human fetuses perfused with corticosterone at midterm. Biochim. Biophys. Acta, 121:433-460.

Pion, R., et al. 1965. Studies on the metabolism of C21 steroids in the human placental unit. I. Formation of αB unsaturated 3 ketones in midterm placentas perfused in situ with pregnenolone and 17α hydroxypregnenolone. Acta Endocr. (Kobenhavn), 48:234-248.

Rivarola, M. A., M. G. Forest, and C. J. Migeon. 1968. Testosterone, androstenedione and dehydroepiandrosterone in plasma during pregnancy and at delivery: Concentration and protein binding. J. Clin. Endocr., 28:34-40.

Ross, N. H. 1960. Electron Microscopy of human foetal adrenal cortex. In Currie, A. R., T. Symington, and J. K. Grant, eds. The Human Adrenal Cortex. Baltimore, The Williams & Wilkins Co., pp. 558-569.

Ryan, K. J. 1965. Estrogens: blood and placental levels and the factors which control them. In Proc. 2nd Int. Congr. of Endocrinology. Amsterdam, Excerpta Medica Foundation ICS, 83:727-731.

——— R. A. Mergs, and Z. Petro. 1966. Biosynthesis of progesterone in the human placenta. Int. Congr. on Hormonal Steroids. Amsterdam, Excerpta Medica Foundation ICS, 663-666.

Schreier, K. 1964. Studien zur Entwicklungsphysiologie des Fettstoffwechsels. I. Mitteilung, über die Serumlipide der Säuglinge., Z. Kinderheilk., 91:157-162.

Seely, J. R. 1961. Adrenal functional in newborns: Methodology and perinatal circulating steroid patterns. Amer. J. Dis. Child., 102:530-533.

——— 1964. Adrenocortical function in newborn humans: Methodology and perinatal circulating patterns. Ph.D. Thesis, University of Utah.

Siiteri, P. K., and P. C. MacDonald. 1966. Placental estrogen biosynthesis during human pregnancy. J. Clin. Endocr., 26:751-761.

Slaunwhite, W. R., and A. A. Sandberg. 1959. Transcortin, a corticosteroid binding protein of plasma. J. Clin. Invest., 38:384-391.

Solomon, S. 1966. The formation and metabolism of neutral steroids in the human fetus and placenta. Int. Congr. on Hormonal Steroids. Amsterdam, Excerpta Medica Foundation ICS, 132:653-662.

——— and H. G. Friesen. 1968. Endocrine Relations between Mother and Fetus. Ann. Rev. Med., 19:399-430.

——— J. T. Lanman, J. Lind, and S. Lieberman. 1958. The biogenesis of Δ4 androstenedione and 17α hydroxyprogesterone from progesterone by surviving human fetal adrenals. J. Biol. Chem., 233:1084-1088.

——— et al. 1967. The formation and metabolism of steroids in the fetus and the placenta. Recent Progr. Hormone Res., 23:297-349.

Swineyard, C. A. 1943. Growth of the human suprarenal glands. Anat. Rec., 87:141-150.

Sybulski, S., and E. Venning. 1961. The possibility of corticosteroid production by human and rat placental tissue under in vitro conditions. Canad. J. Biochem., 39:203-214.

Touchstone, J. C., J. W. Greene, R. C. McElroy, and T. Murawec. 1963. Blood estriol conjugation during human pregnancy. Biochemistry, 2:653-657.

Ulstrom, R. A., E. Colle, J. W. Reynolds, and J. Burley. 1961. Adrenocortical function in newborn infants. IV. Plasma concentrations of cortisol in the early neonatal period. J. Clin. Endocr., 21:414-425.

Uotila, U. V. 1940. The early embryological development of the fetal and permanent adrenal cortex in man. Anat. Rec., 76:183-203.

Van Luesden, H., and C. H. Villee. 1965. The de novo synthesis of steroid and steroids from acetate by preparations of human term placenta. Steroids, 6:31-45.

Velican, C. 1946-47. Embiogenese de la surrenale humaine. Arch. Anat. Micr. Exp., 36:316-333.

Villee, D. B. 1966. The role of progesterone in the development of adrenal enzymes. In Proc. 2nd Int. Congr. on Hormonal Steroids. Amsterdam, Excerpta Medica Foundation ICS, 132:680-686.

———— and C. A. Villee. 1964. Synthesis of corticosteroids in the fetoplacental unit. In Proc. 2nd Int. Congr. of Endocrinology. Amsterdam, Excerpta Medica Foundation ICS, 83:709-714.

———— L. I. Engel, and C. A. Villee. 1959. Steroid hydroxylation in human fetal adrenals. Endocrinology, 65:465-474.

Warrell, D. W., and R. Taylor. 1968. Outcome for the fetus of mothers receiving prednisolone during pregnancy. Lancet, 1:117-118.

Zander, J. 1962. Die Hormonbildung der Placenta und ihre Bedeutung für die Frucht. Arch. Gynaek., 198:113-127.

31

The Anterior Lobe of the Hypophysis

JOSÉ CARA • Department of Pediatrics, Maimonides Medical Center, State University of New York Downstate Medical Center, Brooklyn, N. Y.

Introduction

Cells in the anlage of the anterior lobe of the pituitary differentiate very early in the human fetus. Basophilic cells can be identified by about the eighth week of gestation, and the acidophils are found one to two weeks later (Falin, 1961). The fine structure of the fetal pituitary at about the twelfth week is consistent with a gland which is producing and secreting hormone, and by the eighteenth week the anterior lobe of the pituitary resembles the adult organ (Falin, 1961). The anterior lobe of the pituitary in perinatal life contains five or more distinct cells (Salazar et al., 1969), which secrete at least six independent hormones. The development of more elaborate techniques of histochemistry, immunofluorescence, and electron microscopy has permitted further development of the concept that each major hormone of the pituitary is produced by a distinct cell type, the "one cell one hormone theory" (Purves, 1966). The application of radioimmunoassay techniques in recent years has confirmed and expanded the results of bioassay procedures and has provided important new information concerning the pituitary content and the circulating levels of pituitary hormones in the fetus and in the newborn.

Much research remains to be done to clarify the time of initiation and the mechanisms which maintain the hypothalamus-pituitary-target gland homeostasis in fetal life. We will discuss here the physiologic significance of the anterior lobe of the pituitary in perinatal life, with particular attention to the production and secretion of human growth hormone (HGH), adrenocorticotropin (ACTH), thyrotropin (TSH), follicle stimulating hormone (FSH), luteinizing hormone (LH) or interstitial cell stimulating hormone (ICSH), and prolactin (LTH).

935

Human Growth Hormone (HGH)

Human fetal pituitary cells first show signs of staining with anti-human growth hormone antiserum between the tenth and fourteenth weeks of life, and staining is consistent after the seventeenth week (Ellis et al., 1966; Porteous and Beck, 1968). Acidophils have been reported as early as 9 to 10 weeks of fetal life (Falin, 1961). Porteous and Beck (1968) consider that the probable sequence of differentiation of the acidophils of the fetal pituitary is first the appearance of the human growth hormone (HGH) antigen and later the development of acidophilic cytoplasmic granules. More than 97 percent of the HGH-positive cells are acidophils, the remainder being chromophobes and basophils (Ellis et al., 1966). Presumably, the acidophil granules represent compacted deposits of HGH. Fetal HGH is immunologically indistinguishable from adult HGH in fluorescence tests (Ellis et al., 1966). At birth, the staining reactions of the acidophils are similar to those of corresponding cells in the adult hypophysis (Porteous and Beck, 1968).

PITUITARY CONTENT OF GROWTH HORMONE

Growth hormone is the most abundant hormone in the adenohypophysis. Parlow (1966), using a radioimmunoassay method, studied the HGH content of human pituitaries pooled according to age. He found that HGH was detectable in fetal pituitaries of less than five months of fetal age and progressively increased with age to a maximum at about twelve to eighteen years. There was, however, no significant difference in HGH content in pituitaries from birth to six months of age. Kaplan and Grumbach (1967) found that the HGH content of pituitaries obtained from ten aborted human fetuses between the estimated gestational ages of 70 and 162 days varied from 0.2 to 8.0 μg per mg of gland and correlated well with fetal age and pituitary size. Similarly, the growth hormone content of pituitaries from various animal species continues to increase throughout intrauterine life, reaching a maximum just before birth (Contopoulos, 1967). Gershberg (1957) and Rice and Ponthier (1968), using a bioassay technique, presented data suggesting the presence of biologically active HGH in human fetal pituitaries obtained during the last trimester.

PLASMA LEVEL OF HGH

The plasma concentration of HGH in fetuses and in the newborn is high and shows considerable individual variation (Hunter and Greenwood, 1964; Kalkhoff et al., 1964; Cornblath et al., 1965; Laron and Mannheimer, 1966; Glick, 1968; Westphal, 1968). Kaplan and Grumbach (1967) found that HGH in cord blood from aborted fetuses of estimated gestational age of 70 to 162 days was in the adult acromegalic range, greatly in excess of the plasma HGH of pregnant women at comparable stages of gestation. Early in the third trimester the serum HGH was six times the mean HGH in cord samples from full-term fetuses. At birth, the concentration of HGH is higher in the umbilical artery than in the umbilical vein (Yen et al., 1965). Cornblath et al., (1965) found that the umbilical vein plasma concentration of HGH ranged from 9 to 320 mμg/ml. No differences were found in the levels of HGH between infants born by normal vertex presentation and infants delivered by cesarean section with or without a trial of labor. Furthermore, no correlation was found between the amount of HGH in cord blood and the blood glucose, birth weight, length of gestation or race (Cornblath et al., 1965). HGH remained high in peripheral venous blood during the first 48 hours of life, after which it decreased rather sharply during the first week. In the full-term baby, the decline continued more slowly during the second and third weeks. In the low birth-weight infant the decrease during the first week was less marked, and a secondary rise occurred between the third and fourth weeks of life, declining thereafter. Thus, the serum HGH was higher in low birth-weight infants than in full-term infants in the period between the second and sixth days and again between the second and eighth weeks of life (Cornblath et al., 1965). Male full-term infants and female low birth-weight infants had significantly higher serum HGH than corresponding babies of the opposite sex. Twins sampled at the same age during the neonatal period showed a wide discrepancy in the plasma levels of HGH (Cornblath et al., 1965). Infants of diabetic mothers have been reported to have values of HGH in cord blood in the same range as normal newborns (Glick, 1968). More recently, however, Westphal (1968) found much lower levels of HGH in cord blood in infants of diabetic mothers than in normal newborns.

HGH RESPONSE TO HYPOGLYCEMIA

Insulin-induced hypoglycemia greatly increases the serum HGH in the full-term and in the low birth-weight infant (Cornblath et al., 1965; Westphal, 1968). The response is greater than in older children and adults. The absolute increment is considerably greater on the first day than at the end of the first week of life for full-term infants. In the low birth-weight infant on the other hand, the increment at the end of the first week of life is even greater than during the first 24 hours. In infants of diabetic mothers, the HGH response to insulin-induced hypoglycemia is less pronounced than in normal newborns (Westphal, 1968).

HGH RESPONSE TO HYPERGLYCEMIA

In contrast to the response in adults, hyperglycemia induced by the injection of glucose produces an increase in levels of HGH in the neonate during the first two weeks of life (Cornblath et al., 1965; Westphal, 1968). The increase is greater on the first day of life than at the end of the first week. Like the response to hypoglycemia, the increase is more pronounced in the low birth-weight than in the full-term infant at the end of the first week of life. After the second week the induced hyperglycemia results in inhibition of HGH secretion as it does in older children and adults (Cornblath et al., 1965; Westphal, 1968).

THE PHYSIOLOGIC ROLE OF HGH

The role of HGH in fetal and early postnatal life is not yet clear. Although the human pituitary is capable of producing, storing, and secreting HGH as early as 71 days of gestational age, the precise time of the initiation of hypothalamic-pituitary feedback control is not known. Antigenically, fetal HGH is similar to adult HGH, and it is biologically active although we do not know the exact relationship between levels of immunoreactive HGH and biologically active HGH in blood. However, newborns with the rare syndrome of absence of the pituitary gland and normal skull are born with normal weight and length (Brewer, 1957; Reid, 1960; Dunn, 1966; Steiner and Boggs, 1965). Likewise human cyclopic fetuses, in whom the pituitary is usually absent, are born with normal body weight and length for gestational age (Edmonds, 1950). Human anencephalic monsters in whom the pituitary gland is hypoplastic or reduced to a few cells are born with normal body size in spite of the abnormal hypothalamic-pituitary connections (Nanagas, 1925; Tuchmann-Duplessis, 1959; Erez and King, 1966). The somatotrophs in these abnormal pituitaries are not as numerous and heavily granulated as in normal human fetuses (Salazar et al., 1969), and the level of HGH in cord blood from anencephalics is in the low normal range but higher than in maternal blood (Kaplan and Grumbach, 1967). In cases of isolated deficiency of HGH, either sporadic or familial, affected children are born normal in size even when the mother is HGH-deficient (Rimoin et al., 1966b). Similarly, other abnormalities in the level of HGH in maternal blood do not appear to affect fetal growth. In one rare case of maternal hypophysectomy during the twenty-sixth week of gestation, the body size of the newborn infant was normal for gestational age when delivered at the thirty-fifth week (Little et al., 1958). Gemzell (1964) reported a hypophysectomized woman treated with human gonadotrophins, who conceived and delivered a normal full-term baby in spite of presumably very low or absent levels of HGH in the maternal circulation.

Deprivation of the pituitary in rat fetuses by decapitation in utero resulted in some growth retardation that could be prevented by the injection of growth hormone into the headless fetuses (Heggestad and Wells, 1965). Electrocoagulation of the pituitary in fetal lambs produced some retardation in somatic development (Liggins and Kennedy, 1968). In rabbits, however, decapitated fetuses continued to grow and were born with normal body size and weight (Jost, 1954). Similarly, hypophysectomy of monkey fetuses did not alter their rate of growth, even when the mothers were hypophysectomized at the same time (Hutchinson et al., 1962).

Conversely, infants born of acromegalic mothers are normal in size (Abelove et al., 1954), and pharmacologic doses of growth hormone given to pregnant animals resulted in normal size offspring (Zamenhof et al., 1966). The absence of significance of levels of circulating maternal HGH for fetal growth may be partially explained by absence of placental transfer of HGH, as demonstrated by the injection of radioiodinated HGH into women in labor (Gitlin et al., 1965). Even pharmacologic doses of HGH injected into the mother between 270 and 10 minutes before delivery failed to show placental transfer of HGH into the fetus (Laron et al., 1966b). Children who present the picture of hypopituitarism later in life are usually born with normal weight and length, and no growth retardation is detected during the first few months of life, suggesting that the deficiency of growth hormone is not important for growth during early postnatal life (Brasel et al., 1965). Rimoin et al. (1966b), however, have reported that growth retardation begins shortly after birth in the genetic types of growth hormone deficiency, even though the infant is born with normal weight and length; impaired growth may not become grossly apparent until late infancy or early childhood, however. Treatment of premature and full-term infants with HGH has failed to elicit changes indicating a physiologic effect, suggesting that they were relatively refractory to the metabolic and growth promoting effects of HGH early in life (Ducharme and Grumbach, 1961; Vest et al., 1963, Chiumello et al., 1965). These observations all support the prevailing concept that HGH from either fetal or maternal pituitary is not a major determinant of growth during fetal and early postnatal life (Rimoin et al., 1966b). The high level of HGH found at these times seems paradoxic. The stress of labor is not responsible for the high values immediately after birth since newborns delivered by cesarean section have comparable values (Cornblath et al., 1965). Furthermore, the clearance rate of exogenous HGH in the newborn is more rapid than in the adult (Cornblath et al., 1965). The high levels of HGH in cord blood, associated with rapid clearance, and the higher levels of HGH in umbilical artery than in umbilical vein, indicate active secretion of HGH by the pituitary of the fetus and neonate. Cornblath et al. (1965) have calculated that the newborn produces about 4.2 mg of HGH in 24 hours, a rate comparable to that expected for a 70-kg man. Gitlin et al. (1965), however, consider this conclusion uncertain because of the difficulties in interpreting the serum disappearance rate of labeled HGH. Several hypotheses have been proposed to explain the high values of circulating HGH during the perinatal period (Westphal, 1968). Immaturity of the homeostatic control of HGH secretion has been implicated as responsible for this situation. Diminution of HGH in blood after a few days of life could be interpreted as the result of maturation of feedback control. The lower plasma HGH in infants of diabetic mothers could be considered the result of a more mature feedback control due to the exercise of this mechanism during intrauterine life as a consequence of abnormal maternal glucose homeostasis (Westphal, 1968).

The ineffectiveness of exogenous HGH in newborns has been considered to be due to the saturation of receptor sites by high levels of endogenous HGH. This point could be explored by administering HGH to cyclopic infants or newborns with the genetic type of isolated deficiency of HGH, and then studying its effects, since these infants have low values of endogenous HGH. Another possible explanation for the high levels of HGH and the relative refractoriness to exogenous HGH could be immaturity of the enzymatic systems upon which HGH acts, resulting in turn in an inefficient feedback mechanism. Future elucidation of the primary sites of action of the HGH as well as the neuroendocrine influences upon the production and secretion of HGH in the perinatal period might provide answers to these questions. Although direct evidence is still lacking, a close correlation between the plasma level of HGH and the level of biologically active HGH is assumed.

Laron et al. (1966a), however, have described a genetic type of pituitary dwarfism with clinical and laboratory data suggesting a deficiency of HGH, but with elevated serum levels of immunoreactive HGH. Since these patients responded to the administration of exogenous HGH, the authors postulated an inborn error of metabolism with production and secretion of an abnormal HGH molecule. On the other hand, Merimee et al. (1968a) have reported an unusual variety of endocrine dwarfism with high basal levels of immunologically assayable HGH in plasma and attenuated metabolic response to exogenous HGH, suggesting a defective response to HGH in peripheral tissues. The same group of investigators have described end-organ subresponsiveness to HGH in the African pygmies (Merimee et al., 1968b). These pygmies have normal basal levels of plasma HGH and are able to respond to provocative stimuli with an increase in plasma HGH concentration (Rimoin et al., 1967), but they show less metabolic effect in response to the injection of HGH than normal controls or HGH-deficient subjects (Merimee et al., 1968b). In the above mentioned syndrome as well as in the case of the pygmies the affected infants are born normal in size and weight. Conversely, considerable rate of growth has been reported in children with low plasma levels of immunoreactive HGH (Holmes et al., 1968; Kenny et al., 1968). All these observations have raised new questions regarding the exact relationship between growth and circulating levels of HGH as measured by radioimmunoassay techniques.

Adrenocorticotropin (ACTH)

Special characteristics of the hypothalamic-pituitary-adrenal axis in the human fetus differentiate it from the same axis in extrauterine life and from that of other species during intra- or extrauterine life (Lanman, 1953; Solomon and Friesen, 1968; Gardner, 1969; Villee, 1969). The human fetal adrenal gland at term is about twenty times larger than the adult adrenal in relation to body weight. At birth about 80 percent of the adrenal gland is fetal adrenal cortex (Tahka, 1951; Lanman, 1953; Gardner, 1969). The fetal cortex is a very active steroidogenic organ as evidenced cytologically (Johannisson, 1968); by the large amount of steroids in fetal blood (Eberlein, 1965; Shackleton and Mitchell, 1967) and by the large amount of estriol in maternal urine as a result of the placental transformation of fetal adrenal steroids (Simmer et al., 1966; Reynolds et al., 1968; Solomon and Friesen, 1968; Villee, 1969). Similarly the blood and urine of infants during the first few days of life contain large amounts of steroids of adrenal origin (Gardner, 1956; Bongiovanni, 1962; Eberlein, 1965; Reynolds, 1965; Cathro et al., 1969; Cara, 1969a). Lanman (1962), in a review of available information including his own observations, concluded that the primary adrenocorticotrophic factor for the fetal adrenal gland is ACTH from the fetal pituitary, the large size of the fetal adrenal reflecting strong ACTH stimulation. Increased secretion of ACTH by the fetal pituitary would be secondary to relative inability of the fetal adrenal to synthesize cortisol. The resulting negative feedback would in turn increase stimulation to the hypothalamic-pituitary-adrenal axis in the fetus, with consequent hyperplasia of the adrenal cortex until the needs for cortisol are met (Lanman, 1962). Since most of the steroids secreted by the adrenal gland during late fetal life and during early postnatal life in humans have the Δ 5-3 β-ol configuration, Eberlein (1965) has postulated that the impaired ability of the fetal adrenal to produce cortisol is due to relative deficiency of the Δ 5-3 β-ol hydroxysteroid dehydrogenase system (see Ch. 30).

ACTH has been measured by bioassay in fetal pituitary extract as early as the fourth month of intrauterine life (Taylor et al., 1953), and it seems to increase with advancing fetal age (Ghilain and Schwers, 1957). Stark et al. (1965) cultured in vitro combined pituitary and adrenal tissue from human fetuses of both sexes, ranging in size from 18 cm to 46 cm body length. Their results indicate that the fetal pituitary is able to produce ACTH independently of hypothalamic stimulation, at least for some time, and that the fetal adrenal is able to secrete hydrocortisone. Berson and Yalow (1968), using a radioimmunoassay method, found that at birth plasma ACTH concentrations were significantly higher in cord blood (mean 161 ± 29 $\mu\mu g$/ml) than in maternal venous blood (mean 56 ± 23 $\mu\mu g$/ml) in seven of eight cases. Concentrations above 60 $\mu\mu g$/ml were observed in only two of the mothers but in all the cord blood specimens. The adrenocorticotropic effect of the human fetal pituitary seems to be stronger in the last trimester of pregnancy, the period when the fetal adrenal grows markedly. In human anencephalic monsters with rudimentary pituitary glands, the fetal adrenal is about normal in size during the first four or five months of intrauterine life as if a normal hypothalamic-pituitary system were not necessary for adrenal growth during that period (Nichols, 1956; Tuchmann-Duplessis, 1959; Potter, 1961). After the fifth month of pregnancy, however, atrophy of the fetal adrenal progresses as term approaches (Tuchmann-Duplessis, 1959). At birth the adrenal glands of these anencephalics are almost always atrophic (Benirschke, 1956; Tuchmann-Duplessis, 1959; Frandsen and Stakemann, 1964; Erez and King, 1966) with no ultrastructural evidence of secretory activity (Johannisson, 1968), and steroidogenesis is much reduced as reflected in low levels of steroids in cord blood and in the urine in the newborn period, particularly those steroids with the Δ 5-3 β-ol configuration (Nichols et al., 1958; Eberlein, 1965). Furthermore, the urinary excretion of estriol is diminished in women carrying anencephalic fetuses. Frandsen and Stakemann (1964) studied the urinary excretion of estriol in 17 pregnant women carrying anencephalic fetuses, and found that in 16 cases the values were very low; the anencephalic newborns showed marked adrenal atrophy. In the remaining case the excretion of estriol was normal, and the anencephalic offspring had an almost normal fetal adrenal gland. Since maternal urinary estriol during pregnancy seems to reflect the amount of precursor steroids produced by the fetal adrenal gland, these findings are interpreted as indicating fetal adrenal hypofunction in the anencephalic. Tuchmann-Duplessis and Mercier-Parot (1963) attribute the atrophy of the adrenal glands in anencephalics to abnormal hypothalamic-pituitary connections. One may also speculate that the number of pituitary cells present in cases of anencephaly may not be enough to supply the large amount of ACTH necessary to maintain fetal adrenal function, causing a state of relative deficiency of pituitary ACTH. Interestingly, Kenny et al. (1966b) have reported that the cortisol production rate in anencephalic newborns studied by them was at the lower limit of normal. They postulate that the small amount of pituitary tissue usually present in anencephaly could be sufficient for the stimulation of subnormal cortisol secretion but not for maintenance of the fetal cortex.

In human newborns with congenital absence of the pituitary gland the adrenals have been reported to be absent (Dunn, 1966) or atrophic (Blizzard and Alberts, 1956; Reid, 1960). Brewer (1957) has reported a case with absence of the anterior lobe of the pituitary but with a normal posterior lobe and with atrophic adrenal glands. In cyclopic newborns (Brewer, 1957) and in cases of cebocephaly with absence of the pituitary gland, the adrenals are very small (Haworth et al., 1961). Mosier (1956) has described a case of hypoplasia of the pituitary and of the adrenal glands in a child who died at four days of age. Maternal ACTH did not seem to cross the placenta to compensate for the absence of ACTH from the fetal pituitary in any of these cases. Migeon et al. (1968) have reported six patients with congenital adrenocortical unresponsiveness to ACTH, presumably due to an abnormality at the site of ACTH action on cortisol biosynthesis.

Experimental hypophysectomy of rabbit fetuses (Jost, 1957) and in rat fetuses (Kitchell and Wells, 1952) produces atrophy of the fetal adrenal that can be restored to normal by ACTH given to the fetus. The adrenal atrophy occurs in hypophysectomized fetuses whether the mothers are intact or adrenalectomized, indicating that either no maternal ACTH or insufficient maternal ACTH crossed the placenta to compensate for the lack of fetal ACTH (Jost, 1957). Hypophysectomy of fetuses of rabbits at different gestational ages produces more change in size and histology of the fetal adrenal when it is done between the eighteenth and twentieth days of gestation than when it is done before or after this critical period (Jost, 1957). It is possible that the fetal pituitary-adrenal system may pass through a period of high activity when it exerts its major physiologic role in the fetus. The last trimester of pregnancy seems to be the period of higher activity of the human fetal pituitary-adrenal system.

The hypothalamic-pituitary-adrenal homeostatic mechanism, or at least the pituitary-adrenal feedback mechanism, seems to be operative during fetal life. Cortisone injected intraperitoneally in rat and rabbit fetuses results in reduction in size of the fetal adrenals (Jost, 1957; Wells, 1957). Simultaneous injection of ACTH into the fetus counteracts this effect (Jost, 1957). In rabbits and rats the administration of cortisone to pregnant mothers results in reduction in size of the fetal adrenals, presumably because of the placental passage of the steroid and its effects upon the fetal pituitary (Jost, 1957). On the other hand, adrenalectomy of pregnant animals produces enlargement of the fetal adrenal. This can be prevented if the fetus is hypophysectomized, indicating that the source of ACTH is the fetal pituitary and that maternal ACTH does not cross the placenta in the rat, at least in sufficient amounts to stimulate the fetal adrenal (Jost, 1957; Christianson and Chester Jones, 1957).

In women large amounts of prednisone or hydrocortisone administered during pregnancy and labor caused a marked decrease in cord blood levels of C-19 steroids produced by the fetal adrenal cortex (Simmer et al., 1966). Likewise maternal urinary estrogens, particularly estriol, were lowered, presumably as a result of the decreased production of precursors by the fetal adrenals (Simmer et al., 1966;

Scommegna et al., 1968; Driscoll, 1969). These findings are interpreted as indicating suppression of the fetal pituitary-adrenal axis by the exogenous steroids after crossing the placenta. Although adrenal atrophy has been reported in infants born to mothers treated with large doses of glucocorticoids (Lanman, 1962), in the majority of cases the fetus is apparently not damaged by maternal treatment with corticoids (Bongiovanni and McPadden, 1960; Popert, 1962). In two infants who died a few hours after birth to mothers treated with large doses of glucocorticoids, the adrenals were histologically normal (Simmer et al., 1966). Furthermore Kenny et al. (1966b) have reported normal cortisol production rates in such infants when they were studied at less that 48 hours of life.

Conversely, Dassler (1966) reported that the administration of ACTH to normal pregnant women in the last trimester resulted in a marked increase in the urinary excretion of estriol. Maeyama et al. (1969) have confirmed these observations and found a remarkable increase in estriol excretion following intramuscular ACTH in women carrying twin pregnancies. On the other hand, women pregnant with anencephalic fetuses have abnormally low levels of urinary estriol (Frandsen and Stakemann, 1964), and it increases little or not at all after intramuscular ACTH (Maeyama et al., 1969). These results seem to indicate that maternal ACTH can cross the placenta without loss of activity and act upon the fetal adrenal cortex. However, after the intravenous administration of ACTH to pregnant women Scommegna et al. (1968) found a small increase and Dickey and Thompson (1969) a significant decrease in maternal urinary estriol. The different routes of ACTH administration could be responsible for these conflicting results, but further studies are necessary to elucidate this interesting aspect of the pituitary-adrenal axis in fetal life and the question of placental passage of ACTH from the maternal circulation into the fetus. ACTH injected into pregnant rats has been found to stimulate the fetal adrenal (Jones et al., 1953).

In newborn dogs studied within the first 24 hours after birth the feedback control for the hypothalamic-pituitary-adrenal appears to be functional since plasma cortisol rises after ACTH administration and falls to low levels after dexamethasone injection (Muelheims et al., 1969). In the rat the hypothalamic-pituitary-adrenal axis is relatively unable to respond to experimental stress (Jailer, 1949; Eguchi et al., 1964; Eguchi and Wells, 1965) or to dexamethasone administered during the first few days of life (D'Angelo, 1966).

In the human neonate conflicting results have been reported by different groups of investigators (Aarskog, 1965). Eberlein (1965), however, found that plasma total ketosteroids and particularly plasma Δ 5-3 β-ol-hydroxy steroids rise after delivery, remain elevated during the first week of life, and decline thereafter. Furthermore, these steroids rise in plasma and in urine in response to medical and surgical stresses (Eberlein, 1965; Cathro et al., 1969). Kenny et al. (1966a) have reported that in newborn infants less than five days old the cortisol production rate per square meter of body surface is higher than in older infants, children, and adults. These observations indicate that the pituitary-adrenal axis of the human neonate functions at a higher level and is capable of responding to stress.

The physiologic role of the hypothalamus-pituitary-adrenal system in fetal life has not yet been clearly defined. The adrenocorticotropic function of fetal pituitary is not essential for fetal survival or fetal growth. Anencephalic and cyclopic monsters as well as newborns with absent pituitary glands are born with normal body size. In animals hypophysectomy or adrenalectomy or combined hypophysectomy and adrenalectomy do not affect fetal growth markedly (Jost, 1966). However, in rabbits and rats the pituitary-adrenal axis seems to be necessary for normal glycogen deposition in fetal liver (Jost, 1961; Jacquot and Kretchmer, 1964). In the human fetus the physiologic role if any, of the fetal adrenal, in the normal storage of glycogen deserves more study.

Gardner (1969) considers that the fetal adrenal in man may represent a vestigial remnant. However, the large volume of the adrenal in fetal and neonatal life, and the active steroidogenesis which occurs during fetal life and shortly after birth, suggest that this gland is important. The steroids with a Δ 5-3 β-ol configuration so prominent in the secretion of the fetal adrenal may have biologic effects of which we are not yet aware (Cara, 1969b). Further investigation of the physiologic effects of these steroids may be necessary before we can understand more clearly the role of the fetal adrenal cortex in fetal and in fetomaternal homeostasis.

Thyrotropin (TSH)

The organogenesis of the thyroid gland in early life in rodents does not require the presence of the pituitary gland (Jost, 1953, 1966). However, near the end of intrauterine life, a functional relationship has been established between the pituitary and the thyroid, and fetal hypophysectomy results in retardation of histologic development and growth of the fetal thyroid (Jost, 1953, 1961), a diminution in the uptake of radioactive iodine (Jost et al., 1952), and a decrease in the secretion of thyroxine (Geloso, 1958). The administration of thyroid stimulating hormone (TSH) to the fetus corrects these deficiencies (Sethre and Wells, 1951; Hwang and Wells, 1959; Jost, 1966). Conversely, the administration of thyroxine to the fetus inhibits thyroid growth and the secretion of fetal thyroid hormone, presumably by inhibition of TSH secretion (Hwang and Wells, 1959). In chick embryos the evidence also favors self-differentiation of the thyroid gland in the initial stages of development (Martindale, 1941).

In human fetuses TSH activity has been reported both in serum and in pituitary homogenates as early as the third month of gestation (Costa et al., 1965). In vitro cultures of human fetal anterohypophysis reveal that immunoreactive TSH can be produced as early as 14 weeks of fetal life (Gitlin and Biasucci, 1969a). On the other hand the synthesis of thyroxine and triiodothyronine in the human thyroid in vitro begins at about 11 weeks of gestation (Shepard, 1967), and studies of in vitro cultures of fetal thyroid gland suggest the production of thyroglobulin at or before 29 days of gestation (Gitlin and Biasucci, 1969b). In man, therefore, TSH does not appear to be necessary for organogenesis of the thyroid gland or for the initiation of thyroid function in early fetal life. However, a functional relationship between pituitary and thyroid is well established later in fetal life. In the rare cases of complete absence of the pituitary gland or of the adenohypophysis with normal skull, the thyroid gland is hypoplastic with small follicles, the majority of which are empty (Brewer, 1957; Reid, 1960). The thyroid is also hypoplastic in cases of cebocephaly (Haworth et al., 1961) and cyclopy with absence of the pituitary gland (Brewer, 1957). In anencephaly, however, the thyroid gland is not structurally different from that of the normal newborn in spite of abnormal hypothalamic-pituitary connections (Tuchmann-Duplessis, 1959). Salazar et al. (1969) have identified thyrotrophs, apparently active in the adenohypophysis of two liveborn anencephalics, suggesting that their differentiation and secretion of TSH is not entirely dependent upon hypothalamic activity during fetal life. The fetal thyroid seems to enjoy some degree of autonomy and is less affected than the adrenal gland by the absence of the pituitary in these syndromes. Isolated deficiency of TSH resulting in hypothyroidism in childhood has been described in a few instances (Fink, 1967). Although deficiency of TSH presumably is present before birth, these children are not clinically hypothyroid at birth. Furthermore, the injection of exogenous TSH elicits radioactive iodine uptake by the thyroid, indicating that organogenesis of the gland took place despite the absence of TSH (Fink, 1967).

The time in fetal life at which the fetal pituitary-thyroid feedback system becomes established and its physiologic significance in the rather protected fetal environment are difficult to ascertain in man. Experimentally, it has been established that the fetal pituitary-thyroid axis has the potential of reacting to conditions that disrupt its homeostasis. Unilateral thyroidectomy in rats in late fetal life produces compensatory hypertrophy of the remaining thyroid tissue, presumably through an increase in production of TSH (Eguchi and Morikawa, 1966). The administration of propylthiouracil to pregnant guinea pigs during the last several weeks of gestation resulted in goitrous offspring with increased TSH in both plasma and pituitary. The increased TSH was closely correlated with the appearance of enlarged basophils in the fetal pituitary, containing glycoprotein granulations (D'Angelo, 1967). Fetal goitrogenesis is prevented only if the fetus itself is hypophysectomized (Jost, 1957); maternal hypophysectomy has no effect on the development of the goiter. In the human the administration of propyltriouracil to pregnant women produces enlargement of the thyroid in the fetus as early as the fifth month of pregnancy (Davis and Forbes, 1945). This is indirect evidence of the capability of the fetal pituitary to produce and secrete TSH in response to a block in the synthesis of thyroid hormone. Shepard and Andersen (1969), however, were unable to produce goiter in fetuses of less than 120 gestational days by the administration of propylthiouracil to pregnant women, suggesting that the pituitary-thyroid functional relationship is not well established before this time.

Deficiency or excess thyroid hormone or TSH in maternal circulation have little or no effect upon the pituitary-thyroid axis of the fetus in rodents and in humans. Hypophysectomized women made fertile by the use of human gonadotropins (Gemzell, 1964), as well as women hypophysectomized during pregnancy, have delivered infants without noticeable effects upon the pituitary-thyroid axis in spite of the absence of TSH in maternal circulation (Little et al., 1958). Infants born of mothers with low levels of thyroid hormone due to primary hypothyroidism and with presumably high levels of circulating TSH show no evidence of excessive TSH effects such as hyperthyroidism and/or thyroid enlargement (Hodges et al., 1952).

This and other indirect evidence indicate that maternal TSH does not cross the placenta in the human. More direct evidence is provided by the study of Fisher et al. (1969) which demonstrates a fetomaternal gradient of TSH in blood. In rats (Knobil and Josimovich, 1958) and in guinea pigs (Peterson and Young, 1952) it has been well established that TSH does not cross the placenta. On the other hand, long-acting thyroid stimulator (LATS), an immunoglobulin G of extrapituitary origin, can cross the placenta and appears to be responsible for the majority of cases of hyperthyroidism in newborn infants (Burke, 1968).

Congenital goiter in newborns as a result of placental passage of excessive amounts of iodine has been ascribed to increased production of fetal TSH due to interference with normal pituitary thyroid homeostasis (Croughs and Visser, 1965). Stanbury et al. (1968) have described a child with hypothyroidism without goiter and with high concentrations of TSH in blood who had no thyroid response to exogenous TSH. They postulated impaired ability of the thyroid to respond specifically to stimulation by TSH with cell division and synthesis of thyroglobulin. Here again the patient did not show evidence of hypothyroidism early in life although presumably the defect was present in fetal life.

Production of TSH can be suppressed in the human fetus when exceedingly large amounts of thyroid are administered to the mother (Carr et al., 1959). In this respect triiodothyronine (T_3) appears to be more effective since it crosses the placenta more readily than thyroxine (T_4) because it is more loosely bound to proteins in maternal blood (Raiti et al., 1967; Dussault et al., 1969).

The transitional period from uterus to external environment is marked by abrupt changes in thyroid function (Florshein et al., 1966). In rodents experimental studies indicate that the pituitary-thyroid system functions at a higher level in late fetal life than in early postnatal life. TSH content of the pituitary in newborn guinea pigs is relatively low (D'Angelo, 1967). Unilateral thyroidectomy in late fetal life in rats caused a significant increase in the size of the remaining lobe of the thyroid. In early postnatal life, however, the compensatory hypertrophy was less marked (Eguchi and Morikawa, 1966). Thyroxine administered to normal newborn guinea pigs was effective in suppressing the pituitary-thyroid system and lowering the production of TSH as indicated by reduction in thyroid and pituitary weights and lowered TSH stores in the latter (D'Angelo, 1967). However, the administration of propylthiouracil to rodents during the first two weeks of life failed to induce significant histologic changes in the thyroid or to alter the TSH level in blood or pituitary (D'Angelo, 1967).

In the human fetus at term and in the neonate at birth blood concentration of TSH is high and increases even more after a few minutes of extrauterine life (Utiger et al., 1968). Fisher et al. (1969) found that blood samples obtained from the scalp of human fetuses during the three hours immediately preceding delivery showed a higher TSH concentration than in the respective maternal blood samples. Furthermore, paired maternal-cord blood samples at birth demonstrated a significantly higher free thyroxine and TSH concentration in cord blood. This gradient was also present in paired samples obtained from cesarean deliveries. The authors concluded that the human fetus at term and the newborn immediately after birth have a relative hyperthyrotropinemia that is not accounted for by extrauterine exposure or the stress of birth since the gradient is also present in paired samples obtained from cesarean deliveries (Fisher et al., 1969). Furthermore, a few minutes after birth a large amount of TSH is released from the fetal pituitary. The mean serum TSH increases from 9.5 μU/ml in cord blood to 60 μU/ml and 86 μU/ml at 10 and at 30 minutes after birth respectively. The TSH concentration then falls rapidly between 30 minutes and 3 to 4 hours and more gradually thereafter to 13 μU/ml by 48 hours of extrauterine life. This rapid rise and fall in serum TSH concentration may represent a release of stored pituitary TSH. Maternal serum TSH concentrations are low and stable during labor and in the postpartum period (Fisher and Odell, 1969). The stimulus for this early massive discharge of pituitary TSH is unknown. The early rise is not prevented by warming the newborn infant during the first 3 hours of life. If the newborn infant is exposed to room temperature between the third and fourth hours after birth, however, TSH increases significantly. This second rise in TSH concentration is prevented if the infant is kept warm and is therefore attributed to cooling of the infant. These high blood levels of TSH in the fetus at term and in the neonate would explain previous observations indicating increased thyroid function in the newborn, such as increased PBI concentration (Danowski et al., 1951), increased saturation of the thyroxine binding protein in blood and the high rate of thyroidal radioiodine clearance at 48 hours of life (Fisher and Oddie, 1964; Fisher et al., 1966). It would also explain why nonincubated infants were found to have higher PBI values and greater thyroid radioiodine clearances at 48 hours of life than incubated infants (Fisher et al., 1966).

The physiologic significance of the increased levels of TSH and thyroid hormone in late fetal life and in early extrauterine life is not yet clear. Increased function of the pituitary-thyroid axis is not required for the high rate of growth of the fetus and newborn since the absence of this function does not impair fetal growth. It is possible that the hypothalamic-pituitary-thyroid homeostatic mechanism is not well adjusted during the perinatal period and that the increased production of thyroid hormone does not parallel physiologic needs. However, neither the fetus nor the newborn present clinical evidence of excessive thyroid hormone. Another possibility is that the peripheral tissues in the fetus and in the newborn do not respond to thyroid hormone in the same manner as a more mature organism, and a higher level of circulating hormone might be needed. Investigation of the effects of thyroid hormone in the enzymatic systems in tissues of the fetus and newborn may help elucidate this point.

Gonadotropins

The hypothalamic-pituitary-gonadal axis in mammals varies greatly in its physiologic significance among various species. In rabbits decapitation of the male fetus before differentiation of the genital tract results in such gross developmental abnormalities as reduced prostate and feminine external genitalia. (Jost, 1951, 1957, 1961). This is interpreted as a consequence of elimination of the pituitary, since the interstitial cells of the testis show changes parallel to those of the genital tract, and the genital abnormalities can be prevented if equine gonadotropin is injected into the decapitated fetuses (Jost, 1951, 1961, 1966). The results of fetal decapitation at different times during gestation suggest that in rabbits the fetal pituitary stimulates the testis maximally during a limited period of development which coincides with the most important stage of the organogenesis of the genital tract (Jost, 1966). On the other hand effects of fetal decapitation were almost absent in fetuses of rats (Kitchell and Wells, 1952). Similarly in man the fetal pituitary does not appear to be necessary for differentiation of the gonads and organogenesis of the genital tract. Absence of the pituitary in man is not accompanied by any constant abnormality of the genital tract, although there is a trend toward hypoplasia of the testes and the penis. In a case of congenital absence of the pituitary gland in a male newborn, Blizzard and Alberts (1956) reported hypoplastic external genitalia, cryptorchidism, and complete absence of the interstitial cells of the testis with a marked increase of the interstitial connective tissue. Reid (1960) in another newborn with absence of the pituitary found the testes in the scrotum, although smaller than usual, but the interstitial cells were present and the tubules were well developed. In a case of absence of the anterior lobe of the pituitary the ovaries were normal, with numerous primordial follicles (Brewer, 1957). In anencephaly the gonads are generally normal, and there are no consistent abnormalities of the genital tract (Tuchmann-Duplessis, 1959; Benirschke, 1956; Salazar et al., 1969), although hypoplasia of the penis and of the testes has been described in some cases (Tuchmann-Duplessis, 1959; Erez and King, 1966). Zondek and Zondek (1965b) have reported that the mean number of Leydig cells was significantly lower in anencephaly than in normal controls. Salazar et al. (1969) have described gonadotrophs in pituitaries of anencephalics, suggesting that their differentiation is independent of neurosecretory activity. Perrin and Benirschke (1958) consider that cephalic integrity or hypothalamic control is not essential for the differentiation of genetically determined sex in man.

The gonadotropic activity of the fetal pituitary in man has been studied by Mitskevich and Levina (1965) in 200 pituitaries of both sexes from 8 weeks to 40 weeks of gestation. Luteinizing hormone (LH) was studied by bioassay in mice in 48 human pituitaries from male fetuses and in 51 pituitaries from female fetuses, ranging in age from 13 to 40 weeks of gestation. A definite sex difference was found in the content of LH in fetal pituitary: LH was found only in pituitaries from female fetuses and during a strictly limited period of fetal life, from the eighteenth to the twenty-eighth weeks of gestation. Before and after this period no LH could be detected in pituitaries from female fetuses. In pituitaries from male fetuses no LH could be detected at any time during intrauterine life. The authors consider, however, that the negative results could be due to limitations in the sensitivity of the bioassay method (Mitskevich and Levina, 1965).

The content of prolactin (LTH) was studied in 72 human pituitaries from 16 to 40 weeks of gestation, 38 of these from male fetuses and 34 from female fetuses. Prolactin as measured by the pigeon crop wall bioassay appears in fetal pituitary of both sexes at 19 to 20 weeks of gestation. The prolactin content of fetal pituitaries increases with fetal age, reaching a maximum at term. The period of prolactin production coincides with an increase in the number of acidophils in fetal pituitary, to which the production of prolactin is usually attributed (Miskevich and Levina, 1965). It is interesting to note that the fetus exists in an environment rich in estrogen, and this environment is known to stimulate prolactin secretion. Gitlin and Biasucci (1969a) have studied the ontogenesis of fetal pituitary gonadotropins by incubating human pituitary from 11 fetuses from 29 days to 18 weeks gestation in a medium with C^{14} labeled aminoacids, followed by immunoelectrophoresis and radioautography. They found that FSH synthesis was well established at 14 weeks but absent at 10.5 weeks of gestation. Kaplan et al. (1969) found that in human fetuses the *content* of immunoreactive FSH in the pituitary was 3.3 mμg (1.1 mμg/mg tissue) at 70 days of gestation with a rise to 77.5 mμg (11.7 mμg/mg tissue) at 150 days of gestation. In the neonatal period the FSH content of human pituitaries varies from 118 mμg to 843.3 mμg. The *serum concentration* of immunoreactive FSH in 10 fetuses with a gestational age of 97 to 133 days varies from 312 to 46 mμg per ml. These values are higher than those found by the same group of investigators in serum in prepubertal children (1 to 3 mμg/ml). No sex difference was found in the pituitary content or in the plasma level of FSH in human fetuses or in newborns (Kaplan et al., 1969). Levina (1968), however, using a bioassay procedure reported that FSH was present in pituitaries of female fetuses at about 13 weeks of gestation, whereas it was found irregularly and in lesser amount in pituitaries of male fetuses.

The initiation of the synthesis of gonadotropin by the human fetal pituitary seems to occur too late to account for the initial differentiation and growth of the testis. Leydig cells are already evident in the fetal testis at about the eighth week of gestation, and they increase rapidly in number, reaching a maximum at about 14 to 16 weeks of gestation (Niemi et al., 1967). Histochemically they present maximal evidence of steroidogenic activity at about 12 weeks of gestation with a decline around the nineteenth week of gestation; by the twenty-third week more than half of the interstitial cells are enzymatically unactive, but some fully reactive cells remain visible until the end of gestation (Niemi et al., 1967; Zondek and Zondek, 1965a). Therefore, factors other than gonadotropins from the fetal pituitary should be responsible for the initial development and maintenance of the interstitial cells of the fetal testis. It is generally accepted that chorionic gonadotropin is such a factor. In the placenta the concentration of chorionic gonadotropin rises rapidly to a peak between the eighth and the twelfth weeks of pregnancy, after which it falls sharply (Diczfalusy, 1953). Chorionic gonadotropin can be detected in pregnant women as early as ten days after ovulation (Albert and Berkson, 1951), and it is present in fetal tissues in physiologically significant amounts (Bruner, 1951). Maintenance of the activity of the interstitial cells of the fetal testis after the decline in the production of chorionic gonadotropin suggests that other stimulating factors, perhaps gonadotropin from the fetal pituitary, would act upon the testis in late fetal life (Jost, 1966). This would explain the hypoplasia of the penis and of the interstitial cells observed at birth in cases of absence of the pituitary gland. Eguchi and Morikawa (1968) have reported that in the perinatal age in the rat there appears to be a reciprocal relationship between the pituitary and the testes and that the Leydig cells are maintained largely by the fetal pituitary.

Conversely the fetal ovary is very active in gametogenesis, but its steroidogenic activity is very limited, especially when compared with the fetal adrenal or the fetal testis. This agrees well with the rather insignificant role of the human fetal ovary in the differentiation of either the genital ducts or the external genitalia (Van Wyk and Grumbach, 1968).

Information is scant concerning the role of the central nervous system in the production and release of pituitary gonadotropins by the fetal hypophysis. Extracts from the median eminence of newborn rabbits and rats and from 1- to 2-month-old calves were found to be very active with regard to gonadotropin releasing activity, while extracts obtained from 20-day-old rabbit fetuses showed no evidence of such activity (Campbell and Gallardo, 1966). From their own observations and other evidence Harris and Levine (1966) have concluded that rats of both sexes are born with a sexually undifferentiated central nervous system which is of the female type. This pattern becomes fixed in the female in the first few days of life. In the male during the first few days of life the testicular secretions are fundamental in the organization of normal mechanisms underlying future patterns of sexual behavior and gonadotropin secretion (Harris and Levine, 1965). On the other hand pituitaries from human fetuses of either sex, ranging in age from 13 to 18 weeks of gestation, when implanted in the sellar region of mature hypophysectomized male rats were able to maintain the normal weight and histology of the testes. These results would indicate that in the human fetus the hypothalamus has undergone a sexual differentiation by the age of 13 to 18 weeks of gestation and is responsible for the sexual dimorphism found in the secretion of gonadotropins by the fetal pituitary (Levina, 1968). It is possible that the hypothalamic differentiation may be brought about by the secretion of testicular androgens that starts at about the ninth week of gestation (Levina, 1968). This challenging field of neurophysiologic and psychosexual development in fetal and early postnatal life is being explored actively at present.

Conclusion

The fetal pituitary is able to synthesize growth hormone by the tenth week of gestation, FSH and TSH by the thirteenth to fourteenth weeks, and prolactin around the eighteenth week of gestation. ACTH has been found in fetal pituitary by the fourth month of pregnancy, although indirect clinical evidence indicates that the fetal pituitary can secrete ACTH before the twelfth week of gestation. Absence of the fetal pituitary, however, does not seem to interfere with organogenesis and functioning of target glands early in fetal life, nor with fetal growth during the entire intrauterine life. In the last trimester, however, the fetal pituitary exerts a trophic effect upon the target glands which is very marked for the adrenal cortex, less evident for the thyroid, and questionable for the gonads. The time of initiation and maintenance of the pituitary secretions under feedback control has not been established. Clinical evidence would indicate that the pituitary-adrenal cortex feedback mechanism is well established before the twelfth week of gestation and that the pituitary-thyroid feedback control is operative as early as the fifth month of pregnancy. The role of the hypothalamus in these regulatory

mechanisms is not yet known. In man there appears to be no intrinsic sex difference in the ability of the fetal pituitary to secrete gonadotropins. The hypothalamus
however, seems to undergo a sexual differentiation around the thirteenth week of
gestation and would be responsible for the sexual difference in the secretion of
gonadotropin by the fetal pituitary. It is conceivable that the hypothalamic differentiation may be brought about by the androgens secreted by the fetal testes.

Acknowledgement

The author is indebted to Dr. Howard A. Joos for advice and help in editing the
manuscript.

REFERENCES

Aarskog, D. 1965. Cortisol in the newborn infant. Acta Paediat. Scand., Suppl.
158:9-91.

Abelove, W. A., J. J. Rupp, and K. E. Paschkis. 1954. Acromegaly and pregnancy.
J. Clin. Endocr., 14:32-44.

Albert, A., and J. Berkson. 1951. A clinical bio-assay for chorionic gonadotropin.
J. Clin. Endocr., 11:805-820.

Benirschke, K. 1956. Adrenals in anencephaly and hydrocephaly. Obstet. Gynec.,
8:412-425.

Berson, S. A., and R. S. Yalow. 1968. Radioimmunoassay of ACTH in plasma. J. Clin.
Invest., 47:2725-2751.

Blizzard, R. M., and M. Alberts. 1956. Hypopituitarism, hypoadrenalism and hypogonadism in the newborn infant. J. Pediat., 48:782-792.

Bongiovanni, A. H. 1962. The adrenogenital syndrome with deficiency of 3β-hydroxy-
steroid dehydrogenase. J. Clin. Invest., 41:2086-2092.

———— and A. J. McPadden. 1960. Steroids during pregnancy and possible fetal
consequences. Fertil. Steril., 11:181-186.

Brasel, J. A., J. C. Wright, L. Wilkins, and R. M. Blizzard. 1965. An evaluation
of seventy-five patients with hypopituitarism beginning in childhood. Amer. J.
Med., 38:484-498.

Brewer, D. B. 1957. Congenital absence of the pituitary gland and its consequences.
J. Path. Bact., 73:59-67.

Bruner, J. A. 1951. Distribution of chorionic gonadotropin in mother and fetus at
various stages of pregnancy. J. Clin. Endocr., 11:360-374.

Burke, G. 1968. The long-acting thyroid stimulator of Graves' disease. Amer. J. Med.,
45:435-450.

Campbell, H. J., and E. Gallardo. 1966. Gonadotrophin-releasing activity of the
median eminence at different ages. J. Physiol. (London) 186:689-697.

Cara, J. 1969a. Unpublished data.

———— 1969b. Isolation and identification of 16-OH-pregnenolone (pregn-5-en-3β,
16α-diol-20-one) in urine from a patient with adrenocortical carcinoma. Steroids,
13:519-527.

Carr, E. A., et al. 1959. The effect of maternal thyroid function on fetal thyroid
function and development. J. Clin. Endocr., 19:1-18.

Cathro, D. M., C. C. Forsyth, and J. Cameron. 1969. Adrenocorticol response to stress in newborn infants. Arch. Dis. Child., 44:88-95.

Chiumello, G., A. Vaccari, and F. Sereni. 1965. Bone growth and metabolic studies of premature infants treated with human growth hormone. Pediatrics, 36:836-842.

Christianson, M., and I. Chester Jones. 1957. The interrelationships of the adrenal glands of mother and foetus in the rat. J. Endocr., 15:17-42.

Contopoulos, A. N. 1967. Comparative aspects of growth hormone during fetal life. International Symposium on Growth Hormone, Milan, Italy. Excerpta Medica Foundation, ICS No. 142, p. 35.

Cornblath M., et al. 1965. Secretion and metabolism of growth hormone in premature and full term infants. J. Clin. Endocr., 25: 209-218.

Costa, A., et al. 1965. Thyroid function and thyrotropin activity in mother and fetus. In Cassano, C., and Andreoli M., eds. Current Topics in Thyroid Research. New York, Academic Press, Inc., pp. 738-748.

Croughs, W., and H. K. A. Visser. 1965. Familial iodide-induced goiter. Evidence for an abnormality in the pituitary-thyroid homeostatic control. J. Pediat., 67: 353-362.

D'Angelo, S. A. 1966. Maturation of pituitary TSH and ACTH mechanism in the guinea pig: Effects of propylthiouracil and dexamethasone on fetus and neonate. Second International Congress on Hormonal Steroids, Milan, Italy. Excerpta Medica Foundation, ICS No. 111, p. 84.

———— 1967. Pituitary-thyroid interrelations in maternal, fetal and neonatal guinea pigs. Endocrinology, 81:132-138.

Danowski, T. S., et al. 1951. Protein-bound iodine in infants from birth to one year of age. Pediatrics, 7:240-244.

Dassler, C. G. 1966. Der Einfluss von Corticotrophin auf die Östrogenausscheidung in der Schwangerschaft und bei intrauterinem Fruchttod. Acta Endocr. (Kobenhavn), 53:401-406.

Davis, L. J., and W. Forbes. 1945. Thiouracil in pregnancy. Effect on foetal thyroid. Lancet, 2:740-742.

Dickey, R. P., and J. P. Thompson. 1969. Effect of ACTH and Metyrapone on estriol, 17-hydroxycorticosteroid, 17-ketosteroid, pregnanediol and preganetriol excretion in late pregnancy. J. Clin. Endocr., 29:701-706.

Diczfalusy, E. 1953. Chorionic gonadotrophin and oestrogens in the human placenta. Acta Endocr. (Kobenhavn), (Suppl. 12).

Driscoll, A. M. 1969. Urinary oestriol excretion in pregnant patient given large doses of prednisone. Brit. Med. J., 1:556-557.

Ducharme, J. R., and M. M. Grumbach. 1961. Studies on the effects of human growth hormone in premature infants. J. Clin. Invest., 40:243-252.

Dunn, J. M. 1966. Anterior pituitary and adrenal absence in a live-born normocephalic infant. Amer. J. Obstet. Gynec., 96:893-894.

Dussault, J., V. V. Row, G. Lickrish, and R. Volpe. 1969. Studies of serum triiodothyronine concentration in maternal and cord blood: Transfer of triiodothyronine across the human placenta. J. Clin. Endocr., 29:595-603.

Eberlein, W. R. 1965. Steroids and sterols in umbilical cord blood. J. Clin. Endocr., 25:1101-1118.

Edmonds, H. W. 1950. Pituitary, adrenal and thyroid in cyclopia. Arch. Path. (Chicago), 50:727-735.

Eguchi, Y., and L. J. Wells. 1965. Response of the hypothalamic-typophyseal adrenal axis to stress: Observations in fetal and caesarean newborn rats. Proc. Soc. Exp. Biol. Med., 120:675-678.

———— and Y. Morikawa. 1966. A study of the rat thyroid during perinatal days with observations of compensatory changes following unilateral thyroidectomy. Anat. Rec., 156:415-422.

———— and Y. Morikawa. 1968. Changes in pituitary gonadal interrelations during perinatal days in the rat. Anat. Rec., 161:163-170.

———— K. Eguchi, and L. J. Wells. 1964. Compensatory hypertrophy of right adrenal after left adrenalectomy: Observation in fetal, newborn and week-old rats. Proc. Soc. Exp. Biol. Med., 116:89-92.

Ellis, S. T., J. S. Beck, and A. R. Currie. 1966. The cellular localization of growth hormone in the human fetal adenohypophysis. J. Path. Bact., 92:179-183.

Erez, S., and T. M. King. 1966. Anencephaly: A survey of 44 cases. Obstet. Gynec., 27:601-604.

Falin, L. I. 1961. The development of human hypophysis and differentiation of cells of its anterior lobe during embryonic life. Acta Anat. (Basel), 44:183-205.

Fink, C. W. 1967. Thyrotropin deficiency in a child resulting in secondary growth hormone deficiency. Pediatrics, 40:881-885.

Fisher, D. A., and T. H. Oddie. 1964. Neonatal thyroidal hyperactivity. Response to cooling. Amer. J. Dis. Child., 107:574-581.

———— T. H. Oddie, and E. J. Makoski. 1966. The influence of environmental temperature on thyroid, adrenal and water metabolism in the newborn human infant. Pediatrics, 37:583-591.

———— and W. D. Odell. 1969. Acute release of thyrotropin in the newborn. J. Clin. Invest., 48:1670-1677.

———— W. D. Odell, C. J. Hobel, and R. Garza. 1969. Thyroid function in the term fetus. Pediatrics, 44:526-535.

Florshein, W. H., M. A. Flaircloth, N. L. Corcorran, and P. Rudko. 1966. Perinatal thyroid function in the rat. Acta Endocr. (Kobenhavn), 52:375-382.

Frandsen, V. A., and G. Stakemann. 1964. The site of production of oestrogenic hormones in human pregnancy. III. Further observations on the hormone excretion in pregnancy with anencephalic foetus. Acta Endocr. (Kobenhavn), 47:265-276.

Gardner, L. I. 1956. Adrenocortical metabolism of the fetus, infant and child. Pediatrics, 17:897-924.

———— 1969. Development of the normal fetal and neonatal adrenal. In Gardner, L. I., ed. Endocrine and Genetic Diseases of Childhood. Philadelphia, W. B. Saunders Company, pp. 392-406.

Geloso, J. P. 1958. Récherches préliminaires sur la sécrétion de thyroxine par la thyroide du foetus de rat, en fin de gestation. C. R. Acad. Sci. [D] (Paris), 246:168-171.

Gemzell, C. 1964. Therapy of gynecological disorders with human gonadotropin. Vitamins and Hormones, 22:129.

Gershberg, H. 1957. Growth hormone content and metabolic actions of human pituitary glands. Endocrinology, 61:160-165.

Ghilain, A., and J. Schwers. 1957. Extraction et dosage de l'ACTH dans l'hypophyse foetale humaine. C. R. Soc. Biol. (Paris), 151:1606-1609.

Gitlin, D., and A. Biasucci. 1969a. Ontogenesis of immunoreactive growth hormone, follicle-stimulating hormone, thyroid-stimulating hormone, luteinizing hormone, chorionic prolactin and chorionic gonadotropin in the human conceptus. J. Clin. Endocr., 29:926-935.

————— and A. Biasucci. 1969b. Ontogenesis of immunoreactive thyroglobulin in the human conceptus. J. Clin. Endocr., 29:849-853.

—————J. Kumate, and C. Morales. 1965. Metabolism and maternofetal transfer of human growth in the pregnant woman at term. J. Clin. Endocr., 25:1599-1608.

Glick, S. M. 1968. Normal and abnormal secretion of growth hormone. Ann. N. Y. Acad. Sci., 148:471-487.

Harris, G. W., and S. Levine. 1965. Sexual differentiation of the brain and its experimental control. J. Physiol. (London), 181:379-400.

Haworth, J. C., H. Medovy, and A. J. Lewis. 1961. Cebocephaly with endocrine dysgenesis. J. Pediat., 59:726-733.

Heggestad, C. B., and L. J. Wells. 1965. Experiments on the contribution of somatotrophin to prenatal growth in the rat. Acta Anat. (Basel), 60:348-361.

Hodges, R. E., H. E. Hamilton, and W. C. Keettel. 1952. Pregnancy in myxedema. Arch. Intern. Med. (Chicago), 90:863-868.

Holmes, L. B., et al. 1968. Normal growth with subnormal growth-hormone levels. New Eng. J. Med., 279:559-566.

Hunter, W. M., and F. C. Greenwood. 1964. A radio-immunoelectrophoretic assay of human growth hormone. Biochem. J., 91:43-56.

Hutchinson, D. L., J. L. Westover, and D. W. Will. 1962. The destruction of the maternal and fetal pituitary glands in subhuman primates. Amer. J. Obstet. Gynec. 83:857-865.

Hwang, U. K., and L. J. Wells. 1959. Hypophysis-thyroid system in the fetal rat: Thyroid after hypophyseoprivia, thyroxin, triiodothyronine, thyrotropin and growth hormone. Anat. Rec., 134:125-141.

Jacquot, R., and N. Kretchmer. 1964. Effect of fetal decapitation on enzymes of glycogen metabolism. J. Biol. Chem., 239:1301-1304.

Jailer, J. W. 1949. The pituitary-adrenal relationship in infant rat. Proc. Soc. Exp. Biol. Med., 72:638-639.

Johannisson, E. 1968. Foetal adrenal cortex in human: Its ultrastructure at different stages of development and in different functional states. Acta Endocr. (Kobenhavn), 58 (Suppl. 130):7-107.

Jones, J. M., C. W. Lloyd, and T. C. Wyatt. 1953. A study of interrelationships of maternal and fetal adrenal glands of rats. Endocrinology, 53:182-191.

Jost, A. 1951. Récherches sur la différenciation sexuelle de l'embryon de lapin. IV. Organogenese sexuelle masculine après décapitation du foetus. Arch. Anat. Micr. Morph. Exp., 40:247-281.

————— 1953. Sur le developpement de la thyroide chez le foetus de lapin décapité. Arch. Anat. Micr. Morph. Exp., 42:168-183.

————— 1954. Hormonal factors in the development of the fetus. Cold Spring Harbor Sympos. Quant. Biol., 19:167-180.

————— 1957. The secretory activities of fetal endocrine glands and their effect upon target organs. In Villee, C. A., ed. Gestation. New York, Josiah Macy, Jr., Foundation, pp. 129-171.

————— 1961. The role of fetal hormones in prenatal development. Harvey Lect., 55:201-226.

————— 1966. Anterior pituitary function in foetal life. In Harris, G. W., and B. T. Donovan, eds. The Pituitary Gland. Berkeley, University of California Press, Vol. 2, pp. 299-323.

———— F. F. Morel, and M. Marois. 1952. Nouvelles récherches à l'aide du radioiode I ^{131} sur la fonction thyroidienne du foetus de lapin décapité. C. R. Soc. Biol. (Paris), 146:1066-1070.

Kalkhoff, R., et al. 1964. Diabetogenic factors associated with pregnancy. Trans. Ass. Amer. Physicians, 77:270-780.

Kaplan, S. L., and M. M. Grumbach. 1967. Growth hormone in the human fetus and in anencephaly. International Symposium on Growth Hormone, Milan, Italy. Excerpta Medica Foundation, ICS No. 142, p. 51.

———— M. M. Grumbach, and T. H. Shepard. 1969. Gonadotropins in serum and pituitary of human fetuses and infants. Society for Pediatric Research. Thirty-ninth Annual Meeting Program and Abstracts, p. 8.

———— C. Preeyasombat, J. S. Spaulding, and C. J. Migeon. 1966b. Cortisol production rate. IV. Infants born of steroid-treated mothers and of diabetic mothers. Infants with trisomy syndrome and with anencephaly. Pediatrics, 37:960-966.

Kenny, F. M., C. Preeyasombat and C. J. Migeon. 1966a. Cortisol production rate. II. Normal infants, children and adults. Pediatrics, 37:34-42.

———— A. Drash, L. Y. Carces, and A. Susen. 1968. Iatrogenic hypopituitarism in craniopharyngioma; unexplained catch-up growth in 3 children. J. Pediat., 72:766-775.

Kitchell, R. L., and L. J. Wells. 1952. Functioning of the hypophysis and adrenals in fetal rats: Effects of hypophysectomy, adrenalectomy, castration, injected ACTH and implanted sex hormones. Anat. Rec., 112:561-586.

Knobil, E., and J. B. Josimovich. 1958. Placental transfer of thyrotrophic hormone, thyroxime, triiodothyronine and insulin in the rat. Ann. N. Y. Acad. Sci., 75:895-904.

Lanman, J. T. 1953. The fetal zone of the adrenal gland. Its developmental course, comparative anatomy, and possible physiologic functions. Medicine, 32:398-430.

———— 1962. An interpretation of human foetal adrenal structure and function. *In* Currie, A. R., T. Symington, and J. K. Grant, eds. The Human Adrenal Cortex. Baltimore, The Williams & Wilkins Co., pp. 547-558.

Laron, Z., and S. Mannheimer. 1966. Measurement of human growth hormone. Israel J. Med. Sci., 2:115-119.

———— A. Pertzelman, and S. Mannheimer. 1966a. Genetic pituitary dwarfism with high serum concentration of growth hormone. A new error of metabolism? Israel J. Med. Sci., 2:152-155.

———— et al. 1966b. Lack of placental transfer of human growth hormone. Acta Endocr. (Kobenhavn), 53:687-692.

Levina, S. E. 1968. Endocrine features in development of human hypothalamus, hypophysis and placenta. Gen. Comp. Endocr., 11:151-159.

Liggins, G. C., and P. C. Kennedy. 1968. Effects of electrocoagulation of the foetal lamb hypophysis on growth and development. J. Endocr., 40:371-381.

Little, B., et al. 1958. Hypophysectomy during pregnancy in a patient with cancer of the breast: Case report with hormone studies. J. Clin. Endocr., 18:425-443.

Maeyama, M., T. Nakagawa, Y. Tuchida, and H. Matuoka. 1969. The role of human fetal adrenal in steroidogenesis: Effects of adrenocorticotropin on urinary excretion of estrogens in pregnancy. Steroids, 13:59-67.

Martindale, F. M. 1941. Initiation and early development of thyrotropic function in the incubating chick. Anat. Rec., 79:373-393.

Merimee, T. J., et al. 1968a. An unusual variety of endocrine dwarfism: Subresponsiveness to growth hormone in a sexually mature dwarf. Lancet, 2:191-193.

———— et al. 1968b. Metabolic effects of human growth hormone in the African pygmy. Lancet, 2:194-195.

Michie, E. A. 1966. Oestrogen levels in urine and amniotic fluid in pregnancy with live anencephalic foetus and the effect of intra-amniotic injection of sodium dehydroepiandrosternone sulphate on these levels. Acta Endocr. (Kobenhavn), 51:535-542.

Migeon, C. J., et al. 1968. The syndrome of the congenital adrenocortical unresponsiveness to ACTH: Report of six cases. Pediat. Res., 2:501-513.

Mitskevich, M. S., and S. E. Levina. 1965. Investigation on the structure and gonadotropic activity of anterior pituitary in human embryogenesis. Arch. Anat. Micr. Morph. Exp., 54:129-143.

Mosier, H. D. 1956. Hypoplasia of the pituitary and adrenal cortex; Report of occurrence in twin siblings and autopsy findings. J. Pediat., 48:633-639.

Muelheims, G. H., F. E. Francis, and R. A. Kinsella, Jr. 1969. Suppression of the hypothalamic-pituitary-adrenal axis in the newborn dog. Endocrinology, 85:365-367.

Nanagas, J. C. 1925. A comparison of the growth of the body dimensions of anencephalic human fetuses with normal fetal growth as determined by graphic analysis and empirical formulae. Amer. J. Anat., 35:455-494.

Nichols, J. 1956. Observations on the adrenal of the premature anencephalic fetus. Arch. Path. (Chicago), 62:312-317.

———— O. L. Lescure, and C. J. Migeon. 1958. Levels of 17-hydroxycorticosteroids and 17-ketosteroids in maternal and cord plasma in term anencephaly. J. Clin. Endocr., 18:444-452.

Niemi, M., M. Ikonen, and A. Hervonen. 1967. Histochemistry and fine structure of the interstitial tissue in the human foetal testis. In Wolstenholme, G. E. W., and M. O'Connor, eds. Endocrinology of the Testis. CIBA Foundation Colloquia on Endocrinology. Boston, Little, Brown and Company, Vol. 16, pp. 31-52.

Parlow, A. 1966. The pituitary content of growth and other hormones during fetal and later life. In Blizzard, R. M., ed. Human Pituitary Growth Hormone: Report of the Fifty-fourth Ross Conference on Pediatric Research. Columbus, Ohio, Ross Labs, p. 94.

Perrin, E. V., and K. Benirschke. 1958. Somatic sex of anencephalic infants. J. Clin. Endocr., 18:327-328.

Peterson, R. R., and W. C. Young. 1952. The problem of placental permeability for thyrotrophin, propylthiouracil and thyroxine in the guinea pig. Endocrinology, 50:218-255.

Popert, A. J. 1962. Pregnancy and adrenocortical hormones. Some aspects of their interaction in rheumatic diseases. Brit. Med. J., 1:967-972.

Porteous, I. B., and J. S. Beck. 1968. The differentiation of the acidophil cell in the human foetal adenohypophysis. J. Path. Bact., 96:455-462.

Potter, E. L. 1961. Pathology of the Fetus and the Infant, 2nd ed. Chicago, Year Book Medical Publishers Inc., pp. 331-332.

Purves, H. D. 1966. Cytology of the adenohypophysis. In Harris, G. W., and B. T. Donovan, eds. The Pituitary Gland. Berkeley, University of California Press, Vol. 1, pp. 147-232.

Raiti, S., G. B. Holzman, R. L. Scott, and R. M. Blizzard. 1967. Evidence for the placental transfer of tri-iodothyronine in human beings. New Eng. J. Med., 277:456-459.

Reid, J. R. 1960. Congenital absence of the pituitary gland. J. Pediat. 56:658-664.

Reynolds, J. W. 1965. The excretion of two Δ5-3β-OH, 16α-hydroxysteroids by normal infants and children. J. Clin. Endocr., 25:416-423.

———— S. Mancuso, N. Wiqvist, and E. Diczfalusy. 1968. Physiological role of 16-keto-androstenediol (16-Keto ADL) in the feto-placental unit. Pediat. Res., 2:413-414.

Rice, B. F., and Ponthier, R., Jr. 1968. Luteinizing hormone and growth hormone activity of the human fetal pituitary. J. Clin. Endocr., 28:1071-1072.

Rimoin, D. L., T. J. Merimee, and V. A. McKusick. 1966a. Growth-hormone deficiency in man: an isolated, recessively inherited defect. Science, 152:1635-1637.

———— T. J. Merimee, and V. A. McKusick. 1966b. Sexual ateliotic dwarfism: A recessively inherited isolated deficiency of growth hormone. Trans. Ass. Amer. Physicians, 79:297-311.

———— et al. 1967. Growth hormone in African pygmies. Lancet, 2:523-526.

Salazar, H., M. A. MacAulay, D. Charles, and M. Pardo. 1969. The human hypophysis in anencephaly. I. Ultrastructure of the pars distalis. Arch. Path. (Chicago), 87:201-211.

Scommegna, A., B. R. Nedoss, and S. C. Chattoraj. 1968. Maternal urinary estriol excretion after dehydroepiandrosterone-sulfate infusion and adrenal stimulation and suppression. Obstet. Gynec., 31:526-533.

Sethre, A. E., and L. J. Wells. 1951. Accelerated growth of the thyroid in normal and "hypophysectomized" fetal rats given thyrotropin. Endocrinology, 49:369-373.

Shackleton, C. H. L., and F. L. Mitchell. 1967. The measurement of 3β-hydroxy-Δ5 steroids in human fetal blood, amniotic fluid, infant urine and adult urine. Steroids, 10:359-385.

Shepard, T. H. 1967. Onset of function in the human fetal thyroid: Biochemical and radioautographic studies from organ culture. J. Clin. Endocr. 27:945-958.

———— and H. J. Andersen. 1969. Cited by Shepard, T. H. 1969. Development of the thyroid gland. In Gardner, L. I., ed. Endocrine and Genetic Diseases of Childhood. Philadelphia, W. B. Saunders Company, pp. 200-206.

Simmer, H. H., et al. 1966. Neutral C19-steroids and steroid sulfates in human pregnancy. III. Dehydroepiandrosterone 16α-hydroxydehydroepiandrosterone sulfate, 16α-hydroxydehydroepiandrosterone sulfate in cord blood and blood of pregnant women with and without treatment with corticoids. Steroids, 8: 179-193.

Solomon, S., and H. G. Friesen. 1968. Endocrine relations between mother and fetus. Ann. Rev. Med., 19:399-430.

Stanbury, J. B., P. Rocmans, U. K. Buhler, and Y. Ochi. 1968. Congenital hypothyroidism with impaired thyroid response to thyrotropin. New Eng. J. Med., 279:1132-1136.

Stark, E., A. Gyevai, K. Szalay, and Z. Acs. 1965. Hypophyseal-adrenal activity in combined human foetal tissue cultures. Canad. J. Physiol. Pharmacol., 43:1-7.

Steiner, M. M., and J. D. Boggs. 1965. Absence of pituitary gland, hypothyroidism hypoadrenalism and hypogonadism in a 17-year old dwarf. J. Clin. Endocr., 25:1591-1598.

Tahka, H. 1951. On the weight and structure of the adrenal glands and the factors affecting them, in children of 0-2 years. Acta Paediat. Scand., 40 (Suppl. 81).

Taylor, N. R. W., J. A. Loraine, and H. A. Robertson. 1953. The estimation of ACTH in human pituitary tissue. J. Endocr., 9:334-341.

Tuchmann-Duplessis, H. 1959. Étude des glandes endocrines des anencéphales. Déduction sur les correlations hypophyso-nerveuses du foetus humain. Biol. Neonat., 1:8-32.

———— and L. Mercier-Parot. 1963. Étude comparative de la structure de l'hypophyse et de la surrénale des anencéphales et des hydrocéphales humains. C. R. Soc. Biol. (Paris), 157:977-981.

Utiger, R. D., et al. 1968. TSH secretion in newborn infants and children. J. Clin. Invest., 47:97a (abstract).

Van Wyk, J. J., and M. M. Grumbach. 1968. Disorders of sex differentiation. *In* Williams, R. H., ed. Textbook of Endocrinology. Philadelphia, W. B. Saunders Company, Ch. 8, pp. 537-612.

Vest, M., J. Girard, and U. Buhler. 1963. Metabolic effects of short term administration of human growth hormone in infancy and early childhood. Acta Endocr. (Kobenhavn), 44:613-624.

Villee, D. B. 1969. Development of endocrine function in the human placenta and fetus. New Eng. J. Med., 281:473-384, 533-541.

Wells, L. J. 1957. Effect of fetal endocrines on fetal growth. *In* Ville, C. A., ed. Gestation. New York, Josiah Macy, Jr., Foundation, pp. 187-227.

Westphal, O. 1968. Human growth hormone: A methodological and clinical study. Acta Paediat. Scand., (Suppl. 182).

Yen, S.S.C., O. H. Pearson, and S. Stratman. 1965. Growth hormone levels in maternal and cord blood. J. Clin. Endocr., 25:655-660.

Zamenhof, S., J. Mosley, and E. Schuller. 1966. Stimulation of the proliferation of cortical neurons by prenatal treatment with growth hormone. Science, 152:1396-1397.

Zondek, L. H., and T. Zondek. 1965a. Leydig cells of the foetus and newborn in normal and toxaemic pregnancy. Biol. Neonat., 8:1-22.

———— and T. Zondek. 1965b. Observations on the testis in anencephaly with special reference to the Leydig cells. Biol. Neonat., 8:329-347.

32

Insulin in Fetal and Neonatal Metabolism

JAMES R. TIERNAN • Department of Child Health, Royal Children's Hospital, University of Queensland, St. Lucia, Brisbane, Australia

Introduction

The human fetus uses maternal glucose as its main energy source and receives a constant supply of maternal amino acids. Insulin stimulates glycogen and fat synthesis from glucose and protein synthesis from amino acids and might be expected to play an important part in fetal growth. At birth the placental glucose supply is cut off, and the infant's blood glucose falls to mean levels of 50 to 60 mg/100 ml (Cornblath and Schwartz, 1966). These low levels may persist for 4 to 10 days in the normal term infant and for weeks in the premature infant. Symptoms of hypoglycemia may occur at blood glucose levels below 20 mg/100 ml, and severe neurologic damage may result if adequate treatment is not instituted (Cornblath and Reisner, 1965). These findings have stimulated great interest in the control of blood sugar in newborn infants and in insulin as the prime regulator of blood glucose concentration. However, because of the difficulties involved in measuring insulin it has only recently become possible to obtain direct information concerning the role of this hormone in fetal and neonatal metabolism.

Metabolic Actions and Effects of Insulin

Insulin plays an important role in the regulation of blood glucose concentration, plasma free fatty acid concentration, protein synthesis, energy storage, and fasting metabolism.

REGULATION OF BLOOD GLUCOSE CONCENTRATION

The fasting blood glucose concentration represents a balance between glucose utilization and hepatic glucose output. Insulin stimulates peripheral utilization of

959

glucose by facilitating the entry of glucose into the muscle cell and fat cell. In the absence of insulin these cells exclude glucose. However, the maintenance of a stable fasting blood glucose level probably depends largely on hepatic uptake and release. Glucose can pass freely into the liver cell in the absence of insulin, and glucose balance across the liver would appear to depend on two specific enzymes—glucose-6-phosphatase which stimulates release of free glucose from glucose-6-phosphate and is found only in liver and kidney cells, and glucokinase, a specific glucose phosphorylating enzyme which has been identified in human liver by Brown et al. (1967). The affinity of this enzyme for glucose varies according to the amount of insulin present. Elevated insulin levels increase glucokinase activity, and activity decreases as insulin levels fall. Cahill (1965) has suggested that insulin may regulate glucose balance in the liver cell, and hence control the set of the blood glucose concentration through its action on glucokinase.

ENERGY STORAGE AND FASTING METABOLISM

Insulin facilitates the entry of glucose into the muscle cell and the fat cell. Inside both cells glucose is phosphorylated, under the influence of hexokinase, to glucose-6-phosphate. In the muscle cell glucose is metabolized or converted to glycogen and stored. In the fat cell glucose provides glycero-3-phosphate and fatty acids for triglyceride synthesis. Insulin has a further independent action on fat metabolism whereby it inhibits the breakdown of triglycerides to free fatty acids and glycerol and thus lowers the serum free fatty acid level. Insulin therefore not only initiates a chain of events whereby blood glucose is converted into stored energy but also inhibits release of this energy. In addition, insulin stimulates the uptake of amino acids into muscle and their incorporation into protein. These effects are probably very important in the growing fetus. However, in the immediate newborn period, prior to the establishment of feeding, the infant must rely largely on stored energy, and insulin may play an important role in the regulation of metabolism during this time of relative starvation. Cahill et al. (1966) have suggested that a low, finely regulated level of circulating insulin is necessary for efficient metabolism during fasting. Low serum insulin levels reduce glucose entry into muscle and fat, allow breakdown of triglycerides to free fatty acids and glycerol, and allow breakdown of proteins to amino acids. Thus free fatty acids become available as an energy source for muscle, and glucose is preserved for noninsulin-sensitive tissues such as brain. Glycerol and amino acids are liberated and may be converted to glucose in the liver.

Measurement of Insulin

Many methods have been developed to measure insulin in blood or tissue extracts, and these have been critically reviewed by Berson and Yalow (1966). Those most commonly used now are the epididymal fat pad bioassay and the radioimmunoassay.

BIOASSAY

This is based on the metabolic effects which insulin exerts on isolated insulin-sensitive tissues. Rat diaphragm and rat epididymal fat tissue have been extensively used. The capacity of these tissues to take up glucose from an incubation medium is greatly augmented by insulin. There is a dose-response relationship between the amount of insulin added and glucose uptake from the medium. However, in these systems, plasma shows activity which resembles that of pancreatic insulin in some respects but not in others, and therefore when these methods are used to measure insulin in plasma the results are expressed as plasma insulinlike activity.

RADIOIMMUNOASSAY

Radioimmunoassy is based on the ability of insulin in plasma or other biologic fluids to compete with I^{131}-labeled insulin for binding sites on insulin antibodies. The competitive binding effect of plasma is compared with that produced by known standard solutions of insulin derived from the same species. Because of its greater specificity and sensitivity the immunoassay has proved most useful in the study of insulin levels in the newborn infant. Insulin measured in this system is referred to as *immunoreactive insulin.*

Insulin in Fetal Metabolism

The fetus is primarily concerned with the utilization of glucose, its major metabolic fuel, and would therefore benefit from a plentiful supply of circulating insulin. Adam et al. (1969) have detected immunoreactive insulin in human fetal plasma as early as 11 weeks of gestation. Possible sources of this insulin are the maternal blood and the fetal pancreas. Information regarding the possible role of fetal insulin is derived from studies of newborn infants of diabetic mothers.

SOURCES OF CIRCULATING FETAL INSULIN

Several workers have studied placental transfer of insulin but there is considerable variation in the findings. Buse et al. (1962) administered labeled beef insulin intravenously to pregnant women 7 minutes to 274 minutes prior to delivery and found very low levels of labeled material in the umbilical vein. They concluded that the human placenta at term is relatively impermeable to insulin. Spellacy et al. (1964) found no correlation in immunoreactive insulin concentrations between maternal plasma and umbilical vein plasma at delivery in 30 pregnant women, and again concluded that insulin does not pass the placenta. Josimovich and Knobil (1961) found, in the pregnant rhesus monkey between days 107 and 129 of a 170-day gestation period, significant transfer of labeled beef insulin across the placenta in both directions, but the data do not permit any meaningful quantitative evaluation of placental transfer. Gitlin et al. (1965) administered labeled human insulin intravenously to 9 pregnant women 12 to 86 minutes prior to delivery and found significant levels of labeled insulin in cord blood. They concluded from the data that insulin can cross the human placenta in both directions. However, Adam et al. (1969) found no evidence of placental transfer following a 4 to 6 hour intravenous infusion of human insulin I^{131} in 8 pregnant women between 15 and 16 weeks of gestation. Tobin et al. (1969) studied 6 normal primiparae in labor at term and found no significant transfer of insulin from mother to fetus. Despite a marked elevation of maternal immunoreactive insulin in response to intravenous glucose, there was no corresponding increase in immunoreactive insulin in fetal scalp blood.

Most studies indicate that insulin does not cross the human placenta, and, hence, we may assume that the circulating immunoreactive insulin demonstrated in an 11-week fetus (Adam et al., 1969) is of fetal origin. Islets of Langerhans can be detected histologically in the human fetal pancreas between the tenth and fourteenth weeks of gestation, and Steinke and Driscoll (1965) have extracted insulin, measured by the epididymal fat pad assay, from the pancreas of a 12-week human fetus. Thus, the evidence suggests that the human fetal pancreas can synthesize and release insulin during the first trimester of pregnancy.

THE ROLE OF FETAL INSULIN

Protein synthesis is occurring from the beginning of gestation, and glycogen synthesis in the fetal heart and liver probably begins before 15 weeks, but whether insulin exerts an action on these processes at this time is unknown. McCance and Widdowson (1951) have shown that the marked increase in the rate of fetal growth in the third trimester is largely due to increased fat synthesis. Fee and Weil (1963) showed that this increase is exaggerated to a striking degree in the infant of the diabetic mother, and studies in this group of infants provide valuable information regarding the possible role of insulin in stimulating fat synthesis in the last weeks of fetal life.

In infants of diabetic mothers, the islets of Langerhans are increased in size and number, there is hypertrophy and hyperplasia of the beta cells (the degree corresponding to the birth weight) (Driscoll, 1965), and the extractable insulin content of the pancreas is considerably higher than that of control infants (Steinke and Driscoll, 1965). Baird and Farquhar (1962) observed that the newborn infant of the diabetic mother, following an intravenous glucose load, shows a more rapid glucose disappearance rate and a greater rise in insulinlike activity, as measured by the rat diaphragm assay, than does the normal newborn infant. Immunoreactive insulin values are difficult to interpret in the newborn infant of the insulin-treated diabetic mother because antiinsulin antibodies cross the placenta and interfere with the assay. Studies have been carried out in newborn infants of noninsulin-treated diabetic mothers which indicates a greater immediate immunoreactive insulin response to intravenous glucose (Isles et al., 1968; Jorgensen et al., 1966) and a more prompt release of immunoreactive insulin following oral glucose (Pildes et al., 1969) in the infant of the diabetic mother than in the normal infant. Thus there is a considerable amount of evidence in support of "hyperinsulinism" in the infant of the diabetic mother. However, this widely accepted concept has recently been questioned by King et al. (1969). These authors found that during a constant slow intravenous infusion of glucose, infants of insulin-treated and noninsulin-treated diabetic mothers disposed of the exogenous glucose more slowly than normal newborns. Plasma immunoreactive insulin levels in infants of noninsulin-treated diabetic mothers were similar to those in normal infants.

Shima et al. (1966) found a positive correlation between birth weight and serum immunoreactive insulin levels in the umbilical vein at birth in a group of infants whose gestational ages varied from 36 to 41 weeks. Joassin et al. (1967) confirmed these findings in normal term infants and in infants of gestational diabetic mothers. Since third trimester growth is the main factor influencing birth weight, the correlation between cord insulin levels and birth weight suggests that insulin may play an important role in fetal growth in the third trimester through its action in promoting fat synthesis from glucose.

Insulin in Neonatal Metabolism

At birth the placental glucose source is cut off, and until oral feeding is established, the infant must obtain glucose from endogenous sources. Serial determinations of blood sugar during the early neonatal period have been performed by several workers, and the results have been reviewed by Smith (1959) and Cornblath and Schwartz (1966). Methods of blood collection and blood sugar measurement vary so that it is difficult to compare actual values, but a definite pattern of glycemia is seen in the neonatal period. There is a fall in blood glucose during the first hours of life, followed by a period of instability in which mean levels are low by adult standards.

The fasting blood glucose level represents a balance between hepatic output and peripheral utilization. The normal term infant has a generous supply of glycogen (Shelley and Neligan, 1966), and the enzymes necessary for glycogen breakdown and gluconeogenesis are present in human fetal liver (Villee, 1953; Dawkins, 1966). Cornblath et al. (1961, 1963) and Mulligan and Schwartz (1962) observed glucose release following injection of glucagon in the first hours of life. The neonatal liver thus seems capable of responding to hypoglycemia, but intravenous glucose tolerance tests in newborn infants (Cornblath et al., 1963; Bowie et al., 1963) showed no rebound in the blood glucose after two hours, suggesting a failure of regulation of the hepatic response to low blood glucose levels. The same workers noted a slow rate of glucose disappearance after intravenous glucose injection, suggesting decreased peripheral utilization of glucose in the newborn infant. Measurements of immunoreactive insulin after glucose loading in newborn infants have explained some of these findings.

INSULIN RESPONSE TO GLUCOSE IN THE NEONATAL PERIOD

Normal adults respond to an intravenous glucose load with a rapid rise in immunoreactive insulin levels to a peak 1 to 5 minutes after the end of the injection, followed by a sharp decline (Seltzer et al., 1967). Spellacy et al. (1967) administered glucose, 1 g per kg body weight, via either umbilical vein or umbilical artery catheter, to 12 newborn infants on the first day of life and prior to the first feeding. Blood glucose and plasma immunoreactive insulin were measured at 15, 30, 60, and 120 minutes after glucose injection. There was a definite immunoreactive insulin response, but maximum values occurred at 60 minutes. In another study in a similar group of infants, Jorgensen et al. (1966) measured immunoreactive insulin 5 minutes and 30 minutes after glucose injection and found higher levels at 30 minutes than at 5 minutes.

Isles et al. (1968) studied another group of normal term infants at 2 hours of age. They, too, showed a late immunoreactive insulin peak 60 minutes after an intravenous glucose load, but also observed an early peak at 2 minutes in some infants. This "double peak" immunoreactive insulin response to a glucose load was also observed by Gentz et al. (1969) in 20 of 35 newborn infants whose birth weights were less than 2,300 g. These authors divided the infants into those appropriate for gestational age, who had birth weights above the 10th percentile (Battaglia and Lubchenco, 1967), and those small for gestational age, who had birth weights below the 10th percentile for their period of gestation. The immunoreactive insulin responses were slightly greater in the former group, but the differences were not significant. Gentz et al. (1969) also observed infants who showed only one immunoreactive insulin peak (at 2 minutes) and infants who showed no immunoreactive insulin response to an intravenous glucose load.

The most striking feature of the immunoreactive insulin response to an intravenous or intra-arterial glucose load in the newborn infant as compared to the adult is the wide individual variation seen in the infant (Tiernan et al., 1967). Figure 1 shows the response in the infant of a gestational diabetic mother (O'Sullivan and Mahan, 1964) who shows the pattern seen in the normal adult. Figure 2 shows the "double peak" pattern in a normal infant, with immunoreactive insulin values still above the fasting level 90 minutes after the glucose injection. The shift in the immunoreactive insulin peak from 1 minute, as seen in the adult and the infant of the diabetic mother (Fig. 1), to 60 minutes, as seen in many newborn infants (Fig. 2), provides an explanation for the instability of the blood glucose in many newborn infants. Immunoreactive insulin levels are still elevated in many infants 1 hour after glucose injection, but in the adult the immunoreactive insulin concentration approaches the fasting level by this time. Pildes et al. (1969) have shown that, following an oral glucose load in the newborn infant, there is a slow but sustained immunoreactive insulin response and elevated levels persist for at least 2 hours after the glucose load. This inappropriate immunoreactive insulin response to glucose loading will produce swings in the infant's blood glucose which are unpredictable by reference to normal adult standards and may be responsible for the instability of blood glucose concentration in the neonatal period.

The relationship of the glucose disappearance rate Kt (Ikkos and Luft, 1957) to immunoreactive insulin response is difficult to define, but those infants who have the greatest insulin response tend to have the most rapid glucose disappearance

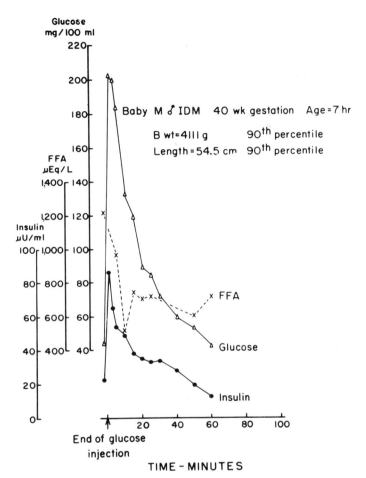

Fig. 1. Changes in glucose, free fatty acid, and immunoreactive insulin levels following intra-arterial glucose, 0.5 g per kg over 2 minutes, at 7 hours of age in the infant of a gestational diabetic mother (IDM).

rates. Bowie et al. (1963) noted a slow rate of glucose disappearance in the first hour after a glucose load in newborn infants but a more rapid rate of glucose disappearance in the second hour. The more rapid rate in the second hour might be expected if maximum insulin values occur at 60 minutes. However, Gentz et al. (1969) found no difference in mean glucose disappearance rates between infants who showed a "double peak" immunoreactive insulin response and those who showed "no response" indicating that glucose disappearance rates may be influenced by factors other than insulin secretion. Also, stimuli other than glucose have been shown to cause insulin release (Buchanan, 1969), and Grasso et al. (1968) have demonstrated a significant rise in immunoreactive insulin in premature infants on the first day of life following administration of an amino acid mixture via the umbilical vein.

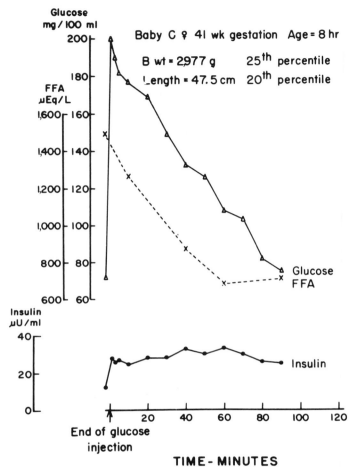

Fig. 2. Changes in glucose, free fatty acid, and immunoreactive insulin levels following intra-arterial glucose, 0.5 g per kg over 2 minutes, at 8 hours of age in a normal term infant.

THE ROLE OF INSULIN IN THE NEONATAL PERIOD

The newborn infant must adapt to nutritional circumstances quite different from those of fetal life. During the fast after birth the infant is dependent on liver glycogen stores and gluconeogenesis to provide glucose for brain metabolism. The normal term infant manages reasonably well, but the premature and the low birth weight for gestational age infant may have difficulty in maintaining an adequate supply of glucose. These infants have decreased amounts of liver glycogen at birth (Shelley and Neligan, 1966), and Cornblath et al. (1963) suggested that the relatively large neonatal brain may utilize 70 to 150 percent of the hepatic glucose output. It would seem highly desirable, at least in the premature and low birth weight for gestational age infant, to restrict glucose utilization to brain only during the period prior to establishment of oral feeding. This requires exclusion of glucose from muscle and fat cells, and hence low levels of circulating insulin. Some newborn infants show a delay in immunoreactive insulin release after a glucose load, and some infants had no significant increase in immunoreactive insulin 60 minutes after glucose injection. These findings suggest an adaptation of the insulin release mechanism in order to keep circulating levels low.

The patterns of insulin release described in newborn infants were seen in infants only a few hours old and are presumably present at birth. If insulin plays an active role in fat synthesis from glucose in fetal life one might expect an active insulin release mechanism in the fetus. If this is so, placental insufficiency may provide an explanation for the adaptation to the sluggish insulin release of some newborn infants. Naeye (1965) found organ changes in a group of newborn infants of low birth weight for gestational age, similar to those found in older infants with alimentary malnutrition, and suggested that the newborn infants had suffered from malnutrition in utero due to inadequate placental function. Cahill et al. (1966) performed glucose tolerance tests in normal adults before and after a period of starvation and found a decrease in the rate of glucose disappearance and in the magnitude of the immunoreactive insulin response after the fast. It may be that the pattern of immunoreactive insulin response in the newborn infant is due to a period of relative starvation in late pregnancy.

The fall in blood glucose to low levels after birth and the persistence of these levels have not yet been fully explained. Infants of diabetic mothers have a rapid initial fall in blood glucose, and values below 20 mg per 100 ml are frequently recorded in these infants during the first 3 hours of life (McCann et al., 1966). The rapid fall in infants of diabetic mothers is almost certainly due to increased levels of circulating insulin. Figure 3 shows the relationship between the glucose disappearance rate, K (calculated by plotting the glucose data semilogarithmically and drawing a regression line visually according to the first order equation), and immunoreactive insulin levels, during the first 90 minutes of life in the infant of a gestational diabetic mother. There is a parallel fall in glucose and immunoreactive insulin levels, and the fall in glucose ceases when insulin reaches the fasting level.

Shelley and Neligan (1966) suggested, on the basis of animal studies (Shelley, 1960), that the fetal blood glucose concentration may be only half the maternal level, that the relatively high levels in cord blood are associated with the stress of delivery, and that the fall after birth represents a return to normal fetal levels. This theory is consistent with the slightly elevated levels of immunoreactive insulin in cord blood (Joassin et al., 1967), but the data available on human fetal blood glucose levels (Adam et al., 1969), do not support it. If low blood glucose levels in newborn infants represent persistence of fetal levels, it will be necessary to explore the factors responsible for the subsequent rise to adult levels. Glucokinase appears gradually after birth in the rat and the guinea pig (Walker, 1963; Ballard and Oliver, 1964; see Ch. 13), and the appearance of this enzyme may be responsible for the set of the blood glucose at adult levels (Cahill, 1965). However, there is as yet no information on the time of appearance of glucokinase in fetal human liver.

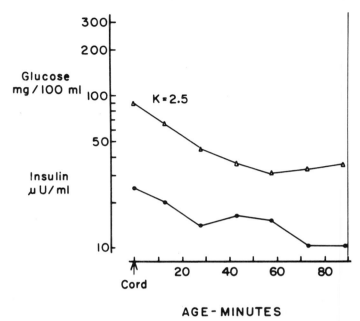

AGE-MINUTES

Fig. 3. Semilogarithmic plot of glucose and immunoreactive insulin concentrations immediately after birth in the infant of a gestational diabetic mother. Glucose disappearance rate, K = 2.5 percent per minute.

Conclusion

The sensitivity of the immunoassay technique has enabled us to demonstrate the presence of circulating insulin in the fetus and the newborn infant and the ability of most newborn infants to release insulin in response to a glucose load. The combination of hyperinsulinism and increased amounts of body fat in the newborn infant of the diabetic mother, and correlations between cord insulin levels and birth weight, suggest that insulin exerts a major influence on fetal growth in the third trimester. The differences in magnitude and timing of the immunoreactive insulin response to glucose loading, in the newborn infant and in the adult, provide explanations for many of the variations in blood glucose which occur in the neonatal period. Diminished and delayed release of insulin is probably responsible for the slow glucose disappearance rate in the first hour after a glucose load, and the instability of blood glucose concentration is probably due to the persistence of elevated levels of insulin for up to 120 minutes after a glucose load. There is as yet no satisfactory explanation for the low mean blood glucose levels in the neonatal period, and further studies of hepatic carbohydrate metabolism in the newborn infant are necessary to clarify this problem.

Acknowledgments

The unpublished work of J. R. Tiernan, M. L. Kemball, and C. A. Smith referred to in this chapter was performed in the Neonatal Research Laboratory, Boston Hospital for Women (Lying-in Division); the Elliott P. Joslin Research Laboratory; and the Departments of Pediatrics and Medicine, Harvard Medical School. These studies were supported by the Association for the Aid of Crippled Children, New York; the Elliott P. Joslin Research Laboratory, Boston; the John A. Hartford Foundation, Inc., New York; and National Institute of Child Health and Human Development Grant 5-TO-HD00050-08 and United States Public Health Service Grant AM-09748-02.

REFERENCES

Adam, P. A. J., et al. 1969. Human fetal insulin metabolism early in gestation: Response to acute elevation of the fetal glucose concentration and placental transfer of human insulin-I-131. Diabetes, 18:409-416.

Baird, J. D., and J. W. Farquhar. 1962. Insulin-secreting capacity in newborn infants of normal and diabetic women. Lancet, 1:71-74.

Ballard, F. J., and I. T. Oliver. 1964. Ketohexokinase, isoenzymes of glucokinase and glycogen synthesis from hexoses in neonatal rat liver. Biochem. J., 90:261-268.

Battaglia, F. C., and L. O. Lubchenco. 1967. A practical classification of newborn infants by weight and gestational age. J. Pediat. 71:159-163.

Berson, S. A., and R. S. Yalow. 1966. Insulin in blood and insulin antibodies. Amer. J. Med., 40:676-690.

Bowie, M. D., P. B. Mulligan, and R. Schwartz. 1963. Intravenous glucose tolerance in the normal newborn infant: The effects of a double dose of glucose and insulin. Pediatrics, 31:590-598.

Brown, J., D. M. Miller, M. T. Holloway, and G. D. Leve. 1967. Hexokinase isoenzymes in liver and adipose tissue of man and dog. Science, 155:205-207.

Buchanan, K. D. 1969. Disorders of carbohydrate metabolism. J. Clin. Path., 22 (Suppl.) No. 2:2.

Buse, M. G., W. J. Roberts, and J. Buse. 1962. The role of the human placenta in the transfer and metabolism of insulin. J. Clin. Invest., 41:29-41.

Cahill, G. F., Jr. 1965. Pathophysiology of diabetes. Med. Clin. N. Amer., 49:881-891

———— et al. 1966. Hormone-fuel interrelationships during fasting. J. Clin. Invest., 45: 1751-1769.

Cornblath, M., and S. H. Reisner. 1965. Blood glucose in the neonate and its clinical significance. New Eng. J. Med., 273:378-381.

———— and R. Schwartz. 1966. Disorders of Carbohydrate Metabolism in Infancy. Philadelphia and London, W. B. Saunders Company, Part I, pp. 33-54.

———— S. H. Wybregt, and G. S. Baens. 1963. Studies of carbohydrate metabolism in the newborn infant. VII. Tests of carbohydrate tolerance in premature infants. Pediatrics, 32:1007-1024.

———— et al. 1961. Studies of carbohydrate metabolism in the newborn infant. III. Some factors influencing the capillary blood sugar and the response to glucagon during the first hours of life. Pediatrics, 27:378-389.

Dawkins, M. J. R. 1966. Biochemical aspects of developing function in newborn mammalian liver. Brit. Med. Bull., 22:27-33.

Driscoll, S. G. 1965. The pathology of pregnancy complicated by diabetes mellitus. Med. Clin. N. Amer., 49:1053-1067.

Fee, B. A., and W. B. Weil, Jr. 1963. Body composition of infants of diabetic mothers by direct analysis. Ann. N. Y. Acad. Sci., 110:869-897.

Gentz, J. C. H., R. Warrner, B. E. H. Persson, and M. Cornblath. 1969. Intravenous glucose tolerance, plasma insulin, free fatty acids and β-hydroxybutyrate in underweight newborn infants. Acta Paediat. Scand., 58:481-490.

Gitlin, D., J. Kumate, and C. Morales. 1965. On the transport of insulin across the human placenta. Pediatrics, 35:65-69.

Grasso, S., A. Messina, N. Saparito, and G. Reitano. 1968. Serum-insulin response to glucose and aminoacids in the premature infant. Lancet, 2:755-756.

Ikkos, D., and R. Luft. 1957. On the intravenous glucose tolerance test. Acta Endocr., 25:312-334.

Isles, T. E., M. Dickson, and J. W. Farquhar. 1968. Glucose tolerance and plasma insulin in newborn infants of normal diabetic mothers. Pediat. Res., 2:198-208.

Joassin, G., M. L. Parker, R. S. Pildes, and M. Cornblath. 1967. Infants of diabetic mothers. Diabetes, 16:306-311.

Jorgensen, K. R., T. Deckert, L. M. Pedersen,.and J. Pedersen. 1966. Insulin, insulin antibody and glucose in plasma of newborn infants of diabetic women. Acta Endocr. (Kobenhavn), 52:154-167.

Josimovich, J. B., and E. Knobil. 1961. Placental transfer of I^{131} insulin in the rhesus monkey. Amer. J. Physiol., 200:471-476.

King, K. C., P. A. J. Adam, G. A. Clemente, and R. Schwartz. 1969. Infants of diabetic mothers: Attenuated glucose uptake without hyperinsulinemia during continuous glucose infusion. Pediatrics, 44:381-392.

McCance, R. A., and E. M. Widdowson. 1951. Composition of the body. Brit. Med. Bull., 7:297-306.

McCann, M. L., et al. 1966. Effects of fructose on hypoglucosemia in infants of diabetic mothers. New Eng. J. Med., 275:1-7.

Mulligan, P. B., and R. Schwartz. 1962. Hepatic carbohydrate metabolism in the genesis of neonatal hypoglycaemia: Effects of the administration of epinephrine, glucagon, and galactose. Pediatrics, 30:125-135.

Naeye, R. L. 1965. Malnutrition: Probable cause of fetal growth retardation. Arch. Path. (Chicago), 79:284-291.

O'Sullivan, J. B., and C. M. Mahan. 1964. Criteria for the oral glucose tolerance test in pregnancy. Diabetes, 13:278-285.

Pildes, R. S., R. J. Hart, R. Warrner, and M. Cornblath. 1969. Plasma insulin response during oral glucose tolerance tests in newborns of normal and gestational diabetic mothers. Pediatrics, 44:76-83.

Seltzer, H. S., E. W. Allen, A. L. Herron, Jr., and M. T. Brennan. 1967. Insulin secretion in response to glycaemic stimulus: Relation of delayed initial release to carbohydrate intolerance in mild diabetes mellitus. J. Clin. Invest., 46:323-335.

Shelley, H. J. 1960. Blood sugars and tissue carbohydrate in foetal and infant lambs and rhesus monkeys. J. Physiol., 153:527-552.

——— and G. A. Neligan. 1966. Neonatal hypogylcaemia. Brit. Med. Bull., 22:34-39.

Shima, K., S. Price, and P. P. Foa. 1966. Serum insulin concentration and birth weight in human infants. Proc. Soc. Exp. Biol. Med., 121:55-59.

Smith, C. A. 1959. The Physiology of the Newborn Infant, 3rd ed. Springfield, Ill., Charles C Thomas, Publisher, pp. 270-279.

Spellacy, W. N., S. A. Gall, and K. L. Carlson. 1967. Carbohydrate metabolism of the normal term newborn: Plasma insulin and blood glucose levels during an intravenous glucose tolerance test. Obstet. Gynec., 30:580-583.

———— F. C. Goetz, B. Z. Greenberg, and J. Ells. 1964. The human placental gradient for plasma insulin and blood glucose. Amer. J. Obstet. Gynec., 90:753-757.

Tiernan, J. R., M. L. Kemball, and C. A. Smith. April, 1967. Endogenous insulin, neonatal blood glucose, hypoglycemia. Soc. Ped. Res. Abstr., p. 169.

Tobin, J. D., J. F. Roux, and J. S. Soeldner. 1969. Human fetal insulin response after acute maternal glucose administration during labor. Pediatrics, 44:668-671.

Steinke, J., and S. G. Driscoll. 1965. The extractable insulin content of pancreas from fetuses and infants of diabetic and control mothers. Diabetes, 14:573-578.

Villee, C. A. 1953. Regulation of blood glucose in the human fetus. J. Appl. Physiol., 5:437-444.

Walker, D. G. 1963. On the presence of two soluble glucose phosphorylating enzymes in adult liver and the development of one of these after birth. Biochim. Biophys. Acta, 77:209-226.

33

Thyroid Hormones

JAMES F. MARKS ● **Department of Pediatrics, University of Texas, Southwestern Medical School, Dallas, Texas**

Introduction

Various tests of thyroid function will be referred to during the course of this discussion. These will be defined at the beginning. These tests fall into several groups: 1, direct measurements of thyroidal hormone in the serum; 2, measurements of thyroid-binding proteins; 3, in-vitro and in-vivo isotope studies; and 4, measurements of unbound circulating thyroid hormones.

In the first category of direct measurements of thyroidal hormone in serum fall the PBI (protein-bound iodine), BEI (butanol extractable iodine), and thyroxine iodine. The last mentioned test may be performed by one of several techniques involving either column chromatography or dialysis procedure depending on the properties of thyroxine-binding proteins.

In the next group of studies are measurements of thyroid-binding globulin or thyroid-binding globulin capacity. There are three basic proteins that participate in the binding of thyroid hormone in the plasma. They are albumin, thyroid-binding prealbumin (TBPA), and thyroid-binding globulin (TBG).

The in-vitro I^{131} triiodothyronine uptake is in a sense an indirect measurement of thyroid-binding globulin capacity. In these techniques a labeled amount of I^{131} is incubated in vitro with either whole blood or serum mixed with a resin sponge. In either case the red cells or the resin act as inert surfaces that pick up labeled triiodothyronine which is not absorbed by the plasma. Thus, an elevated triiodothyronine uptake correlates with a low thyroid-binding globulin capacity, while a decreased triiodothyronine uptake correlates with a high thyroid-binding globulin capacity.

The standard I^{131} in-vivo uptake has been done using various dosages in the perinatal period. Thyroxine turnover studies using in-vivo radioisotopes have also been used, and these will be referred to specifically where applicable further in the discussion.

The "free thyroxine" (T_F) is used to refer to that fraction of the circulating thyroxine iodine that is not bound to the plasma proteins. This is felt by some investigators to represent the critical or biologically active portion of circulating

973

thyroid hormones. It has been measured by a number of techniques involving chromatographic and dialysis procedures.

New techniques are being developed for the measurements of triiodothyronine in the plasma. Such a measurement is held by some to be a more critical assessment of circulating thyroid hormones than is the measurement of thyroxine. One of these techniques has now been applied in the study of the perinatal period. During the course of this discussion, there has been no mention of some old standby techniques, such as the serum cholesterol and the basal metabolic rate. These studies appear to be of very little value in assessing thyroid function in the perinatal period.

Maternal Thyroid Function

It is known that the protein-bound iodine and similar measurements of circulating thyroid hormone are elevated in the pregnant woman. In 1956, Dowling et al. demonstrated that the thyroid-binding globulin capacity of maternal serum was elevated in comparison to that of the nonpregnant adult. It could be postulated then that the elevation of thyroid-binding globulin could explain the elevation of protein-bound iodine in the pregnant woman without invoking any basic alteration of thyroid function. The work of these authors has been subsequently confirmed by other investigators using different techniques. In addition, Hamolsky et al. (1957) had shown that the in vitro I^{131} triiodothyronine uptake is depressed in the pregnant woman, which would be consistent with the elevation found in thyroid-binding globulin capacity.

Clark and Horn (1965) have used the product of the PBI times the erythrocyte triiodothyronine uptake as a rough measure of free thyroxine. Using this technique they demonstrated that the free thyroxine index is the same for both the pregnant woman and nonpregnant normal adults. Sterling and Hegedus (1962), Ingbar et al. (1964), Lee et al. (1964), and Marks et al. (1966), using more specific techniques in measurement of free thyroxine, have clearly demonstrated that the free thyroxine in the pregnant woman is essentially the same as that found in the normal nonpregnant adult.

It has been postulated that some thyroid function tests might be of prognostic value during pregnancy. Nicoloff et al. (1962) have suggested that the measurements of thyroxine-binding globulin capacity would be helpful. They have shown in a group of patients that an abrupt fall in thyroxine-binding globulin capacity correlates with a sudden unexpected termination of pregnancy.

In the normal pregnant woman, using the conventional thyroid function techniques, one would expect the protein-bound iodine or similar measurements of circulating thyroid hormone to be elevated. The triiodothyronine measured by either the resin or red cell technique would be depressed. Free thyroxine measured by any of the conventional techniques would be within the normal range. Thyroxine turnover rates in the normal pregnant woman are equivalent to those in the normal nonpregnant adult (Dowling, 1967).

Development of the Fetal Thyroid

Many studies have shown that the human fetal thyroid will pick up iodine at about 12 weeks of fetal life. There is a great deal of variation in many species of mammals with regard to this. The rat will not pick up iodine until nearly the end of gestation, whereas the monkey will pick up iodine at about the beginning of the second trimester of gestation.

The most recent definitive study in humans was performed by Shepard (1967), who studied thyroxine synthesis in human fetal organ cultures using I^{125} incubation medium. Fetuses with a length from 22 to 142 mm and with a gestational age from 45 to 112 days were studied. In those fetuses of less than 68 mm no organic iodine, central colloidal cavity, or tissue binding of I^{125} could be noted. At 68 mm or 74 gestational days and in all later stages, a full spectrum of iodinated thyroidal materials could be found, including monoiodotyrosine, diiodotyrosine, thyroxine, and triiodothyronine. In addition, I^{125} tissue binding was apparent on radioautographs. The exact sequences of the biochemical events could not be specifically delineated in the human tissue.

In the same study, Shepard (1967) demonstrated that the 20-day gestational rat fetuses would accumulate I^{125}, and they would show a gradual reduction of monoiodotyrosine and diiodotyrosine occurring over an 18-hour period. Puromycin inhibited organic binding of I^{125}, but cyanide did not.

Gitlin and Biasucci (1969) have shown that synthesis of immunoreactive thyroglobulin is present by the 29th day of human fetal development.

Thus, by several different types of methodology, the time of onset of thyroid activity in the human fetus can be demonstrated. Questions, of course, remain unanswered. First, what is the exact sequence in the origination and organization of biochemical events in the human fetal thyroid? Secondly, what is the significance of the development of hormonogenesis in the human fetus on the overall pattern of fetal development? Third, what is the significance of differences in hormonogenesis among various mammalian species?

Fetal-Maternal Relationships

There is a small amount of species variability as to the ways which various substances related to thyroid biologic activity exchange themselves between mother and fetus. Iodine, TSH, the thiourea drugs, thyroxine, and a long acting thyroid stimulator (LATS) will be considered.

In the rat, guinea pig, rabbit, and monkey, among other species as well as man, iodine transfer from mother to fetus has been demonstrated. A number of investigators have shown that radioactive iodine administered to mothers prior to therapeutic abortion has appeared localized in the thyroid of human fetuses from about the twelfth gestational week. Ample clinical evidence exists as to the toxic effects on the newborn infant of iodine administered to the mother during pregnancy. Thus, there is no question that the human placenta is freely permeable to iodine at least during the second and third trimesters of pregnancy.

In no species studied has there been any demonstration of placental passage of TSH. When Peterson and Young (1952) gave TSH to guinea pig mothers, the fetal thyroid was not hyperplastic. On the other hand such animals given propylthiouracil have shown fetal thyroid hyperplasia which was blocked by concomitant thyroid administration to the mother. Knobil and Josimovich (1959) have shown in the rat that the offspring of hypophysectomized mothers will develop goiter formation from propylthiouracil due entirely to the fetal production of TSH and that this effect is similarly blocked by maternal administration of triiodothyronine or thyroxine with suppression of fetal TSH production. Thus, although there is no placental permeability to TSH, the fetal pituitary can respond to environmental stimuli produced by maternal administration of other materials which do appear to cross the placenta.

Many investigators (Peterson and Young, 1952; Knobil and Josimovich, 1959) have clearly shown that the placenta is freely permeable to the thiourea drugs. Transplacental passage of these drugs produces goiter formation not only in experimental animals but also in the human fetus. This will be discussed later in more detail.

The problems of placental passage of thyroxine and triiodothyronine form the most interesting aspect of the fetal-maternal thyroid relationship. The type of indirect evidence cited above in the discussion of TSH and the thiourea drugs seems to suggest that thyroxine or triiodothyronine is able to cross the placenta in experimental animals to the extent that it at least partially blocks the TSH stimulation which produces goiters in the offspring of thiourea-treated animals. Direct studies have been done in a number of species including man.

Grumbach and Werner (1956) studied the transfer of thyroid hormones across the human placenta at term. They blocked the thyroid with stable iodine and then gave I^{131}-labeled triiodothyronine or thyroxine and measured the total serum precipitable radioactive iodine. They concluded that the human placenta was capable of allowing some transfer of small but significant amounts of thyroxine but that the barrier was slow. Their work is subject to criticism since they did not chromatograph fetal serum, and by their own admission, they could not rule out a sequence of breakdown, transfer, and resynthesis.

Pickering (1964), in work on the macaque monkey, has studied the placental transfer of I^{131}-labeled thyroxine to the pregnant monkey at various stages from 50 to 150 days' gestation in an animal whose normal gestational age is 167 days. Determinations of thyroxine and triiodothyronine I^{131} were made in maternal serum, fetal serum, and fetal and placental tissues. Significant amounts of thyroxine of maternal origin were found in these tissues during that period of fetal life which was studied.

Studies in the rhesus monkey by Schultz et al. (1965) on placental transfer of I^{131}-labeled triiodothyronine show that the majority of maternal-to-fetal placental transfer of radioactivity was in the form of iodine and a chemically unrecognized compound. Only traces of triiodothyronine and thyroxine were detected. In fetal-to-maternal studies Schultz et al. (1965) felt that the triiodothyronine was more readily transferred into the maternal circulation. Again small amounts of iodine and a similar unknown compound which they felt to be a sulphate conjugate of triiodothyronine appeared on chromatography. In their studies there was a considerably greater concentration gradient from the fetus to the mother than from the mother to the fetus. They suggested that maternal thyroid hormones were not readily available for fetal needs in the later part of pregnancy. In the human, Myant (1958) has shown that I^{131}-labeled triiodothyronine and thyroxine injected into mothers scheduled for therapeutic abortion at 10 to 18 weeks cannot be readily identified in fetal tissues. Fisher et al. (1964) have studied the effects of administration of intravenous loads of sodium L-thyroxine on the BEI, triiodothyronine, and thyroxine resin uptakes in 15 mothers with uncomplicated pregnancies and their infants. Following such loading, newborn BEI and triiodothyronine uptakes increased progressively with increasing maternal thyroid dose and increasing time. However, such increases were much less than those parallel in the maternal serum even at a maximum load and time. These data suggested that the maternal transport was limited by maternal thyroid-binding proteins as well as perhaps by an inherent placental permeability defect with regard to thyroxine. They suggested the primary gradient in thyroxine transport in the human was from fetus to mother rather than the other way around.

Dussault et al. (1968), using the technique of Nauman et al. (1967), have shown that both total and free triiodothyronine levels in human maternal and infant cord blood are equal to each other. The free triiodothyronine values are slightly depressed below normal adult values. With maternal administration of extremely large doses of triiodothyronine, both the maternal and cord levels of total triiodothyronine rise, although the rise is much less marked in cord blood. The values of free triiodothyronine in both of these groups are equal but elevated above the normal adult levels. These data suggest that triiodothyronine does cross the placenta but at a gradient which appears conditioned by the high levels of maternal thyroid-binding protein.

Thus, a few conclusions appear applicable with regard to placental transport of triiodothyronine and thyroxine. First, these materials probably do cross the placenta but cross it slowly. Secondly, there is most probably a better gradient from fetus to mother than from mother to fetus in the human. Whether sufficient amounts cross the placenta to be of consequence to a fetus unable to make its own thyroxine is still a matter of conjecture.

Another interesting substance that should be considered is long acting thyroid stimulator (LATS). This material is a protein, a 7-S gammaglobulin. The work of Kriss et al. (1964) suggests that this material is an antibody to some component of thyroid tissue. It does cross the placenta readily. It is found in infants of mothers with Graves' disease and has been found in those situations of congenital thyrotoxocosis in which it has been sought. This particular area will be discussed in more detail in the section on neonatal thyroid pathology.

Thus the series of compounds relating to thyroid activity have been considered. Iodine apparently crosses quite readily with evidence of maternal-fetal passage as early as the twelfth gestational week in the human fetus. Propylthiouracil and the other thiourea drugs also cross quite readily. Thyroxine and triiodothyronine seem to cross, although certainly less well than the above compounds. It appears that the gradient from fetus to mother is greater than that from mother to fetus. Long acting thyroid stimulator, a 7-S gammaglobulin, crosses quite readily.

Neonatal Thyroid Function

In both the full-size and low birth weight infant the various serum protein-bound measures of thyroid hormone are increased in the first week of life. In 1951, Danowski et al. showed that the PBI became elevated shortly after birth, reaching its peak in the first three days of life. Man et al. (1952) have demonstrated similar data using the BEI. The PBI is essentially back to adult values by three months of age, although statistically the mean level in the three-month-old is slightly greater than that in the older child or adult. The PBI returns completely to normal by one year of age. In their initial report, Danowski et al. (1951) suggested possible reasons for this. One was an increase in actual circulating thyroid hormone. Others were related to changes in blood volume in the infant or alteration in thyroid-binding proteins in the infant.

In 1956, Dowling et al. showed that the level of thyroid-binding globulin in human cord blood was higher than that in normal nonpregnant adults but lower than that in mothers at term. They suggested that the thyroid-binding globulin capacity was elevated but to a lesser degree in the normal full-size infant than in the mother. In 1961, Marks et al. showed that the triiodothyronine uptake was elevated during the first week of life in normal full-size infants and normal low birth weight infants. These data relating to the elevated triiodothyronine uptake correlated well with the demonstration of Dowling et al. of an increased thyroid-binding globulin capacity. They indicated that the increase in protein-bound iodine was independent of a change in thyroid-binding globulin capacity.

If they had been related one would have expected the binding capacity and the triiodothyronine uptake to decrease when the PBI rose, whereas in fact the reverse occurs.

In 1965, Clark and Horn made an algebraic approximation of the free thyroxine index by using a multiple of the PBI and T_3 uptake. Following their example, Marks (1965) recalculated his data and showed that the free thyroxine index was increased during the first week of life. Subsequently, Marks et al. (1966) indicated that the free thyroxine level, using the chromatographic technique described by Lee et al. (1964), was elevated during the first week of life in comparison to both mothers at term and normal nonpregnant adults and normal children. These data were accumulated on normal, full-size infants. DeNayer et al. (1966) showed that the free thyroxine of cord blood was equivalent to the mother's serum level at term. The cord blood TBPA was lower than the maternal.

A number of workers have shown that the I^{131} uptake in the newborn full-size infant is increased above values for older children and adults. It has been shown by Fisher and Oddie (1963) that the thyroxine excretion rate during infancy is markedly increased above the normal adult values. They demonstrated a thyroxine secretion rate of 18.6 $\mu g/kg/day$ or 246 $\mu g/m^2/day$. This is a marked increase above an adult value of 178 μg/day for the average, 1.73m² adult. On a weight basis it represents a sevenfold increase in thyroxine turnover in the infant. On a body surface area basis it represents a twofold increase in the thyroxine secretion rate.

Utiger (1969) and Fisher et al. (1969) have shown a rise in plasma TSH during the first 24 hours of life. Fisher showed the cord TSH to be substantially greater than the maternal TSH. There was a significant increase from the cord level of 9.1 μU/ml to a value of 85 μU/ml at 30 minutes of age. This level fell rapidly to 3 to 4 hours and then fell more gradually to 10 μU/ml at 48 hours of age. Although delayed cooling will also stimulate TSH, at least in the newborn infant, warming does not prevent the release of TSH as demonstrated by Fisher et al. (1969).

Neonatal Thyroid Pathology

In this section a few relevant areas of clinical pathologic states in normal full-size and low birth-weight infants will be considered. Congenital goiters, congenital hyperthyroidism, and hypothyroidism in the infant will be discussed. Emphasis will be placed on those conditions which involve alterations in the maternal-fetal biologic unit.

Congenital goiters of multiple etiologies have been described in the newborn infant. Among the causes are 1, maternal iodide administration; 2, maternal thiourea administration; 3, congenital thyrotoxicosis; 4, congenital defects of thyroxine synthesis; 5, hematomas of the thyroid; and 6, neoplastic change within the thyroid. Iodine-induced goiter in the newborn appears to be a not uncommon problem as indicated from the pediatric literature. There are reports of infants with strangulation from excessively large goiters of this type. Since the suppression of infantile TSH secretion by exogenous thyroxine or triiodothyronine is not rapid enough to reduce glandular enlargement in these infants, surgery is a necessity in those infants in whom significant signs of airway obstruction exist. In the asthmatic on iodine the substitution of other modes of therapy during pregnancy would be of great advantage to the unborn infant. Thiourea drugs also may give rise to significant thyroidal enlargement and respiratory embarrassment. It is uncommon that such infants will have a derangement of thyroid function. It is believed by Herbst and Selenkow (1965) that the concomitant administration of thyroxine as well as propylthiouracil to the mother will minimize the morbidity and mortality in such newborns.

Goiter has been reported in infants with enzymatic deficiencies of thyroid function at birth; however, it is much more common for such patients to develop goiters later on in infancy and in early childhood. Among the tumors reported to produce thyroidal enlargement in the newborn are hamartomas, hemangiomas, lymphomas, and teratomas.

There are now at least 35 reports of congenital thyrotoxicosis. The author has an additional 5 unreported cases and feels sure that the real incidence of this condition is much higher than reported. Although the goiter found in congenital thyrotoxicosis may be present at birth, it is not infrequent to see this occurrence as late as a week following birth.

Congenital hyperthyroidism is seen in a small proportion of infants of mothers with treated and untreated thyrotoxicosis. In those cases in whom it has been studied, concomitant LATS titres have been found in both the mother and the child. Since LATS may persist in maternal serum for a prolonged period of time beyond the surgical or medical treatment of thyrotoxicosis, it is not unusual to find neonatal thyrotoxicosis in infants of mothers previously successfully treated for Graves' disease. As noted previously, LATS is a 7-S gammaglobulin which freely crosses the placenta in the human from mother to fetus. The work of Kriss (1968), who has isolated LATS with light chains of both the kappa and lambda variety, would seem to indicate that this material is an antibody and not a genetically determined abnormal protein. Sunshine et al. (1965) have demonstrated LATS in the plasma of a thyrotoxic infant up to 21 days. Just what is the exact relationship of this material to thyrotoxicosis in general and specifically to thyrotoxicosis in the newborn is at present unclear. It is apparent, however, that LATS has been found in the sera of those newborn thyrotoxic infants in whom it has been sought.

Congenital thyrotoxicosis is an acute, frequently severe, self-limiting disease. According to the survey of Sunshine et al. (1965) it has about 20 percent mortality rate. Significant symptoms may last up to six weeks to three months of age. Goiter may frequently be present at birth but usually does not appear until three to five days of age and may occur as late as seven or eight days of age. Exophthalmos is present early and will persist beyond the actual period of thyrotoxicosis, frequently being apparent up to a year of age. In general, the hypermetabolic state associated with congenital thyrotoxicosis has subsided by three months of age. Treatment consists of keeping up with the increased fluid and caloric demands of the infant, an attempt at suppression of the thyrotoxicosis with iodine, and treatment of congestive cardiac failure when present. There have been mixed reports on the use of the thiourea drugs in this disease. It does appear on theoretic grounds, however, that they would be extremely useful since their onset of action is too slow for this relatively short-lived disease. There are sporadic reports (Mahoney et al., 1964) on the use of reserpine and guanethidine in managing some of the autonomic aspects of thyroid hormone action during this disease. These reports are still too scattered in the newborn form of Graves' disease to be evaluated accurately.

Hypothyroidism in the newborn period should be considered briefly. Basically there are four types of hypothyroidism that are seen in infancy. These are 1, congenital athyrotic cretinism; 2, congenital goitrous cretinism; 3, iodine lack cretinism; and 4, cretinism secondary to some type of intrauterine insult. These varieties are discussed quite adequately in Wilkins' (1965) excellent consideration of thyroid problems in children. Several points should be mentioned. Although it is very difficult to make a diagnosis of hypothyroidism in the first weeks or months of life, a diagnosis at that time would save a great amount of future morbidity in the affected patient. As mentioned above, infants with congenital goitrous cretinism usually do not have a large palpable goiter in the neonatal period. With the popularity of I^{131} as a treatment for Graves' disease, one must be alert to the possibility of hypothyroidism in the offspring of mothers treated during pregnancy. Almost invariably these are mothers who are unknowingly pregnant at the actual time of their therapy. It is the author's opinion that the infant of any mother who had received I^{131} at the twelfth week of gestation or beyond should be considered hypothyroid and should be so treated.

Conclusion

A number of significant parameters clearly indicate an increase in thyroid function in the newborn period above that seen in older children and adults. To what extent this contributes to the maintenance of day-to-day homeostasis in a small infant with an unfavorable weight-to-body surface area ratio and to the rapid rate of growth found in the normal newborn infant are questions that at this stage remain unanswered.

Three major aspects of neonatal thyroid pathology in the human infant have been considered: 1, goiter; 2, congenital hyperthyroidism; and 3, congenital hypothyroidism.

REFERENCES

Barker, S. B., M. J. Humphrey, and M. H. Soley. 1951. The clinical determination of protein bound iodine. J. Clin. Invest., 30:55.

Chapman, E. M., G. W. Lorner, D. Robinson, and R. D. Evans. 1948. The collection of radioactive iodine by the human fetal thyroid. J. Clin. Endocr., 8:717.

Clark, R., and D. B. Horn. 1965. Assessment of thyroid function by the combined use of the protein-bound iodine and the resin uptake of 131 I-triiodothyronine. J. Clin. Endocr., 25:39.

Danowski, T. S., et al. 1950. Increases in serum thyroxine during uncomplicated pregnancy. Proc. Soc. Exp. Biol. Med., 74:323.

———— et al. 1951. Protein bound iodine in infants from birth to one year of age. Pediatrics, 7:240.

DeNayer, P., et al. 1966. Free thyroxine in maternal and cord blood. J. Clin. Endocr., 26:233.

Dowling, J. T., W. G. Appleton, and J. T. Nicoloff. 1967. Thyroxine turnover during human pregnancy. J. Clin. Endocr., 27:1749.

———— N. Freinkel, and S. H. Ingbar. 1956. Thyroxine binding by sera of pregnant women, newborn infants and women with spontaneous abortion. J. Clin. Invest., 35:1263.

Dussault, J. H., V. V. Row, G. Lickerish, and R. Volpe. 1968. Total triiodothyronine concentration in the serum of pregnant and newborn human subjects: The effect of maternal triiodothyronine administration before parturition. Third International Congress of Endocrinology, Mexico City, 1968.

Evans, T. C., R. M. Kretzchmar, R. E. Hodges, and C. W. Song. 1967. Radioiodine uptake studies in human fetal thyroid. J. Nucl. Med., 8:157.

Fisher, D. A., and T. H. Oddie. 1963. Thyroxine secretion rate during infancy. Effects of estrogen. J. Clin. Endocr., 23:811.

———— H. Lehman, and C. Lackey. 1964. Placental transport of thyronine. J. Clin. Endocr., 24:393.

———— T. H. Oddie, and J. C. Burroughs. 1962. Thyroidal radioiodine uptake rate measurements in infants. Amer. J. Dis. Child., 103:738.

———— and W. D. Odell. 1969. Acute release of thyrotropin (TSH) in the newborn. Pediat. Res., 3:378.

———— C. J. Hoebel, and W. D. Odell. 1969. The fetal-maternal gradient of thyroid function. Pediat. Res., 3:375.

Fisher, P. M. S. 1951. Hyperthyroidism in the first year of life. S. Afr. Med. J., 25:217.

Fisher, W. D., M. L. Voorhess, and L. I. Gardner. 1963. Congenital hypothyroidism in infant following maternal I-131 therapy with a review of hazards of environmental radioisotope contamination. J. Pediat., 62:132.

Galina, M. P., N. L. Annet, and A. Einhorn. 1962. Iodides during pregnancy. New Eng. J. Med., 26:1124.

Gitlin, D., and A. Biasucci. 1969. Ontogenesis of immunoreactive thyroglobulin in the human conceptus. J. Clin. Endocr., 29:849.

Grumbach, M. M., and S. C. Werner. 1956. Transfer of thyroid hormone across the human placenta at term. J. Clin. Endocr., 16:1392.

Hamolsky, M. W., A. Godoletz, and A. S. Freedberg. 1959. The plasma protein-thyroid hormonal complex in man. III. Further studies of the in vitro red blood cell uptake of I^{131}-I-triiodothyronine as a diagnostic test of thyroid function. J. Clin. Endocr., 19:103.

———— M. Stein, and A. S. Freedberg. 1957. The thyroid hormone-plasma protein complex in man. II. A new in vitro method for study of "uptake" of labeled hormonal components in human erythrocytes. J. Clin. Endocr., 17:33.

Herbst, A. L., and H. A. Selenkow. 1965. Hyperthyroidism during pregnancy. New Eng. J. Med., 273:627.

Hodges, R. E., T. C. Evans, J. T. Bradbury, and W. C. Keetel. 1955. The accumulation of radioactive iodine by human fetal thyroids. J. Clin. Endocr., 15:661.

Ingbar, S. H., L. E. Braverman, D. Dawber, and A. Y. Lee. 1964. A simple method for measuring free thyroxine in serum. Clin. Res., 12:271.

Knobil, E., and J. B. Josimovich. 1959. Placental transfer of thyrotropic hormone, thyroxine, triiodothyronine and insulin in the rat. Ann. N. Y. Acad. Sci., 75:895.

Kriss, J. 1968. Inactivation of LATS by anti-kappa and anti-lambda anti-sera. American Society for Clinical Investigation, 60th Meeting, Atlantic City, 1968.

———— V. Pleshakov, and J. R. Chien. 1964. Isolation and identification of the long acting thyroid stimulation and its relation to hyperthyroidism and circumscribed pretibial myxedema. J. Clin. Endocr., 24:1005.

Lee, N. D., R. J. Henry, and O. J. Golub. 1964. Determination of the free thyronine content of serum. J. Clin. Endocr., 24:486.

Lindegren, L., and P. Starr. 1966. Neonatal thyroidology: Correlations of PBI, TBG, bone age and growth. Acta Endocr. (Kobenhavn), 51:77.

Mahoney, C. P., G. E. Pyne, S. J. Stamm, and J. L. Bakke. 1964. Neonatal Graves' disease. Amer. J. Dis. Child., 107:516.

Malkasian, A. D., and W. N. Tauxe. 1965. Uptake of L-triiodothyronine I^{131} by erythrocytes during pregnancy. J. Clin. Endocr., 25:923.

Man, E. B., D. E. Pickering, J. Walker, and R. E. Cooke. 1952. Butanol extractable iodine in the serum of infants. Pediatrics, 9:32.

Marks, J. F. 1965. Free thyroxine index in the newborn. J. Clin. Endocr., 25:852.
———— M. Hamlin, and P. Zack. 1966. Neonatal thyroid function. II. Free thyroxine in infancy. J. Pediat., 68:559.
———— J. Wolfson, and R. Klein. 1961. Neonatal thyroid function. Erythrocyte T uptake in early infancy. J. Pediat., 58:32.
Martin, N. M., and R. D. Rento. 1962. Iodine goiter with hypothyroidism in two newborn infants. J. Pediat., 61:94.
McKenzie, J. M. 1964. Neonatal Graves' disease. J. Clin. Endocr., 24:660.
Mosier, H. D., M. K. Armstrong, and M. A. Schultz. 1963. Measurements of the early uptake of radio-active iodine by the thyroid gland: A method requiring reduced irradiation. Pediatrics, 31:426.
Murphy, B. E. P., and C. J. Pattee. 1964. Determination of thyroxine utilizing the property of protein-binding. J. Clin. Endocr., 24:187.
Myant, N. B. 1958. Passage of thyroxine and tri-iodo-thyronine from mother to fetus in pregnant women. Clin. Sci., 17:75.
Nataf, B. M., E. M. Rivera, and I. L. Chaikoff. 1965. Role of thyrotropic hormone in iodine metabolism of embryonic rat thyroid glands in organ culture. Endocrinology, 76:35.
Nauman, J. A., A. Nauman, and S. C. Werner. 1967. Total and free triiodothyronine in human serum. J. Clin. Invest., 46:1346.
Nicoloff, J. T., R. Nicoloff, and J. T. Dowling. 1962. Evaluation of vaginal smear, serum gonadotropin, protein-bound iodine and thyroxine-binding as measures of placental adequacy. J. Clin. Invest., 41:1998.
Peterson, R. P., and W. C. Young. 1952. The problem of placental permeability for thyrotropic, propylthiouracil and thyroxine in the guinea pig. Endocrinology, 50:218.
Pickering, D. E. 1964. Maternal thyroid hormone in the developing fetus. Amer. J. Dis. Child., 107:567.
Pileggi, V. J., N. D. Lee, O. J. Golub, and R. J. Henry. 1961. Determination of iodine compounds in serum. I. Serum thyroxine in the presence of some iodine contaminants. J. Clin. Endocr., 21:1272.
Schultz, M. A., J. B. Forsander, R. A. Chez, and D. L. Hutchinson. 1965. The bidirectional placental transfer of I^{131} 3:5:3' triiodothyronine in the rhesus monkey. Pediatrics, 35:743.
Shepard, T. H. 1967. Onset of function in the human fetal thyroid: Biochemical and radioautographic studies from organ culture. J. Clin. Endocr., 27:945.
Singh, V. N., and I. L. Chaikoff. 1966. Effects of 1-methyl-2-mercaptoimidazole and perchlorate on the insulin-mediated enhancement of I^{131} incorporated into iodoamino acids by fetal thyroid glands in organ culture. Endocrinology, 78:339.
Spafford, N. R., E. A. Carr, G. A. Lowrey, and W. H. Beierwaltes. 1960. I^{131} labeled triiodothyronine erythrocyte uptake of mothers and newborn infants. Amer. J. Dis. Child., 100:844.
Sterling, K., and A. Hegedus. 1962. Measurements of free thyroxine concentration in human serum, J. Clin. Invest., 41:1031.
Sunshine, P., H. Kusumoto, and J. P. Kriss. 1965. Survival time of circulating longacting thyroid stimulator in neonatal thyrotoxicosis. Implications for diagnosis and therapy of the disorder. Pediatrics, 36:869.
Tanaka, S., and P. Starr. 1959. The binding of thyroxine analogues by human serum protein. Acta Endocr. (Kobenhavn), 31:161.

Utiger, R. D. 1968. Plasma TSH in health and disease: Immunoassay studies. Third International Congress of Endocrinology, Mexico, City, 1968.

Van Middelsworth, L. 1954. Radioactive iodine uptake of normal newborn infants. Amer. J. Dis. Child., 88:439.

White, C. 1912. A foetus with congenital hereditary Graves' disease. J. Obstet. Gynaec. Brit. Emp., 21:231.

Wilkins, L. 1965. The Diagnosis and Treatment of Endocrine Disorders in Childhood and Adolescence, 3rd ed. Springfield, Ill., Charles C Thomas, Publisher, Ch. 6-8.

Part VII

HYPOXIA NEONATORUM

34

Characteristic Metabolic and Functional Responses to Oxygen Deficiency in the Central Nervous System

LUBOR JÍLEK, ELIANA TRÁVNÍČKOVÁ, and STANISLAV TROJAN ● **Institute of Physiology, Faculty of Medicine, Charles University, Prague, Czechoslovakia**

Introduction

Hypoxia is the most frequent cause of brain damage in the perinatal period, and it contributes considerably to the mortality of newborn infants as well as to their morbidity. World statistics indicate hypoxia as the cause of death and of permanent disorders in the function of the central nervous system (CNS) in 70 to 80 percent of injured newborns (Potter and Adair, 1949; Potter, 1952; Nesbett, 1947; Štembera et al., 1964; Štembera, 1967).

The mortality of newborns has decreased significantly during the last few years, but the relative importance of hypoxia as a cause of brain damage in the fetus and newborn is increasing. While the treatment of other potentially lethal states is successful, it is a disturbing fact that only partial success has been attained in combating hypoxic damage of the brain. Consequently, this problem increasingly attracts the attention of obstetricians, neurologists, pediatricians, and physiologists.

This chapter deals mainly with pathophysiologic problems, which have been studied in animal experiments. A more detailed clinical discussion of this topic can be found in obstetric and pediatric monographs (Lesný, 1959; Horský and Štembera, 1967). For initial orientation, some physiologic data will be discussed first (for more details see Ch. 23).

Physiologic Data

SUPPLY OF THE BRAIN WITH BLOOD, OXYGEN, AND NUTRIENTS DURING THE PERINATAL PERIOD

Physiologic data on this topic are still very scanty. The fraction of the cardiac output that goes into the fetal brain is not known. It probably depends upon the development of the weight ratio between the brain and the rest of the body and upon the intensity of energy metabolism in the nervous tissue. It is assumed that the brain of the newborn infant, representing 10 to 11 percent of the total body weight (340 to 360 g), consumes about 50 percent of the total oxygen intake (Diemer, 1968). The brain of adults (weight 1,400 g) represents 2 percent of the body weight and uses approximately 20 percent of the total oxygen consumption under normal conditions and 15 to 20 percent of the cardiac output (Kety, 1955; Hoff et al., 1956).

OXYGEN

The Po_2 in the brain tissue of the newborn lies in the range of 17 to 20 mm Hg (Fig. 1). This assumption follows from the fact that the Po_2 in the umbilical vein is approximately 30 mm Hg and in the umbilical artery 10 to 15 mm Hg (Beer et al., 1955; Wulf, 1967). In adult brain tissue the Po_2 is 50 to 60 mm Hg (Po_2 in arterial blood is 100 mm Hg, in venous blood 45 mm Hg). The oxygen saturation of the blood flowing to the fetal brain in the period just preceding birth is 40 to 50 percent, which means that it contains 8 to 10 percent by volume oxygen (Barcroft, 1946). The relatively high oxygen content in fetal blood under the conditions of low Po_2 is caused by the specific properties of fetal erythrocytes and fetal hemoglobin (Allen et al., 1953; Minkowski and Swierczewski, 1959; Braun, 1960; Slomko and Glowinska, 1961; Huehns et al., 1964) (Fig. 2).

GLUCOSE

Glucose seems to be the main energy substrate for the nervous tissue from the earliest stages of fetal development (Himwich, 1951). The fetal blood glucose level (Nelson method) is approximately 80 mg/100 ml; in adults it is 100 mg/100 ml (Štembera, 1966). Post partum, it frequently decreases to values as low as 20 to 40 mg/100 ml, which is a level that in adults causes serious functional and structural disturbances of the CNS. It is assumed that this decrease is caused by the exhaustion of carbohydrate stores before breast feeding is established and by a still insufficient gluconeogenic mechanism (Znamenáček, 1968).

AMINO ACIDS AND LIPIDS

The concentration of the α-amino-N in the blood of the newborn is about 5 mg/100 ml in contrast to 3 mg/100 ml in the maternal blood (Clementson, 1954).

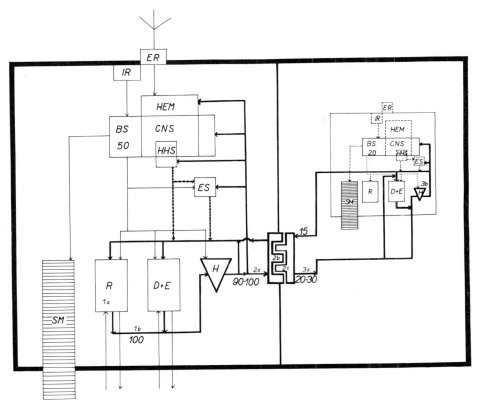

Fig. 1. Scheme of interrelationships in oxygen supply between mother and fetus. CNS, central nervous system; HEM, hemispheres; BS, brain stem; ER, exteroreceptors; IR, interoreceptors; HHS, hypothalamohypophyseal system; ES, endocrine system; SM, skeletal musculature; R, respiratory system; D+E, digestive and excretory system; H, heart. Heavy line, circulation; light line, reflex regulation; heavy and light, humoral regulation. Large numbers, Po₂. Small numbers with the index a, b, c indicate the cause of hypoxia (see p. 993). Interrupted lines, immature regulating systems. Left, mother; right, fetus.

The concentration of FFA is about 0.3 mEq/liter in the newborn and 1.8 mEq/liter in the mother (Šabata et al., 1964). Although the normal structural development of the CNS depends upon these substrates, it is not yet clear whether they take part also in the energy metabolism of fetal nervous tissue under physiologic conditions. This possibility is not generally accepted (Himwich, 1951; Jílek, 1966). The level of these substances in blood is determined mainly by their placental transport (Snoeck, 1958; Villee, 1960; Garmesheva, 1959, 1967).

Transport of nutrients into the brain also depends on the properties of the blood-brain barrier. The blood-brain barrier is more permeable in the immature brain, which holds true especially for amino acid transport (Stern and Peyrot, 1927; Bakay, 1953; Dobbing, 1961; Kassil, 1963; Vernadakis and Woodbury, 1965).

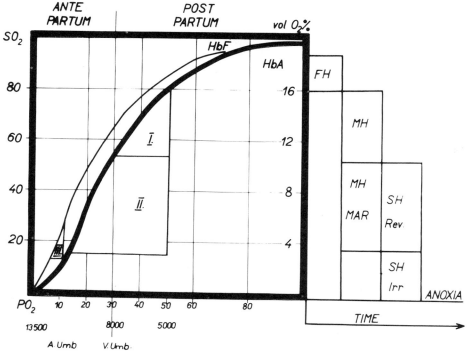

Fig. 2. Scheme of interrelationships between oxygen offer and intensity of hypoxia in the brain. HbA, O_2 absorption curve of adult hemoglobin; HbF, O_2 absorption curve of fetal hemoglobin; Po_2, partial pressure of oxygen; So_2, blood saturation; volume O_2, amount of oxygen in percent. FH, functional hypoxia; MH, metabolic hypoxia; MAR, metabolic adaptive reactions; SH Rev., structural hypoxia, reversible changes; SH Irr., structural hypoxia, irreversible brain damage (see p. 995). A. Umb., umbilical artery; V. Umb., umbilical vein; I, oxygen reserve in adults; I+II, oxygen reserve in newborns; III, oxygen reserve in fetus.

CHARACTERISTICS OF CEREBRAL METABOLISM

The more immature the nervous tissue, the higher is the proportion of anaerobic glycolysis in energy metabolism (Koch and Koch, 1913; Himwich, 1951; Feldberg and Malcolm, 1954; Richter, 1955). The importance of aerobic glycolysis, i.e., the utilization of glucose in the presence of oxygen, which is several times more effective than anaerobic glycolysis in terms of energy production, steadily increases during development. The metabolism of proteins and lipids and also enzyme activities show developmental changes. The development of the metabolism runs parallel to the development of structure and function (see Ch. 23).

METABOLIC RATE IN THE BRAIN

The metabolic rate increases steadily during development (Himwich, 1951; Mysliveček and Jílek, 1953; Richter, 1955). The energy generated during intrauterine life is, in general, used for structural build up, i.e., for proteosynthesis and lipogenesis (myelinization). Postnatally the energy produced is used for further structural maturation, but some additional energy is required for neuronal activity.

In adults functional energy processes predominate. The highest energy requirements are connected with the maintenance of physiologic conditions for the bioelectric and metabolic processes of the excitable membranes (McIlwain, 1955; Jílek, 1966) (Fig. 3).

The metabolic rate in different parts of the brain depends upon the stage of their ontogenetic development. In the immature brain the highest oxygen consumption is in the tissues of the brain stem, whereas in the adult brain it is in the prosencephalon, especially in the cerebral cortex and basal ganglia.

PHYSIOLOGIC CHANGES IN THE SUPPLY OF THE BRAIN WITH OXYGEN AND NUTRIENTS DURING DELIVERY

The blood glucose level of the mother increases during labor by 30 to 40 mg/100 ml (Štembera, 1966), most probably as a result of the activation of the sympathoadrenal system. This mechanism favors the supply of the fetus with glucose. On the other hand, the oxygen supply of the fetus is hampered, mainly in consequence of uterine contractions, which reduce or even temporarily interrupt the uteroplacental circulation.

At the same time, the lactic acid in maternal blood increases and may even exceed the lactate concentration in the umbilical artery (Vedra, 1967). In this case the lactic acid flows from the mother to the fetus. An analogous situation

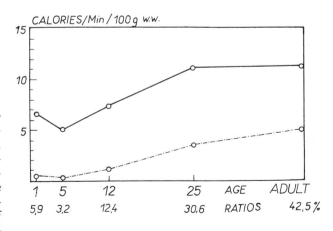

Fig. 3. Development of energy metabolism in brain. Abscissa, age of rats in days. Ordinate, calories / minute / 100g wet weight. Solid curve, in vitro metabolism under aerobic conditions, i.e., resting metabolism. Dashed curve, in vivo metabolism under anaerobic conditions, i.e., basal anaerobic metabolism (see p. 1012). Values given under each age represent the ratio between these two types of metabolism (resting metabolism = 100 percent). (From Jílek. 1966.)

CALORIES/Min / 100 g w.w.

| AGE | 1 | 5 | 12 | 25 | AGE | ADULT |
| RATIOS | 5,9 | 3,2 | 12,4 | 30,6 | RATIOS | 42,5% |

exists also in respect to pyruvic acid and to FFA (Hodr and Štembera, 1959; Hodr et al., 1963). The decreasing supply of oxygen and increasing supply of glucose, lactic acid, and possibly also of other nutrients during labor is quite physiologic. The acid-base balance shifts toward acidosis.

The temporary lack of oxygen, for example during normal uterine contractions, is compensated for by the oxygen stores of the fetus. However, these are small since the oxygen content of the fetal blood, and especially its absolute Po_2, is low. The oxygen reserve is about 50 percent of the Po_2 in the umbilical artery, which means approximately 5 mm Hg Po_2, or 2 percent by volume of oxygen. In adults the Po_2 reserve is 20 mm Hg, that is, around 6 percent by volume O_2. Another compensation for fetal hypoxia can be achieved by an increase of the fetoplacental blood flow which can be up to 30 percent higher (Štembera et al., 1967) (Fig. 2).

The handicap in oxygen supply during labor may be partially compensated for by an increasing supply of glucose and eventually of lactic acid and other nutrients (see p. 991).

The adverse influence of labor on the supply of the fetal brain with oxygen is most marked in primiparas. In subsequent pregnancies the duration of labor decreases, and the possibility of its unfavorable influence on the brain of the fetus diminishes.

The small oxygen reserve of the fetus is one of the causes of brain hypoxia. During intrauterine development the homeostasis of the fetus is ensured mainly by the complex of maternal homeostatic mechanisms. These ensure optimal conditions for the development of fetal tissues, including the nervous tissue, at a time when the fetal regulatory mechanisms are not yet developed. On the other hand, failure of these homeostatic relationships between the fetus and the mother may lead rather quickly to a disturbance in the supply of oxygen, and possibly also of nutrients, to the fetus. If this does occur in the perinatal period in humans, it is the nervous system which suffers the most, since at this time it is already advanced in maturation and consequently more sensitive to changes in the inner environment. Hence, the perinatal period is a time when the CNS is exposed to an unusually high danger of hypoxic damage.

The Main Causes of Perinatal Hypoxia of the CNS

Hypoxia may be caused essentially by disorders of the following functions: 1, homeostasis of Po_2 in the maternal organism; 2, placental transport of oxygen, including disturbances of the uteroplacental and fetoplacental circulation; 3, oxygen transport in the blood; 4, respiratory functions of the newborn.

DISORDERS OF THE Po_2 HOMEOSTASIS IN THE MOTHER

Hypoxic (aerogenic) hypoxia. This is caused by low Po_2 in the environment, e.g., altitude hypoxia; lung diseases, e.g., pneumonia, bronchopneumonia, TB, silicosis, asthma, and so on. They are often combined with hypercapnia. Inhalation anesthesia (NO_2, cyclopropane, and so forth) (1a in Fig. 1).

Anemic hypoxia. Severe anemia, as, for instance, pernicious anemia, hemorrhage, etc. (1b in Fig. 1).

Hypoxia from excessive oxygen consumption. For instance convulsions or exhausting physical activity during the second stage of labor.

DISORDERS OF OXYGEN TRANSPORT IN THE PLACENTA

Disorders of the uteroplacental circulation. These are caused by severe heart failure of the mother, that causes also a disorder of PO_2 homeostasis of the mother; circulatory failure, including the hypotensive orthostatic syndrome; hypertension disease, accompanied by sclerotic changes in the vessels; and vascular spasm in toxemia, prolonged tetanic contractions, diabetes, epilepsy, etc. (2a in Fig. 1).

Disorders of oxygen diffusion through the placental membrane. These disorders are caused by fibrinoid degeneration of the villi in toxemia, prolonged pregnancy, and diabetes; and reduction of the diffusion surface, e.g., premature separation of placenta (2b in Fig. 1).

Disorders of the fetoplacental circulation. These are caused by umbilical cord accidents, e.g., premature clamping of the cord, prolapse of the cord, and so on; spasm of the umbilical vessels (caused by certain drugs); and diminished fetoplacental blood flow, e.g., decrease of the fetal blood pressure (2c in Fig. 1).

DISORDERS OF THE OXYGEN TRANSPORT IN THE FETUS AND NEWBORN

Anemia. Disorders of oxygen transport can be caused by increased destruction or decreased production of erythrocytes, i.e., blood group incompatibility (hemolytic disease of the newborn infant) and anemia accompanying infections and toxemia. Blood loss caused by placental hemorrhage, i.e., placenta previa, premature separation of the placenta; hemorrhage from the umbilical cord, i.e., rupture of the cord, velamentous insertion of the umbilical vessels, varices or aneurysms of the umbilical vessels, excessively short cord; fetomaternal transfusion, i.e., a transplacental backflow of fetal blood into the maternal circulation; blood loss from one twin into the other. Hemorrhage into the organs or body cavities of the newborn. This type occurs during the few first days after birth, and it may be caused by trauma or possibly by disorders in blood coagulation (3a in Fig. 1).

Malformations of the Heart. (3b in Fig. 1).

DISORDERS OF THE RESPIRATORY FUNCTION OF THE NEWBORN

Inhibition of the respiratory center. This often occurs as a consequence of intrauterine hypoxia, the so-called early asphytic syndrome; the inhibiting influence of certain drugs, e.g., morphine, barbiturates, and some other sedatives.

Defective development of lung tissue. This is found especially in premature infants as the so called late asphyctic syndrome.

Disorders of ventilatory functions. These disorders are of the hyaline membranes, aspiration, malformations, and so forth.

This list gives the most important causes of hypoxia (Ylppö, 1924; Potter and Adair, 1949; Wintrobe, 1956; Nesbett, 1957; Lesný, 1959; Lehndorff, 1962; Betke, 1963; Kendall, 1963; Oehlert, 1963; Ullery and Hollenbeck, 1965; Měrka and Horanský, 1966; Opatrný and Tišer, 1966, Hickl, 1967; Štembera, 1967). As a rule, several of the above mentioned factors are frequently combined. The most frequent cause of perinatal hypoxia is toxemia (30 to 40 percent), which creates a combination of disorders of the uteroplacental circulation and of placental transport. Further factors of importance are prolonged pregnancy, placental dysfunction, diabetes of the mother, disorders of parturition, umbilical cord accidents, hemolytic disease, and transplacental hemorrhage.

The Characterization of Hypoxia

Metabolic, functional, and structural changes in the nervous tissue caused by hypoxia are determined by 1, the type of hypoxia; 2, the intensity of hypoxia; 3, the duration of hypoxia; and 4, the stage of maturation of the nervous tissue.

THE TYPE OF HYPOXIA

Hypoxic Hypoxia (Aerogenic)
Cause: Lack of oxygen (low P_{O_2}) in the external environment; disorders in the diffusion of oxygen between the external and internal environments.
Clinical conditions: Disorders of the diffusion of oxygen through the placental membrane (e.g., degenerative changes of the placenta, premature separation of of the placenta); hypoxia of the mother, since the internal environment of the mother is the external environment of the fetus.

Anemic Hypoxia:
Cause: Lowered capacity of the blood to transport oxygen, e.g., decrease of the hemoglobin content of the blood.
Clinical conditions: Hemorrhage, anemia, hemolytic disease, and so forth.

Stagnant Hypoxia:
Cause: Insufficient supply of oxygen and nutrients to the nervous tissue caused by circulatory disorders. It is accompanied by insufficient elimination of catabolites.
Clinical conditions: Umbilical cord accidents, circulatory disorders of the fetus, disorders of the fetoplacental circulation, malformations of the heart, circulatory failure of the newborn, and so on.

Histotoxic Hypoxia:
Cause: Blocking of oxidative enzymes (respiratory chain).
Clinical conditions: Poisoning by CO, cyanides, certain drugs, and so on (Barcroft, 1925; Peters and Van Slyke, 1931).

Hypoxia from Excessive Oxygen Consumption:
Cause: The oxygen consumption in the tissues is increased to such an extent
that it cannot be compensated for by the available sources of oxygen.
Clinical conditions: For instance in the brain by convulsions and in the maternal
organism in protracted second stage of labor (Himwich, 1951).

The most common cause of hypoxic damage to the fetal brain is the combination
of stagnant and hypoxic, and possibly anemic, hypoxia.

THE INTENSITY OF HYPOXIA

From the point of view of intensity, hypoxia can be divided into four groups.
Functional Hypoxia. It is the mildest degree of hypoxia. The organism
maintains O_2 homeostasis by a complex of reflex and hormonal reactions, mainly
by increasing the cardiac output and the respiratory minute volume, by redistribu-
tion of blood, and by activation of the sympathoadrenal and hypothalamohypophyseal systems.
Metabolic Hypoxia. In hypoxia of medium degree of severity, Po_2 and oxygen
supply to the tissues is decreased. The homeostatic systems are no longer capable
of maintaining the Po_2 equilibrium in the internal environment so that hypoxidosis
develops. As a consequence the nervous tissue responds with metabolic changes.
These are, however, not accompanied by structural changes, regardless of whether
the metabolic changes are of a reactive or adaptive character. The changes are
either substantially or completely reversible.
Structural Hypoxia (Destructive). The most severe degree of hypoxia. Metabolic changes exceed the stage of reversibility. Structural changes occur which
are usually irreversible.

The individual parts of the brain are not equally injured by hypoxia. Decisive
factors are their oxygen and nutritional requirements, the rate of metabolic function,
and other characteristics of the metabolism, such as the ratio of aerobic to anaerobic
metabolism. However, it may take a number of minutes to several hours for the
hypoxic changes to appear (Jílek, 1958a, b; Fischer and Jílek, 1958).
Anoxia or absence of oxygen. The functional, metabolic, and structural changes
proceed very quickly, and all parts of the brain suffer at the same time. The biochemical disturbance and the destruction of neurons take place in seconds or
within a few minutes.

THE DURATION OF HYPOXIA

The extent of hypoxic damage is determined not only by the intensity of hypoxia
but also by its duration. The longer the hypoxia, the more severe and pronounced
are its consequences. For instance, long continued functional hypoxia leads to
adaptive changes which can be of functional or metabolic type (Adolph, 1964;
Barbashova, 1964; Dahl and Balfour, 1964; Trávníčková, 1966; Trávníčková et
al., 1967; Trojan et al., 1968a). Prolonged metabolic hypoxia can cause structural
damage in the nervous tissue. If the duration of structural hypoxia exceeds a certain

time limit, the histopathologic changes become irreversible (Jílek, 1958b). The most rapid destruction of the nervous tissue takes place in anoxia.

THE DEGREE OF MATURATION OF THE NERVOUS TISSUE

The developmental stage of the nervous tissue, characterized by its specific metabolic, functional, and morphologic properties, is another important factor which determines the extent of hypoxic changes caused by a certain intensity and duration of hypoxia. In general, the less mature a certain structure of the CNS is, the more able it is to tolerate longer periods of hypoxia without irreversible tissue damage. For example, hypoxia of a certain intensity and duration that leads to structural changes in the tissue of the adult brain, would cause only metabolic changes in the developmentally immature brain. Therefore, the limits of age-specific hypoxia tolerance shift during ontogeny and the time factor becomes increasingly important with maturation. The development of the metabolic rate and of other characteristics of metabolism are of great importance, such as the ratio between aerobic and anaerobic metabolism and the mutual relationships between energy metabolism, proteosynthesis, and biophysical functions (i.e., polarization of excitable membranes).

The present stage of our knowledge and the limited diagnostic procedures do not yet allow an evaluation of the mutual relationship of all these factors that play a decisive role in perinatal hypoxia. This makes both a precise diagnosis and the prognosis of the hypoxia of the CNS very difficult. Hence, the prevention as well as the treatment of hypoxia is still more empiric than causative.

The Tolerance of the CNS of the Fetus and Newborn to Hypoxia and Anoxia

The fate of the organism exposed to hypoxia or anoxia is determined by the reaction of its CNS. This holds true for postnatal life and most probably also for the late stages of intrauterine life. The function of the heart is always less impaired by severe bouts of hypoxia than is the function of the CNS (Jílek and Trojan, 1960c). The relatively high hypoxia tolerance of the reticular formation of the medulla oblongata is very important since it regulates vital functions such as respiration, circulation, digestion, and excretion. With increasing differentiation and maturation the medulla becomes more integrated into the regulatory system of the CNS but along with this change, this tissue loses its hypoxia tolerance.

Thus we can conclude that the degree of maturity of the nervous tissue determines its resistance to hypoxia during the perinatal period. This is well documented by clinical experience as well as by experiments in animals. In the newborn infant the brain stem is relatively advanced in maturation while the higher brain centers are functionally, biochemically, and morphologically immature. The human newborn can survive anoxia lasting 10 to 15 minutes without permanent consequences, whereas the survival time of the adult CNS is 2 to 3 minutes (Smith, 1959; Štembera, 1967; Horský and Štembera, 1967). We might also say that the CNS of the newborn infant is approximately five times more hypoxia-resistant than is that of the adult.

The mammals born with a less mature CNS than man survive longer. For example, the newborn rat or rabbit survives 20 times longer than does the adult, i.e., 40 to 45 minutes. On the contrary, the mammals which are capable of independent life immediately after birth are much more sensitive to hypoxia. For example, the newborn guinea pig is only twice as resistant as the adult. But its intrauterine development lasts 3 times as long as that of the rat (Fazekas et al., 1941; Himwich, 1951; Jílek, 1957; Jílek and Trojan, 1960c; Naiman and Williams, 1964) (Fig. 4).

The decrease of the resistance parallels the course of development of the CNS (Fig. 5).

The high resistance of the immature CNS to hypoxia of certain newborns goes along with (and is at the expense of) a long period of direct dependence on the mother; that is the so-called suckling period.

The interrelationship between the duration of intrauterine development, the degree of the maturity of the CNS at birth, and the duration of the suckling

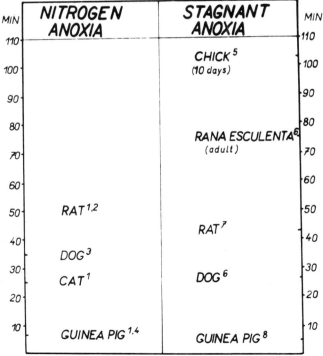

Fig. 4. Survival time of different newborn animals in hypoxic and stagnant anoxia. Ordinate, survival time in minutes. (Data from 1. Fazekas et al., 1941; 2. Hahn, 1953b; 3. Kabat, 1940; 4. Málek, 1947; 5. Jílek and Trojan, 1968; 6. Jílek and Trojan, 1966; 7. Jílek and Trojan, 1960c; 8. Trojan and Jílek, 1968c.)

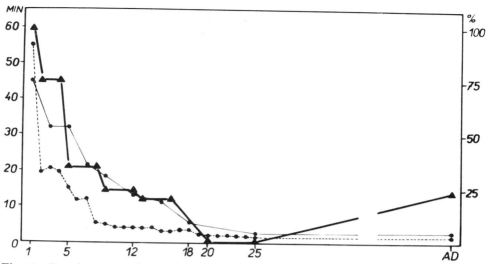

Fig. 5. Development of resistance of rats to stagnant hypoxia (ligature of both a. carotis, thick line), stagnant anoxia (acceleration of 10 *g*, thin line), and aerogenic anoxia (nitrogen anoxia, dotted line). Abscissa, age of rats in days; AD, adults. Ordinate, left, survival time in minutes; right, percent of surviving rats in stagnant hypoxia. (Data from Jílek, 1957; Jílek and Trojan, 1960c; Hahn, 1953b; Mourek, 1958.)

period are complicated, and they are genetically specific for each animal species. We can assume that the CNS of the fetus or of the premature infant will be more resistant to hypoxia than will the CNS of the full-term newborn.

The first reaction of the tissue to hypoxia is found to occur on a biochemical level, but functional and structural changes are inseparable.

Biochemical Responses of the Nervous Tissue to Hypoxia

A more detailed research of metabolic changes produced by hypoxia in the CNS of the human fetus and newborn is quite difficult. Much of our knowledge is gained from animal experiments. However, ontogenic and phylogenic differences among species and in particular between mammals and the human infant have to be taken into consideration, and that makes it quite difficult to extract basic principles pertinent to human pathology.

Most experimental animals, such as the rat, rabbit, dog, and cat, are born with a less mature CNS than the newborn human infant. The brain of a 10- to 12-day-old rat can be compared in some respect to the developmental stage of the brain of a newborn infant (McIlwain, 1955; Jílek, 1966; see also Ch. 23). At this time rapid myelinization starts in the higher parts of the CNS in both of them, neuroblasts are maturing into neurons, and synaptic connections are developing. Anatomic and functional interrelationships are established between the higher and lower parts of the brain, and spontaneous rhythmic EEG activity begins. It is possible to say that in the rat the development of the CNS from birth until the tenth day of life roughly corresponds to the time span from day 210 post conception to birth in man. The developmental period of the rat brain from days 10 to 20 corresponds approximately to the period between birth and 4 months of life in the human infant. These comparisons are, of course, very approximate, and therefore the interpretation of animal experiments in respect to man must be done with great caution.

The heterogeneity of the nervous tissue renders more difficulties in analysis and interpretation of animal experiments. Although the basic characteristics of the metabolism in different neurons and in different parts of the CNS are similar, there are some specific topical differences. For example, the neuroendocrine function and the metabolism of proteins of some centers in the hypothalamus are different from those of the cerebral cortex. The question of the metabolic and functional relationship between glial and nervous elements (Hydén, 1960) and the related problems of the blood-brain barrier are still unsolved in adults and even more open for discussion in developmental physiology.

Furthermore, the difficulties of interpretation are increased by a considerable variability of results since they are obtained by the use of different experimental methods for producing hypoxia or anoxia. This presentation is mainly concerned with investigations of stagnant hypoxia and anoxia, i.e., of oligemia and ischemia of the brain.

Isolated stagnant hypoxia of the brain was produced by ligation of both common carotid arteries (Jílek, 1957). As was shown by Mitchell and Himwich (1966) the rat brain derives approximately 85 percent of its blood via the carotid arteries. The remaining 15 percent is supplied by the a. vertebralis. Stagnant anoxia (ischemia) of the brain was achieved by a positive radial acceleration of 10 g (in the head-tail direction) on a special centrifuge (Jílek and Trojan, 1960c). This procedure stops the venous return and consequently the entire circulation. Under these conditions the blood is concentrated in the lower parts of the body.

Stagnant hypoxia and anoxia interrupt not only the oxygen supply but also the supply of nutrients, such as glucose, amino acids, fatty acids, and so on. In addition, the supply of water and electrolytes becomes restricted, and at the same time the catabolites, such as CO_2 and lactic acid, cannot be removed. Similar events take place in disorders of the uteroplacental and fetoplacental circulations and in disorders of placental transport, and these are the most frequent causes of perinatal hypoxia. Hence, the experimental stagnant hypoxia simulates a pathologic situation frequently found in perinatal hypoxia; however, the experimental procedure does not simulate all etiologic factors.

The majority of our experiments which will be discussed here were performed in white rats of an inbred Wistar strain, kept under standard conditions. The biochemical investigations were performed in brain samples taken from the prosencephalon, which includes the telencephalon (cerebral cortex and basal ganglia) and the diencephalon (thalamus and hypothalamus).

ENERGY METABOLISM, OXYGEN CONSUMPTION, AND HIGH-ENERGY PHOSPHATES

The energy metabolism of the brain can be graded according to its intensity: 1, Functional metabolism. The metabolic rate at a normal level of physiologic activity of neurons and nervous tissue; 2, Resting metabolism. The metabolic rate in the nervous tissue, whose functional activity is inhibited, e.g., by certain drugs, hypothermia, or in in-vitro experiments; 3, Basal metabolism. The metabolic rate that is necessary for the maintenance of the biochemical and biophysical ultrastructure within the limits of reversibility.

In-vivo and in-vitro experiments have shown that immature nervous tissue has a lower functional and resting metabolism than does mature tissue. This fact was demonstrated by measurements of oxygen and glucose utilization. In rat brain the O_2 consumption in vitro increases twice from birth to maturity (Himwich, 1951; Mysliveček and Jílek, 1953). Hypoxia causes a further decrease of the intensity of oxidative metabolism in immature brain tissue. After 4 hours of stagnant hypoxia the water content in the prosencephalon did not change in the young animals. In adults the water content increased slightly but not significantly (Jílek, 1958d; Mourek et al., 1965; Mourek, 1966) (Figs. 6 and 7).

The absolute amount of energy that is necessary for the maintenance of the ultrastructure within the limits of reversibility in the perinatal period is very low under anoxic conditions. It represents only a fraction of the total energy metabolism of the adult brain (Jílek et al., 1965, 1967). During anoxia or hypoxia the immature nervous tissue has not only a low functional and resting metabolism, but also a very low basal anaerobic metabolism.

The changes in energy metabolism during hypoxia can be considered in terms of changes in high-energy phosphates. During aerogenic anoxia the amount of creatine phosphate, ATP, and ADP decreases in the immature nervous tissue much more slowly than in adult brain (Albaum and Chinn, 1953; Samson et al., 1958; Lolley and Samson, 1962; Dahl and Balfour, 1964; Oja, 1966).

These results show that the intensity of energy metabolism in the CNS is of

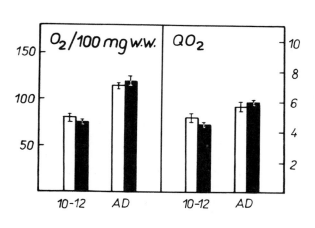

Fig. 6. Oxygen consumption in prosencephalon after 2 hours of stagnant hypoxia (in vitro, Warburg method). Abscissa, age of rats. Ordinate, oxygen consumption in μl. Left, oxygen consumption/100 mg wet weight/hour, right, QO$_2$ =oxygen consumption/ mg dry weight/hour (From Jílek. 1958d. *Sborn. Lék.* 60:242-248.)

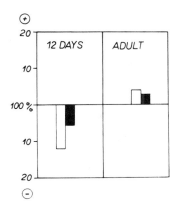

Fig. 7. Relative changes in oxygen consumption of brain tissue after 2 hours of stagnant *hypoxia*. Ordinate, changes in percent. White columns, O$_2$/100 mg wet weight black columns, QO$_2$ (From Jílek, 1958d. *Sborn. Lék.* 60:242-248.)

considerable importance for hypoxia tolerance especially under anoxic conditions. However, the low metabolic rate is not the sole cause of the high tolerance of the nervous tissue to hypoxia in the perinatal period. This is indicated by the fact that the rate of aerobic metabolism in the rat brain doubles postnatally while the hypoxia tolerance decreases more than twenty-fold. Therefore, other specific factors must be involved.

During stagnant hypoxia produced by occlusion of the carotids for 4 hours the concentration of ATP and ADP in the prosencephalon of 12-day-old rats is not decreased, but, on the contrary, it shows a moderate rise. In adult animals these compounds decrease significantly. A similar situation exists during the early stages of stagnant anoxia (Antošová et al., 1967) (Figs. 8 and 9).

From this we conclude that immature nervous tissue, when it is exposed to hypoxia, is able to maintain a balanced energy metabolism, which is necessary for sustaining the ultrastructure within the limits of reversibility. The immature nervous tissue can do that better and for a longer time than can the mature tissue of the adult brain. This is related not only to the low metabolic rate, but also and primarily to a specific metabolic response of the immature nervous tissue to hypoxia (see p. 996).

CARBOHYDRATE METABOLISM. ANAEROBIC GLYCOLYSIS

Glucose is the main substrate for energy metabolism in the nervous tissue during the whole ontogeny. During hypoxia the intensity of anaerobic glycolysis in the nervous tissue increases more in the immature tissues than in the mature and has been called "reversed Pasteur effect." This is indicated by the relatively greater increase in lactic acid in immature nervous tissue in comparison to that in adult tissues (Jílek et al., 1961b, 1962b, 1966b, c; Krulich et al., 1962) (Figs. 10 and 11). The change in pyruvic acid concentration in the immature brain tissue during hypoxia is inconclusive.

The ratio of lactate to pyruvate (L/P) and the so-called lactate excess (XL= $(L_E - L_C) - (P_E - P_C) (L_C/P_C)$ (Huckabee et al., 1962) during hypoxia are much

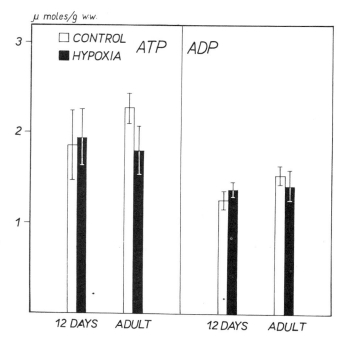

Fig. 8. Changes of ATP and ADP in prosencephalon after 4 hours of stagnant hypoxia (ligature of both carotids) in 12-day-old and adult rats. Ordinate, changes in μ moles/g wet weight. (Data from Antošová et al., 1967.)

lower in immature than in mature nervous tissue (Vorel et al., 1968). Even if we look upon those L/P ratios and XL values critically and cautiously they clearly show that immature nervous tissue suffers less during hypoxia than does mature tissue.

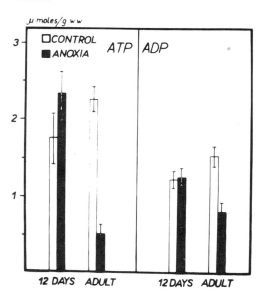

Fig. 9. Changes of ATP and ADP in prosencephalon after 2 minutes of stagnant anoxia (acceleration 10 g) in 12-day-old and adult rats. Ordinate, changes in μ moles/g wet weight. (Data from Antošová et al., 1967.)

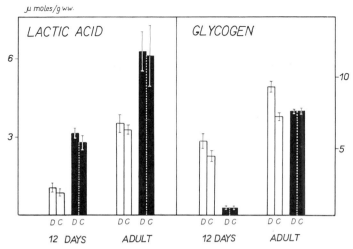

Fig. 10. Glycogen and lactic acid content in brain tissue after 4 hours of stagnant hypoxia in 12-day-old and adult rats. Ordinate, lactic acid (left) and glycogen (right) in μmole/g wet weight. D, diencephalon; C, cerebral cortex. (From Krulich et al. 1962. *Physiol. Bohemoslov.*, 11:58-63.)

Experimental results show that under hypoxic conditions the immature nervous tissue utilizes tissue glycogen more than free glucose. This holds true for both stagnant and aerobic hypoxia (Krulich et al., 1962; Jílek et al., 1966b). The utilization of glycogen is energetically more advantageous than that of glucose since the gain of high-energy bonds is one third higher for the former. However, the glycogen stores in the brain are relatively low in comparison to those in other organs, especially liver and heart. The glycogen content increases rapidly during the period of maturation of the higher parts of the CNS, that is, in rats after the tenth day of life.

The concentration of free glucose in the brain decreases during stagnant hypoxia by approximately 50 percent. This seems to be due to the decreasing supply of

Fig. 11. Relative rise in lactic acid concentration and fall in glycogen content after 4 hours of stagnant hypoxia in 12-day-old and adult rats. Ordinate, relative changes in percent (controls = 100 percent). Black columns, glycogen; white columns, lactic acid. D, diencephalon; C, cerebral cortex. (From Krulich et al. 1962. *Physiol. Bohemoslov.*, 11:58-63.)

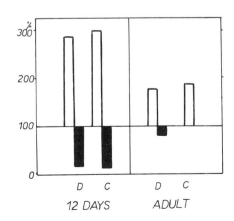

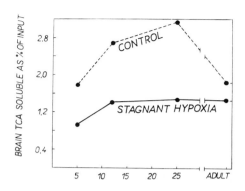

Fig. 12. Penetration of glucose into prosencephalon in control animals and under conditions of stagnant hypoxia (ligature of the carotids). Abscissa, age in days. Ordinate, total soluble TCA, plotted as percentage of original radioactive input (i.p.). (From Haber et al. 1968. *In Ontogenesis of the Brain.* Charles University.)

glucose (Haber et al., 1968) (Fig. 12); furthermore, hypoxia increases the activity of lactate dehydrogenase (LDH) in the prosencephalon, while the activity of succinate dehydrogenase (SDH) is unchanged. This is indicative of an increase of anaerobic glycolysis (Janata et al., 1968). After four hours of stagnant hypoxia the spectrum of LDH isoenzymes is unchanged (Krásný et al., 1967). In the adult the activity of both enzymes is significantly decreased, especially that of SDH, as shown in Figure 13.

The importance of anaerobic glycolysis for the high hypoxia tolerance of the

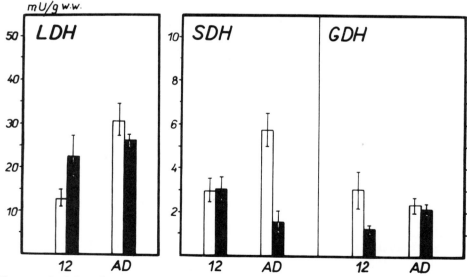

Fig. 13. Activity of lactate (LDH), succinate (SDH), and glutamate (GDH) dehydrogenase in prosencephalon after 4 hours of stagnant hypoxia in 12-day-old and adult rats. Ordinate, enzyme activity in U/minute/g wet weight. White columns, controls; black columns, hypoxia. (Data from Janata et al., 1967.)

immature CNS has been shown in experiments where animals have been treated with monoiodoacetate. This agent blocks the phosphoglyceraldehyde dehydrogenase and thus the Embden-Meyerhof pathway of glycolysis. Newborn animals treated with monoiodoacetate lose their high hypoxia tolerance and become almost as sensitive as adults (Himwich, 1951; Trojan and Jílek, 1960b; Trojan and Jílek, 1962b) (Fig. 14).

This seems to indicate that during hypoxia the immature nervous tissue can increase the intensity of anaerobic glycolysis and that the brain of newborns is able to use thus obtained energy more efficiently than is the mature brain. This, in conjunction with the absolute low rate of energy metabolism, can fulfill the basic energy needs of the immature nervous tissue, including proteosynthesis and the maintenance of the biochemical ultrastructure within the limits of reversibility.

The final response depends of course on both the intensity and the duration of hypoxia. The less intense the hypoxia and/or the shorter the exposure, the more effectively these mechanisms can function.

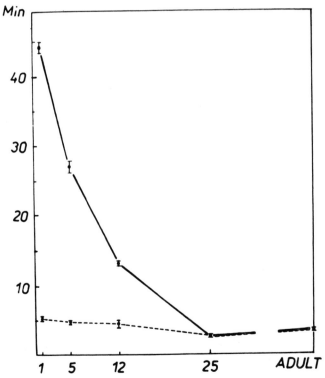

Fig. 14. Influence of monoiodoacetic acid on resistance of rats to stagnant anoxia. Abcissa, age in days. Ordinate, survival time in minutes. Solid curve, control animals; dashed curve, animals treated with monoiodoacetic acid.

AMINO ACID METABOLISM

The total content of free amino acids in the brain increases during ontogeny. This is especially true for glutamic acid (Glu). The other amino acids show minor changes only or decrease during development (Roberts et al., 1950; Ansell and Richter, 1954; Vernadakis and Woodbury, 1962; Agrawal et al., 1966).

Glutamic acid is the most abundant amino acid in the brain. In the perinatal period the pool of Glu, Gln, Asp, and γ-aminobutyric acid (GABA) is relatively small. Hypoxia has no significant effect on the concentration of these amino acids. Only the concentration of Asp decreases slightly, but significantly, during stagnant hypoxia, while the concentration of GABA increases (Dravid and Jílek, 1965) (Fig. 15).

The intermediary metabolism of amino acids, especially Ser, Ala, Asp, Glu, and Gly, is closely related to carbohydrate metabolism (Krebs cycle, oxidative deamination) and naturally to protein metabolism (transamination, proteosynthesis). These relationships change during development. In 5-day-old rats only 15 percent of the carbon of C^{14}-glucose was incorporated into the free amino acids of the brain, while in adults it was 75 percent (Haber et al., 1968). In the immature nervous tissue the incorporation of C^{14}-glucose remained almost unaffected during hypoxia, but in adults it decreased markedly (Fig. 16).

The concentration of free amino acids in immature nervous tissue seems to depend on plasma amino acids. The level of a-NH$_2$-N in the blood plasma of the fetus and newborn is relatively high (Clementson, 1954). At this time the blood-brain barrier is more permeable for amino acids than in the adult (Himwich et al., 1957; Dobbing, 1961).

Figure 17 shows that the activity of glutamic-oxalacetic transaminase (GOT)

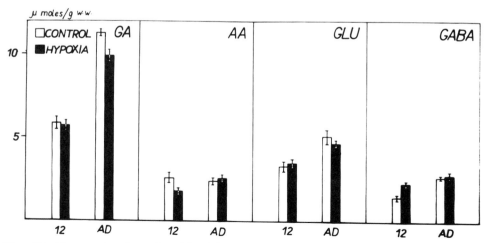

Fig. 15. Changes in glutamic acid (GA), aspartic acid (AA), glutamine (GLU), and GABA levels after 4 hours of stagnant hypoxia in 12-day-old and adult (AD) rats. White columns, hypoxia. (From Dravid and Jílek. 1965. *J. Neurochem.,* 12:837-843.)

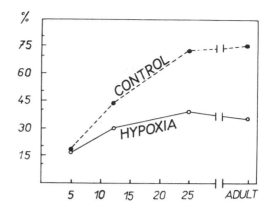

Fig. 16. Conversion of glucose to ninhydrine-positive components in the rat prosencephalon. Abscissa, age in days. Ordinate, NH₃ fraction as percent of input. (From Haber et al. 1968. *In* Ontogenesis of the Brain. Charles University.)

and glutamic-pyruvic transaminase (GPT) in the brain of immature rats is low. During hypoxia the GPT activity increases but the GOT activity does not change. In adult brain the GOT activity is markedly decreased during hypoxia (Janata et al., 1968). Glutamate dehydrogenase activity is decreased during hypoxia in the brains of 12-day-old rats. From these experiments we would like to conclude that during hypoxia the metabolism of amino acids in immature brain is only slightly affected. Furthermore, it seems that aspartic acid is of considerable importance in immature tissue, as was shown by its decrease during stagnant hypoxia. This decrease could affect RNA synthesis, since aspartic acid forms orotic acid, a component for RNA synthesis. The ratio of free Asp to Glu is 1:2 in immature brain tissue, while it is 1:5 in the adult brain.

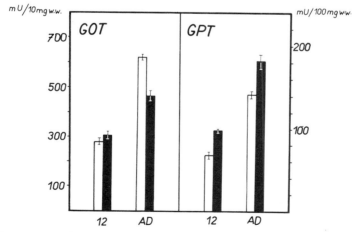

Fig. 17. The activity of glutamic-oxalacetic transaminase (GOT) and glutamic-pyruvic transaminase (GPT) after 4 hours of stagnant hypoxia in 12-day-old and adult (AD) rats. Ordinate, enzyme activity, left, mU/10 mg wet weight; right, mU/100 mg wet weight. (Data from Janata et al., 1960.)

NUCLEIC ACID METABOLISM AND PROTEOSYNTHESIS

Stagnant hypoxia does not change the concentrations of RNA, DNA, or protein in immature nervous tissue, at least not during the first four hours. In adults, on the contrary, the concentration of RNA as well as of protein decreases (Fig. 18).

Stagnant hypoxia increases significantly the rate of proteosynthesis in immature nervous tissue, as shown in vivo by the incorporation of H³-uridine into the cytoplasmic and nuclear RNA. This important effect has been verified by in vitro experiments using the incorporation of C¹⁴-leucine into proteins (in the cell-free system of *E. coli*) (Sirakova et al., 1968). In adults proteosynthesis is markedly depressed by hypoxia (Figs. 19 and 20).

LIPID METABOLISM

The effect of hypoxia on the metabolism of neutral fat, phospholipids, and other lipids has not yet been studied sufficiently. It seems that under hypoxic conditions the concentration of phospholipids decreases in rat brain (Czetverikov, 1966). There it was assumed that the released inorganic phosphate may be used in other metabolic reactions. Whether this also holds true for the immature brain is not yet known.

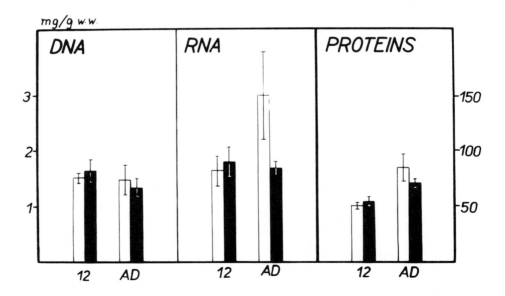

Fig. 18. DNA, RNA, and protein content in the prosencephalon after 4 hours of stagnant hypoxia in 12-day-old and adult (AD) rats. (Data from Sirakova et al., 1968.)

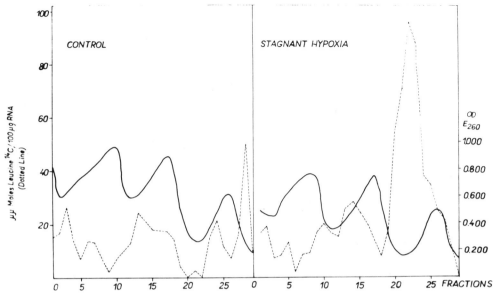

Fig. 19. Template activity of cytoplasmic RNA (fractionated on sucrose density gradient) in a cell-free proteosynthetic system of *E. coli* in 12-day-old rats. Ordinate, OD₂₆₀ = optical density at 260 mµ (solid line). Left, control animals; right, after 4 hours of stagnant hypoxia. (Data from Sirakova et al., 1968.)

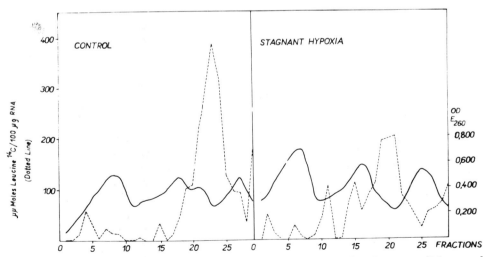

Fig. 20. Template activity of cytoplasmic RNA in adult animals. Same conditions and presentation as in Figure 19. (Data from Sirakova et al., 1968.)

PENTOSE PHOSPHATE PATHWAY (PENTOSE SHUNT)

This alternate pathway of glycolysis and its importance during hypoxia have not been investigated. An increase in the activity of glucose-6-P dehydrogenase (G-6-PDH) during hypoxia shows that this pathway might be more actively used in the immature nervous system of 5-day-old rats (Janata et al., 1968). The changes found in lipid metabolism and the pentose phosphate pathway during hypoxia could be of importance, especially in respect to the rapid postnatal myelinization of the CNS.

PERSPECTIVES

These results show that immature nervous tissue reacts to hypoxia in a specific manner which is distinctly different from the reaction of mature differentiated nervous tissue of adults. Immature tissue adapts metabolically to new conditions of the internal environment. Of prime importance is the decrease in energy requirements, which are already low at this time, and the increase in the proportion of anaerobic glycolysis. Glucose seems to be used as the main substrate for energy production, and the utilization of glycogen is advantageous in terms of effectiveness (ATP yield). Consequently, the energy balance remains positive for a relatively long time during hypoxia, and the concentration of high-energy phosphates remains unchanged. This energy is sufficient to maintain the ultrastructure, as well as to increase proteosynthesis. The activity of some enzymes, such as LDH and GPT, aid and further ensure this complex adaptive process.

In this manner a favorable vital circle is established that ensures a new energy steady state and thus the longer survival of immature nervous tissue in hypoxia. This also facilitates an extensive reversibility of hypoxic changes (see below). This metabolic response has the features of a reaction as well as of an adaptation and has been called the "metabolic adaptive reaction" of immature nervous tissue (Jílek et al., 1968a) (Fig. 21).

On the contrary, the metabolic changes in the adult brain are predominantly passive. The differentiated, mature tissue is unable to maintain an energy homeostasis during hypoxia. Consequently proteosynthesis decreases, enzyme activities diminish, the cellular ultrastructure undergoes destruction, irreversible changes develop quickly, and the neuron dies (Fig. 22).

The metabolic changes which are characteristic for the metabolic adaptive reaction in immature nervous tissue are completely reversible. They are not accompanied by evident disorders of reflex activity. After restitution of normal circulation and normal oxygen supply to the CNS, all experimental animals developed normally, and they did not disclose any permanent neurologic disorders.

In adult rats the biochemical changes were accompanied by clonic-tonic seizures, and 30 percent of the animals died during the hypoxia experiments. The surviving animals had lasting disorders of CNS functions, especially of higher CNS parts.

The metabolic adaptive reaction is most probably initiated by the lack of oxygen; however, the catabolites of anaerobic glycolysis may participate actively since the

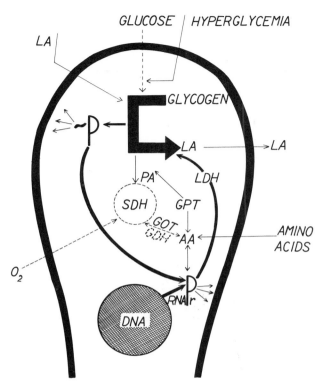

Fig. 21. Scheme of biochemical changes in *immature nervous tissue,* i.e., in 12-day-old rats during stagnant hypoxia. LA, lactic acid; PA, pyruvic acid; AA, amino acids; Pr, proteins; $\sim$P, high-energy phosphate bonds. LDH, lactate- SDH, succinate- GDH, glutamate dehydrogenase. GOT, glutamic-oxalacetic; GPT, glutamic-pyruvic transaminase. Thick lines, increased activities; thin lines, unchanged; interrupted lines, decreased activities.

injection of lactic acid or lactate increased the resistance of immature nervous tissue to stagnant anoxia (ischemia). Lactate treatment had no effect in hypoxic adult animals (Dahl and Balfour, 1964; Jílek et al., 1964). Therefore, it seems to be possible that the increasing amount of lactate that is transferred from the mother to the fetus during labor may have a protective function. This increased transport of lactate is especially marked during protracted labor, when the fetus is most endangered by hypoxia.

The metabolic adaptive reaction was investigated and shown to occur especially under the conditions of hypoxia (oligemia). However, the question remains as to whether similar metabolic processes are also effective during anoxia (ischemia) of the CNS. A study of the concentration of high-energy phosphates shows that this possibility exists in the early stage of anoxia in the immature nervous system (Antošová et al., 1967). It is evident that the metabolic adaptive mechanism needs more time to become effective than there is in the beginning of anoxia. Therefore, it seems that the high tolerance to anoxia (ischemia) in newborns is primarily due

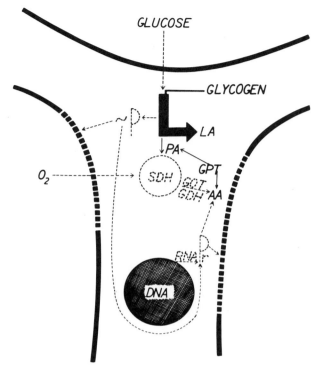

Fig. 22. Scheme of biochemical changes *in mature nervous tissue*, i.e., in adult animals, during stagnant hypoxia. Same abbreviations and presentation as in Figure 21.

to their extremely low rate of the so-called anaerobic basal metabolism of the brain (Jílek, 1966; Jílek et al., 1965, 1967). The immature tissue is able to maintain its biochemical ultrastructure within the limits of reversibility for a relatively long time even at a very low metabolic rate. Both factors are complementary. The active metabolic adaptation is of prime importance during hypoxia, while the passive decrease in the metabolic rate to the lowest possible level predominates during anoxia.

Metabolic, functional, and structural immaturity is the basic condition of the metabolic adaptive reaction. The nervous tissue of the youngest individuals is capable of coping with much broader variations of the internal environment than is the highly differentiated mature brain tissue. In the youngest individuals certain homeostatic mechanisms (reflex and humoral regulations) are not yet developed. Newborns react to changes in the external environment by much greater changes in their internal environment than do the mature organisms.

In the course of ontogenetic and phylogenetic development the reaction and adaptation shifts from the cellular level to the level of the organism as a whole. Immature nervous tissue reacts to the changes of the internal environment more flexibly than do the functionally and metabolically specialized tissues of adult individuals.

During intrauterine life the homeostasis of the fetus is secured by the maternal organism. During labor and in the neonatal period, however, the organism is exposed to big environmental variations which primarily affect the highly sensitive nervous tissue. Under these conditions, the most effective protection is provided by a metabolic adaptation at the cellular level. This mechanism disappears in the course of development along with increasing structural differentiation and functional specialization, and it becomes replaced by the more effective system of reflex and humoral regulations.

That adaptation is part of the mechanism operating in hypoxia confirms the fact that stagnant hypoxia (oligemia) increases the resistance of immature nervous tissue to stagnant anoxia (ischemia). In adults, on the contrary, previous oligemia lowers the resistance (Trojan and Jílek, 1960a, 1962a) (Fig. 23).

The direct, metabolic adaptation of immature nervous tissue to changes in the internal environment, especially to hypoxia, has a broader biologic meaning. The resistance to anoxia (ischemia) is increased during stagnant hypoxia, aerogenic hypoxia (Jílek et al., 1968b), anemic hypoxia (Trávníčková et al., 1962), and histotoxic hypoxia. The last can be induced experimentally by inhibitors of aerobic reactions, such as malonate, arsenitate, arsenate, and cyanate (Jílek et al., 1963). Pretreatment with these types of hypoxia lowers the anoxia tolerance in adults.

The hypoxia and anoxia tolerance of immature nervous tissue is primarily due to its ability to adapt metabolically to new environmental conditions on the cellular level, and, furthermore, it is facilitated by the basically low level of energy metabolism and the relatively high contribution of anaerobic glycolysis.

The question remains whether immature human nervous tissue has similar properties.

Functional Responses of Immature Nervous Tissue to Hypoxia

The functional changes during hypoxia are closely related to metabolic changes. The functional status of the nervous tissue depends directly on the supply of energy.

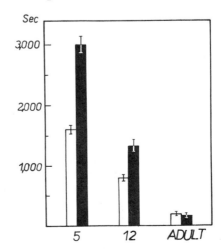

Fig. 23. Influence of 4 hours of stagnant hypoxia (ligature of both carotids) on resistance of the CNS to stagnant anoxia (acceleration 10 g). Abscissa, age of rats in days. Ordinate, resistance in seconds of survival time. (Data from Jílek et al. 1968a.)

Primarily, energy is needed for the maintenance of the membrane mechanisms, such as the polarization of the membranes, and consequently normal excitability and function of the neurons. The energy requirements for the function of the neurons are very high. Neuronal function stops as soon as the level of energy metabolism drops below a certain limit. However, the disappearance of function does not indicate that the neuron has been destroyed. The basal metabolism is able to maintain the ultrastructure of the neuron within the limits of reversibility for a relatively long time, even after function has discontinued. This is especially true for immature nervous tissue. Hence, disappearance or disorders of the function of a certain part of the CNS during hypoxia depend on the stage of its developmental maturity. The more mature a certain brain region is, the more it will suffer from hypoxia. The metabolic, functional, and structural maturity of the CNS are closely related. The functional development of the CNS simulates the phylogenetic evolution to a certain extent (Himwich, 1951; Volochov, 1951). In the perinatal period the lower, phylogenetically older parts of the CNS are more differentiated and functionally developed than the higher, newer parts of the brain. Therefore, they also make greater demands on energy supply. This makes them more sensitive to oxygen deficiency.

The signs and symptoms of hypoxic disorders of the CNS during the prenatal period in man are still uncertain and not completely understood. Only the changes in heart function and the changes of intestinal motility, such as alterations of the heart rate and sounds and meconium that appears in the amniotic fluid during hypoxia, are accessible for diagnostic purposes (Huffman, 1960; Eastman and Hellman, 1966; Tenney and Little, 1961; Reid, 1962; Ullery and Hollenbeck, 1965; Horský and Štembera, 1967). However, no uniform opinion exists on how to evaluate such findings. Marked alterations of heart action need not be accompanied by any manifest changes of the function of the CNS, and, on the contrary, in some cases of severe hypoxic damage to the CNS no alerting intrauterine symptoms were found. A direct influence of hypoxia on the cardiac conductive system and/or on the heart muscle, or on the intestinal smooth muscles, in addition to disorders of reflex regulations, has to be considered in such cases, and it might explain some discrepancies.

One of the reasons for these diagnostic difficulties is our limited knowledge of the functional development of the human CNS during the perinatal and early postnatal periods.

The nervous system of experimental animals is much more simply organized than is the human brain. The interpretation of experimental research on functional changes due to hypoxia is in general more difficult than the interpretation of biochemical changes. The basic metabolic characteristics of the nervous system are more similar among different species than are functional characteristics. Nervous regulatory functions develop in the course of ontogeny and phylogeny in a more complicated manner than does metabolism. The highest stage of integration among different regulatory systems has been attained in man. This integration permits the most accurate adaptation to environmental changes, and, in addition, enables the human being to actively transform and change his environment. Furthermore, it forms the basis for mental functions.

For the evaluation of disorders of the CNS that have been caused by hypoxia, it is necessary to remember that only the reflex mechanisms which are already mature and thus functioning are accessible to neurologic examination. For instance, hypoxia may cause damage to the immature cerebral cortex of newborn infants, but this damage remains at first latent, since, at that time, the cerebral cortex is not yet fully operating (Windle, 1940, 1967; Preston, 1945; Campbell et al., 1950).

This damage may, however, disclose its fatal consequences later in life. The development of the CNS proceeds according to the genetic information, but at the time when the integration of the injured or destroyed brain areas becomes a necessary condition for the normal course of reflex regulatory functions, a disintegration of the central regulations ensues. In the perinatal period the function of the lower parts of the CNS, that is, the brain stem and spinal cord, is largely independent and relatively simple. Later in life and in the course of further brain differentiation and specialization functional development requires the establishment of interrelations between higher and lower parts of the brain. If the higher brain centers are damaged by hypoxia or other factors, a developmental conflict occurs that hampers the organism seriously or may even lead to death.

From these facts we conclude that in the perinatal period it is very difficult to assess the extent of damage to the somatic or autonomic functions of the CNS caused by hypoxia. In pediatrics several indices for the estimation of the intensity of hypoxic brain damage are in use, such as changes of muscle tone, intensity of the baby's cry, type of respiration, skin color, and so forth. These signs are in use for several systems of evaluation (Apgar et al., 1955). However, in human infants the consequences of perinatally acquired brain damage do not usually appear to the full extent before the third or fourth month of life. This fact restricts the efficiency of all therapeutic measures. Mental retardation and motoric disorders appear even later.

Perinatal hypoxia may eventually lead to "late death," as it is known from clinical experience and from experimental observations in animals (Jílek, 1957).

Functional hypoxic disorders can be divided into two main groups: 1, instantaneous disorders, which appear during hypoxia and which are more or less reversible; 2, lasting disorders which are caused by irreversible damage of certain parts of the CNS during the perinatal period.

INSTANTANEOUS FUNCTIONAL DISORDERS OF THE CNS

In the perinatal period, the brain stem, and especially the reticular formation, dominates reflex regulatory activity, whereas in adults the higher parts of the brain dominate, especially the cerebral cortex. In newborn rats (from birth until day 10) stagnant hypoxia injures mainly the coordinating functions of the brain stem, that is, the reticular formation of the medulla oblongata and pons. This is evident from disorders of the sucking reflex and of the primitive righting reflexes. Starting from days 10 to 12, hypoxia causes an increase in spontaneous motor activity, opisthotonus, and rotation around the longitudinal axis. From days 14 to 16, when the rats open their eyes, clonic-tonic seizures appear, which resemble experimental

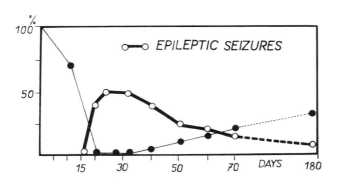

Fig. 24. Development of susceptibility to epileptic seizures, caused by stagnant hypoxia of the brain in rats. Abscissa, age in days. Ordinate, percent of animals with epileptic seizures (thick line); thin line, development of resistance to ligation of the carotids. (From Jílek. 1958b. *Physiol. Bohemoslov.*, 7:356-362.)

epilepsy. The frequency of the seizures reaches its maximum in the transitory period of life, that is, the time when the animals become capable of an independent life, the so-called weaning period (Fig. 24). In adults, hypoxia-induced seizures are less frequently observed, and disorders of cortical functions dominate. Hence it is obvious that during the perinatal period hypoxia damages particularly those parts of the brain that are most mature at that time, that is, the brain stem (Jílek, 1958b). This observation has been confirmed by histopathologic examinations. In the brains of 10- to 12-day-old rats the most profound changes are found in the medulla oblongata, in the pons, and in the corpus striatum, while in adults the lesions are preponderant in the cerebral cortex. The gradient of functional and structural damage shifts during development from the phylogenetically older parts to the higher, developmentally younger parts of the brain (Himwich, 1951; Fischer and Jílek, 1958, 1965; Fischer et al., 1962) (Fig. 25).

Disorders of central regulatory functions occur apparently not only in the somatic sphere, but also in the autonomic sphere. Isolated stagnant hypoxia of the brain causes a rise of blood glucose and lactate and an increase of the activity of LDH in blood plasma. Hyperglycemia and hyperlactacidemia increase the resistance of immature nervous tissue to hypoxia and anoxia. The cause of the favorable influence of hyperlactacidemia on the resistance to hypoxia is not clear. Perhaps it can

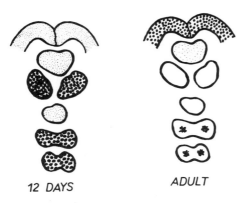

12 DAYS   **ADULT**

Fig. 25. Gradient of histopathologic damage caused by ligation of both carotids for 8 hours. From top to bottom, cerebral cortex, thalamus, corpus striatum, hypothalamus, pons, and medulla oblongata. The darker the area, the greater the damage. (From Fischer and Jílek. 1958. *Sborn. Lék.*, 60: 346-354.)

stimulate in an unspecific way the development of the metabolic adaptive reaction (Vorel et al., 1969).

THE DYNAMICS OF HYPOXIC CHANGES

Functional, structural, and biochemical changes have particular dynamics which depend on the stage of development of the nervous tissue. Irreversible changes do not develop immediately but develop gradually in the course of exposure to hypoxia or anoxia. Therefore, it is possible to distinguish between revival time and survival time of brain functions. A certain reflex activity disappears or becomes defective sooner or later after onset of hypoxia. But even after it has disappeared, complete restitution is possible if the supply of oxygen or nutrients is resumed in time, that is, during the revival time. The survival time includes the occurrence of irreversible brain damage.

Therefore, we distinguish among initial functional disorders, the full development of functional changes, and the onset of irreversible brain damage. An analysis of the consequences of temporary oligemia reveals that in immature nervous tissue (12-day-old rats) the initial changes, the full development of the reflex disorders, and the terminal changes appear almost simultaneously. In adults, on the other hand, a relatively long time interval was observed between initial symptoms and the onset of irreversible damage (Jílek, 1958a, c).

In the perinatal period the first warning symptoms of disorders due to hypoxia appear shortly before the onset of changes which are either irreversible or which can be restored only to a small extent. This is due to specific properties of the immature CNS. As a rule the first disturbances of brain functions appear in the brain stem. At this period of life the brain stem is relatively mature, and at the same time it is also a very important regulatory system for other brain functions. Hence, the first signs of hypoxic damage appear late, because the warning by rapidly developing cortical symptoms is absent. In adults, these cortical symptoms make it possible to apply a more or less effective treatment in time.

The occurrence of irreversible changes in the immature brain is substantially slower than in adults. The metabolic adaptive reaction maintains hypoxic changes within the limits of reversibility for a long time. The duration of this time limit depends on the intensity of hypoxia and on the stage of brain development. The brains of 12-day-old rats survive oligemia for 4 hours without any consequences, while under the same conditions 30 percent of adults die; the surviving adult animals have a diminishing ability to develop conditioned reflexes (Jílek et al., 1968a). Newborn rats survive ischemia of 44 minutes without any consequences; in adults exposure for only 2 minutes causes permanent cortical damage (Jílek et al., 1962).

Immaturity of the CNS has, from the clinical and biologic standpoint, advantages as well as disadvantages. On one hand, immaturity is the cause of the high resistance of the CNS to different changes in the internal environment; on the other hand, it greatly limits the diagnostic exploration. Therefore, a rapid and objective diagnosis of imminent hypoxic damage must be of prime interest to the experimenter, as well as to the clinician.

Stagnant hypoxia and anoxia lead to changes which often recede a long time after normal circulation in the brain has been reestablished. The dynamics of the functional, metabolic, and structural changes do not run parallel. In 12-day-old rats, for instance, the metabolic changes caused by ischemia return to normal within 4 hours (measuring brain glycogen and lactic acid), but during the following 48 hours the concentration of lactic acid in the brain increases significantly again. The structural changes, on the contrary, show signs of an extensive repair at the same time (Fig. 26). Functional disorders, however, are permanent and become manifest in a markedly diminished ability to learn (development of conditioned reflexes). In adults the order of changes during hypoxia is completely different (Jílek et al., 1966c).

The duration of biochemical and structural changes after acute hypoxia and their dynamics are of practical significance from the standpoint of repeated attacks of hypoxia. Repeated exposure of the brain to hypoxia is not rare in clinical practice. Repeated hypoxia may lead to an accumulation of hypoxic changes and to an increase in severity of hypoxic damage. This depends on the time intervals between the hypoxic exposures and on the intensity of the foregoing hypoxic damage (Jílek and Trojan, 1967a; Trojan and Jílek, 1968a, b).

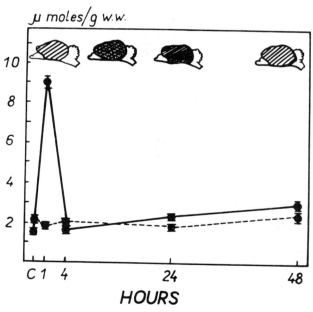

Fig. 26. Dynamics of biochemical and structural changes in hemisphere due to stagnant anoxia of 12 minutes in 12-day-old rats. Abscissa, C, control animals, 1, immediately after ischemia; 4, 24, 48 hours after ischemia. Ordinate, μmoles/g wet weight. Solid curve, lactic acid; dashed curve, glycogen. Schematic drawings of the brain demonstrate intensity of histopathologic changes; the darker the area the greater the changes.

HISTOPATHOLOGIC CHANGES

Analysis of the histopathologic changes showed that there are specific structural differences between mature and immature nervous tissue, and also among the consequences of different intensities of hypoxia. It is very difficult to foresee the further fate of the nervous tissue from only the extent and type of histopathologic changes. For instance, extensive structural changes in immature tissue, such as vacuolization and edema, are for a great part reversible, while the prima vista much smaller changes in adults are a sign of the death of the neuron (Fischer and Jílek, 1958, 1965).

PERMANENT EFFECTS OF BRAIN HYPOXIA AND ANOXIA

The permanent effects of brain hypoxia and anoxia are the most serious clinical problem of perinatal brain damage. The immature nervous system is very resistant to acute hypoxia, but permanent, i.e., irreversible changes develop if the intensity and/or duration of hypoxia exceeds a certain limit. The more developed the brain is, and the more intensive and longer the hypoxia lasts, the more serious are the permanent brain damages.

Very immature nervous tissue is not permanently damaged even by relatively intensive hypoxia or long-lasting anoxia. All newborn rats survived the permanent ligature of the carotid arteries. At the age of 12 days more than 30 percent of the animals survived. The surviving individuals had no disorders of unconditioned reflex activity 3 months after oligemia, and they developed conditioned reflexes as well as did the controls. However, the differentiation and extinction of conditioned reflexes were disturbed. The predominance of excitation over inhibition in the sphere of conditioned reflexes was the only lasting effect in these animals (Jílek and Fischer, 1959) (Fig. 27).

Histopathologic analysis showed in these experiments only a moderate decrease of the number of cortical neurons. We observed no changes in other parts of the brain. It is of interest that during acute hypoxia, significantly smaller changes occurred in the brain cortex than in the brain stem. However, three months later the histopathologic deficits, mainly the decrease of the neuronal population, were

Fig. 27. Conditioned reflexes, differentiation, and extinction in adult rats (3 months old), which have survived the ligation of both common carotids at age of 12 days. White columns, controls; black columns, after ligation. (From Jílek and Fischer. 1959. *Activ. Nerv. Sup.* (*Praha*), 1:223-227.)

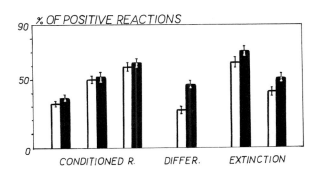

evident only in the cerebral cortex, whereas the lesions in the brain stem were repaired practically ad integrum. It seems that the cerebral cortex is the most vulnerable part of the brain in the entire course of ontogeny. The higher parts of the brain are first in order to be subjected to permanent damage by intensive and/or long-lasting hypoxia. The functional and structural reversibility of hypoxic effects seems to be less in the higher than in the lower parts, although the brain stem suffers more in acute hypoxia. A similar situation exists in stagnant anoxia, i.e., in ischemia. One-day-old rats survive stagnant anoxia 20 times longer than adults, and 5-day-old rats survive 10 times longer. In addition, such a long-lasting anoxia does not change the ability to develop extinct conditioned reflexes in newborn rats. Permanent effects of anoxia start to appear after day 12, if the duration of ischemia was at least 12 minutes (Jílek et al., 1962a) (Fig. 28).

Immature nervous tissue can survive not only longer and more intensive hypoxia than the mature tissue, but also the damaging effects of hypoxia in this tissue are much smaller.

EARLY CEREBRAL PALSY (THE ASPHYCTIC SYNDROME)

In the perinatal period permanent brain damage in man becomes manifest clinically as so-called early cerebral palsy. This syndrome has four basic types: hemiparetic, convulsive, hyperkinetic, and apathic. Most frequent is the paretic type which turns into a spastic type after the second year of life. The topics of these disorders, i.e., their localization in the brain, are not yet fully clear. Pathologists localize these lesions mainly in the brain stem, in the basal ganglia, and in the cerebral cortex. The complete analysis of these functional disorders is the task of

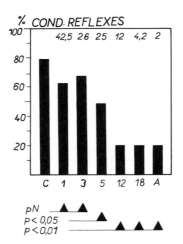 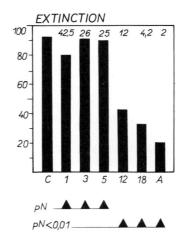

Fig. 28. Conditioned reflexes and extinction in rats which were exposed to stagnant anoxia at different ages (days of life) and which were tested 3 months later. Abscissa, age in days for hypoxia treatment; A, adults. Numbers over the columns indicate duration of brain ischemia in minutes; C, control values. Ordinate, percent of positive reactions. (From Jílek et al. 1962a. *Čas. Lék. Česk.*, 101:656-659.)

the neurologist and pathologist. Statistics show that hypoxia is the cause of perma-nent brain damage in 75 to 85 percent of all cases. The CNS may be injured by hypoxia in the prenatal, intranatal, and postnatal periods.

Prenatal and/or intranatal hypoxia can damage the respiratory center and thus produce the so-called early asphyctic syndrome, caused by insufficient respiratory function after birth, which leads to aerogenic (hypoxic) hypoxia. In these patients a vicious cycle of effects can be established and finally cause permanent injury of central regulatory functions.

In man the cerebral cortex with its mental functions is especially vulnerable. Consequently perinatal hypoxia reaches not only into the domain of the pediatrician (the asphyctic syndrome) and neurologist (early cerebral palsy) but also into the domain of the psychiatrist and educator (perinatal encephalopathy).

Every year several hundred thousand newborn infants in the world are perma-nently injured by perinatal hypoxia. Medical science now helps save the lives of the majority of them but very often at the price of permanent somatic and mental disability. Therefore, the early diagnosis of cerebral injury due to hypoxia is of great importance. However, because of functional immaturity at birth, the neurolo-gist cannot detect permanent brain disorders with certainty earlier than several weeks or even months after the damage has occurred. It can be expected that an early and reliable diagnosis of brain injury will undoubtedly be improved by the further development of electrophysiologic diagnostic methods, such as prenatal and postnatal EEG, EKG, evoked potentials, changes of tissue impedance and polariza-tion, and so forth.

Adaptation of Immature Nervous Tissue to Hypoxia and Anoxia

Immature nervous tissue can adapt to changing conditions of the inner environ-ment either directly and immediately (the metabolic adaptive reaction), or by true adaptation.

The metabolic adaptive reaction is a process whose main components are met-abolic changes which develop directly under the influence of hypoxia, or subse-quent to other changes of the internal environment. These changes outlast the influence of hypoxia for only a short time, and metabolism returns relatively quickly to the normal state. The adaptive reaction is conditioned by the immaturity of the nervous tissue, and it is based on metabolic changes at the cellular and molecular level. This does not occur in mature tissue. True adaptation is a complex process with metabolic, functional, and possibly also structural components. It develops under the conditions of repeated and/or long-lasting hypoxia. It outlasts the stressor for a relatively long time. It is not limited by the developmental stage and therefore it can occur in the immature as well as in the mature nervous system (Adolph, 1956, 1964; Barbashova, 1964, 1967; Trávníčková, 1966, 1968; Trojan and Jílek, 1968b).

As can be expected, the adaptation of the developmentally immature organism to hypoxia will be different from the adaptation in adults. During early developmental stages metabolic components are probably predominant, while in adults the main components are functional.

The fetal CNS develops and grows under conditions that are hypoxic only from the standpoint of the adult organism. Under certain pathologic circumstances, however, the fetal CNS can be exposed to a long-lasting and intensive hypoxia, or to some other long-lasting changes of the internal environment. For example, this occurs in hemolytic disease, in diabetes of the mother, toxemia, tuberculosis of the mother, and so forth. Some of these conditions exist also in postnatal life, as for instance in congenital heart disease, in anemias, and so on.

According to animal experiments immature nervous tissue is capable of adapting to repeated and/or long-lasting changes of the internal environment.

Repeated stagnant anoxia (ischemia, acceleration of 10 g) markedly increases the resistance of immature nervous tissue to this stressor (Fig. 29). The intervals between the individual exposures to anoxia are of great importance. If the intervals are too long (24 hours in the rat), adaptation does not develop. If they are too short, and thus the stressors too frequent (2-hour intervals, 4 times daily), the effects accumulate and lead to irreversible brain damage. Hence, there is not only a time limit for the duration of anoxia (i.e., revival time) but also an optimal time interval (4 to 6 hours) for the development of adaptation.

The younger the nervous tissue developmentally, the more pronounced are the adaptive changes. In newborn rats adaptation has significantly more favorable effects than in older animals, that is, after 12 days of age (Trojan and Jílek, 1964; Jílek and Trojan, 1967a).

Repeated stagnant hypoxia (oligemia, acceleration of 5 g) also causes an adaptation but not as marked as in the case of repeated anoxia (Trojan and Jílek, 1968a, b).

Repeated hemorrhage (i.e., a long-lasting decrease of the Hb content, post-

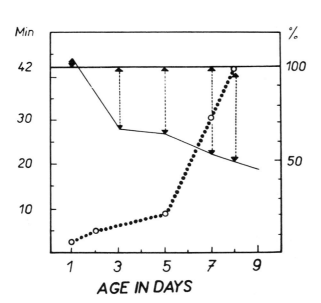

Fig. 29. Survival time and mortality of rats exposed to repeated stagnant anoxia lasting 42 minutes from first day of life. Abscissa, age in days. Ordinate, left, survival time in minutes (solid line); right, mortality in percent (dotted line). Arrows indicate the differences in survival time in minutes. (From Trojan and Jílek. 1964. *Physiol. Bohemoslov.*, 13:473-477.)

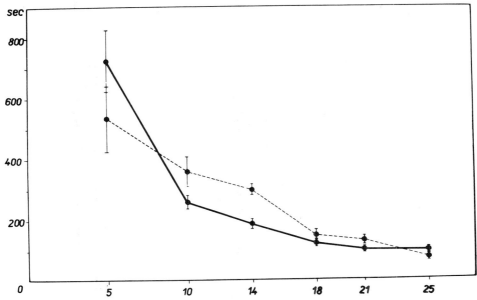

Fig. 30. Influence of repeated blood loss on resistance to hypoxic (nitrogen) anoxia. Abscissa, age of rats in days. Ordinate, survival time in seconds. Solid curve, controls; dashed curve, after repeated blood loss. (From Trávníčková et al. 1962. *Physiol. Bohemoslov.*, 11:231-235.)

hemorrhagic anemia, anemic hypoxia) performed 6 times within the period of days 1 to 12 of age significantly increases the tolerance of the CNS to hypoxia and stagnant anoxia. It is remarkable that the great increase in resistance coincides in time with the absolutely greatest decrease of the Hb content in the blood. The adaptive changes outlast the last hemorrhage by 13 to 23 days (Trávníčková, 1962, 1966; Trávníčková et al., 1964) (Figs. 30 and 31). EEG studies showed that the development of adaptation in the reticular formation of the medulla oblongata precedes that in the cerebral cortex, but the adaptive changes in the cerebral cortex last longer (Trávníčková et al., 1967) (Fig. 32).

Adaptation to anemic hypoxia becomes manifest not only in the CNS but also in changes in the synthesis of hemoglobin. In bled animals the synthesis of fetal hemoglobin (HbF) is prolonged into postnatal life (Trávníček et al., 1966) (Fig. 33).

The long-lasting histotoxic hypoxia that can be produced by repeated injections of sodium arsenite or sodium arsenate in early postnatal life also significantly increases the tolerance of nervous tissue to anoxia (Trojan and Jílek, 1967b; Trojan et al., 1967a, b).

The basic factor of adaptation in the immature brain is a metabolic change. Functional and endocrine factors do not participate. It seems that similar metabolic processes occur in adaptation and in the adaptive reaction. These are a decrease in oxidative metabolism as measured in vitro (Trojan et al., 1968b), an increase of glycolysis, as found in vivo (Trávníčková, 1968), and an unchanged level of

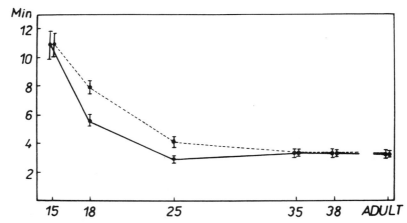

Fig. 31. Influence of repeated blood loss on resistance to stagnant anoxia. Abscissa, age
of rats in days. Ordinate, survival time in minutes. Solid curve, controls; dashed
curve; rats after repeated blood loss. (From Trávníčková et al. 1962. *Physiol.
Bohemoslov.*, 11:231-235.)

free amino acids, as observed in the brain of adapted animals (Trávníčková, 1968).

These observations lead to the conclusion that a true metabolic adaptation occurs
in immature nervous tissue that is exposed to various changes of the inner environment. Our knowledge, however, is sparse at the present time, and future research
has to elucidate the mechanisms essential for these adaptational processes.

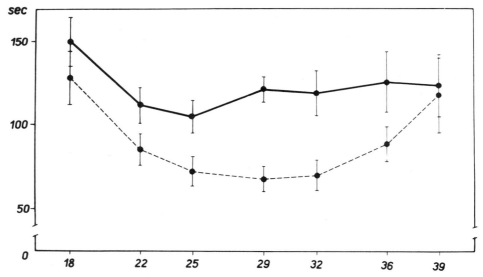

Fig. 32. Duration of electric silence caused by altitude hypoxia (simulated altitude of
12,000 m) in control rats (solid curve) and after repeated blood loss (dashed
curve). Abscissa, age in days. Ordinate, duration of electric silence in seconds.
(From Trávníčková et al. 1967. *Physiol. Bohemoslov.*, 16:153-159.)

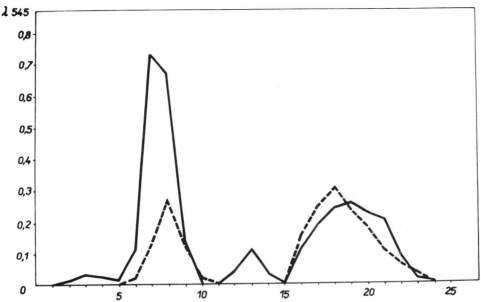

Fig. 33. Fractionation of hemoglobin on CM-sephadex in 21-day-old rats. Ordinate, extinction at wave length 545 mμ. Solid curve, controls; dashed curve, rats after repeated blood loss. (From Trávníček et al. 1966. *Physiol. Bohemoslov.*, 15: 175-178.)

None of the factors mentioned interferes with the development of unconditioned reflex activity or with the ability of learning, providing that they lead to the development of adaptation (Trávníčková, 1966; Trojan et al., 1968, 1969).

Some Problems of Prevention and Therapy of Perinatal Hypoxia and Anoxia

PHYSIOLOGIC PREVENTION

The danger of hypoxic damage to the CNS during labor is closely related to several physiologic factors, such as the restriction of the uteroplacental and fetoplacental circulations during uterine contractions, restriction of brain circulation caused by pressure on the head during dilation of the cervix, and so on. The organism tries to compensate for these dangers by mechanisms which either originate in the maternal organism or are due to immaturity of the fetal CNS.

INFLUENCE OF THE MATERNAL ORGANISM ON THE RESISTANCE OF THE CNS DURING PARTURITION

The level of glucose and lactate in the maternal blood increases during labor. In the fetal blood the level of these compounds increases accordingly (Inavodo-Garcia et al., 1966; Štembera, 1966; Vedra, 1967). It is known that hyperglycemia has a beneficial effect on cerebral tolerance to any type of hypoxia and anoxia during the whole course of ontogeny (Büsing, 1940; Selle, 1941; Britton and Kline, 1945; Hiestand and Nelson, 1946; Van Middlesworth, 1946; Smith and Oster, 1946; Trojan and Jílek, 1961). The increased levels of lactic acid and lactate also have a favorable effect on the resistance of immature nervous tissue (Jílek et al., 1964). It was shown that the influence of lactic acid is not due to pH changes. In adults the application of lactic acid decreases resistance. Accumulation of lactic acid might be one of the stimuli leading to the development of adaptive metabolic reactions (see p. 1017).

The estrogen level is increased in the blood of the mother near term. Estrogens increase the cerebral tolerance to anoxia (Trojan and Jílek, 1967a) since they might act by inhibiting the energy metabolism of the brain.

Several other changes in the internal environment of the mother could also be of importance, as for instance, the increase of the plasma level of corticoids or epinephrine.

THE IMMATURITY OF THE FETAL CNS

The immaturity of the nervous tissue of the fetus and of the newborn is the major reason for its high tolerance to hypoxia and anoxia (see p. 996). It may be important that near term the oxygen content of the fetal blood decreases. This is most probably due to the increasing disproportion among the size of the fetus, its metabolic needs, and the placental oxygen transport (Westin, 1955; Bartels and Moll, 1964; Štembera, 1967). This prenatal gradual decrease of the oxygen supply may stimulate the development of adaptive processes in the CNS. The partially adapted metabolism increases the tolerance for acute, and eventually intensive, hypoxia or anoxia during labor.

CLINICAL PREVENTION AND THERAPY

Prevention of hypoxia is the basic requirement for a successful fight of hypoxic damage of the CNS.

The basic principles of clinical prevention are: 1, Organizational measures: prenatal care for pregnant women, deliveries in hospitals with adequate equipment, eugenic measures, and so forth; 2, efforts to shorten labor, and the use of analgesia; 3, the termination of gestation before term (induction) or of labor (cesarean section) in cases of imminent, obvious danger of hypoxic damage to the fetus, e.g., in toxemia, diabetes, and prolonged gestation. If all these measures cannot prevent the hypoxic damage to the nervous tissue, an effective therapy has to be searched for. For details the reader is referred to monographs and other appropriate literature (Nikolajev, 1952; Delafresnaye and Oppé, 1953; Hughes et al., 1954; Caldeyro-Barcia and Alvarez, 1957; Nesbett, 1957; Pugovischnikova, 1959; Horský and Štembera, 1967).

ATTEMPTS TO INFLUENCE THE COURSE OF CEREBRAL HYPOXIA AND ANOXIA EXPERIMENTALLY

An increase of hypoxia and anoxia tolerance can be achieved by a prolongation of the revival and survival times by: 1, substitution of oxygen and adequate nutrients; 2, lowering of the metabolic rate of the organism, including the nervous tissue; and 3, providing optimal conditions for the development of metabolic adaptive reactions.

SUBSTITUTION OF THE DECREASED SUPPLY OF OXYGEN AND OF NUTRIENTS

An increase in the maternal arterial Po_2 during the antenatal or intranatal period by breathing of oxygen leads not only to an increase of the Po_2 in the fetus but also to an increase of the oxygen content of its blood. This can be achieved since the oxygen saturation of the fetal blood is only 50 percent due to the low Po_2 at the placental membrane. After birth, the main factor is an increase of the amount of oxygen dissolved in plasma and an increase in Po_2, i.e., an increase of the diffusion gradient.

Hyperbaria (2 atm) has a significantly favorable effect in cases of stagnant hypoxia of the nervous tissue during the perinatal period as well as in adults. It increases the number of surviving animals after occlusion of both carotids (Doležal et al., 1967). The increased P_{N_2}, or rather its inhibitory effect on the activity of the CNS, could also be of some benefit during hyperbaria.

Hyperoxia by breathing of pure oxygen for eight hours has an effect which is similar to that of hyperbaria. In the course of eight hours, however, the toxic effects of pure oxygen on lung tissue, especially pulmonary edema, mitigate the beneficial effects of hyperoxia. This may be the reason why the effect of hyperoxia is less favorable than the effect of hyperbaria (Doležal et al., 1967). Hyperoxia also causes vasoconstriction in the brain, especially in the youngest animals (Jílek and Trojan, 1960a).

The beneficial effect of *hyperglycemia* is commonly used in clinical practice and has been demonstrated in many experiments (Britton and Kline, 1945; Hiestand and Nelson, 1946; Trojan and Jílek, 1961; Jílek and Trojan, 1963, 1964).

The increased concentration of glucose in the internal environment increases the tolerance to stagnant and hypoxic hypoxia and also to stagnant anoxia (Fig. 34). At the present time hyperglycemia appears to be the most effective method in fighting damaging effects of hypoxia during the entire perinatal period. However, the mechanism of this effect is not quite clear. Glucose is a very important source of energy for the nervous tissue, but in addition, it seems to have a stimulatory effect on anaerobic glycolysis. This is shown by the fact that the beneficial effect of glucose is abolished by monoiodoacetic acid, which is an inhibitor of glyceraldehyde phosphate dehydrogenase (Trojan and Jílek, 1960b, 1962c).

The effect of hyperglycemia can be potentiated by insulin (Jílek et al., 1966). The effect of insulin on glucose transport through the blood-brain barrier during development is, however, not yet clear.

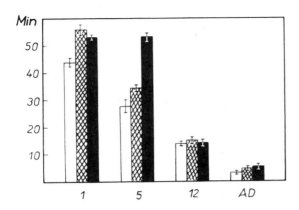

Fig. 34. Influence of hyperglycemia (220 to 240 mg/100 ml) and fasting of 8 hours on resistance to stagnant anoxia. Abscissa, age in days; AD, adults. Ordinate, survival time in minutes. White columns, controls; black columns, hyperglycemia; shaded columns, fasting. (From Trojan and Jílek. 1961. *Physiol. Bohemoslov.*, 10:467-473.)

Some experiments have shown that injected *ATP* increases the resistance of the CNS to hypoxic hypoxia. The mechanism of this effect is not clear. The administered ATP cannot serve as, or substitute a source of energy, but it might have a vasodilatatory effect similar to ADP and adenylic acid (Hahn, 1953a). Therefore, ATP can only increase the tolerance to oligemia, but not to ischemia, where an effect on the circulation is irrelevant (Jílek and Trojan, 1967c). The beneficial effect of ATP injections in perinatal hypoxia has been confirmed in clinical practice (Znamenáček, 1966; Znamenáček and Přibylová, 1966).

Many experiments have shown that immature nervous tissue reacts with a metabolic adaptive reaction not only to hypoxia but also to several other changes in the internal environment. We observed, for instance, that the survival time of gasping after decapitation, i.e., stagnant anoxia, can be prolonged in newborn rats in many different ways, such as i.p. injection of distilled water, saline solution, acetic acid, sodium acetate, lactic acid, malonate, arsenate, cyanate, lactate, and so on. Therefore, it seems that this type of reaction of immature nervous tissue is a common biologic phenomenon, since it reacts in a similar manner to many different factors (Jílek, 1966). Thus, it is necessary to evaluate the influence of various factors on the tolerance of the immature CNS to hypoxia and anoxia in respect to these facts.

LOWERING OF THE METABOLIC RATE OF THE CNS

Attempts to lower the metabolic rate of the CNS are based on the assumption that this procedure lowers the requirements for oxygen and nutrients and thereby increases the hypoxia tolerance. This assumption is undoubtedly true in adults, because the metabolic rate in their CNS is the determining factor for tissue survival in hypoxia. However, in hypoxia immature nervous tissue reacts in a specific and different way than the mature, adult brain. Many factors which can be beneficial in adulthood have an unfavorable influence in the perinatal period.

The metabolic rate of the brain can be reduced by: 1, lowering the temperature of the CNS (general hypothermia); 2, inhibition of metabolic processes and/or of the function of the CNS (pharmacologically); and 3, combination of both. This is the usual practice, since both routes are mutually dependent.

Stagnant hypoxia is favorably affected only by very mild *hypothermia*, that is, by a decrease of 2 to 3 °C of the rectal temperature (Fig. 35). Marked hypothermia has, on the contrary, a definitely unfavorable effect. It seems that hypothermia inhibits the metabolic adaptive reaction, and it may also have an adverse effect on the circulation by lowering the heart rate and the minute volume. Furthermore, it shifts the Hb dissociation curve to the left. It must also be taken into account that the temperature of the cerebral cortex in the youngest animals is higher than the rectal temperature (Jílek and Trojan, 1960a); in adults it is just reverse.

In general, hypothermia increases the tolerance to anoxia. The degree of its protective effect is directly related to the degree of cooling (Trojan and Jílek, 1965). The survival time in anoxia depends primarily on the intensity of the metabolic rate (Table 1). This is true for the entire course of ontogeny.

THE INFLUENCE OF AGENTS WHICH INHIBIT THE FUNCTION AND THE METABOLISM OF THE CNS

Chlorpromazine (10 mg/kg) does not affect the tolerance to stagnant hypoxia, but pentobarbital (20 mg/kg) increases the tolerance significantly (Jílek, 1960). Both drugs have a favorable effect on the tolerance to stagnant anoxia. In the newborn, chlorpromazine has a greater effect than pentobarbital. In adults it is reversed (Fig. 36). The effect of pentobarbital increases with increasing intensity of aerobic metabolism, which is in agreement with the fact that pentobarbital inhibits both the activity of the CNS and oxidative metabolism. An analysis of simultaneous changes of the rectal temperature showed the direct inhibitory effect of these drugs

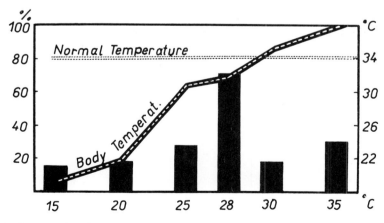

Fig. 35. Influence of environmental and body temperature on the resistance of 12-day-old rats to stagnant hypoxia of the brain (ligature of carotids lasting for 8 hours). Abscissa, temperature of environment in °C. Ordinate, left, survival of rats in percent (black columns); right, rectal temperature of rats after 8 hours of stagnant hypoxia. (From Jílek and Mareš. 1961. *Česk. Pediat.*, 16:115-121.)

TABLE 1. The Influence of Hypothermia on the Resistance to Stagnant Anoxia in Rats[a]

Age (days)	Rectal temperature during ischemia[b]	Resistance (sec)	Rectal temperature during ischemia	Resistance (sec)	Increase of resistance (percent)	Rectal temperature during ischemia[c]		Resistance (sec)	Increase of resistance (percent)
						Initial	After ischemia		
1	31,5±0,3	2,070±30	30,0±0,1	2,580±60	25	31,3±0,4	22,0±0,3	2,655±45	29
3	32,0±0,2	1,155±45	30,1±0,2	1,575±90	36	31,9±0,3	22,0±0,2	1,650±30	43
5	32,5±0,3	1,110±30	30,0±0,1	1,350±30	21	32,6±0,3	22,0±0,3	1,620±60	46
7	33,2±0,4	870±45	30,0±0,1	1,155±45	32	33,0±0,2	22,0±0,2	1,290±30	48
9	33,2±0,3	780±30	30,2±0,2	975±30	25	33,2±0,3	22,0±0,3	1,125±45	44
12	33,9±0,4	495±45	30,1±0,1	690±30	39	33,9±0,2	23,0±0,3	795±45	60
25	37,2±0,3	165±15	30,2±0,2	225±15	36	37,4±0,4	28,3±0,4	172±10	4
Adults	37,1±0,1	180±10	30,2±0,2	235±20	31	37,1±0,2	32,2±0,3	187±7	4

[a] Acceleration 10 g.
[b] Corresponds to rectal temperature of control animals.
[c] The experiments were conducted in the environmental temperature 22°C. Cooling was achieved within 2 to 3 minutes.

Fig. 36. Influence of chlorpromazine (10 mg/kg i.p.) and pentobarbital (30 mg/kg i.p.) on resistance to stagnant anoxia (ischemia). Abscissa, age of rats in days; AD, adults. Ordinate, survival time in minutes. White columns, controls; shaded columns, treatment with chlorpromazine; black columns, treatment with pentobarbital. (From Trojan and Jílek. 1961. *Physiol. Bohemoslov.*, 10:467-473.)

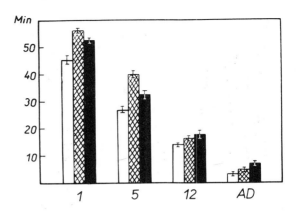

on metabolism. The latter is decisive and not secondary by decreasing the body temperature, i.e., hypothermia (Trojan and Jílek, 1961).

Some of the neuroplegics, such as perathiepin and octoclothepin, increase the anoxia tolerance only in the immature nervous tissue but not in adults where they have the opposite effect (Jílek and Trojan, 1967).

Great caution is necessary in using some of the circulatory stimulants, such as adrenalin derivatives, which are relatively often used in treating newborns suffering from hypoxia. These drugs stimulate the CNS and thereby increase the sensitivity of the nervous tissue to hypoxia by increasing oxygen consumption (Presl, 1960).

An experimental analysis of the effect of drugs showed that their influence depends on the following factors: 1, the developmental maturity of the CNS; 2, the intensity of hypoxia; 3, the type of hypoxia; 4, the type of the drug; 5, the dose of the drug; 6, the time relation between application of the drug and exposure to hypoxia or anoxia; 7, the concentration of the drug in the individual parts of the CNS; and 8, the maturational stage of the blood-brain barrier.

The same compound may even have opposite effects under different conditions, e.g., the effect of chlorpromazine on tolerance to hypoxia and anoxia (Trojan and Jílek, 1962b; Jílek and Trojan, 1963; Jílek et al., 1964).

Heparin was claimed to prevent some damage due to anoxia. In our experiments we did not find any increase in tolerance to stagnant anoxia after injection of even large doses of heparin (600 IU i.p.) (Karásek and Mourek, 1959; Trojan and Jílek, 1961).

Fasting by deprivation of food and water for eight hours has a significantly favorable effect on the resistance to ischemia in very immature animals (Jílek and Trojan, 1960b; Trojan and Jílek, 1960a; Mourek, 1960, 1965). This may be due to the depression of brain metabolism due to poor nutrition or dehydration. This leads to the speculation that the physiologically late onset of lactation is a biologic factor that increases the hypoxia tolerance of the CNS.

OPTIMAL CONDITIONS FOR THE DEVELOPMENT OF THE METABOLIC ADAPTIVE REACTION

Rehydration and Realimentation: The adaptive mechanism can be hampered secondarily by some somatic and/or autonomic disturbances which develop in consequence of cerebral hypoxia, as for instance a defective sucking reflex. It has been shown that under these conditions rehydration and realimentation increase the survival of the immature individual (Jílek, 1966).

Hormonal Influences: Some hormonal factors which affect the metabolism of the CNS may also contribute to the development of the metabolic adaptive reaction.

In the adult organism hypoxia stimulates the secretion of adrenocortical hormones. However, during the perinatal period, the adrenals are not functional. Nevertheless, aldosterone treatment increases the tolerance of the CNS to ischemia in newborn rats (Londonová et al., 1968).

The preventive administration of antifibrinolytics also increases cerebral tolerance to hypoxia in the perinatal period. This effect may be explained by the hypothesis that in some cases of hypoxia circulatory disorders in the brain are caused by the release of fibrinolytic factors from the nervous tissue (Ludwig, 1968).

The entire topic of perinatal hypoxia and anoxia in the CNS and the sequential results of damage is obviously very complex. Although our present knowledge is incomplete, nevertheless, it seems to be possible to arrive at some general conclusions concerning the specific reactions of the nervous tissue due to changes of the internal environment. The outlying considerations will help the clinician in his search for developing methods for the prevention and therapy of perinatal hypoxia. Furthermore, this challenging field of study needs more profound analysis of all processes involved. Experimental as well as clinical investigations will be needed for creating a solid basis for treating hypoxic damage of the CNS, which is the most frequent injury of the organism during the perinatal period.

REFERENCES

Abramson, H. 1960. Resuscitation of the Newborn Infant. St. Louis, The C. V. Mosby Co.

Adolph, E. F. 1956. General and specific characteristics of physiological adaptations. Amer. J. Physiol., 184:18-28.

——— 1964. Perspectives of adaptation: Some general properties. *In* Dill, D. B., ed. Adaptation to the Environment. Handbook of Physiology. Washington, D. C., American Physiological Society, Sect. 4, pp. 27-35.

Agrawal, H. C., J. M. Davis, and W. A. Himwich. 1966. Postnatal changes in free amino acid pool of rat brain. J. Neurochem., 13:607-615.

Albaum, H. G., and H. I. Chinn. 1953. Brain metabolism during altitude acclimatization. Amer. J. Physiol., 174:141-145.

Allen, D. W., J. Wyman, Jr., and C. A. Smith. 1953. The oxygen equilibrium of fetal and adult human hemoglobin. J. Biol. Chem., 203:81-87.

Ansell, G. B., and D. Richter. 1954. A note on the free amino acid content of rat brain. Biochem. J., 57:70-73.

Antošová, E., J. Wagner, and L. Jílek. 1967. The changes of ATP, ADP and AMP in the brain caused by ischemia during ontogeny of the rat. Fourth Meeting of FEBS, Oslo. Abstracts, p. 26.

Apgar, V., B. R. Girdany, R. McIntosh, and H. C. Taylor. 1955. Neonatal anoxia. I. A study of the relation of oxygenation at birth to intellectual development. Pediatrics, 15:653-662.

Avery, M. E. 1964. The Lung and its Disorders in the Newborn Infant. Philadelphia, W. B. Saunders Company.

Bakay, L. 1953. Studies on the blood-brain barrier with radioactive phosphorus: Embryonic development of the barrier. Arch. Neurol. (Chicago), 70:30-35.

Barbashova, Z. I. 1964. Cellular level of adaptation. In Dill, D. B., ed. Adaptation to the Environment. Handbook of Physiology. Washington, D. C., American Physiological Society, Sect. 4, pp. 37-54.

———— 1967. Studies on the mechanisms of resistance to hypoxia. Int. J. Biometeor., 11:243-254.

Barcroft, J. 1925. The Respiratory Function of the Blood. Part I. Lessons from High Altitude. Cambridge, Cambridge University Press.

———— 1946. Research on Prenatal Life. Oxford, Blackwell Scientific Publications.

Bartels, H., and W. Moll. 1964. Passage of inert substances and oxygen in the human placenta. Pflueger. Arch. Ges. Physiol., 280:165-177.

Beer, R., H. Bartels, and H. A. Raczkowski. 1955. Die Sauerstoffdissoziationskurve des fetalen Blutes und der Gasaustausch in der menschlichen Placenta. Pflueger. Arch. Ges. Physiol., 260:306-319.

Betke, K. 1963. Blutverluste und Blutungsanämien bei Neugeborenen. Zbl. Gynaek., 85:113-120.

Braun, W. 1960. Das Vorkommen des fetalen Hämoglobins im Säuglings- und Kindersalter. Kinderaerztl. Prax., 28:561-564.

Britton, S. W., and R. F. Kline. 1945. Age, sex, carbohydrate, adrenal cortex and other factors in anoxia. Amer. J. Physiol., 145:190-202.

Büsing, K. H. 1940. Der Einfluss von Kreislaufmitteln, Vitaminen und Traubenzucker auf die Höhenfestigkeit. Luftf. Med. Abh., 3:43-47.

Caldeyro-Barcia, R., and H. Alvarez. 1957. Physiology of Prematurity. New York, Josiah Macy Foundation.

Campbell, W. A. B., E. A. Cheeseman, and A. W. Kilpatrick. 1950. The effects of neonatal asphyxia on physical and mental development. Arch. Dis. Child., 25:351-359.

Clementson, C. A. B. 1954. The placental transfer of amino-acids in normal and toxaemic pregnancy. J. Obstet. Gynec., 61:364-371.

Czetverikov, D. A. 1966. Obmen fosfolipidov golovnovo mozga krys pri ostrom kislorodnom golodanii. Probl. Neirochim. (Moskva), pp. 141-147.

Dahl, N. A., and W. M. Balfour. 1964. Prolonged anoxic survival time due to anoxia pre-exposure brain ATP, lactate and pyruvate. Amer. J. Physiol., 207:452-456.

Delafresnaye, J. F., and T. E. Oppé, eds. 1953. Anoxia of the Newborn Infant. Oxford, Blackwell Scientific Publications.

Diemer, K. 1968. Grundzüge der postnatalen Hirnentwicklung. In Linneweh, F., ed. Fortschr. Paedol., 2:1-25.

Dobbing, J. 1961. The blood-brain barrier. Physiol. Rev., 41:130-188.

Doležal, V., F. Vorel, L. Jílek, and S. Trojan. 1967. Vliv hyperbarie na odolnost krys proti stagnační hypoxii mozku béhem ontogenese. Cesk. Fysiol., 16:262-263.

Dravid, A. R., and L. Jílek. 1965. Influence of stagnant hypoxia (oligemia) on some free amino acids in rat brain during ontogeny. J. Neurochem., 12:837-843.

Eastman, N. J., and L. M. Hellman. 1966. Williams Obstetrics, 13th ed. New York, Appleton-Century-Crofts.

Fazekas, J. F., F. A. D. Alexander, and H. E. Himwich. 1941. Tolerance of the newborn to anoxia. Amer. J. Physiol., 134:281-284.

Feldberg, W., and J. L. Malcolm. 1954. Chemistry in relation to the development of the nervous system. Nature (London), 174:455-457.

Fischer, J., and L. Jílek. 1958. Morphological changes of the CNS after ligature of the carotids in the course of postnatal life in the rat. Sborn. Lék., 60:346-354.

——— and L. Jílek. 1965. Neurohistopathologische Veränderungen nach Hypoxie und Anoxie in der Ontogenese. Eine experimentelle Studie. Proceedings of the Vth International Congress of Neuropathology, Zurich. Amsterdam, Excerpta Medica Foundation ICS, No. 100, pp. 1034-1039.

——— L. Jílek, and S. Trojan. 1962. Reversibility of histopathological changes of the CNS, caused by stagnant anoxia in the ontogeny of rats. Cas. Lék. Cesk., 101: 650-654.

Garmasheva, N. L., ed. 1959. Pathophysiology of Intrauterine Development. Leningrad, State Publishing Office for Medical Literature (in Russian).

——— 1967. The Placental Circulation. Leningrad, State Publishing Office for Medical Literature (in Russian).

Haber, B., A. R. Dravid, and L. Jílek. 1968. Effect of stagnant hypoxia on glucose U-C^{14} utilisation by rat brain during ontogeny. In Jílek, L., and S. Trojan, eds. Ontogenesis of the Brain. Prague, Charles University, pp. 169-175.

Hahn, P. 1953a. Einfluss der Adenosintriphosphorsäure und von Kationen auf die Resistenz gegen Höhenanoxie. Cesk. Fysiol., 2:178-182.

——— 1953b. Änderungen der Widerstandsfähigkeit gegen Höhenanoxie in der Ontogenese. Cesk. Fysiol., 2:307-315.

Hickl, E. I. 1967. Die Früherkennung der fetalen Asphyxiegefährdung (Hypoxie und Azidose). München. Med. Wschr., 109:31-37.

Hiestand, W. A., and J. W. Nelson. 1946. Survival of the isolated respiratory center in the young rat as influenced by adrenaline, ephedrine, insulin and glutathione and the relation to glycemia changes. Amer. J. Physiol., 146:241-245.

Himwich, H. E. 1951. Brain Metabolism and Cerebral Disorders. Baltimore, The Williams & Wilkins Co.

Himwich, W. A., J. C. Petersen, and M. L. Allen. 1957. Hematoencephalic exchange as a function of age. Neurology, 7:705-710.

Hodr, J., and Z. K. Štembera. 1959. Vliv porodu na glycidový metabolismus rodičky. Cesk. Gynek., 24:616-622.

——— Z. K. Štembera, V. Šabata, and M. Novák. 1963. Změny v energetickém metabolismu v průbehu porodní činnosti. Cesk. Gynek., 28:482-485.

Hoff, E. C., J. J. Petterson, Jr., and R. G. Grenell. 1956. Circulation through the Brain. In Fulton, J. F., ed. A Textbook of Physiology. Philadelphia, W. B. Saunders Company, pp. 796-805.

Horský, J., and Z. K. Štembera, eds. 1967. Intra-uterine Dangers to the Foetus. Amsterdam, Excerpta Medica Foundation.

Huckabee, W. E., J. Metcalfe, H. Prystowsky, and D. H. Barrow. 1962. Insufficiency of oxygen supply to pregnant uterus. Amer. J. Physiol., 202:198-204.

Huehns, E. R., et al. 1964. Human embryonic haemoglobins. Nature (London), 201: 1095-1097.

Huffman, J. W. 1960. Obstetrics and Gynecology. Philadelphia, W. B. Saunders Company.

Hughes, E., C. W. Lloyd, and C. V. Ledergerber. 1954. La Prophylaxie en Gynécologie et Obstetrique. Basel Georg.

Hydén, H. 1960. The Neuron. *In* Brachet, J., and A. E. Mirský, eds. The Cell. London, Academic Press, Inc., Vol. 4, pp. 215-323.

Inavodo-Garcia, E., C. Chanez, and A. Minkowski. 1966. Lactacidemia and pyruvicemia during ischemic foetal anoxia in rats. Biol. Neonat., 10:209-226.

Janata, V., et al. 1968. The influence of stagnant hypoxia on the activities of some dehydrogenases and transaminases in the brain of rats during ontogenesis. Fifth Meeting of FEBS, Prague.

———— 1957. Reaction of the organism to cerebral ischemia in the course of ontogenesis: The development of resistance to cerebral ischemia in the rat. Sborn. Lék., 59:188-195.

———— 1958a. Reaction of the organism to ischemia of the brain during ontogenesis. II. The development of functional changes in the central nervous system following ligature of the carotids during postnatal life in rats. Physiol. Bohemoslov., 7: 282-291.

———— 1958b. Epileptic seizures in rats following ligature of the carotids. Physiol. Bohemoslov., 7:356-362.

———— 1958c. Response of the rat to temporary ischemia of the CNS. Sborn. Lék., 60:235-241.

———— 1958d. Contribution to the research on changes of the cerebral metabolism after ligature of the carotids during the ontogenesis of rats. Sborn. Lék., 60:242-248.

———— 1966. Stagnant Hypoxia and Anoxia of the Brain During Ontogeny. Praha, SZdN. (in Czech).

———— and J. Fischer. 1959. Repair of changes in the CNS caused by ligature of the the carotids in the early stages of development in rats. Activ. Nerv. Sup. (Praha), 1:223-227.

———— and S. Trojan. 1960a. Temperature changes in the cerebral cortex of the rat during asphyxia, nitrogen hypoxia and O_2 inhalation in the course of ontogeny. Physiol. Bohemoslov., 9:186-195.

———— and S. Trojan. 1960b. The effect of starvation and hyperglycaemia on the surviving of spinal reflexes and the activity of the respiratory center after decapitation of rats in the course of ontogenesis. Sborn. Lék., 62:272-279.

———— and S. Trojan. 1960c. The development of resistance to positive and negative radial acceleration during ontogeny of the rat. Physiol. Bohemoslov., 9:528-533.

Jílek, L. 1960. Effect of chlorpromazine, urethane and pentobarbital on the resistance to cerebral oligemia in rats during postnatal life. Acta Univ. Carol. [Med.] (Praha), 7:749-771.

———— and P. Mareš. 1961. The effect of body temperature on the resistance of young rats to cerebral oligaemia. Cesk. Pediat., 16:115-121.

———— and S. Trojan. 1963. Influencing the resistance of the organism to oligemia and CNS ischaemia during ontogenesis. Cesk. Pediat., 18:26-32.

———— and S. Trojan. 1964. The effect of repeated intraperitoneal glucose administration during early postnatal development on resistance of the central nervous system to anoxia. Physiol. Bohemoslov., 13:504-509.

———— and S. Trojan. 1966. Development of the resistance to general stagnant anoxia (ischemia) in dogs. Physiol. Bohemoslov., 15:62-67.

———— and S. Trojan. 1967a. Adaptation of the central nervous system to repeated acceleration. *In* Morávek, M., and J. Dvořák, eds. Some Problems of Aviation and Space Medicine. Prague, Charles University, pp. 101-103.

———— and S. Trojan. 1967b. The effect of perathiepin and octoclothepin on cerebral ischemia in rats during ontogeny. Activ. Nerv. Sup. (Praha), 9:627-628.

———— and S. Trojan. 1967c. Unpublished results.

———— and S. Trojan. 1968. Unpublished results.

———— J. Mourek, and S. Trojan. 1961a. The influence of malonate on resistance to nitrogen anoxia and on the persistance of certain reflexes during ontogeny of the rat. Physiol. Bohemoslov., 10:267-274.

———— et al. 1961b. On the questions of development of phenomena of adaptation in CNS during ontogenesis. Plzen. Lék. Sborn., Suppl. 3:105-112.

———— E. Trávníčková, and S. Trojan. 1962a. Changes in higher nervous activity after hypoxic brain damage in the early postnatal period. Cas. Lék. Cesk., 101:656-659.

———— S. Trojan, L. Krulich, and J. Fischer. 1962b. Entwicklung der Reaktion und der Adaptation des zentralen Nervensystems auf Stagnationshypoxie und Anoxie während der Ontogenese. Z. Aerztl. Fortbild. (Jena), 56:388-394.

———— L. Krulich, and S. Trojan. 1963. The effect of sodium arsenate on the survival of spinal reflexes and the activity of the respiratory centre after decapitation in rats during their postnatal development. Physiol. Bohemoslov., 12:242-247.

———— S. Trojan, and E. Trávníčková. 1965. The reaction and adaptation of the organism to anoxia. Activ. Nerv. Sup. (Praha), 7/2: 132-134.

———— S. Trojan, and E. Trávníčková. 1966a. Lactic acid and glycogen changes in the rat brain due to aerogenic (altitude) hypoxia during ontogenesis. Physiol. Bohemoslov., 15:532-537.

———— S. Trojan, L. Krulich, and J. Mourek. 1966b. Unpublished results.

———— S. Trojan, E. Trávníčková, and J. Fischer. 1966c. Dynamika zmen metabolismu glycidů v mozku krys po ischémii v průbůhu ontogenese. Cesk. Fysiol., 15:482.

———— E. Trávníčková, and S. Trojan. 1967. The metabolic reaction of the nervous tissue to hypoxia and anoxia during ontogeny. In Horský, J., and Z. K. Štembera, eds. Intra-uterine Dangers to the Foetus. Amsterdam, Excerpta Medica Foundation, pp. 115-120.

———— E. Trávníčková, and S. Trojan. 1968a. Unpublished results.

———— et al. 1968b. The metabolic adaptive reaction of the immature nervous tissue to stagnant hypoxia. In Jílek, L., and S. Trojan, eds. Ontogenesis of the Brain. Prague, Charles University, pp. 143-157.

———— J. Fischer, L. Krulich, and S. Trojan. 1964. The reaction of the brain to stagnant hypoxia and anoxia during ontogeny. In Himwich, W. A., and H. E. Himwich, eds. The developing brain, Progr. Brain Res., 9:113-131.

Kabat, H. 1940. The greater resistance of very young animals to arrest of the brain circulation. Amer. J. Physiol., 130:588-599.

Karásek, F., and J. Mourek. 1959. The action of heparin on resistance to anoxia. Sborn. Lek., 61:97-100.

Kassil, G. N. 1963. Gemato-encephalitcheskii barier. Izd. Akad. Nauk. S.S.S.R.

Kendall, N. 1963. Anemia in the newborn infant. Pediat. Clin. N. Amer., 10:613-621.

Kety, S. S. 1955. Changes in cerebral circulation and oxygen consumption which accompany maturation and aging. In Waelsch, H., ed. Biochemistry of the Developing Nervous System. New York, Academic Press, Inc. pp. 208-217.

Koch, W., and M. L. Koch. 1913. Contributions to the chemical differentiation of the central nervous system. III. The chemical differentiation of the brain of the albino rat during growth. J. Biol. Chem., 15:423-448.

Krásný, J., B. Večerek, and L. Jílek. 1967. The influence of stagnant hypoxia of the brain on the activity of isoenzymes of lactic dehydrogenase. Fourth Meeting of FEBS, Oslo. Abstracts, p. 25.

Krulich, L., L. Jílek, and S. Trojan. 1962. The effect of oligaemia on the content of glycogen and lactic acid in the brain of the rat during ontogeny. Physiol. Bohemoslov., 11:58-63.

Laitl, J. 1963. An Experimental Study of the Resistance of the Organism to Anoxia during Ontogeny and its Influencing by Chlorpromazine. Dissertation. Institute of the Care of Mother and Child, Prague.

Lehndorff, H. 1962. Anämische Zustände bei Neugeborenen. Wien. Med. Wschr., 112:533-534.

Lesný, I. 1959. Raná dětská mozková obrna. Praha, SZdN.

———— V. Vojta, and V. Jelínek. 1960. Pituitary implantation in cerebral palsied children. Cereb. Palsy J., 2:167-169.

Lolley, R. N., and F. E. Samson. 1962. Cerebral high-energy compounds—changes in anoxia. Amer. J. Physiol., 202:77-79.

Londonová, A., S. Trojan, and L. Jílek. 1968. Unpublished results.

Lucas, W., T. Kirschbaum, and N. S. Assali. 1966. Cephalic circulation and oxygen consumption before and after birth. Amer. J. Physiol., 210:287-292.

Ludwig, H. 1968. Mikrozirkulationsstörungen und Diapedesenblutungen im fetalen Gehirn bei Hypoxie. Basel, S. Karger.

Málek, J. 1947. Vliv sníženého tlaku vzduchu na těhotná morčata. Cesk. Gynek., 12 (26):454-470.

McIlwain, H. 1955. Biochemistry and the Central Nervous System. London, J. and A. Churchill., Ltd.

Měrka, J., and V. Horanský. 1966. Syndrôm anémie a šoku novorodencov v dosledku fetálnych hemorágií. Cesk. Pediat., 21:153-156.

Minkowski, A., and E. Swierczewski. 1959. The organ capacity of the human foetal blood. In Walker, J., and A. Turnbull, eds. Oxygen Supply to the Human Foetus. Oxford, Blackwell Scientific Publications, pp. 237-253.

Mitchell, W. K., and W. A. Himwich. 1966. Hemodynamic studies in the circle of Willis in the rat. Experientia, 22:673-677.

Mourek, J. 1958. The development of resistance to nitrogen anoxia during ontogenesis of the normal and decorticated rat. Sborn. Lék., 60:211-216.

———— 1960. Body weight loss and its after-effects during ontogeny of the rat (II.). Physiol. Bohemoslov., 9:196-201.

———— 1965. The influence of fasting and the development of the organism during the early stages of ontogenesis (with special reference to the development of the central nervous system). Acta Univ. Carol. [Med.] (Praha), 11:493-520.

———— 1966. Vývoj oxydačního metabolismu v centrálním nervovém systému savců. Praha, SZdN.

———— V. Pružková, J. Slavíček, and M. Trojanová. 1965. Some problems of oxidative metabolism of the nervous system in the ontogenesis of mammals. Activ. Nerv. Sup. (Praha), 7:128-129.

Mysliveček, J., and L. Jílek. 1953. Razvitie potreblenia kisloroda v nekotorych tkaniach krysy. Cesk. Fysiol., 2:363-366 (in Russian).

Naiman, J. G., and H. L. Williams. 1964. Effects of diphenylhydantoin on the duration of respiratory activity during anoxia. J. Pharmacol. Exp. Ther., 145:34-41.

Nesbett, R. E. L. 1957. Perinatal Loss in Modern Obstetrics. Philadelphia, F. A. Davis Co.

Nikolajev, A. P.   1952.   Profilaktika i terapia vnutriutrobnoi asfiksii ploda. Izd. Akad. Nauk. S.S.S.R.

Oehlert, G.   1963.   Die Neugeborenenanämie. Geburtsh. Frauenheilk., 23:685-695.

Oja, S. S. 1966. Postnatal changes in the concentration of nucleic acids, nucleotides and amino acids in the rat brain. Ann. Acad. Sci. Fenn. [Med.], p. 125.

Opatrný, E., and H. Tišer. 1966. Perinatální encefalopatie z porodnického hlediska. Prac. Lek. pp. 522-525.

Persianinoff, A. S.   1961.   Asfiksia ploda i novorozdenogo. Moscow, Medgiz.

Peters, J. P., and D. D. Van Slyke. 1931. Quantitative Clinical Chemistry. Baltimore, The Williams & Wilkins Co.

Potter, E. L. 1952. Pathology of the Fetus and Newborn. Chicago, Yearbook Medical Publishers, Inc.

——— and F. L. Adair. 1949. Fetal and Neonatal Death. Chicago, University of Chicago Press.

Presl, J. 1960. The influencing of the resistance to oxygen debt. In Mourek, J., ed. Hypoxia of Newborn Mammals. Prague, SZdN. (in Czech).

Preston, M. I. 1945. Late behavioral effects found in cases of prenatal, natal and post-natal anoxia. J. Pediat., 26:353-366.

Pugovischnikova, M. A. 1959. Patofiziologia vnutriutrobnogo razvitia. Moscow, Medgiz.

Reid, D. E.   1962.   A Textbook of Obstetrics. Philadelphia, W. B. Saunders Company.

Richter, D. 1955. The metabolism of the developing brain. In Waelsch, H., ed. Biochemistry of the Developing Nervous System. New York, Academic Press, Inc., pp. 225-250.

Roberts, E., S. Frankel, and P. J. Harman. 1950. Amino acids of nervous tissue. Proc. Soc. Exp. Biol. Med., 74:383-387.

Šabata, V. Z. K. Štembera, J. Hodr, and M. Novák. 1964. Die Wirkung von Glucoseinfusionen auf den Lipid- und Hydratstoffwechsel der Gebährenden und der Frucht. Z. Geburtsh. Gynaek., 162:253-264.

Samson, F. E., Jr., W. M. Balfour, and N. A. Dahl. 1958. The effect of age and temperature on the cerebral requirement in the rat. J. Geront., 13:241-247.

Selle, W. A. 1941. Influence of glucose on the gasping pattern of young animals subjected to acute anoxia. Amer. J. Physiol., 123:441-447.

Sirakova, I., L. Sirakov, L. Jílek, and I. Rychlík. 1968. Changes in nucleic acid metabolism in the brain caused by stagnant hypoxia during ontogeny in the rat. In Lodin, Z., and S. Rous, eds. Macromolecules and the Function of the Neuron. Amsterdam, Excerpta Medica Foundation, Monograph Series, pp. 330-334.

Slomko, Z., and D. Glowinska. 1961. Hemoglobina plodova w krvi pepowinowej. Pol. Tyg. Lék., 16:244-246.

Smith, C. A. 1959. The Physiology of the Newborn Infant. Oxford, Blackwell Scientific Publications.

Smith, D. C., and R. H. Oster. 1946. Influence of blood sugar levels on resistance to low oxygen tension in the cat. Amer. J. Physiol., 146:26-32.

Snoeck, J.   1958.   Le Placenta Humain. Paris, Masson et Cie.

Štembera, Z. K. 1966. The relationship between the blood levels of glucose, lactic acid and pyruvic acid in the mother and in both umbilical vessels of the healthy fetus. Biol. Neonat., 10:227-238.

——— 1967. Hypoxia of the Foetus. Prague, SZdN. (in Czech).

——— J. Hodr, and J. Janda. 1967. Differences in the metabolism of healthy and hypoxic foetuses rated according to the arterio-venous difference in oxygen, glucose, lactic acid and pyruvic acid contents in the umbilical vessels and to the amount of blood flowing through the umbilical cord. *In* Horský, J., and Z. K. Štembera, eds. Intra-uterine Dangers to the Foetus. Amsterdam, Excerpta Medica Foundation, pp. 77-83.

———— et al. 1964. Asfyxie a perinatální úmrtnost (antenatální a intranatální). Cesk. Gynek., 29:485-492.

Stern, L., and R. Peyrot. 1927. Le fonctionnement de la barrière hemato-encephalique aux divers stades de development chez les diverses espèces animales. C. R. Soc. Biol. (Paris), 96:1124-1126.

Tenney, B., and B. Little. 1961. Clinical Obstetrics. Philadelphia, W. B. Saunders Company.

Trávníček, T., E. Trávníčková, and K. Šulc. 1966. Changes in haemoglobin fractions separated on CM-sephadex in normal newborn rats and in newborn rats after repeated blood losses. Physiol. Bohemoslov., 15:175-178.

Trávníčková, E. 1962. Changes of the blood count and of somatic development of young rats after repeated loss of blood. Sborn. Lek., 64:145-154.

———— 1966. The Development of the Reaction and Adaptation of the Organism on the Blood Loss during Ontogeny. Prague, SZdN., Babákova sbírka sv. 44 (in Czech).

———— 1968. The influence of repeated blood loss on the developing organism. *In* Jílek, L., and S. Trojan, eds. Ontogenesis of the Brain. Prague, Charles University, pp. 177-192.

———— L. Jílek, and S. Trojan. 1964. A propos de la question d'adaptation du système nerveux central aux pertes de sang répétées pendant l'ontogenèse. J. Physiol. (Paris), 56:663.

———— L. Jílek, and S. Trojan. 1967. EEG changes caused by altitude hypoxia after repeated blood loss in young rats. Physiol. Bohemoslov., 16:153-159.

———— J. Mourek, and S. Trojan. 1962. The effect of repeated blood loss on resistance to nitrogen and stagnation anoxia during postnatal development of the rat. Physiol. Bohemoslov., 11:231-235.

Trojan S., and L. Jílek. 1960a. Surviving of spinal reflexes and the activity of the respiration center after decapitation of rats in the course of ontogenesis. Sborn. Lék., 62:263-271.

———— and L. Jílek. 1960b. The effect of malonate and monoiodacetic acid on the survival of spinal reflexes and the function of the respiratory center after decapitation of rats in the course of ontogenesis. Sborn. Lék., 62:350-357.

———— and L. Jílek. 1961. Procedures affecting the resistance of rats to positive acceleration during ontogeny. Physiol. Bohemoslov., 10:467-473.

———— and L. Jílek. 1962a. Changes in the resistance of rats to stagnant anoxia after ligature of the carotid arteries in the course of ontogeny. Sborn. Lék., 64:188-192.

———— and L. Jílek. 1962b. Differences in the effect on hypoxia and anoxia of the central nervous system in the course of ontogenesis. Sborn. Lék., 64:304-310.

———— and L. Jílek. 1962c. The effect of monoiodacetic acid on resistance to stagnant anoxia during development of the rat. Physiol. Bohemoslov., 11:142-148.

———— and L. Jílek. 1964. The consequences of repeated exposure to stagnation anoxia during early postnatal development of the rat. Physiol. Bohemoslov., 13:473-477.

———— and L. Jílek. 1965. Influence of hypothermia on the resistance of the central nervous system against ischemia during ontogenesis of the rat. Sborn. Lék., 67: 127-132.

———— and L. Jílek. 1967a. Vliv estrogenů na odolnost proti positivnímu zrychlení v průběhu ontogenese. Cesk. Fysiol., 16:41.

———— and L. Jílek. 1967b. Influence of repeated administration of sodium arsenate on the reflex activity of rats. Sborn. Lék., 69:175-180.

———— and L. Jílek. 1968a. Adaptation of rats to repeated oligemia of the central nervous system produced by positive radial acceleration of 5 g. Physiol. Bohemoslov., 17:153-159.

———— and L. Jílek. 1968b. Adaptation of the central nervous system to repeated hypoxia and anoxia in the early postnatal life period. *In* Jílek, L., and S. Trojan, eds. Ontogenesis of the Brain. Prague, Charles University, pp. 193-203.

———— and L. Jílek. 1968c. Unpublished results.

———— L. Jílek, and J. Mourek. 1967a. The effect of repeated administration of sodium arsenite upon oxygen consumption in brain and liver of rats during development. Sborn. Lék., 69:361-365.

———— L. Jílek, and E. Trávníčková. 1967b. Effect of arsenic compounds on resistance of the central nervous system of the rat to hypoxia and anoxia during ontogenesis. Physiol. Bohemoslov., 16:538-542.

———— D. Škvorová, and L. Jílek. 1968. Influence of repeated stagnation hypoxia, caused by acceleration of 5 g, on the somatic and functional development of the rat and the activity of its adrenals. Sborn. Lék., 70:216-221.

———— L. Jílek, J. Mourek, and M. Trojanová. 1969. Influence of repeated oligemia and ischemia, induced by positive acceleration on the oxygen consumption in the brain and diaphragm of the rat during ontogeny. Sborn. Lék., 71:29-36.

———— L. Jílek, K. Schauerová, and D. Škvorová. 1969. Vliv opakované stagnační anoxie, způsobené positivním zrychlením 10g na somatický a funkční vývoj krysy a stav jejích nedledvin. Sborn. Lék., 70:345-351.

Ullery, J. C., and Z. J. R. Hollenbeck. 1965. Textbook of Obstetrics. St. Louis, The C. V. Mosby Co.

Van Middlesworth, L. 1946. Glucose ingestion during severe anoxia. Amer. J. Physiol., 146:491-495.

Vedra, B. 1967. Two different mechanisms of intrauterine asphyxia during labor. *In* Horský, J., and Z. K. Štembera, eds. Intra-uterine Dangers to the Foetus. Amsterdam, Excerpta Medica Foundation, pp. 98-102.

Vernadakis, A., and D. M. Woodbury. 1962. Electrolyte and amino acid changes in rat brain during maturation. Amer. J. Physiol., 203:748-752.

———— and D. M. Woodbury. 1965. Cellular and extracellular spaces in developing rat brain. Arch. Neurol. (Chicago), 12:284-293.

Villee, C. A., ed. 1960. The Placenta and Fetal Membranes. Baltimore, The Williams & Wilkins Co.

Volochov, A. A. 1951. Zakonomernosti ontogeneza nervnoi deiatelnosti. Moscow, Academy of Medical Science (in Russian).

Vorel, F., L. Jílek, and S. Trojan. 1968. The influence of stagnant hypoxia of the brain on glycemia, lactacidemia and the LDH activity in blood plasma. Physiol. Bohemoslov., 17:911-915.

———— L. Jílek, Z. Makoč, and S. Trojan. 1968. The relationships between lactate and pyruvate in the brain of the rat during stagnant hypoxia in the course of ontogeny. Proceedings of the Czechoslovak Physiological Society (In press).

Wenner, J. 1960. Untersuchungen über die Hypoxie des Gehirns bei Säuglingen mit angeborenen Herzfehlern. 59. Tg. D. Ges. Kinderheilk., Kassel.

Westin, B. 1955. Oxygen and carbon dioxide tension in the umbilical vessels of the human fetus in prolonged asphyxia. Acta Physiol. Scand., 35:26-30.

Windle, W. F. 1940. Physiology of the Fetus. Philadelphia, W. B. Saunders Company.

———— 1967. Brain damage in the newborn resulting from asphyxiation at birth. *In* Horský, J., and Z. K. Štembera, eds. Intra-uterine Dangers to the Foetus. Amsterdam, Excerpta Medica Foundation, pp. 110-114.

Wintrobe, M. M. 1956. Clinical Hematology. Philadelphia, Lea & Febiger, pp. 760-769.

Wulf, H. 1967. A comparative study of actual blood gases and acid-base metabolism in maternal and fetus blood during parturition. *In* Horský, J., and Z. K. Štembera, eds. Intra-uterine Dangers to the Foetus. Amsterdam, Excerpta Medica Foundation, pp. 89-93.

Ylppö, A. 1924. Zum Entstehungsmechanismus der Blutungen bei Frühgeburten und Neugeborenen. Ztschr. Kinderh., 23: 685-695.

Znamenáček, K. 1966. Die Bedeutung der ATP in der Neugeborenenperiode. Z. Kinderheilk., 96:349-353.

———— 1968. Asphyxia and Resuscitation of the Newborn Infant. Prague, SZdN. (in Czech).

———— and H. Přibylová. 1966. Die ATP zur Verbeugung des asphyktischen Neugeborenen-Syndroms. Z. Kinderheilk., 96:354-364.

35

Metabolic Effects in Hypoxia Neonatorum

UWE STAVE ● Fels Research Institute, Yellow Springs, Ohio and HELMUT WOLF ● University Children's Hospital, Göttingen, Germany

Introduction

Hypoxia of a certain degree and duration is a normal phenomenon in every delivery. During the passage of the fetus through the birth canal the umbilical vessels become temporarily compressed or even occluded. Retroplacental bleeding can occasionally begin before the expulsion of the baby is completed, thus causing a reduction of placental gas exchange. Finally, the first gasp is normally preceded by a short period of primary apnoea. However, as long as the *respiration* is established within 60 seconds after complete birth, the *skin color* is expected to be rosy; and if the *heart rate, reflex irritability,* and *muscle tone* are normal, the hypoxia sub partu has apparently not affected the newborn. These five observations mentioned are used for the Apgar scoring system (Apgar, 1953). Even the highest Apgar scores of 8 to 10 can be achieved by newborns with an arterial oxygen saturation below 10 percent (James et al., 1958). At birth, the infant's arterial oxygen saturation is found between 0 and 70 percent, and there is no or very little correlation between the newborn's arterial oxygen saturation and the 1-minute Apgar score (James et al., 1958; Apgar et al., 1958). The antenatal decrease of blood oxygenation and the subsequently developing tissue hypoxia are known to be well tolerated by the fetus and the newborn as long as this situation does not exceed a certain degree and duration. However, we still cannot define the upper limit for hypoxia tolerance in human newborns, and we still know very little about the metabolic mechanisms involved in hypoxia tolerance.

As soon as the acceptable limit of physiologic hypoxia sub partu is exceeded, and the hypoxia tolerance is exhausted (see Ch. 2), the damaging effects of oxygen deficit will take place. Clinically, we are then dealing with mild, moderate, or severe hypoxia neonatorum. Frequently, the terms "anoxia" or "asphyxia" are used instead, but true anoxia is very rare and asphyxia neonatorum has included a variety of conditions leading to deficient oxygenation of the blood, or it just means the delayed establishment of spontaneous respiration after birth (Thorn,

1969). Most frequently the term "asphyxia" is used to denote a simultaneous decrease both in the intake of oxygen and in the elimination of carbon dioxide, i.e. hypoxia plus hypercapnia (James et al., 1958). However, the etymology of the word "asphyxia" leads to the impression that the circulation is failing (asphyxia means no pulse) and thus, to avoid confusion, the term "asphyxia" will be avoided in this chapter.

The ability of newborn animals to withstand prolonged anoxia or hypoxia as compared with adults is a well-known fact (Mott, 1961), but it does not seem to be justified to seek the sole explanation for the newborn's hypoxia tolerance in its ability to utilize anaerobic glycolysis to a much greater extent than can the adult organism (Himwich et al., 1942). Details concerning underlying metabolic processes and the regulatory functions during periods of oxygen deficit are still sketchy for the newborn mammal, including man. In the preceding chapter the effect of oxygen deprivation on the central nervous system has been discussed. As shown there, the CNS is most sensitive to lack of oxygen. The survival of the hypoxic newborn or adult is dependent upon the functional state of the CNS. If hypoxemia is complicated by a failing circulation, self-poisoning of the tissues will take place; hence, the prognosis will be worse in such cases (Miller and Miller, 1966).

This may show most clearly how the blood and circulatory system link the sensitive brain tissue and the rest of the body. The latter has to provide the circulation (heart), oxygen (lungs), nutrients (from various depots and by metabolism), and hormones, and it has to eliminate metabolic end-products. Himwich (1958) stressed the point that more simultaneous observations of different variables in hypoxic newborns are likely to provide a sounder interpretation of the metabolism. Furthermore, such a more complex picture will disclose that not only the brain but also the rest of the body is affected by the toleration of prolonged hypoxia.

Hypoxia neonatorum denotes a clinical symptom caused by inadequate supply of oxygen to tissues. For pathogenetic reasons we distinguish *hypoxia fetalis* and *hypoxia neonatorum*. In cases of hypoxia fetalis the hypoxic condition develops in the fetus and can persist until after birth. After the first gasp has occurred a persisting hypoxia as well as a newly developing condition leading to hypoxia should be called "hypoxia neonatorum." The symptom of hypoxia can pertain to quite different diseases and abnormalities, of which disturbances of the pulmonary gas exchange and of the respiratory center are the most frequent causes. Details about the pathogenesis of hypoxia fetalis and neonatorum are discussed in Chapter 34. Usually, the postnatally developing hypoxemia and hypoxia is pathogenetically easier to define and metabolically better investigated. Furthermore, most experiments with newborn animals have been performed after respiration was established.

The old knowledge of medical science that newborn babies tolerate anoxia and hypoxia much better than do adults has also long been confirmed by animal experiments. In 1670 Boyle (cited in Mott, 1961) mentioned the high resistance to anoxia in his pneumatic experiments with one-day-old kittens, but not until the twenties of this century did the phenomenon of anoxia survival in newborns become the topic of numerous physiologic and biochemical investigations (Reiss and Haurowitz, 1929; Fazekas et al., 1941; Villee et al., 1958; reviews by Cooke, 1958; Mott, 1961; Dawkins, 1966; Dawes, 1968). The experimental procedures used to produce anoxia or hypoxia in newborn animals varied considerably among researchers, and also, the definition of survival did not always agree. Survival of experimental anoxia or hypoxia without impairment of any function is of great importance for the human baby; however, in animal experiments the necessary thorough examinations and follow-up studies after anoxia treatment have mostly been avoided. Furthermore, different criteria have been used for measuring the time of anoxia survival, such as the last gasp or heart arrest. In vitro experiments with newborn animals were mostly performed by transferring them into an atmosphere of pure nitrogen for producing anoxia, or by exposure to hypobaric or low-oxygen environments for hypoxia studies. In vitro experiments, such as those performed in human fetal tissues by Villee et al. (1958), provided important insights into the metabolic capabilities of different tissues in anaerobic environments. However, the nervous and humoral regulatory mechanisms seem to be most important in the hypoxic newborn, and those together with metabolic interactions between organs and tissues must be investigated in the intact animal.

Metabolic studies during anoxic or hypoxic states in newborn human infants are, for practical and ethical reasons, very much restricted to blood analyses. These will be surveyed in the following sections in preference to data from other newborn mammals. However, in animal experiments certain conditions can be kept constant, thus allowing observations which rarely can be studied in human infants. In animal experiments tissue analyses and changes in blood constituents can be studied simultaneously and, therefore, some pertinent data for blood and tissues will be discussed on page 1065.

Oxygen Consumption and Body Temperature During Hypoxia

The different pathogenic factors which are involved in the etiology of hypoxia neonatorum render conclusions based on various clinical observations rather difficult. Careful provisions for an appropriate environment have to be provided and adequate methods for measurements must be selected. As shown in Chapter 16, the oxygen consumption of newborn infants increases if the environmental temperature decreases, or more precisely, if the temperature gradient between skin and environment increases. In order not to confuse the effects of cold and oxygen deficiency, the following data will be restricted to observations where the oxygen consumption was measured while the infants were kept in a neutral temperature environment. In healthy newborn infants a moderately hypoxic environment of 13 to 15 percent oxygen does not alter the oxygen consumption compared with that in those breathing room air (Oliver and Karlberg, 1963; Cross et al., 1966).

Some observations are available of newborns breathing 12 percent oxygen. Eventually, these infants disclosed cyanosis and somnolence and hence the possible hazards of inducing hypoxia of more severe degree naturally forbids such studies in human infants (Cross et al., 1966). However, measurements in newborn babies suffering from respiratory distress or severe heart failure have been reported. Severe respiratory distress in premature infants of less than 60 hours of age depresses the oxygen consumption significantly. Miller et al. (1962) found a mean oxygen consumption of 6.0 ml O_2 per kg per minute (S.D. ±1.34 ml) in 10 infants with respiratory distress syndrome (RDS) compared with a normal mean of 8.4 ml O_2 per kg per minute (S.D. ±0.9 ml) measured in 37 healthy or recovered premature infants. Levison et al. (1964) reported low oxygen consumption in 28 infants with RDS during the first 40 hours of life, and subsequently during recovery these babies increased their O_2 consumption above normal values. It is of special interest to note that the latter authors found that depressed oxygen consumption was not always correlated with arterial hypoxemia. Thus, systemic metabolic demand for oxygen was considered to be a major factor in changes of oxygen consumption during prolonged periods of respiratory distress.

Chronically hypoxic infants suffering from cardiovascular or cardiopulmonary disease showed, at least in most cases, normal values for oxygen consumption (Brück et al., 1962; Levison et al., 1965). However, individual values are scattered over a wide range, and 5 infants out of 16 studied by Levison et al. (1965) exhibited a marked acidosis together with low oxygen consumption. From measurements of the arterial partial pressure of O_2 (P_aO_2) the same authors concluded that "the search for some universal critical figure for P_aO_2 in regard to levels of oxygen consumption is probably illusory in the varied clinical situations" and that "a critical P_aO_2 is only meaningful under a given constant set of conditions." Circulatory peculiarities of congenital heart disease prevent or limit comparisons of the energy metabolism. Infants suffering from cyanotic heart failure showed a diminished increase of their oxygen consumption in a cool environment, but this insufficiency could also be based on their inability to increase the heart output sufficiently (Brück et al., 1962).

Investigating healthy and hypoxic infants up to 6 months of age, Varga (1967) came to a similar conclusion that severe arterial hypoxemia depresses oxygen consumption, but no linear correlation was found between P_aO_2 and O_2 consumption. Furthermore, this author observed that once the organism is adapted to chronic hypoxia, the oxygen consumption approaches normal values.

Studies in experimental hypoxia in newborn dogs (Moore, 1956), kittens (Hill, 1959; Moore, 1959), lambs (Cross et al., 1959), rabbits (Blatteis, 1964), mice (Cassin, 1963), and monkeys (Dawes et al., 1960) show slightly reduced oxygen consumption in 10 percent oxygen, and in some species marked reductions were demonstrated during more severe oxygen deprivation (Dawes, 1961). Mott (1963) pointed out that not only the environmental temperature but also regional changes of oxygen uptake, and in addition, the especially slow increase in minimum oxygen consumption during the first day of life (lambs) have to be considered as determining factors. Newborn rats are more immature at birth than the other mammals listed above (see Ch. 34). Therefore, it was no surprise to find a different behavior of the regulatory system in the early postnatal period of rats. On the first day of life rats reduce their oxygen consumption on breathing 18 percent oxygen and more in 15 percent oxygen. However, three- to four-day-old rats maintain normal oxygen consumption in an environment containing 15 percent oxygen (Taylor, 1960).

The increment of oxygen consumption observed during exposure to a cold environment (see Ch. 16) is particularly susceptible to hypoxia. This cold-induced increase can be depressed by reducing the environmental oxygen concentration to 10 percent in kittens (Hill, 1959), rabbits (Dawes and Mott, 1959; Blatteis, 1964), lambs (Cross et al., 1959) and monkeys (Dawes et al., 1960). However, the extra heat produced in response to cold does not seem to be uniquely depressed by hypoxia (Hill, 1959), and moreover, this mechanism is not uniform with time since a prolonged exposure to both cold and hypoxia leads gradually toward the original basal oxygen consumption. In rabbits this process is accompanied by the development of shivering (Blatteis, 1964). The effect of acclimatization has thus been shown to occur in newborn mammals as well as in the human infant (see above).

The *rectal temperature* of *human* newborns who suffered anoxia or hypoxia during labor or sub partu is significantly lower from birth on (Burnard and Cross, 1958). Similarly, infants suffering from hypoxia because of respiratory distress frequently disclose rectal temperatures below the normal range (Miller et al., 1962; Varga, 1967); however, hypoxemic infants who metabolize oxygen at a normal rate rarely show decreased rectal temperatures (Miller et al., 1962). In 10 healthy infants the mean rectal temperature was 37.0°C, in 11 hypoxemic infants with normal oxygen consumption the rectal temperature averaged 36.8°C, but in 5 severely hypoxemic infants with reduced oxygen consumption the mean rectal temperature was 35.1°C (Levison et al., 1964).

Animal experiments disclosed the same correlations between oxygen consumption and body core temperature. In 12-hour-old rabbits, a short-term exposure to 5 percent oxygen reduced the rectal temperature by 2°C, but two- to eight-day-old rabbits showed only a very small drop of rectal temperature after 4 hours of exposure to 10 percent oxygen in an environment of 35°C (Blatteis, 1964). Newborn rabbits which were exposed to 6.5 percent oxygen during the entire first day of extrauterine life in a chamber kept at 30.5°C by radiant heat reduced their rectal temperature to 35.9±0.85°C compared with control rabbits in room air which showed 36.7±0.70°C (18 animals in each group; mean ± standard deviation). This difference was statistically significant (Stave, 1969).

In connection with more recent attempts to use hypothermia for preventing brain damage during hypoxia in infants suffering from RDS (Westin et al., 1962; Miller et al., 1964a), it is of interest to note that survival times (last gasp) in five different mammalian species exposed to 95 percent N_2 with 5 percent CO_2 increase with artificial reduction of body temperatures and that for the species tested a body temperature of approximately 15°C is optimal for survival under these conditions. Newborn puppies cooled to 15°C body temperature made their last gasp in this anoxic environment after 105 minutes, whereas puppies kept at normal body temperature survived only 14 minutes. Miller and Miller (1966) concluded that "exposure to hypoxia-hypercapnea during cooling enhances the protective effects of hypothermia against asphyxia." The prevention of generalized arterial vasoconstriction and an increase in blood flow seem to provide a greater supply of nutrients for the tissues and a more effective removal of waste material from the tissues; both are very important factors for prolonged anoxia survival achieved by an overall reduction of the energy metabolism due to drastic cooling.

Effect of hypoxia on blood gases and metabolites

Important information on the metabolic situation of newborn infants can be quickly provided by blood analyses. Only arterial blood is representative for the general supply of nutrients available for the tissues, whereas the blood obtained from different peripheral veins carries varying amounts of unused nutrients and metabolic end-products with great regional differences. Depending on clinical circumstances information from venous blood samples might suffice for certain purposes, but during periods of hypoxemia or impaired circulation the analysis of arterial blood is highly desirable, especially for information on the amount of oxygen carried to the tissues. If no catheter was left in the umbilical cord vessels and no puncture of an artery is possible, "arterialized" capillary blood can be obtained for measuring the P_aO_2 and oxygen saturation (Smith and Kaplan, 1942; Gambino, 1961), but in a series of simultaneous determinations on the first day of life, Berg and Dörrler (1969) found the capillary Po_2 lower by 21 mm Hg than the arterial pressure.

The analysis of cord blood at birth is of only limited significance because of impaired placental functions which frequently occur prior to cord clamping and blood sampling. The oxygen content of blood taken from the umbilical vein is related to the gas exchange in the placenta, and hence it bears little relation to the oxygenation of the newborn's tissues (Caldwell et al., 1957; Pennoyer et al., 1956). This latter situation is better reflected by the oxygen level in the blood obtained from the umbilical arteries (Ch. 6).

OXYGEN

The normal full-term human infant discloses a wide range in oxygen blood levels in both the umbilical vein and arteries (see Ch. 3). The range of oxygen saturation found in the umbilical vein is 10 to 84 percent, and in the umbilical arteries it is 0 to 70 percent (James et al., 1958). In approximately one third of all newborns the arterial oxygen saturation (S_aO_2) was found to be below 10 percent, and in 7 out of 63 infants no oxygen was measurable. In 43 vigorous newborns with Apgar scores between 8 and 10, James et al. (1958) calculated a mean S_aO_2 of 22.2 percent. Crawford (1965) reported in newborns selected as "clinically acceptable ideal cases" mean values for S_aO_2 between 30 and 34 percent with differences for primi- and multigravida. Figures 1A and 1B demonstrate the postnatal changes for P_aO_2 and S_aO_2.

The analysis of capillary fetal scalp blood during the final stages of expulsion showed a slight decrease in oxygen saturation from 42.3 to 30.4 percent (Hochuli and Schneider, 1966). In the same series of measurements which were performed

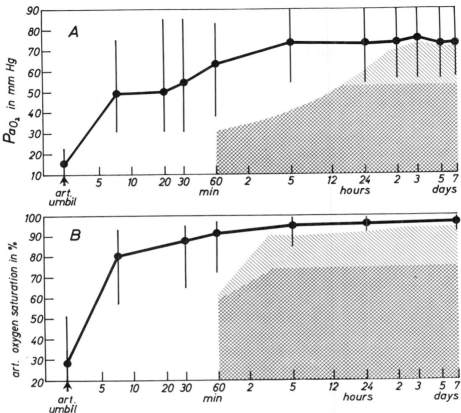

Fig. 1. Postnatal changes of: A. oxygen partial pressure ($P_{a}O_2$) B. oxygen saturation in arterial blood. Abscissa, Logarithmic time scale. Vertical bars represent the range. The lightly shaded areas designate the range for values measured frequently in infants suffering from mild or moderate hypoxemia; the darker shade represents the range for values found in cases of severe hypoxia. (Normal values with ranges from Koch and Wendel, 1968. Hypoxia ranges according to data from Weisbrot et al., 1958; Kerpel-Fronius et al., 1965; Prod'hom et al., 1965; Moss et al., 1965; Boston et al., 1966; Orzalesi et al., 1967; Gupta et al., 1967.)

according to Saling (1962), the authors calculated a mean for oxygen saturation in the umbilical artery of 20.2 percent. Prematurely born infants tend to have slightly lower values than term born infants (MacKinney et al., 1958), but after 3 hours of age normal premature infants had no lower $S_{a}O_2$ than term born infants (Orzalesi et al., 1967). Babies with poor clinical status at birth, i.e., Apgar scores below 6, showed significantly lower oxygen saturation in arterial cord blood (James et al., 1958; MacKinney et al., 1958). Cohnstein and Zuntz (1884) first measured the oxygen saturation of cord blood in mammals, and since that time numerous publications have confirmed that at onset of respiration the newborn suffers from marked hypoxemia that "appears to occur as a normal phenomenon in almost every delivery" (James et al., 1958).

Factors contributing to this subpartal hypoxemia are 1, cord compression; 2, changes in uterine blood flow; 3, impaired placental function; and 4, disturbances of maternal respiratory gas exchange and/or acid-base state (details are discussed in Ch. 34). Analgesia and anesthesia during labor and expulsion have varying and occasionally marked effects on the newborn's arterial oxygen saturation (James et al., 1958; Rooth, 1963); this depression might well last through the first hour of life (Pennoyer et al., 1956). In the majority of normal newborns the arterial oxygen saturation and partial pressure rise quickly after respiration has been established; within the first hour S_aO_2 and P_aO_2 become useful for evaluating the infant's oxygen supply (Figs. 1A and 1B).

ACID-BASE STATUS

The acid-base status constitutes an essential part of homeostasis. The accumulation of acid or the loss of base lead to acidosis since either will lower the blood pH. The opposite pathologic condition, alkalosis, is due to accumulation of base or loss of acid. The arterial blood pH, however, reflects the combined influence of respiratory and nonrespiratory disturbances. Respiratory acid-base disturbances are due to any deviation from the normal CO_2 tension, whereas nonrespiratory acid-base disturbances are reflected by any deviation from the normal content of base in blood. Disturbances can occur as either primary or compensatory (see Ch. 3). The following definitions are according to Astrup et al. (1960). "Buffer base" designates the sum of buffering bicarbonate, hemoglobin, and protein in blood. "Standard bicarbonate" is defined as the plasma bicarbonate concentration when whole blood is equilibrated with CO_2 at 40 mm Hg at 38°C and when the hemoglobin is fully oxygenated. "Base excess" directly expresses the amount of base present in mEq per liter of blood, when the normal mean is arbitrarily fixed at zero; positive values designate an excess of base, and negative values express a deficit of base, which is an excess of acid. For comparison and better understanding of the acid-base status in newborn infants, the normal 95 percent ranges of healthy adults are listed: in arterial blood, pH 7.35 to 7.42; Pco_2 34 to 45 mm Hg; standard bicarbonate 21.3 to 24.8 mEq per liter; base excess -2.3 to $+2.3$ mEq per liter.

The effect of oxygen deficiency is reflected by the acid-base status (see also Ch. 3 and 20). The physiologically occurring mild respiratory and metabolic acidosis sub partu subsides soon after birth (Figs. 2A, 2B, and 2C).

However, in newborns suffering from persistent hypoxemia, e.g., respiratory distress, the acidosis becomes either more severe or, at least, no change occurs toward normalization. The acidosis, which is enhanced by persistent postnatal hypoxemia and hypoxia, further hampers oxygen uptake and CO_2 discharge (see Ch. 10), and this vicious circle becomes more severe as more organic acids accumulate. Thus, the mixed respiratory plus metabolic acidosis at birth slowly changes into a predominantly metabolic acidosis if respiratory distress and

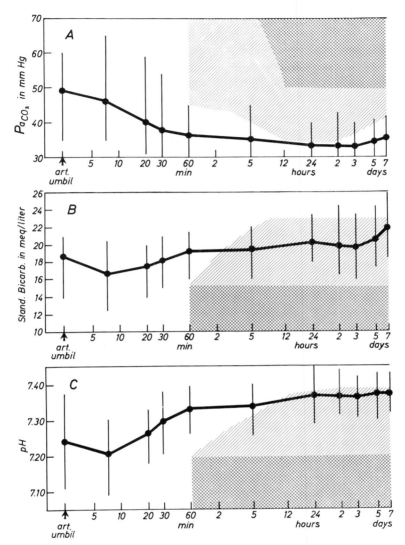

Fig. 2. Postnatal changes and hypoxia ranges of: A. partial pressure of CO_2, B. standard bicarbonate. C. pH in arterial blood. Presentation as in Figure 1. (Normal values from Koch and Wendel, 1968. Hypoxia ranges according to data from Weisbrot et al., 1958; Strang and MacLeish, 1961; Warley and Gairdner, 1962; Keuth and Adenauer, 1963; Kerpel-Fronius et al., 1964; Prod'hom et al., 1965; Moss et al., 1965; Boston et al., 1966; Blennemann, 1966, Gupta et al., 1967; Orzalesi et al., 1967.)

consequently hypoxia persists (James et al., 1958; Kildeberg, 1964; Prod'hom et al., 1965; James, 1967).

In prematurely born infants the postnatal changes of the metabolic acid-base status appear not to differ significantly from those observed in full-term babies (Keuth and Adenauer, 1963; Kildeberg, 1964; Orzalesi et al., 1967; Gupta et al., 1967). Table 1 provides some data which demonstrate the changes which occur

TABLE 1.   Arterial Blood Values of Normal and Distressed Premature Infants

	$P_{a}O_2$ mm Hg	$S_{a}O_2$ %	pH	$P_{a}CO_2$ mm Hg	Base Excess mEq/liter
Normal[a] age 4 h (n=4)	60	91	7.33	47	−3.7
Normal[a] age 15 h (n=21)	68	95	7.45	28	−3.7
Mild RDS[a] age 15 h (n=4)	53	90	7.38	33	−5.3
Severe RDS[b] average age 6 h (n=16)	39[c]		7.10	86[d]	−9.4

[a]Data from Orzalesi et al., 1967.
[b]Data courtesy of Dr. U. Keuth, Neunkirchen-Kohlhof, Germany.
[c]Average O_2 concentration in hood air was 62 percent by volume.
[d]Determination according to Astrup method.

in prematurely born infants suffering from various degrees of respiratory distress. In mild cases of RDS, the deviations are still relatively minor, obviously due to a rather small drop in arterial oxygen saturation. More severe cases of RDS, with consequently higher degrees of hypoxia, show a drastic decrease of pH and buffer base and a high retention of $P_{a}CO_2$. Figures 2B and 2C comprise the normal ranges of values for pH and standard bicarbonate during the first seven days of life. Most of the data published for unaffected premature infants are consistent with those shown for healthy full-term infants (Keuth and Adenauer, 1963; Blenne-mann, 1966). The lightly and heavily shaded areas designate the ranges for values which were frequently measured in moderately or severely hypoxic infants. Such changes which are due to hypoxia of varying degrees undoubtedly can occur before the age of 60 minutes, but the wide scatter of normal values and the small amount of information on hypoxic babies of less than 60 minutes of age prevented us from showing hypoxia values for this age group. Moreover, no strict distinction can be made between moderate and severe cases, although many pediatricians agree that a plasma pH of less than 7.20 (after 60 minutes of age) designates severe acidosis and calls for immediate and intensive treatment.

GLUCOSE

Methodologic differences for measuring blood glucose concentrations render comparisons between older and more recent studies difficult (Wolf, 1960; Baens et al., 1963; Hjelm and Sjölin, 1965; Ek and Daae, 1967). Older methods often referred to "blood sugar" and were based on measurements of the total reducing power, e.g., the Hagedorn-Jensen method. Improved procedures for protein precipitation and different color reactions, such as the Somogyi-Nelson method, diminished the interference by other reducing substances. The true glucose in blood was first determined by the glucose oxidase method (Keilin and Hartree, 1948). However, for measuring blood glucose concentrations in newborns, the oxidase method yields lower values than the highly specific method employing the hexokinase reaction (Wolf, 1969).

During labor the maternal and fetal blood glucose concentrations increase steadily. Raivio and Teramo (1968) found that, during an average expulsion period of six hours, both the maternal and the fetal blood glucose levels increased by approximately 18 percent. One to ten minutes before birth the glucose level in fetal scalp blood (arterialized capillary blood) varied between 61 and 83 mg/100 ml (mean: 72 mg/100 ml), and at birth in the arteria umbilicalis the values ranged between 62 and 84 mg/100 ml (mean: 71 mg/100 ml) (Raivio and Teramo, 1968).

Figure 3A shows the normal postnatal changes of blood glucose concentration obtained by employing a $ZnSO_4$ precipitation of protein preceding the glucose measurement with glucose oxidase (Hjelm and Sjölin, 1965). The range shown covers approximately 90 percent of all measurements obtained from full-term and prematurely born healthy infants (Baens et al., 1963). Immediately after birth the blood glucose level decreases, and the lowest concentrations usually occur between 24 and 60 hours of age (Fig. 3A). This postnatal decline of blood glucose concentration must occur because of one or a combination of the following three mechanisms:

1. *Great need for glucose and thus higher turnover rate of carbohydrates.* The calculation of glucose turnover rates according to Dost et al. (1968) revealed, however, that glucose utilization is markedly lower in one- and two-day-old infants. During the first two days after birth the glucose transfer was found to be between 0.11 and 0.16 g per hour per kg body weight (Gladtke et al., 1968). Transfer designates the amount of a substance that is exchanged between two or more communicating compartments per unit of time. It was calculated that the amount of glucose transfer could provide approximately one fourth to one third of the newborn's total energy requirements. Toward the end of the first week, healthy infants increase their hourly glucose transfer to an average of 0.36 g per kg. The postnatal delay of carbohydrate utilization has been observed by several authors (Bowie et al., 1963; Von Euler et al., 1964), and hence it is unlikely that an increased rate of carbohydrate utilization is responsible for the postnatal hypoglycemia.

2. *Inadequate function of the enzymatic reactions involved in glycogen mobilization.* The most drastic changes of glycogen content occur in the perinatal liver. At birth the human liver contains approximately 50 mg glycogen per g wet weight, and 24 hours later this deposit is reduced to less than 5 mg per g (Shelley, 1969). This fact provides proof that the enzymes engaged in glycogen mobilization are present in neonatal liver, but some of the enzyme activities were found to be lower on the first day of life than after one week or in adult liver (see Ch. 13 and 17). Thus, the postnatal hypoglycemia will be more pronounced if the normal increase

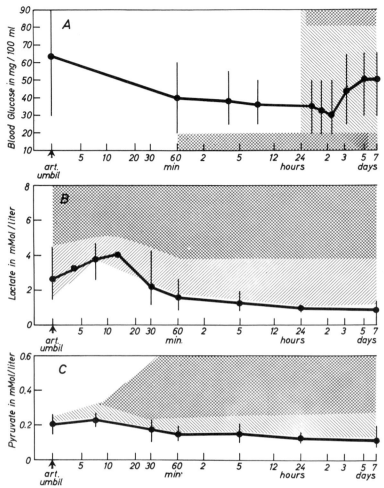

Fig. 3. Postnatal changes and hypoxia ranges for: A. Glucose. B. Lactate. C. Pyruvate
in arterial blood. Presentation as in Figure 1. A. Normal values with range from
Hjelm and Sjölin (1965) complemented by data from Cornblath et al. (1961).
For hypoxia range, from Kerpel-Fronius et al. (1964) and Raivio and Hallman
(1968). B. and C. Normal values with ranges from Koch and Wendel (1968)
complemented by data from Vedra and Ulrych (1960), Štembera and Hodr (1966),
and Daniel et al. (1966). For hypoxia range data from Vedra (1963), Gomez
and Graven (1964), and Daniel et al., (1966).

of glycogenolytic enzyme activities in the liver does not proceed adequately in
newborns. Such a delay of enzyme development has been observed in dysmature
rats (Hommes and Wilmink, 1968). In addition, small-for-date and prematurely
born infants have stored smaller than normal amounts of glycogen (Shelley, 1964;
Shelley and Neligan, 1966). Therefore, the insufficient enzymatic potential and
the small glycogen deposits are additive, and thus they aggravate the hypoglycemia.

Furthermore, the hormonal control mechanisms, the amount of cofactors, and the environmental conditions for glycogenolytic reactions, e.g., severe acidosis, may affect in a negative manner the amount of glucose liberated.

3. *Premature exhaustion of glycogen reserves.* At completion of gestation a full-term infant of 3,500 g body weight has stored approximately 34 g carbohydrates, of which 76 percent is located in the skeletal muscle, 22 percent in the liver, and the remaining 2 percent in heart, brain, kidney, and other tissues (Shelley, 1960). A prematurely born infant of 2,000 g body weight has accumulated not more than a total of 9 g carbohydrates (Widdowson, 1964). Theoretically, the oxidation of 34 g carbohydrates, which would provide 136 calories, could not even cover the energy requirements for basal metabolism for 24 hours; in the premature, the amount of 9 g glycogen would last for less than 12 hours. In fact, however, only a fraction of the total body carbohydrate is mobilized immediately after birth, and it seems that the hepatic glycogen mobilization is by far more decisive than the glucose liberation from other organs (see p. 1069). According to this calculation an amount of approximately 6.6 g hepatic glycogen is available for the full-term baby on the first day of life and considerably less for the prematurely born infant. These calculations by Widdowson (1964) elucidate the vulnerability of the carbohydrate metabolism in the immediate postnatal period. Considering the normal variations of glycogen storage, the markedly lower amounts of available carbohydrates in prematures, and especially the low values found in small-for-date babies (Shelley and Neligan, 1966) the postnatal hypoglycemia can well be related to a premature exhaustion of carbohydrate reserves.

Screening tests for blood glucose revealed that approximately five percent of newborns show hypoglycemic values within the first week of life. (Cornblath et al., 1966; Raivio and Hallman, 1968). Hypoglycemia has been defined as sequential blood glucose values of less than 30 mg/100 ml in full-term newborns and of less than 20 mg/100 ml in prematurely born infants after a 3.5- to 4.5-hour fast (Cornblath et al., 1966). Symptomatic and idiopathic forms of hypoglycemia need to be distinguished by appropriate clinical analyses and tests (Broberger and Zetterström, 1961; Neligan et al., 1963; Cornblath et al., 1966; Antony et al., 1967; Raivio and Hallman, 1968; Gentz et al., 1969a). In discussing the pathogenesis of neonatal hypoglycemia most authors have focused on fetal malnutrition, damage or abnormalities in the central nervous system, genetic factors, and hormonal dysfunction; this latter includes a variety of functional abnormalities related to pancreatic and other endocrine status (Antony et al., 1967). However, case histories of neonatal hypoglycemia revealed that hypoxia insults, placental malfunction, and maternal toxemia are rather frequent findings (Cornblath et al., 1959; Brown and Wallis, 1963; Neligan et al., 1963; Zetterström, 1963). Thus, oxygen deficiency during expulsion and sub partu is a potential factor involved in producing or aggravating hypoglycemia.

Raivio and Hallman (1968) found that the incidence of significant hypoglycemia was 20 percent in small-for-date infants, 16 percent in infants of diabetic mothers, and 15 percent in critically ill babies dying within ten days after birth. In small-for-date infants the fetal malnutrition seems to be correlated with placental dysfunction (Strand, 1966), but the extent of hypoxia involved and the effects on the fetus due to placental malfunction have hardly been touched by investigators (Dancis, 1965) (see also Ch. 1). It should be taken into account that the small-for-date infants frequently show high hematocrit values, and thus their blood glucose level is expected to be lower (Haworth et al., 1967). Similar considerations can be applied to chronic hypoxic infants with high hemoconcentration.

Prematurely born infants suffering from hypoxia disclose widely scattered values with even more extreme glucose concentrations (between 0 and 150 mg/100 ml) as death approaches (Kerpel-Fronius et al., 1964). Usher (1961) reported a mean blood glucose level of 25 mg/100 ml in RDS infants on the first day of life with several patients showing values under 5 mg/100 ml. Baens et al. (1963) found a lower mean for blood glucose in infants suffering from RDS and in infants affected with anoxia bouts, but the difference between this group and unaffected prematures was not statistically significant. In Figure 3A it is marked that blood glucose levels below 20 mg/100 ml and above 80 mg/100 ml occur in newborn babies suffering from severe hypoxia, but most pediatricians will agree that severe hypoxia neonatorum is not accompanied by characteristic changes of the blood glucose concentration; mild or moderate hypoxia causes hyperglycemia in some cases but to a lesser extent. The necessity of early treatment with glucose and short intervals between small meals will, in addition, not permit observations of truly fasting infants. The effect of prolonged hypoxia on fasting newborn animals is discussed below (p. 1068).

LACTATE AND PYRUVATE

Discrepancies between oxygen supply and the requirement of the cell metabolism for oxygen seem to be well detectable by calculating the amount of *excess lactate* from measurements of plasma lactate and pyruvate concentrations. Huckabee (1958b) has shown that excess lactate refers to that fraction of the total lactate change that corresponds closely to the magnitude of tissue oxygen debt. In this respect excess lactate values are thought to be superior to the lactate/pyruvate ratio (L/P).

Pyruvate is a very active metabolite which participates in a great number of intermediary reactions of which the formation of lactate is only one. This latter reaction is catalyzed by lactate dehydrogenase (LDH, see formula), and lactate accumulates in this dead-end pathway as soon as the utilization of pyruvate along the main route is hampered, for instance during anaerobiosis.

$$\text{Pyruvate} + \text{NADH} + \text{H}^+ \xrightarrow{\text{LDH}} \text{Lactate} + \text{NAD}^+$$

The LDH reaction is coupled with one of the basic oxidation-reduction systems in which oxidized NAD represents the lowest potential in the hydrogen ion carrier system. The significance of the dependence of lactate production upon pyruvate and the ratio of reduced and oxidized NAD is depicted in the following formula which is derived from the mass action form of the LDH reaction.

$$[Lactate] = [Pyruvate] \times K \times \frac{[NADH + H^+]}{[NAD^+]}$$

From this formula in which K represents a constant Huckabee (1958a, b) derived the following equation:

$$XL = (L_n - L_o) - (P_n - P_o) \times \frac{L_o}{P_o}$$

This formula allows the calculation of excess lactate (XL) from measurements of lactate and pyruvate blood concentrations under resting (steady state) conditions (L_o and P_o) and blood values obtained after tissue hypoxia has occurred (L_n and P_n).

The concept of using the amount of excess lactate as an expression of tissue oxygen debt has been questioned by Olson (1963), Thomas et al. (1965), Alpert (1965), and others on different bases, but its application can be valuable in all age groups. However, the metabolic situation of the fetus sub partu and of the newborn immediately after birth is extremely different from that of the experimental model (Huckabee, 1958a; Daniel et al., 1966). During the immediate perinatal period the fetal homeostasis ceases to exist, and the postnatal homeostasis needs some time to become established (see Ch. 2); consequently there exists no steady state to which the oxidation-reduction status of the newborn's tissues can be referred (Daniel et al., 1966) Hence, the blood values for excess lactate of newborns cannot be calculated according to Huckabee's (1958a) original concept. Nevertheless, by introducing some additional physiologic measurements the *anaerobic metabolic rate* has been calculated in certain tissue masses. The pregnant uterus, for instance, has been used by Huckabee et al., (1962a, b) for considerations concerning movements of excess lactate in relation to tissue oxygenation.

Both lactate and pyruvate can pass the placenta freely in either direction (Friedman et al., 1960). Since the placenta is revealed to have a high capability of metabolizing lactate (Villee, 1953; DiPietro et al., 1967) even under moderate hypoxic conditions (Huckabee et al., 1962b), the concentration gradient of lactate and pyruvate between maternal and fetal blood does not seem to be a matter of diffusion but is regulated by the placental metabolism (Huckabee et al., 1962b; Vedra, 1963; Daniel et al., 1966). Several authors suggest that some of the cord blood lactate originates from the maternal circulation (Vedra, 1963; Derom, 1964; Štembera and Hodr, 1966).

In human fetuses at gestational ages 34 through 44 weeks (including one fetus at 16 weeks)the umbilical vein had a higher lactate concentration than the arterial blood of the mother, but this holds true only by comparing the mean values of the series; individual values showed no particular pattern (Otey et al., 1967). Otey et al. (1967) found that excess lactate is lost from fetal blood in the placenta and that it does not appear in maternal blood. Furthermore, the simultaneously determined oxygen saturation and the rates of blood flow may yield information on the oxygen supply to the tissues; but, as discussed above, these values do not permit conclusions about the adequacy of oxygen supply to meet the requirements of particular tissues.

Investigations in pregnant goats of interrelationships between maternal and intrauterine lactate and pyruvate concentrations disclosed that "the data as a whole show that these metabolites may be transferred into or out of the placenta on either side in amounts which seem to be independent of each other and in independent directions" (Huckabee et al., 1962a). Furthermore, there is no concentration gradient known along which lactate and pyruvate ions diffuse. Normal goat fetuses at gestational ages between 68 and 139 days were found to have lower lactate and pyruvate concentrations in both umbilical vessels than did the mother in her arterial or uterine venous blood (Kaiser and Cummings, 1958). Studying pregnant goats and their fetuses of gestational ages between 27 and 139 days during periods of hypoxemia, Huckabee et al. (1962b) found highly heterogenous values for blood lactate and pyruvate in individual animals. However, a characteristic pattern became obvious when the exchanges of excess lactate on each side of the placenta were viewed as determinant. As long as the mother's arterial oxygen saturation remained above 90 percent no anaerobic metabolism could be observed in the pregnant uterus, but severe maternal hypoxemia induced anaerobic metabolic reactions in the uterus as a whole. Most important information, however, was gained from experiments with mild to moderate degrees of maternal hypoxemia. Under these conditions the fetus produced marked amounts of excess lactate which were reoxidized by the placenta, and consequently, the uterus as a whole did not present a net anaerobic metabolism. Even fetuses with no measurable amounts of oxygen in cord blood survived without signs of deleterious effects. Jurado-García et al. (1966) confirmed the relative independence of maternal and fetal lactate metabolism in rats and rat fetuses. From their experiments Huckabee et al. (1962b) concluded that the energy metabolism of the fetus cannot be separated from that of the placenta. The fetoplacental unit has a superior efficiency for managing hypoxia situations compared with the isolated fetus. Moreover, these in vivo experiments seem to render in vitro experiments with fetal tissues irrelevant since the vitally important interaction between fetus and placenta is disregarded in such studies.

The fetoplacental unit has also shown to be of great importance for the elimination of bilirubin (Ch. 18) and for the synthesis of steroid hormones (Ch. 30). Parturition leads to destruction of this fetoplacental unit. Consequently, from birth on the burden of managing metabolic problems, such as hypoxia, bilirubin elimination, and steroid synthesis, is transferred to the newborn. This also holds true for the amount of lactate which had increased in the newborn's blood and tissues during labor and expulsion.

Figures 3B and 3C show the range of lactate and pyruvate concentration in arterial blood at birth and through the first seven days after birth. It should be noted again that only arterial blood represents the organism as a whole (Huckabee, 1958a, b; Lundsgaard-Hansen, 1966). Compared with lactate concentrations of one-week-old infants, the lactate level in cord blood is three times higher and the pyruvate level 67 percent higher. The arterial blood concentrations of both metabolites rise immediately after birth (Thalme, 1967), but already within 30 minutes after parturition the levels decrease below cord values. On the second day of life lactate and pyruvate concentrations reach a steady level which is within the normal range of values for older infants and children (Znamenáček and Přibylová, 1964; Acharya and Payne, 1965; Koch and Wendel, 1968).

As discussed above, to apply the concept in calculating excess lactate is not justified for the newborn on the first day. However, Znamenáček and Přibylová (1964) calculated XL from lactate and pyruvate concentrations in capillary blood of newborns up to age 72 hours. The XL values were found to increase for 15 minutes after birth, and thereafter they decreased steadily until they leveled off at the third day; for the calculation of XL the third day values were taken as representative for the resting state (L_o and P_o).

In the cytoplasm the L/P ratio reflects the oxidoreduction state of the NAD system (Hohorst et al., 1965). However, the contribution of tissues and organs to arterial blood lactate and pyruvate concentrations differs considerably (Lundsgaard-Hansen, 1966), and thus the blood L/P ratio represents an integrated value. In addition, the blood levels of lactate and pyruvate are affected by other factors such as renal excretion and delayed diffusion from tissues (see also Alpert, 1965). Nevertheless, the L/P ratio of arterial blood has frequently been used as an indicator for hypoxic conditions. The mean L/P ratio was found to be 17.4 in the umbilical vein (Marx and Greene, 1965) and 13.5 in the umbilical artery (Koch and Wendel, 1968). Ten minutes after birth the L/P ratio increases to 16.5, and thereafter it decreases slowly, e.g., 12.9 at 30 minutes, 8.7 at 5 hours, and 7.7 at 24 hours of age; later on an average of 7.5 is considered normal for arterial blood.

Intravenous loading tests with lactate confirmed that newborns, very soon after birth, develop an increasing ability to metabolize lactate efficiently (Ciampolini and Franchini, 1966). In the newborn the liver seems to be the dominant site for lactate oxidation whereas in adults the skeletal and cardiac muscle, in addition to the liver, metabolize significant amounts of lactate (Alpert, 1965).

In neonatal skeletal muscle the activity of LDH is not more than 10 percent of the adult activity (see Ch. 26); the cardiac muscle of newborns has also a markedly lower LDH activity than that of adults (Stave, 1964; Mager et al., 1968). The immediate postnatal increase of liver LDH activity and its increase in response to hypoxia (Stave, 1967; Mager et al., 1968) provide evidence that the newborn liver develops an increasing capability to metabolize lactate. If some oxygen deficiency persists after parturition the relatively high blood lactate level of the first 15 minutes after birth may not begin to decrease, as in normals. In cases of more severe hypoxia, the lactate level will rise as the oxygen debt increases (Fig. 3B).

As depicted in Figures 3B and 3C hypoxia or anoxia neonatorum is accompanied by elevated lactate concentrations in cord blood and to a minor degree by higher pyruvate values (Eastman and McLane, 1931; James and Burnard, 1961; Vedra, 1963; Räihä, 1963; Daniel et al., 1966; Otey et al., 1967). After birth, the concentrations of both metabolites first increase before they begin to decline within the first half hour after birth, thus running parallel with the normal postnatal changes but on a higher level (James and Burnard, 1961; Daniel et al., 1966).

Elevated lactate and, to a lesser degree, pyruvate concentrations have been frequently observed in newborn infants suffering from RDS, various forms of pneumonia, Wilson-Mikity syndrome, or cerebral hemorrhages affecting the respiratory center. Mild or moderate cases of respiratory distress eventually show minor increases of blood lactate concentrations (Gomez and Graven, 1964; Graven et al., 1965), but frequently the values remain within the upper normal range (Fig. 3B); the pyruvate concentration increases similarly, although mostly delayed and to a minor degree (Fig. 3C). The L/P ratio was found to vary within a wide range (Wang et al., 1963; Marx et al., 1965; Frenzel et al., 1968), and thus the L/P ratio is not a reliable indicator in cases of mild or moderate respiratory distress.

Severe hypoxemia during respiratory distress causes high blood lactate concentrations and often excessively high increases are found in fatal cases. Pyruvate increases also, and the L/P ratio reaches values above 20 (Graven et al., 1965; Payne and Acharya, 1965; Frenzel et al., 1968). During the course of RDS a high L/P ratio was claimed to be of better prognostic significance than lactate alone or even blood pH (Frenzel et al., 1968).

Animal experiments confirmed these findings. Respiratory distress in lambs (Stahlman et al., 1964; Reynolds et al., 1965) and in monkeys (Adamsons et al., 1963) was accompanied by increased blood lactate concentrations. During anoxia very high lactate concentrations were observed in newborn rats (Stafford and Weatherall, 1960), monkeys (Dawes et al., 1960), and lambs (Dawes et al., 1963). Prolonged exposure to low oxygen concentrations (6.5 percent O_2 in nitrogen) caused moderate increases of blood lactate and pyruvate in newborn rabbits (Stave, 1970; see also Fig. 6, p. 1069). The fetuses of severely hypoxic rats were revealed to have a slightly higher blood lactate concentration after 30 minutes than did the mother animals (Thalme, 1967).

FATTY ACIDS, GLYCEROL, AND KETONE BODIES

Calculations of the total glucose transfer in healthy human newborns revealed that only one third to one fourth of the total energy required can be derived from glucose oxidation during the first and second days of life (see p. 1053). Hence, additional metabolic fuel is needed for maintaining the body temperature and for other energy-requiring functions. For example, fatty acids serve as the source for energy production in the ventricular muscle although to a much smaller extent in the newborn than in adults (Wittels and Bressler, 1965; Breuer et al., 1968). Although glucose represents the main metabolic fuel for brain tissue (Himwich, 1951), some other metabolites, such as glycerol (Sloviter et al., 1966), free fatty acids (Geiger, 1958), and ketone bodies (Drahota et al., 1965) may also serve this function to a limited extent (see also Ch. 34). The utilization of fatty acids and ketone bodies in brain tissue has been demonstrated indirectly by the presence of enzyme activities such as β-hydroxybutyrate dehydrogenase (E. C. 1.1.1. 30) in newborn rats (Klee and Sokoloff, 1967) and β-hydroxyacyl-CoA dehydrogenase (E. C. 1.1.1.35) in newborn rabbits (Stave, 1969).

At birth the human infant possesses a considerable supply of lipids, mainly triglycerides, which were deposited during the last few weeks of gestation (see Ch. 15). A full-term newborn of 3,500-g birth weight contains approximately 550 g lipids (Widdowson, 1964) or, differently expressed, lipids represent one sixth of the newborn's body weight. The hydrolysis of neutral fat yields fatty acids and glycerol, both of which can be oxidized for energy production. Soon after birth the utilization of neutral fat increases considerably as indicated by the rising level of plasma fatty acids (Van Duyne and Havel, 1959; Melichar et al., 1962; Chen et al., 1965; Keele and Kay, 1966; Novák et al., 1961) and of plasma glycerol (Persson and Gentz, 1966; Novák et al., 1964). The half-life time of plasma free fatty acids (FFA) was measured to be of about 2 to 3 minutes in healthy adults (Laurell, 1957; Fredrickson et al., 1967). The flux of FFA from the plasma ranged from 0.09 to 1.5 mEq per minute (Fredrickson and Gordon, 1958). The turnover rate of fatty acids appears to be in the same order of magnitude in newborns, as was shown by intravenous loading tests with triglyceride emulsions (Wolf and Melichar, 1970). The turnover rate of FFA was derived from plasma measurements during the presence of artificial triglycerides. Because of this assumed high turnover rate, a minor degree of lipolysis would not even be recognizable by changes of FFA plasma level, and thus marked changes must be indicative of a more marked lipid mobilization. Under normal conditions the fetus does not seem to oxidize lipids to any significant extent (Robertson and Sprecher, 1968), but during periods of oxygen deprivation, e.g., during birth complicated by hypoxia, a certain degree of lipolysis seems to occur. Under the latter conditions a reduction of glucose transfer through the human placenta was observed (Lumley and Wood, 1967). A high cord blood arteriovenous difference of FFA and especially the higher concentrations in the arteria umbilicalis revealed that the fatty acids originate from the fetus and not from the mother. The values in the arteria umbilicalis were found to be approximately twice as high in hypoxia fetalis as in normal cases. The rise in the FFA level is more pronounced in mild than in more severe hypoxia (Šabata et al., 1968a). It can be speculated that the failure of glucose transfer in a mild hypoxic state is the trigger for the mobilization of FFA in the fetus at term. The amount of normal placental transfer of FFA has been claimed to be small (Šabata et al., 1968b; Hagerman and Villee, 1960; Whaley et al., 1966) (see also Ch. 15). New perfusion experiments in human placenta showed a much greater transfer than was expected formerly (Szabo et al., 1969). The other component of neutral fat hydrolysis, glycerol, is also found in markedly elevated concentrations in the arteria umbilicalis during intrauterine hypoxia (Šabata et al., 1970). These observations provide ample evidence that neutral fat can be hydrolyzed prenatally, and hence, that the fetal adipose tissue possesses lipase activity and that the plasma contains lipoproteinlipases (Högstedt and Lindquist, 1963; Gürson and Etili, 1968; Vízek and Hahn, 1968; Persson et al., 1966). At the present time no precise description of the mechanism for FFA mobilization in the fetal organism is available, but it seems possible that adrenaline and noradrenaline stimulate the release of free fatty acids in adipose tissue. An increased production of catecholamines was observed in respiratory distress (Cheek et al., 1963). However, it should be noted that adrenaline is not as effective in newborn lambs during the first postnatal hours as in older lambs (Dawkins, 1964; Van Duyne et al., 1965). The same seems to be true for human newborns (Kaye et al., 1961; Melichar and Novák, 1970; Desmond et al., 1963).

Both adrenaline and noradrenaline stimulate lipolysis and fatty acid oxidation in vitro (Novák et al., 1968b; Novák and Melichar, 1970). Hypoxia or anoxia produces a more pronounced increase of plasma glycerol than of free fatty acids. This effect is explained as being caused by the higher rate of fatty acid oxidation directly at the location of lipolysis according to measurements in brown adipose tissue of the newborn rabbit (Dawkins and Hull, 1964) and in white adipose tissue obtained from human infants (Novák and Melichar, 1970). However, a stimulation that causes adrenaline or noradrenaline secretion does not necessarily lead to elevated plasma FFA concentrations, since a considerable amount of the liberated fatty acids is oxidized in the adipose tissue for heat production and thus does not enter the blood stream. The yield of energy generated from lipid oxidation in adipose tissue does not subside during hypoxia (see p. 1075) or cold stress (see Ch. 16). A certain degree of cold stress after birth is considered normal in every newborn baby, and so is the increased secretion of adrenaline (Schiff et al., 1966; Desmond et al., 1963).

Somatotropic hormone (STH) also stimulates lipolytic reactions. This effect is longer lasting than that of catecholamines (Weil, 1965). In newborns the blood level of STH is higher than in older infants and children (Cornblath et al., 1965; Laron et al., 1967; Stubbe and Šabata, 1970; Westphal, 1968). Small-for-date or hypotrophic newborns were found to have increased lipolytic reactions (Melichar and Wolf, 1968; Gentz et al., 1969b), and their STH blood levels were approximately three to four times higher than in full-term controls (Stubbe and Šabata, 1969). In this context it is of interest to note that blood samples obtained post mortem from prematurely born infants, i.e., under anoxic conditions, contained extremely high STH concentrations and very high amounts of glycerol (Stubbe and Wolf, 1970). However, in newborns who have suffered from hypoxia fetalis, the cord blood contained lower STH concentrations than that of healthy newborns (Stubbe and Šabata, 1970), although the glycerol and FFA values were elevated after hypoxia fetalis (see p. 1061). From these studies it was assumed that prenatally occurring lipolysis is stimulated by catecholamines rather than by STH.

The newborn utilizes the oxidation of fatty acids mainly for heat production. Under normal conditions, i.e., in a neutral thermal environment, approximately 70 percent of the total caloric requirement is covered by fatty acid oxidation. Wolf and Melichar (1970) calculated this value for the newborn of a few days of age from loading tests with triglycerides. We speculate that this already high rate of FFA utilization increases further during hypoxia while glucose utilization decreases. As shown above (p. 1056), the glucose concentration can eventually rise markedly during prolonged hypoxia, whereas the FFA concentrations frequently remain low or fall below the normal range in hypoxic prematures (Melichar and Wolf, 1967). Hence, both glucose and FFA blood level are not indicative of tissue hypoxia or at least they are not sufficiently reliable indicators. The glycerol concentration in blood seems to be more suitable for pursuing the extent of lipolysis since glycerol phosphorylation is very minor and slow in peripheral fat tissues (Novák et al., 1968a). In fact, hypothermic prematures and hypoxic prematures (Melichar and Wolf, 1967) with slightly increased FFA plasma levels were revealed to have significantly elevated plasma glycerol concentrations (Fig. 4B). Thus, the diagnostic significance of glycerol determinations for studying lipid

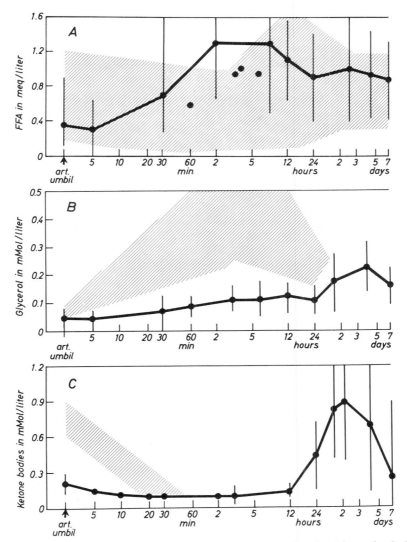

Fig. 4. Postnatal changes and hypoxia ranges for: A. FFA. B. Glycerol. C. Ketone bodies in arterial blood. Presentation as in Figure 1. A. Normal values with ±S.D. or range, respectively from Novák et al. (1964), Keele and Kay (1966), and Persson and Gentz (1966). The extra dots in A represent mean values from Novák et al. (1964) and Keele and Kay (1966) obtained by different analytic methods. Hypoxia range according to data from Šabata et al. (1968a) and Melichar and Wolf (1967). B. Normal values ±1 S.D. according to Novák et al. (1964); and for the second through seventh days, Stubbe and Wolf (1969). Hypoxia range according to data from Melichar and Wolf (1967) and Šabata et al. (1970). C. Normal values and ±2 S.D. or range from Åkerblom et al. (1965), Melichar et al. (1965), and Persson et al., (1966)—information for hypoxia range is still insufficient. The decrease occurring immediately after birth was observed by Persson et al. (1969) and Šabata et al. (1967).

mobilization is superior to FFA blood analyses. Roux and Romney (1967) could not find a significant correlation between FFA cord blood values of healthy and hypoxic newborns. Persson et al. (1970), however, observed a simultaneous increase of FFA and glycerol concentrations in cord blood of newborns who were suffering from prenatal hypoxia. Within two hours after birth the glycerol level was found to be six to eight times above the normally rather low levels of healthy newborns, and the FFA level was only three to four times higher than in controls. Although these findings need to be confirmed, they are in good agreement with blood analyses performed in prematures suffering from respiratory distress. In addition, these results demonstrate that lipolytic reactions occur quite early in the course of prolonged oxygen deficiency. In healthy newborns the ratio of FFA/glycerol (using their molar plasma concentrations) is in the order of 1:10 (Novák et al., 1964), but during postnatal hypoxia it was found to be approximately 1:3 (Melichar and Wolf, 1967).

This molar ratio does not reflect the ratio expected to occur after complete lipolysis in vitro. In addition to different rates of peripheral utilization, FFA and glycerol have different distribution spaces and also different elimination rates. Glycerol dissolves in total body water and has an elimination half-life time of 20 to 30 minutes in newborns (Wolf et al., 1968). Plasma FFA are bound to albumin and thus are distributed in a much smaller compartment; consequently, the half-life time is much shorter (see p. 1061). These factors ought to affect the FFA and plasma glycerol levels quite significantly.

The lipolytic activity can further be pursued by measuring the occurrence of metabolites which are derived from oxidative degradation of lipolytic products. Before birth the capacity for ketone body formation has been detected in liver tissue (Hahn et al., 1964), and postnatally acetoacetate and β-hydroxybutyrate are present in the blood (Melichar et al., 1965; Åkerblom et al., 1965; Schröter et al., 1967; Persson and Gentz, 1966). On the third and fourth days after birth the ketone body concentration reaches markedly high values which decrease toward the end of the first week of life (Fig. 4C). Under normal conditions the fetal tissues at term do not seem to produce ketone bodies. The ketone bodies found in cord blood seem to be transferred from the maternal circulation to the newborn. A rather constant correlation of 2:1 was found between the maternal and fetal ketone body blood levels (Paterson et al., 1967 Rubaltelli, 1967; Šabata et al., 1967, 1968b). The prenatally accumulated amount of ketone bodies is eliminated soon after birth. In newborns suffering from hypoxia fetalis Persson et al. (1970) found elevated concentrations of β-hydroxybutyrate in cord blood. In newborns who remained hypoxemic after birth the normally observed decrease of plasma ketone body concentrations was neither hampered nor enhanced (Fig. 4C). These observations lead to the conclusion that ketone bodies are not produced in measurable amounts during hypoxia.

EVALUATION AND SIGNIFICANCE OF BLOOD ANALYSES

The continuous recording of blood oxygen saturation and pH in anoxic puppies clearly demonstrated that the blood pH decreases steadily and continues to do so after the blood has been completely deprived of oxygen (James, 1967). As shown in this chapter a wide range of values are obtained for oxygen partial pressure or saturation in human cord blood and in arterial blood within the first hour of life; thus, these values are of little predictive significance because of their fluctuations. This situation is taken into account in Figures 1A and 1B (p. 1049) by marking only the hypoxia range for newborns of more than one hour of age. The heavily shaded areas designate the danger zones, and the lightly shaded range covers values of mild to moderate hypoxemia. The acid-base status can certainly be evaluated from different points of view, but for quick orientation and for monitoring the course in high-risk or hypoxic infants, pH measurements are clearly superior. In infants older than one hour pH blood values of less than 7.20 are alarming and indicative of imminent danger. The values derived from pH and CO_2 measurements, such as standard bicarbonate or base excess, are indicative of certain functional deficits. However, hypercapnia alone is far less dangerous than acidosis, and often it occurs only temporarily.

Blood glucose concentrations below 20 mg/100 ml, if verified by a second determination, are eventually dangerous and may demand immediate treatment. Hypoglycemia in newborns without symptoms of hypoxemia is less alarming, especially in newborns of diabetic mothers. Hypoglycemia is occasionally found during severe hypoxia, but it is neither a frequent nor a typical sign of hypoxemia. Elevated blood glucose level may occur more frequently in the beginning of hypoxia, but extremely high glucose concentrations are seen only occasionally in fatal cases of severe hypoxemia.

The blood lactate level is a very sensitive indicator either for the extent of physical activity or for oxygen deficiency. However, the evaluation of lactate together with pyruvate in arterial blood can indicate a dangerous metabolic situation, i.e., metabolic acidosis, if the upper normal range is surpassed (Figs. 3B and 3C). The L/P ratio serves an auxiliary though important function since its calculation prevents the misinterpretation of high lactate levels; as long as the ratio remains below 20 the metabolic acidosis is only moderate; repeated measurements of higher values yielding an L/P ratio of more than 20 should be considered indicative of a dangerous situation resulting from severe oxygen deprivation.

The postnatal changes of plasma FFA and ketone bodies seem to be unaffected by respiratory distress, although both metabolites were found to be higher in cord blood of newborns suffering from hypoxia fetalis. Blood glycerol levels, however, were always found to be significantly elevated in hypoxic newborns.

Among the ten different measurements in blood selected here for discussion the analysis of blood oxygen is important for confirming the existence of a certain degree of hypoxemia, but imminent danger is more reliably indicated by low pH values, rising L/P ratios, and increasing glycerol levels.

Significance of Glycogen Storage

Thus far the human newborn has been the main topic of this chapter. We described the metabolic reactions of the fetus during oxygen deficiency before birth, and we have discussed several metabolic changes which can be measured and investigated when hypoxemia occurs perinatally. Body temperature, gas metabolism, and blood chemistry can, where necessary, be routinely investigated or even continuously recorded; additional information may be obtained from electrocardio-, encephalo-, or myograms, as well as from urine analyses and function tests using combinations of the procedures mentioned. However all of these measurements can provide only indirect information about mechanisms and changes of the cell metabolism, and hence, many questions remain unanswered. This gap can be partially filled by animal experiments. Some of the metabolic principles deduced from in-vitro studies with fetal or newborn tissues might be directly applicable to the human fetus and newborn, but it must be kept in mind that differences among mammalian species are great. Such variations are genetically determined. One of those variations is expressed as the degree of maturation at birth.

The in vitro investigation of immature tissues has certainly contributed valuable information, but its discussion would lead beyond the scope of this chapter. However, the extensive studies of human fetal tissues under aerobic and anaerobic conditions by Villee et al. (1958) must be mentioned for their unique source of information. These authors concluded that the anoxia resistance of the fetal and newborn mammal seems to depend upon the "quantitative differences in the rates of certain enzymatic reactions common to fetal and adult tissues." They found a fourfold greater rate of glycolysis in fetal liver preparations of midway gestation under anaerobic conditions than under aerobic conditions; in the same preparations lipogenesis was decreased during anaerobiosis.

The importance of glycolysis for anoxic survival was shown most impressively by Himwich et al. in 1942. Newborn rats which had been pretreated with iodoacetate survived in an atmosphere of pure nitrogen for only 2 to 3 minutes, whereas poisoning of the respiratory chain enzymes with cyanide did not affect their normal anoxic survival of approximately 40 minutes. These results were later confirmed by Hicks (1953), who also found that after 50 minutes of immersion in pure nitrogen, newborn rats lost all their glycogen from the cardiac muscle and most of their hepatic glycogen.

Since the continuous supply of the fetus with glucose from the maternal circulation via placenta ceases at parturition, the newborn has to mobilize its own carbohydrate reserves which were stored during the last stage of pregnancy. The prenatal deposition of glycogen and its postnatal mobilization are discussed in Chapter 13. The normal newborn has a vital need for carbohydrates for operating the brain and the cardiac muscle, but the hypoxic fetus and newborn apparently depends on these glycogen reserves to an even higher degree. In order to prove the thesis that the amount of carbohydrate reserves constitutes the limiting factor for anoxic survival in newborns, Dawes et al. (1959) measured the glycogen contents of several organs of fetal lambs in mid- and late gestation, and the changes after timed anoxia. The older lamb fetuses lost almost all glycogen from brain and kidneys but none from lung or skeletal muscles during asphyxiation. However, the initially high amounts of glycogen in liver and cardiac muscle were only partially depleted. Dawes et al. (1959) concluded from their experiments that the amount of available *cardiac glycogen* is most critical for anoxia survival. The early exhaustion of cardiac glycogen after asphyxiation as compared with that of other organs has been observed in newborn rats (Hicks, 1953), rabbits (Gaspar, 1957), and guinea pigs (Miller et al., 1964b). However, prolonged exposure to an atmosphere of low oxygen content was revealed to have little or no effect on the glycogen content of cardiac muscle. During the first 24 hours of life the cardiac glycogen of fasting piglets was reduced from 1.1 g per 100 g wet tissue to 0.6 g per 100 g when kept in air, while animals kept in 8 percent oxygen were found to have 0.4 g glycogen per 100 g (Widdowson, 1961). Newborn rabbits kept in a 6.5 percent oxygen-containing atmosphere did not show any difference in their cardiac glycogen as compared with controls (see Fig. 9, p. 1072).

Mäenpää and Räihä (1968) measured the glycogen concentration in one-day-old rats. After 20 minutes of anoxia the glycogen concentration decreased in the liver from 128 to 76 μmoles/g wet weight and in cardiac muscle from 72.5 to 25.9 μmoles/g. In rat fetuses however, the liver glycogen did not change, and the cardiac glycogen concentration decreased from 116 to 74.0 μmoles/g after 20 minutes of anoxia. This observation in fetuses seems to be important since it leads us to speculate that during intrauterine hypoxia the fetus either does not need, or is unable to mobilize, its own hepatic glycogen since the mother provides sufficient glucose, and she even produces more during hypoxia; furthermore, placental glycogen mobilization might suffice the need of fetal organs. This latter mechanism again points to the importance of the fetoplacental unit, and it perhaps provides evidence as to the mechanism by which the placenta can protect the fetal organism.

Gelli et al. (1968) studied the effect of glucose infusions in pregnant rabbits on fetal glycogen deposition. Two days before term, this treatment caused an increase of the fetal cardiac glycogen, and the by sectio delivered fetuses showed significantly prolonged survival during immersion in saline solution at 37°C.

Furthermore, it should be noticed that the cardiac muscle of newborn rats possesses an approximately ten times higher rate of glucose oxidation than the adult ventricular muscle (Wittels and Bressler, 1965). The activities of phosphoglucomutase (E. C. 2.7.5.1) in newborn rabbit heart (Stave, 1964), of hexokinase (E. C. 2.7.1.1) in newborn rabbit and rat heart (Stave, 1964; Walpurger, 1967), and of phosphofructokinase (E. C. 2.7.1.11) in newborn rat heart are significantly higher than in adult cardiac muscle; these are key enzymes for the glycogenolytic and glycolytic pathways (see Ch. 17). Breuer et al. (1967) studied the cardiac carbohydrate metabolism by analyzing the coronary blood of one-to three-week-old puppies. The myocardium of puppies released more lactate and pyruvate and extracted more glucose from the blood than did the cardiac muscle of adult dogs. This information provides evidence that the newborn heart possesses a high capability for utilizing glycogen and glucose, and furthermore it seems probable that the cardiac carbohydrate is mainly utilized directly by the ventricular muscle to provide energy for the maintenance of the circulation during anoxia or hypoxia (Shelley, 1969).

The central nervous system is very dependent upon a sufficient supply of glucose (see Ch. 34). In the immediate postnatal period the mobilization of *hepatic glycogen* provides most of the glucose that enters the blood stream, thus replacing the maternal glucose supply. A close relationship among the rate of hepatic glycogen

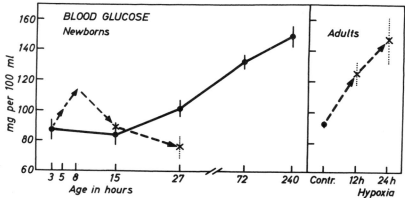

Fig. 5. Glucose concentration in arterial blood of newborn (solid curve) and adult
rabbits (Contr., control animals). Newborns up to 27 hours of age were unfed,
older animals examined after 24-hour fast. Dashed arrows and crosses designate
changes and values after 2, 5, 12 and 24 hours of hypoxia (6.5 percent O_2 for newborns, 8.5 percent for adult animals). Means from 10 to 14 newborns or 12 to 24
adults, vertical bars show S.E.M.

mobilization, the blood glucose level, and survival in anoxia has been demonstrated
in newborn rats (Stafford and Weatherall, 1960). If the amount of liver glycogen
had been prematurely exhausted by insulin treatment, the anoxia survival was only
half as long as without previous glycogen depletion.

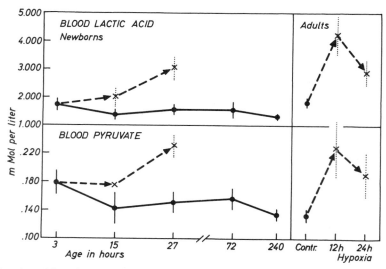

Fig. 6. Lactic acid and pyruvate concentration in arterial blood of newborn and adult
rabbits. Normal postnatal changes and effect of 12 and 24 hours of hypoxia upon
newborn and adult animals. Same group of animals and same presentation as in
Figure 5. Before blood was obtained from adult rabbits they were kept in light
sodium pentobarbital anesthesia for 45 minutes. (Lactate determination according
to Hohorst, 1963; pyruvate according to Bücher et al., 1963.)

The effect of prolonged exposure of newborn rabbits to a low-oxygen atmosphere may exemplify the advantages of simultaneous blood and tissue analyses (Stave, 1969). Three-hour-old unfed rabbits were transferred into an incubator which was kept at 30°C with radiant heat. For producing hypoxia the atmosphere in the incubator contained 6.5 percent oxygen with 5 percent CO_2 in nitrogen; for control animals humidified room air was passed through the incubator (Stave, 1967). The effects of 12- and 24-hour hypoxia upon blood and tissues must be evaluated in relation to normal postnatal changes and, in addition, in comparison with adult animals which also have been subjected to hypoxia (8 to 8.5 percent oxygen) for the same periods of time. The glucose level in arterial blood increases in hypoxic newborns for approximately 5 hours, and subsequently it decreases steadily for as long as 24 hours; at this time the hypoxic newborns have reached a significantly lower level as compared with controls. In adult animals the blood glucose level increases continuously (Fig. 5). The arterial lactate and pyruvate concentrations increase in hypoxic newborn rabbits; the highest values were obtained after 24 hours of hypoxia. In adults, both blood lactate and pyruvate concentrations were found to have the greatest increase after 12 hours of hypoxia, and less after 24 hours of hypoxia (Fig. 6). In the liver of newborns, the lactate and pyruvate concentrations were found within the range of normal values after 12 hours of hypoxia, but after 24 hours of oxygen deprivation, both metabolites increased significantly. Adult animals had begun to accumulate lactate in the liver

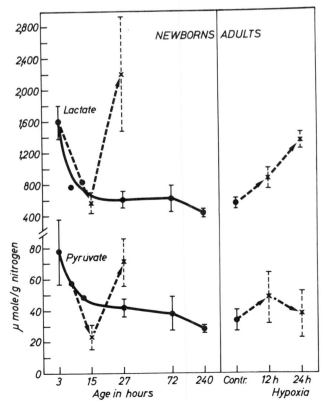

Fig. 7. Lactate and pyruvate concentrations in newborn and adult rabbit liver; postnatal changes and the effect of 12 and 24 hours of hypoxia. Same presentation as in Figure 5. Means calculated from 5 to 12 analyses in each group. Newborns were kept in sodium pentobarbital anesthesia for 10 minutes and adult animals for 45 minutes before laparotomy. Methods for lactate and pyruvate determination as mentioned in Figure 6.

12 hours after the beginning of hypoxia treatment, and they continued this process for 24 hours; the changes of pyruvate concentrations in adult liver were not significant (Fig. 7). Finally, the glycogen concentrations in liver (Fig. 8) and in cardiac muscle and skeletal muscle were studied in the same animals (Fig. 9). In newborn rabbits, hypoxia treatment accelerates the normal postnatal depletion of hepatic glycogen, but after 24 hours of hypoxia, a minimum level of liver carbohydrates was found in both hypoxic and normal newborns. The decline of blood glucose and the exhaustion of available hepatic glycogen during prolonged hypoxia in newborns is clearly illustrated by those results. The cardiac muscle glycogen remains unchanged in newborns and increases in adults after 24 hours of hypoxia. The relatively high concentration of skeletal muscle glycogen in newborns does not decrease markedly, but in adults a statistically significant amount of skeletal muscle glycogen was mobilized. In hypoxic adult rabbits a rough calculation of carbohydrate transfer revealed that approximately 2.5 g glycogen was mobilized from the skeletal musculature, and an amount of the same order had been deposited in liver and cardiac muscle. This process, however, began after 12 hours of hypoxia, and hence we suppose that adaptation to hypoxia was induced after a lag period of more than 12 hours. Although our experiments in newborn rabbits provided evidence that the glycogen of skeletal muscle is not utilized in any appreciable amount during prolonged periods of hypoxia, it has been shown by Bocek and Beatty (1967) that skeletal muscle glycogen can be mobilized under extremely long anoxia conditions. In the latter experiments fetal and neonatal skeletal muscle from Rhesus monkeys were studied in vitro; after 2 hours of anoxia

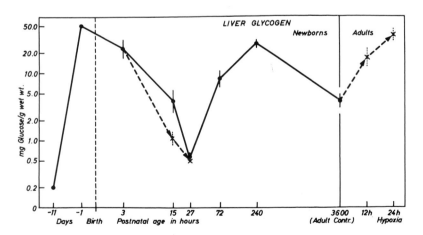

Fig. 8. Developmental changes and the effect of 12 and 24 hours of hypoxia upon rabbit liver glycogen concentration. Presentation on a double logarithmic scale. Dashed arrows and crosses designate changes due to hypoxia treatment (see text). Means calculated from 9 to 15 animals in each group; vertical bars show S.E.M. Glycogen analysis: after alcohol precipitation the glycogen was hydrolyzed and measured as glucose by the glucose oxidase method.

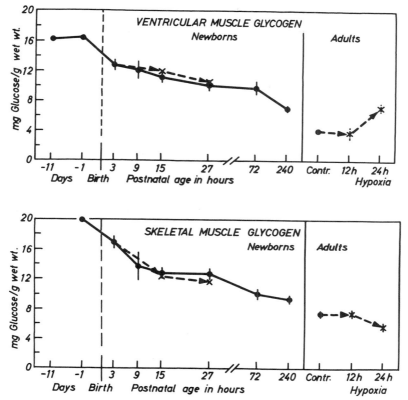

Fig. 9. Developmental changes and the effect of 12 and 24 hours of hypoxia treatment upon cardiac and skeletal muscle glycogen concentrations in rabbits. Same presentation as in Figure 8 but linear scales.

the magnitude of glycogenolysis was greatest in muscle samples from fetuses near term. However, these in vitro experiments do not take into account the neural and humoral control mechanisms which are operative in the whole animal.

Several tissue enzyme activities have been measured in newborn rabbits after prolonged exposure to hypoxia (Stave, 1967). In newborn liver, kidney, and cardiac muscle an increase of glycolytic enzymes was observed after 12 hours of oxygen deprivation; however, after 24 hours of hypoxia the enzyme activities were not found to be elevated as compared with controls. This effect is depicted in Figure 10 for liver glyceraldehydephosphate dehydrogenase, which enzyme represents the central group of the Embden-Meyerhof pathway (see Ch. 17). It should be noticed that in adult liver this enzyme activity increased significantly after 24 hours of hypoxia. The low levels of lactate and pyruvate in newborn liver after 12 hours of hypoxia provide additional proof that the metabolism was still operating aerobically, but after 24 hours of hypoxia large amounts of lactate had accumulated in newborn liver (see Fig. 7).

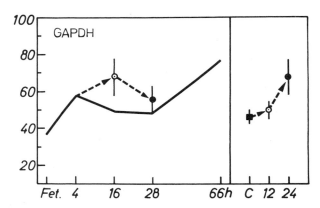

Fig. 10. Perinatal changes of glyceraldehydephosphate dehydrogenase (GAPDH) activity in rabbit liver (solid curve) and the effect of 12 and 24 hours of hypoxia upon this enzyme in newborn and adults. Solid curve constructed from means of 8 to 17 animals in each age group. Dashed arrows and dots, changes after 12 and 24 hours of hypoxia. Vertical bars designate S.E.M. C, control group of adult rabbits; 12 and 24, time of hypoxia. (From Stave. 1967. *Biol. Neonat.* 11:310-327.)

ADENOSINE PHOSPHATES IN TISSUES

In Chapter 34 it was discussed that during *anoxia* the concentration of ATP decreases markedly slower in newborn rat brain than in adult brain. A similar delay of the ATP breakdown during anoxia has been found to occur in liver and cardiac muscle of guinea pig fetuses (Räihä, 1964). The fetuses were made anoxic by clamping of the cord in the intact amniotic sac, and in adult guinea pigs the trachea was clamped in pentobarbital anesthesia. Not only the ATP concentration but also the ATP/ADP ratio decreased much slower in fetal than in adult liver. In a more recent series of experiments Mäenpää and Räihä (1968) studied the effect of increasing periods of anoxia by immersing fetal, neonatal, and adult rats in nitrogen. The concentrations of adenosine phosphates and the ratios of ATP/ADP and ATP/AMP in liver and cardiac muscle are presented in Table 2. The slow decrease of ATP concentrations and ATP/ADP ratios (representing energy potentials) in fetal and newborn tissues, especially in perinatal heart, is quite obvious. Comparisons with tissues from adult rats were limited to 2 to 5 minutes since older animals do not survive longer periods of anoxia. In discussing their experimental findings Mäenpää and Räihä (1968) speculated that the utilization of energy-rich phosphates proceeds less rapidly in tissues of fetuses and newborns than in tissues of adults during anoxia. The low activity of ATPase in fetal tissues (Dawkins, 1959) seems to favor such explanation.

The effect of *hypoxia* upon tissue ATP concentrations is distinct from anoxia effects. Twenty-four hours of exposure to hypoxia did not cause marked changes of liver ATP concentrations in newborns and adult rabbits (Stave, 1970). Furthermore, the ATP/ADP and ATP/AMP ratios did not decrease after 24 hours of hypoxia in both newborn and adult liver (Table 3).

The prolonged reduction of oxygen supply, e.g., 24 hours, opens the way for reactive and adaptive changes in the tissue enzyme pattern. The oxidative phosphorylation represents the major source for ATP synthesis from ADP and inorganic phosphate, while the gain of ATP from glycolytic reactions is considerably smaller. Some information on the capacity of oxidative phosphorylation can be obtained from measurements of tissue enzyme activities involved in the oxidoreduction of

TABLE 2. Effect of Anoxia on Adenosine Phosphates of Fetal, Neonatal, and Adult Rat Tissues[a]

		Control	Time of anoxia			
			2 min	5 min	10 min	20 min
			Liver			
ATP[b]	Fetus	1.88		1.11	0.84	0.74
	1 day	2.24		1.53	1.00	0.65
	Adult	2.84	1.68	—	—	—
ATP/ADP	Fetus	3.9		2.2	2.0	2.3
	1 day	5.6		2.7	1.7	1.5
	Adult	3.7	1.9	—	—	—
ATP/AMP	Fetus	4.7		1.5	1.1	0.9
	1 day	12.5		2.6	1.2	0.8
	Adult	6.6	2.8	—	—	—
			Heart			
ATP[b]	Fetus	2.38		2.39	2.03	2.01
	1 day	2.30		2.33	2.35	1.71
	Adult	4.28	2.09	1.19	—	—
ATP/ADP	Fetus	7.9		7.4	6.3	6.1
	1 day	7.1		6.5	5.7	3.4
	Adult	5.8	1.5	1.2	—	—
ATP/AMP	Fetus	11.9		10.4	9.2	7.7
	1 day	11.5		10.6	10.7	7.4
	Adult	17.8	2.3	0.7	—	—

[a]From Mäenpää and Räihä. 1968. *Ann. Med. Exp. Biol. Fenn.*, 46:306-317.
[b]In μmoles/g wet weight; means of 5 to 10 experiments.

TABLE 3. Effect of Prolonged Hypoxia (6.5 percent O_2) on Adenosine Phosphates of Newborn and Adult Rabbit Liver

	Age Group	Controls	12 hr Hypoxia	24 hr Hypoxia
ATP[a]	3 hr	1464.	—	—
	27 hr	1594.	1360.	1398.
	Adults	1766.	1548.	1729.
ATP/ADP	3 hr	4.7	—	—
	27 hr	3.1	3.9	3.5
	Adult	4.1	4.0	4.1
ATP/AMP	3 hr	8.5	—	—
	27 hr	7.0	8.7	11.7
	Adult	12.0	12.8	13.6

[a]In μmoles/g tissue nitrogen; means of 4 to 12 experiments.

cytochromes and by measuring the amount of cytochromes in tissues. In the perinatal period four enzyme activities engaged in the oxidoreduction of cytochrome c were found to be very low in rat liver and cardiac muscle as compared with adult tissues (Dawkins, 1959; Lang, 1965). In fetal and newborn rabbit, however, only slightly lower activities of respiratory chain enzymes were measured in cardiac muscle, liver, and kidney than in the respective tissues of adult animals (Fig. 11). Thus, species differences are quite large for those enzyme activities in the perinatal period. The newborn rabbits, who are developmentally more mature than newborn rats, show higher activities of respiratory enzymes than the rats. The developmental changes in cytochrome c tissue concentrations proceed in concordance with changes observed for respiratory enzyme activities. At birth the concentrations of cytochrome c in tissues of guinea pigs and rats are very low; in guinea pigs the cytochrome c concentration reaches adult levels on the second day after birth, while in rats this increase occurs over several days in cardiac muscle and requires weeks in liver (Dallman and Schwartz, 1964).

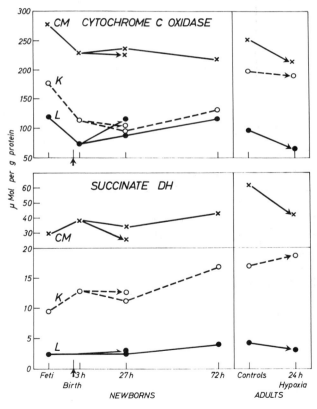

Fig. 11. Perinatal changes of cytochrome c oxidase (E. C. 1.9.3.1) and succinate dehydrogenase (E.C. 1.3.99.1) activity in cardiac muscle (CM, crosses), kidney (open circles, dashed curve), and liver (L). The changes due to 24 hours of hypoxia are marked by arrows for newborn and adult rabbits. Mean values from 5 to 7 fetuses and newborns, and 9 to 12 adults.

The effect of prolonged exposure to hypoxia upon respiratory chain enzymes was studied in tissues of newborn and adult rabbits (Stave, 1970). In general the changes found after 24 hours of hypoxia are minor and not statistically significant, as shown in Figure 11. However, in newborn liver the activity of cytochrome c oxidase increased significantly after 24 hours of hypoxia, whereas in adult liver a decrease was observed. We are moved to speculate that the vital need for supporting the process of oxidative phosphorylation in newborn liver is expressed in its capability to increase the activity of a key enzyme of the respiratory chain.

The rate of ATP synthesis on one side and the utilization or the need for ATP on the other side both affect the ATP level. As long as ATP synthesis and utilization are in balance no change of the concentration can be observed. The overall reduction of metabolic reactions in hypoxic newborns has been documented by their reduced oxygen consumption and decreased body temperature (see p. 1047). Thus, the slowdown of the energy metabolism would explain the smaller need for ATP, but in addition the newborn liver seems to be able to increase its capability to synthesize ATP. The turnover of high energy phosphates needs further investigation.

Lipolysis and Lipogenesis

In newborn rabbits brown adipose tissue constitutes approximately 5 percent of the body weight (Dawkins and Hull, 1964); this tissue is the principal site of heat production in these animals (Hull and Segall, 1965). Exposure to cold as well as infusions of noradrenaline increase the oxygen consumption of newborn rabbits; the increase in heat production, especially in the brown adipose tissue was shown by subcutaneous temperature measurements over the fat pads (Dawkins and Hull, 1964) and by the steep increase of blood flow and oxygen consumption in adipose tissue (Heim and Hull, 1966a). In newborn rabbits the local heat production in brown adipose tissue during exposure to cold was abolished by hypoxia (Dawkins and Hull, 1964) as shown by a decline of oxygen consumption in adipose tissue (Heim and Hull, 1966a). However, the increase in blood flow in brown adipose tissue caused by noradrenaline infusion did not become reduced during hypoxia (Heim and Hull, 1966a). Further investigations of the calorigenic response of newborn rabbits to infusions of catecholamines, propranalol (adrenaline antagonist), glucagon, corticotropin, and to cold exposure revealed that noradrenaline is released at sympathetic nerve endings in brown adipose tissue and thus activates metabolic reactions in situ; the increase in blood flow caused by noradrenaline is secondary to these metabolic actions (Heim and Hull, 1966b). Heim and Hull (1966b) further suggested the possibility that glucagon and corticotropin act directly on brown adipose tissue by increasing its heat-producing metabolic reactions. This condition might be applicable in cases of anoxia which trigger an alarm reaction (see Ch. 2), but in newborn mammals this situation has not been investigated as yet.

Considerable controversy still exists as to whether the adrenal medulla discharges hormones during hypoxia in adults (Goldring et al., 1962; Van Liere and Stickney,

1963). Comline and Silver (1966) reviewed the stimulating effect of anoxia on the adrenal medulla in perinatal calfs and lambs. During severe hypoxia both adrenaline and noradrenaline are secreted by the adrenals in the perinatal period, but the authors found marked differences among the species studied.

In resting human adults the blood levels of adrenaline and noradrenaline are in the same range and average between 0.20 and 0.40 μg per liter; breathing of 10 or 11 percent oxygen did not affect the catecholamine blood levels (Goldring et al., 1962; Flohr et al., 1966). In the human full-term infant the plasma level of adrenaline does not differ from that of the adult. In prematures however, the mean level is 0.86 μg per liter (Cheek et al., 1963). The noradrenaline level averages 2.39 μg per liter in full-term infants and 3.24 μg per liter in prematures (Cheek et al., 1963). Cheek et al. (1963) found that in premature infants suffering from respiratory distress the adrenaline blood level increased fourfold, but the noradrenaline did not change significantly. Short-term exposure of healthy infants to 10 percent oxygen did not affect the urinary excretion of catecholamines (Stern et al., 1964), but the initial voiding of newborns delivered by outlet forceps contained significantly higher amounts of catecholamines than did that of spontaneously born infants (Howard et al., 1964). Less catecholamines were found in the first urine samples of newborns delivered from toxemic mothers and of newborns suffering from placental malnutrition. These conflicting results dealing with catecholamines in plasma and urine of newborns call for further investigation.

The anaerobic lipogenesis in *fetal* tissues has been frequently investigated and discussed since Räihä (1954) suggested that the synthesis of fatty acids could provide the fetal tissues with a means for decreasing their metabolic requirements for oxygen. In this sense fatty acid synthesis provides a "hydrogen sink" (Villee et al., 1958) which is of special need during periods of oxygen deprivation. In vitro experiments with human *fetal* tissues, however, revealed that "the rate of anaerobic lipogenesis is substantially less than that under aerobic conditions," and furthermore "that lipogenesis is of no significance in the ability of the human fetus one half way through gestation to withstand hypoxia" (Villee et al., 1958). Anoxia experiments in *neonatal* rats disclosed a change of this situation. After 45 minutes of anoxia (nitrogen atmosphere) carbon ^{14}-labeled pyruvate was incorporated into carcass and liver fat to the same extent as in untreated newborn rats (Kimmelstiel and Villee, 1956).

Prolonged exposure to a low-oxygen atmosphere affects the lipid tissue metabolism of newborn animals in a different manner. The mean fat content in the liver of 3-hour-old rabbits was 302 mg per g wet weight, and after 24 hours of hypoxia (6.5 percent oxygen) the fat concentration was reduced to 235 mg per g liver as compared with 197 mg per g in controls kept in room air (Stave, 1970). This may be interpreted as indicating a reduced mobilization of hepatic fat during hypoxia. However, a certain amount of neutral fat seems to be synthetized in the liver during hypoxia as evidenced by experiments with newborn rats. After 6 hours of hypoxia (10 percent oxygen) the newborns had incorporated less labeled carbon from glucose or fructose into the hepatic neutral fat than control animals, but when labeled acetate was used the incorporation of C^{14} into neutral fat was almost three times higher after hypoxia than in controls (Schreier, 1966).

It would be premature to draw conclusions from these still insufficient data on the mechanism and significance of lipid metabolism during hypoxia in the newborn. However, evidence is now accumulating that the lipid metabolism and its perinatal regulatory changes are of great importance, not only for the healthy newborn but also for the newborn suffering from oxygen deprivation.

Conclusions

During the expulsion period the fetus experiences oxygen deficiency of varying degree and duration, but permanent damage to the tissues occurs very rarely because hypoxia tolerance is seldom surpassed. Within the immediate postnatal period a prolonged respiratory distress challenges the ability of the newborn organism to tolerate hypoxia in a different way because of the many changes that occur in connection with the process of establishing homeostasis for extrauterine life. Hypoxia fetalis and hypoxia neonatorum cause a progressive metabolic acidosis. Blood analyses performed during the last stage of expulsion and in the newborn baby provide important information for therapeutic measures, but at the present time treatment is still limited to symptomatic corrections. In order to achieve a treatment which protects the organism and prevents the development of tissue damage due to hypoxia, further investigations are needed about the underlying cell metabolic reactions and also about the regulatory changes of the endocrine, circulatory, and nervous systems during perinatal development. Many of these mechanisms can be studied in animal experiments. The hypoxia tolerance of newborn mammals seems to involve the entire organism and many cell metabolic pathways. The energy requirements of the cell metabolism during oxygen deprivation can be supplied not only by an increase in glycolysis, but also by the utilization of fatty acids and amino acids. The markedly slower decrease of tissue ATP concentrations in anoxic newborns than in anoxic adult animals exemplifies the overall efficiency of the newborns' energy metabolism; however, the mechanism for maintaining high ATP tissue levels is still obscure. The overall reduction of energetic processes in hypoxic newborns is well documented by their reduced oxygen consumption and decreased body temperature. Since humoral and nervous regulations seem to play an important role in the management of the cell metabolism during oxygen deprivation, future investigations will have to concentrate on whole animal experiments.

Acknowledgment

The authors gratefully acknowledge the generous support of the Samuel S. Fels Fund, Philadelphia, Pa. Dr. Stave's unpublished data were collected during an investigation supported in part by Public Health Service Research Grant HD 00431 from the National Institute of Child Health and Human Development and by additional funds from General Research Support Grant FR 05537 from the National Institutes of Health. Dr. Wolf's unpublished data were obtained during investigations supported by the Deutsche Forschungsgemeinschaft, grant No. Wo 69.

REFERENCES

Acharya, P. T., and W. W. Payne. 1965. Blood chemistry of normal full-term infants in the first 48 hours of life. Arch. Dis. Child., 40:430-435.

Adamsons, K., Jr., et al. 1963. The treatment of acidosis with alkali and glucose during asphyxia in foetal Rhesus monkeys. J. Physiol. (London), 169:679-689.

Åkerblom, H., T. Ahola, and O. Somersalo. 1965. Acetone bodies in blood of infants and children of various ages. Ann. Paediat. Fenn., 11:108–113.

Alpert, N. R. 1965. Lactate production and removal and the regulation of metabolism. Ann. N.Y. Acad. Sci., 119:995-1011.

Antony, G. J., L. E. Underwood, and J. J. VanWyk. 1967. Studies in hypoglycemia of infancy and childhood. Amer. J. Dis. Child., 114:345-369.

Apgar, V. 1953. A proposal for a new method of evaluation of the newborn infant. Anesth. Analg. (Cleveland), 32:260.

————— D. A. Holaday, L. S. James, and I. M. Weisbrot. 1958. Evaluation of the newborn infant. Second report. J.A.M.A., 168:1985-1988.

Astrup, P., K. Jørgensen, O. Siggard Andersen, and K. Engel. 1960. The acid-base metabolism: A new approach. Lancet, 1:1035-1039.

Avery, M. E. 1962. Cardiopulmonary changes in respiratory distress: Clinical observation and physiological exploration. Pediatrics, 30:859-861.

Baens, G. S., E. Lundeen, and M. Cornblath. 1963. Studies of carbohydrate metabolism in the newborn infant. VI. Levels of glucose in blood in premature infants. Pediatrics, 31:580-589.

Berg, D., and J. Dörrler. 1969. Vergleich zwischen arteriellem und 'arterialisiertem' Capillarblut bei Neugeborenen am ersten Lebenstag. Mschr. Kinderheilk., 117:525-527.

Blatteis, C. M. 1964. Hypoxia and the metabolic response to cold in newborn rabbits. J. Physiol. (London), 172:358-368.

Blennemann, H. 1966. Untersuchungen zur postpartalen Säure-Basen-Situation Frühgeborener. Z. Kinderheilk., 97:101-113.

Bocek, R. M., and C. H. Beatty. 1967. Glycogen metabolism in fetal, neonatal, and infant muscle of the Rhesus monkey. Pediatrics, 40:412-420.

Boston, R. W., F. Geller, and C. A. Smith. 1966. Arterial blood gas tension and acid-base balance in the measurement of the respiratory distress syndrome. J. Pediat., 68:74-89.

Bowie, M. D., P. B. Mulligan, and R. Schwartz. 1963. Intravenous glucose tolerance in the normal newborn infant: The effects of a double dose of glucose and insulin. Pediatrics, 31:590-598.

Breuer, E., E. Barta, L. Zlatoš, and E. Pappová. 1968. Developmental changes of myocardial metabolism. II. Myocardial metabolism of fatty acids in the early postnatal period in dogs. Biol. Neonat., 12:54-64.

————— E. Barta, E. Pappová, and L. Zlatoš. 1967. Developmental changes of myocardial metabolism. I. Peculiarities of cardiac carbohydrate metabolism in the early postnatal period in dogs. Biol. Neonat., 11:367-377.

Broberger, O., and R. Zetterström. 1961. Hypoglycemia with an inability to increase the epinephrine secretion in insulin-induced hypoglycemia. J. Pediat., 59:215-222.

Brown, R. J. K., and P. G. Wallis. 1963. Hypoglycemia in the newborn infant. Lancet, 1:1278-1282.

Brück, K., F. H. Adams, and M. Brück. 1962. Temperature regulation in infants with chronic hypoxemia. Pediatrics, 30:350-360.

Bücher, T., R. Czok, W. Lamprecht, and E. Latzko. 1963. Pyruvate. In Bergmeyer, H. U., ed. Methods of Enzymatic Analysis. Weinheim, Verlag Chemie and New York, Academic Press, pp. 253-259.

Burnard, E. D., and K. W. Cross. 1958. Rectal temperature in the newborn after birth asphyxia. Brit. Med. J., 2:1197-1199.

Caldwell, B. M. et al. 1957. The utility of blood oxygenation as an indicator of post-natal condition. J. Pediat., 50:434.

Cassin, S. 1963. Critical oxygen tensions in newborn, young, and adult mice. Amer. J. Physiol., 205:325-330.

Cheek, D. B., M. Malinek, and J. M. Fraillon. 1963. Plasma adrenaline and nor-adrenaline in the neonatal period and in infants with respiratory distress syndrome and placental insufficiency. Pediatrics, 31:374-381.

Chen, C. H. et al. 1965. The plasma free fatty acid composition and blood glucose of normal and diabetic pregnant women and of their newborns. Pediatrics, 36:843-855.

Ciampolini, M., and F. Franchini. 1966. Modifications of lactate metabolism in the first month of life: Intravenous loading tests of DL-lactate in premature new-born infants. Ann. Paediat. (Basel), 207:335-344.

Cohnstein, J., and N. Zuntz. 1884. Untersuchungen über das Blut, den Kreislauf und die Athmung beim Säugethier-Fötus. Pflueger. Arch. Ges. Physiol., 34:173.

Comline, R. S., and M. Silver. 1966. Development of activity in the adrenal medulla of the foetus and newborn animal. Brit. Med. Bull., 22:16-20.

Cooke, R. E. 1958. Physiology of asphyxia neonatorum. In Windle, W. F., ed. Neuro-logical and Psychological Deficits of Asphyxia Neonatorum. Springfield, Ill., Charles C Thomas Publishers, pp. 88-104.

Cornblath, M., G. B. Odell, and E. Y. Levin. 1959. Symptomatic neonatal hypogly-cemia associated with toxemia of pregnancy. J. Pediat., 55:545-562.

——— et al. 1961. Studies of carbohydrate metabolism in the newborn infant. III. Some factors influencing the capillary blood sugar and the response to glucagon during the first hours of life. Pediatrics, 27:378-389.

——— et al. 1965. Secretion and metabolism of growth hormone in premature and full-term infants. J. Clin. Endocr., 25:209-218.

——— G. Joassin, B. Weisskopf, and K. R. Swiatek. 1966. Hypoglycemia in the newborn. Pediat. Clin. N. Amer., 13:905-920.

Crawford, J. S. 1965. Maternal and cord blood at delivery. Biol. Neonat., 8:131-172.

Cross, K. W., G. S. Dawes, and J. C. Mott. 1959. Anoxia, oxygen consumption and cardiac output in new-born lambs and adult sheep. J. Physiol. (London), 146:316-343.

——— D. D. Flynn, and J. R. Hill. 1966. Oxygen consumption in normal newborn infants during moderate hypoxia in warm and cool environments. Pediatrics, 37:565-576.

Dallman, P. R., and H. C. Schwartz. 1964. Cytochrome c concentrations during rat and guinea pig development. Pediatrics, 33:106-110.

Dancis, J. 1965. The role of the placenta in fetal survival. Pediat. Clin. N. Amer., 12:477-492.

Daniel, S. S., K. Adamsons, and L. S. James. 1966. Lactate and pyruvate as an index of prenatal oxygen deprivation. Pediatrics, 37:942-953.

Dawes, G. S. 1961. Oxygen consumption and hypoxia in the newborn animal. In

Wolstenholme, G. E. W., and M. O'Connor, eds. Somatic Stability in the Newly Born. London, Churchill Ltd., pp. 170-182.

Dawes, G. S. 1968. Foetal and Neonatal Physiology. Chicago, Year Book Medical Publishers, Inc.

———— and J. C. Mott. 1959. Reflex respiratory activity in the new-born rabbit. J. Physiol. (London), 145:85-97.

———— J. C. Mott, and H. J. Shelley. 1959. The importance of cardiac glycogen for the maintenance of life in foetal lambs and newborn animals during anoxia. J. Physiol. (London), 146:516-538.

———— H. N. Jacobson, J. C. Mott, and H. J. Shelley. 1960. Some observations on foetal and newborn Rhesus monkeys. J. Physiol. (London), 152:271-298.

———— J. C. Mott, H. J. Shelley, and A. Stafford. 1963. The prolongation of survival time in asphyxiated immature foetal lambs. J. Physiol. (London), 168: 43-64.

Dawkins, M. J. R. 1959. Respiratory enzymes in the liver of the newborn rat. Proc. Roy. Soc. [Biol.], 150:284-298.

———— 1964. Changes in blood glucose and non-esterified fatty acids in the foetal lamb after injection of adrenaline. Biol. Neonat., 7:160-166.

———— 1966. The hazards of birth. Advances Reprod. Physiol., 1:217-264.

———— and D. Hull. 1964. Brown adipose tissue and the response of new-born rabbits to cold. J. Physiol. (London), 172:216-238.

Derom, R. 1964. Anaerobic metabolism in the human fetus. I. The normal delivery. Amer. J. Obstet. Gynec., 89:241-251.

Desmond, M. M. 1953. Observations related to neonatal hypoglycemia. J. Pediat., 43:253-262.

———— et al. 1963. The clinical behaviour of the newly born. I. The term baby. J. Pediat., 62:307-325.

DiPietro, D. L., J. Gutierrez-Correa, and J. H. Thaidigsman. 1967. Glucose metabolism by human placental villi. Biochem. J., 103:246-250.

Dost, F. H., E. Gladtke, M. von Hattingberg, and H. Rind. 1968. Biokinetische Normwerte bei der intravenösen Glucosebelastung. Klin. Wschr., 46:503-505.

Drahota, Z., P. Hahn, J. Mourek, and M. Trojanová. 1965. The effect of acetoacetate on oxygen consumption of brain slices from infant and adult rats. Physiol. Bohemoslov., 14:134.

Eastman, N. J., and C. M. McLane. 1931. Foetal blood studies. II. The lactic acid content of umbilical cord blood under various conditions. Bull. Hopkins Hosp., 48:261-268.

Ek, J., and L. N. W. Daae. 1967. Whole blood glucose determination in newborn infants, comparison and evaluation of five different methods. Acta Paediat. Scand., 56:461-466.

Fazekas, J. F., F. A. D. Alexander, and H. E. Himwich. 1941. Tolerance of the newborn to anoxia. Amer. J. Physiol., 134:281-287.

Flohr, H., H. Klensch, R. Felix, and P. Geisler. 1966. Plasmakatecholaminkonzentrationen in akuter Hypoxie. Fluorimetrische Messungen im arteriellen und mischvenösen menschlichen Blut. Pflueger. Arch. Ges. Physiol., 290:225-230.

Fredrickson, D. S., and R. S. Gordon, Jr. 1958. The metabolism of albumin-bound C[14] labeled unesterified fatty acids in normal human subjects. J. Clin. Invest., 37:1504-1515.

———— R. I. Levy, and R. S. Lees. 1967. Fat transport in lipoproteins. New Eng. J. Med., 276:34-44.

Frenzel, J., G. Rogner, and B. Maak. 1968. Veränderungen des Lactat/Pyruvat-Quotienten bei hypoxischen Neugeborenen unter der Puffertherapie. Mschr. Kinderheilk., 116:547-552.

Friedman, E. A. et al. 1960. The distribution and metabolism of C^{14}-labeled lactic acid and bicarbonate in pregnant primates. J. Clin. Invest., 39:227-235.

Gambino, S. R. 1961. Collection of capillary blood for simultaneous determinations of arterial pH, CO_2 content, P_{CO_2} and oxygen saturation. Amer. J. Clin. Path., 35:175.

Gaspar, Z. N. 1957. Investigation of the physiologically different glycogen fractions in newborn rabbit. Experientia, 13:113.

Geiger, A. 1958. Correlation of brain metabolism and function by the use of a brain perfusion method in situ. Physiol. Rev., 38:1-20.

Gelli, M. G., G. Enhörning, E. Hultman, and J. Bergström. 1968. Glucose infusion in the pregnant rabbit and its effect on glycogen content and activity of foetal heart under anoxia. Acta Paediat. Scand., 57:1-6.

Gentz, J., B. Persson, and R. Zetterström. 1969a. On the diagnosis of symptomatic neonatal hypoglycemia. Acta Paediat. Scand., 58:449-459.

———— R. Warrner, B. E. H. Persson, and M. Cornblath. 1969b. Intravenous glucose tolerance, plasma insulin, free fatty acids and hydroxybutyrate in underweight newborn infants. Acta Paediat. Scand., 58:481.

Gladtke, E., F. H. Dost, M. von Hattingberg, and H. Rind. 1968. Glucoseumsatz beim Neugeborenen. Deutsch. Med. Wschr., 93:684-686.

Goldring, R. M. et al. 1962. The catecholamines in the pulmonary arterial pressor response to acute hypoxia. J. Clin. Invest., 41:1211-1221.

Gomez, M. F., and S. N. Graven. 1964. The use of fibrinolysin in the treatment of respiratory distress syndrome. Pediatrics, 34:877-880.

Graven, S. N., D. Criscuolo, and T. M. Holcomb. 1965. Blood lactate in the respiratory distress syndrome. Amer. J. Dis. Child., 110:614-617.

Gupta, J. M., G. W. Dahlenburg, and J. A. Davis. 1967. Changes in blood gas tensions following administration of amine buffer THAM to infants with RDS. Arch. Dis. Child., 42:416-427.

Gürson, C. T., and L. Etili. 1968. Relation between endogenous lipoprotein lipase activity, free fatty acids, and glucose in plasma of women in labor and of their newborns. Arch. Dis. Child., 43:679-683.

Hagerman, D. D., and C. A. Villee. 1960. Transport function of the placenta. Physiol. Rev., 40:313-330.

Hahn, J., E. Vavroušková, J. Jirásek, and J. Uher. 1964. Acetoacetate formation by livers from human fetuses aged 8-17 weeks. Biol. Neonat., 7:348-353.

Haworth, J. C., L. Dilling, and M. K. Younoszai. 1967. Relation of blood glucose to hematocrit, birth weight, and other body measurements in normal and growth-retarded newborn infants. Lancet, 2:901-905.

Heim, T., and D. Hull. 1966a. The blood flow and oxygen consumption of brown adipose tissue in the newborn rabbit. J. Physiol. (London), 186:42-55.

———— and D. Hull. 1966b. The effect of propranalol on the calorigenic response in brown adipose tissue of new-born rabbits to catecholamines, glucagon, corticotrophin, and cold exposure. J. Physiol. (London), 187:271-283.

Hicks, S. P. 1953. Developmental brain metabolism: Effects of cortisone, anoxia, fluoroacetate, radiation, insulin, and other inhibitors on the embryo and adult. Arch. Path. (Chicago), 55:302-327.

Hill, J. R. 1959. The oxygen consumption of new-born and adult animals, its dependence on the oxygen tension in the inspired air and on the environmental temperature. J. Physiol. (London), 149:346-373.

Himwich, H. E. 1951. Brain Metabolism and Cerebral Disorders. Baltimore, The Williams & Wilkins Co.

———— 1958. Introduction to the second round table discussion. *In* Windle, W. F., ed. Neurological and Psychological Deficits of Asphyxia Neonatorum. Springfield, Ill., Charles C Thomas Publishers, pp. 141-142.

———— et al. 1942. Mechanisms for the maintenance of life in the newborn during anoxia. Amer. J. Physiol., 135:387-391.

Hjelm, M., and S. Sjölin. 1965. The concentration of glucose in whole blood, plasma, and erythrocytes during the first week of life determined by different methods, and evaluation of the reliability of the methods. Acta. Paediat. Scand., 54:3-16.

Hochuli, E., and D. Schneider. 1966. Fetale Zustandsdiagnostik mittels Amnioscopie, Mikroblutuntersuchung sub partu and Nabelschnurblutanalyse. Schweiz. Med. Wschr., 96:1291-1301.

Högstedt, R., and B. Lindquist. 1963. Lipoprotein lipase in plasma of the normal newborn. Acta Paediat. Scand., 52:61.

Hohorst, H.-J. 1963. L-(+)-Lactate determination with lactic dehydrogenase and DPN. *In* Bergmeyer, H. U., ed. Methods of Enzymatic Analysis. Weinheim, Verlag Chemie and New York, Academic Press, pp. 266-270.

———— et al. 1965. L-(+)-Lactic acid and the steady state of cellular red/ox-systems. Ann. N. Y. Acad. Sci., 119:974-992.

Hommes, F. A., and C. W. Wilmink. 1968. Developmental changes of glycolytic enzymes in rat brain, liver and skeletal muscle. Biol. Neonat., 12:181-193.

Howard, W. F., P. I. McDevitt, and R. W. Stander. 1964. Catecholamine content of the initial voided urine of the newborn. Amer. J. Obstet. Gynec., 89:615-618.

Huckabee, W. E. 1958a. Relationships of pyruvate and lactate during anaerobic metabolism. I. Effects of infusions of pyruvate or glucose and of hyperventilation. J. Clin. Invest., 37:244-254.

———— 1958b. Relationships of pyruvate and lactate during anaerobic metabolism. III. Effect of breathing low-oxygen gases. J. Clin. Invest., 37:264-271.

———— J. Metcalfe, H. Prystowsky, and D. H. Barron. 1962a. Movements of lactate and pyruvate in pregnant uterus. Amer. J. Physiol., 202:193-197.

———— J. Metcalfe, H. Prystowsky, and D. H. Barron. 1962b. Insufficiency of O_2 supply to pregnant uterus. Amer. J. Physiol., 202:198-204.

Hull, D. 1965. Oxygen consumption and body temperature of new-born rabbits and kittens exposed to cold. J. Physiol. (London), 177:192-202.

———— and M. M. Segall. 1965. The contribution of brown adipose tissue to heat production in the new-born rabbit. J. Physiol. (London), 181:449-457.

James, L. S. 1967. Scientific basis for current perinatal care. Arch. Dis. Child., 42:457-466.

———— and E. Burnard. 1961. Biochemical changes occuring during asphyxia at birth and some effects on the heart. *In* Wolstenholme, G. E. W., and M. O'Connor, eds. Somatic Stability in the Newly Born. London, Churchill Ltd., pp. 75-91.

———— et al. 1958. The acid base status of the human infant in relation to birth asphyxia and the onset of respiration. J. Pediat., 52:379-394.

Jurado-García, E., C. Chanez, and A. Minkowski. 1966. Lactacidemia and pyruvicemia during ischemic foetal anoxia in rats. Biol. Neonat., 10:209-226.

Kaiser, I. H., and J. N. Cummings. 1958. pH, carbon dioxide, oxygen, hemoglobin and plasma electrolytes in blood of pregnant goats and their fetuses. Amer. J.

Physiol., 195:481-486.

Kaye, R. et al. 1961. The response of blood glucose, ketones and plasma non-esterified fatty acids to fasting and epinephrine injection in infants and children. J. Pediat., 59:836-847.

Keele, D. K., and J. L. Kay. 1966. Plasma free fatty acid and blood sugar levels in newborn infants and their mothers. Pediatrics, 37:597-604.

Keilin, D., and E. F. Hartree. 1948. The use of glucose oxidase (Notatin) for the determination of glucose in biological material and for the study of glucose-producing systems by manometric methods. Biochem. J., 42:230-238.

Kerpel-Fronius, E., F. Varga, and G. Bata. 1964. Blood gas and metabolic studies in plasma cell pneumonia and in newborn prematures with respiratory distress. Arch. Dis. Child., 39:473-480.

Keuth, U., and F. Adenauer. 1963. Untersuchungen zur Wirksamkeit von Alkali-Glucose-Infusionen bei der protrahierten Acidose der Früh- und Neugeborenen. Z. Kinderheilk., 88:244-254.

Kildeberg, P. 1964. Disturbances of hydrogen ion balance occuring in premature infants. Acta Paediat. Scand., 53:505-516.

Kimmelstiel, R., and C. A. Villee. 1956. Metabolism of carbon^{14}-labeled pyruvate by the newborn rat. Amer. J. Physiol., 184:63-68.

Klee, C. B., and L. Sokoloff. 1967. Changes in D (—)-β-hydroxybutyric dehydrogenase activity during brain maturation in the rat. J. Biol. Chem., 242:3880-3883.

Koch, G., and H. Wendel. 1968. Adjustment of arterial blood gases and acid base balance in the normal newborn infant during the first week of life. Biol. Neonat., 12:136-161.

Lang, C. A. 1965. Respiratory enzymes in the heart and liver of the prenatal and postnatal rat. Biochem. J., 95:365-371.

Laron, Z., S. Mannheimer, M. Nitzan, and J. Goldmann. 1967. Growth hormone, glucose and free fatty acid levels in normal, diabetic and toxaemic pregnancies. Arch. Dis. Child., 42:24-28.

Laurell, S. 1957. Turnover rate of unesterified fatty acids in human plasma. Acta Physiol. Scand., 41:158.

Levison, H., M. Delivoria-Papadopoulos, and P. R. Swyer. 1964. Oxygen consumption in newly born infants with the respiratory distress syndrome. Biol. Neonat., 7:255-269.

———— M. Delivoria-Papadopoulos, and P. R. Swyer. 1965. Variations in oxygen consumption in the infant with hypoxaemia due to cardiopulmonary disease. Acta Paediat. Scand., 54:369-374.

Lumley, J. M., and C. Wood. 1967. Influence of hypoxia on glucose transport across the human placenta. Nature (London), 216:403-404.

Lundsgaard-Hansen, P. 1966. Regional differences of the lactate/pyruvate response to progressive arterial hypoxemia. Pflueger. Arch. Ges. Physiol., 292:60-75.

MacKinney, L. G., I. D. Goldberg, F. E. Ehrlich, and K. C. Freymann. 1958. Chemical analysis of blood from the umbilical cord of the newborn: Relation to fetal maturity and perinatal distress. Pediatrics, 21:555-564.

Mäenpää, P. H., and N. C. R. Räihä. 1968. Effects of anoxia on energy-rich phosphates, glycogen, lactate and pyruvate in the brain, heart and liver of the developing rat. Ann. Med. Exp. Biol. Fenn., 46:306-317.

Mager, M., W. F. Blatt, P. J. Natale, and C. M. Blatteis. 1968. Effect of high altitude on lactic dehydrogenase isozymes of neonatal and adult rats. Amer. J. Physiol., 215:8-13.

Marx, G. F., and N. M. Greene. 1965. Lactate/pyruvate ratio of umbilical vein blood. Amer. J. Obstet. Gynec., 92:548-554.

———— B. E. Smith, and N. M. Greene. 1965. Umbilical vein blood biochemical data and neonatal condition. J. Pediat., 66:989-996.

Melichar, V. and M. Novák. 1970. Einfluss von Adrenalin und Glucagon auf den Kohlenhydrat- und Fettstoffwechsel bei Neugeborenen. In Joppich, G., and H. Wolf, eds. Metabolism of the Newborn. Stuttgart, Hippokrates-Verlag, pp. 360-368.

———— and H. Wolf. 1967. Postnatal changes in blood serum content of glycerol and free fatty acids in premature infants. Biol. Neonat., 11:50-60.

———— and H. Wolf. 1968. Glycerin und freie Fettsäuren im Blutplasma bei hypotrophen Neugeborenen. Klin. Wschr., 46:549-555.

———— M. Novák, P. Hahn, and O. Koldovský. 1962. Changes in serum unesterified fatty acid levels and in adipose tissue in newborns. (In Czech.) Cesk. Fysiol., 11:461.

———— Z. Drahota, and P. Hahn. 1965. Changes in the blood levels of acetoacetate and ketone bodies in newborn infants. Biol. Neonat., 8:348-352.

Miller, H. C. et al. 1962. Oxygen consumption in newborn premature infants. Amer. J. Dis. Child., 103:39-64.

Miller, J. A., and F. S. Miller. 1966. Interactions between hypothermia and hypoxia-hypercapnia in neonates. Fed. Proc., 25:1338-1341.

———— F. S. Miller, and B. Westin. 1964a. Hypothermia in the treatment of asphyxia neonatorum. Biol. Neonat., 6:148-163.

———— R. Zakhary, and F. S. Miller. 1964b. Hypothermia, asphyxia and cardiac glycogen in guinea pigs. Science, 144:1226-1227.

Moore, R. E. 1956. The effect of hypoxia on the oxygen consumption of new-born dogs. J. Physiol. (London), 131:27P.

———— 1959. Oxygen consumption and body temperature in new-born kittens subjected to hypoxia and reoxygenation. J. Physiol. (London), 149:500-518.

Moss, A. J. et al. 1965. Postnatal circulatory and metabolic adjustments in normal and distressed premature infants. Biol. Neonat., 8:177-197.

Mott, J. C. 1961. The ability of young mammals to withstand total oxygen lack. Brit. Med. Bull., 17:144-153.

———— 1963. Oxygen consumption of the newborn. Fed. Proc., 22:814-817.

Neligan, G. A., E. Robson, and J. Watson. 1963. Hypoglycaemia in the newborn: A sequel of intrauterine malnutrition. Lancet, 1:1282.

Novák, M., and V. Melichar. 1970. Die Veränderungen der Fettsäureutilisation im subcutanen Fettgewebe des Neugeborenen. In Joppich, G., and H. Wolf, eds. Metabolism of the Newborn. Stuttgart, Hippokrates-Verlag, pp. 150-162.

———— V. Melichar, and P. Hahn. 1964. Postnatal changes in the blood serum content of glycerol and fatty acids in human infants. Biol. Neonat., 7:179-184.

———— P. Hahn, and V. Melichar. 1968a. Incorporation of glycerol 1-, 3-^{14}C into triglycerides of subcutaneous adipose tissue in the newborn. Biol. Neonat., 12:287-291.

———— V. Melichar, and P. Hahn. 1968b. Changes in the reactivity of human adipose tissue in vitro to epinephrine and norepinephrine during postnatal development. Biol. Neonat., 13:175-180.

———— V. Melichar, P. Hahn, and O. Koldovský. 1961. Levels of lipids in the blood of newborn infants and the effect of glucose administration. Physiol. Bohemoslov., 10:488-491.

Oliver, T. K., and P. Karlberg. 1963. Gaseous metabolism in newly born human infants. Amer. J. Dis. Child., 105:427-435.

Olson, R. E. 1963. "Excess lactate" and anaerobiosis. Ann. Intern. Med., 59:960-963.

Orzalesi, M. M. et al. 1967. Arterial oxygen studies in premature newborns with and without mild respiratory disorders. Arch. Dis. Child., 42:174-180.

Otey, E., V. Stenger, D. Eitzman, and H. Prystowsky. 1967. Further observations on the relationships of pyruvate and lactate in human pregnancy. Amer. J. Obstet. Gynec., 97:1076-1081.

Paterson, P., J. Sheath, P. Taft, and C. Wood. 1967. Maternal and fetal ketone concentrations in plasma and urine. Lancet, 1:862.

Payne, W. W., and P. T. Acharya. 1965. The effect of abnormal birth on blood chemistry during the first 48 hours of life. Arch. Dis. Child., 40:436-441.

Pennoyer, M. M., F. K. Graham, and A. F. Hartmann, Sr. 1956. The relationship of paranatal experience to oxygen saturation in newborn infants. J. Pediat., 49:685-698.

Persson, B., and J. Gentz. 1966. The pattern of blood lipids, glycerol and ketone bodies during the neonatal period, infancy and childhood. Acta Paediat. Scand., 55:353-362.

————— P. B. Björntorp, and B. Hood. 1966. Lipoprotein lipase activity in human adipose tissue. I. Conditions for release and relationship to triglycerides in serum. Metabolism, 15:730.

————— D. Copher, and R. Tunell. 1970. Aspects of lipid metabolism in the immediate neonatal period in the newborn infant. In Joppich, G., and H. Wolf, eds. Metabolism of the Newborn. Stuttgart, Hippokrates-Verlag, pp. 163-178.

Prod'hom, L. S., H. Levison, R. B. Cherry, and C. A. Smith. 1965. Adjustment of ventilation, intrapulmonary gas exchange, and acid base balance during the first day of life. Pediatrics, 35:662-676.

Räihä, C.-E. 1954. Tissue metabolism in the human fetus. Cold Spring Harbor Sympos. Quant. Biol., 19:143.

Räihä, N. C. R. 1963. Organic acids in fetal blood and amniotic fluid. Pediatrics, 32:1025-1032.

————— 1964. Effect of anoxia on lactate/pyruvate and ATP/ADP ratios in adult and fetal guinea pig liver. Ann. Paediat. Fenn., 10:151-157.

Raivio, K. O., and N. Hallman. 1968. Neonatal hypoglycemia. I. Occurrence of hypoglycemia in patients with various neonatal disorders. Acta Paediat. Scand., 57:517-521.

————— and K. Teramo. 1968. Blood glucose of the human fetus prior to and during labor. Acta Paediat. Scand., 57:512-516.

Reiss, M., and F. Haurowitz. 1929. Ueber das Verhalten junger und alter Tiere bei Erstickung. Klin. Wschr., 7:743.

Reynolds, E. O. R. et al. 1965. The effect of immaturity and prenatal asphyxia on the lungs and pulmonary functions of newborn lambs: The experimental production of respiratory distress. Pediatrics, 35:382-392.

Robertson, A. F., and H. Sprecher. 1968. A review of human placental lipid metabolism and transport. Acta Paediat. Scand., (Suppl.183).

Rooth, G. 1963. Influence of nitrous oxide on the acid-base balance of the cord blood. Amer. J. Obstet. Gynec., 85:48-51.

————— S. Sjöstedt, and F. Caligara. 1961. Hydrogen concentration, carbon dioxide tension and acid-base balance in blood of human umbilical cord and intervillous space of placenta. Arch. Dis. Child., 36:278-285.

Roux, J. F., and S. L. Romney. 1967. Plasma free fatty acids and glucose concentrations in the human fetus and newborn exposed to various environmental conditions. Amer. J. Obstet. Gynec., 97:268-276.

Rubaltelli, F. F. 1967. Maternal and foetal ketone levels. Lancet, 1:1103.

Šabata, V., P. Hahn, and Z. Drahota. 1967. The role of glucose and of keto-substances in the metabolism of foetuses of mothers suffering from diabetes. *In* Horský, J., and Z. K. Štembera, eds. Intrauterine Dangers to the Fetus. Amsterdam, Excerpta Medica Monograph, pp. 140-144.

———— Z. K. S. Štembera, and M. Novák. 1968a. Levels of unesterified and esterified fatty acids in umbilical blood of hypoxic fetuses. Biol. Neonat., 12:194-200.

———— H. Wolf, and S. Lausmann. 1968b. The role of free fatty acids, glycerol, ketone bodies and glucose in the energy metabolism of the mother and fetus during delivery. Biol. Neonat., 13:7-17.

———— H. Wolf, and S. Lausmann. 1970. Glycerol levels in the maternal and umbilical cord blood under various conditions. Biol. Neonat., 15:123-127.

Saling, E. 1962. Neues Vorgehen zur Untersuchung des Kindes unter der Geburt. Arch. Gynaek., 197:108.

Schiff, D., L. Stern, and J. Leduc. 1966. Chemical thermo-genesis: Catecholamines and plasma free fatty acids. Pediatrics, 37:577.

Schreier, K. 1966. Ueber den Einfluss des Sauerstoffmangels auf den Kohlenhydrat-, Fett- und Eiweissstoffwechsel während der Postnatalperiode. Z. Kinderheilk., 96:268-290.

Schröter, W., G. Vogler, and M. Jensen. 1967. Die Wirkung von Glucose auf die Acetacetat-Konzentration im Serum Neugeborener. Mschr. Kinderheilk., 115:600.

Shelley, H. J. 1960. Blood sugars and tissue carbohydrate in foetal and infant lambs and Rhesus monkeys. J. Physiol. (London), 153:527-552.

———— 1964. Carbohydrate reserves in the newborn infant. Brit. Med. J., 1:273-275.

———— 1969. The metabolic response of the fetus to hypoxia. J. Obstet. Gynaec. Brit. Comm., 76:1-15.

———— and G. A. Neligan. 1966. Neonatal hypoglycemia. Brit. Med. Bull., 22:34-39.

———— and B. Thalme. 1969. Some aspects of lipid and carbohydrate metabolism in foetal and newborn rabbits. *In* Joppich, G., and H. Wolf, eds. Metabolism of the Newborn. Stuttgart, Hippokrates-Verlag, pp. 178-199.

Sloviter, H. A., P. Shimkin, and K. Suhara. 1966. Glycerol as a substrate for brain metabolism. Nature (London), 210:1334-1336.

Smith, C. A., and E. Kaplan. 1942. Adjustment of blood oxygen levels in neonatal life. Amer. J. Dis. Child., 64:843-859.

Stafford, A., and J. A. C. Weatherall. 1960. The survival of young rats in nitrogen. J. Physiol. (London), 153:457-472.

Stahlman, M. et al. 1964. Pathophysiology of respiratory distress in newborn lambs. Amer. J. Dis. Child., 108:375-393.

Stave, U. 1964. Age-dependent changes of metabolism. I. Studies of enzyme patterns of rabbit organs. Biol. Neonat., 6:128-147.

———— 1967. Age-dependent changes of metabolism. III. The effect of prolonged hypoxia upon tissue enzyme activities of newborn and adult rabbits. Biol. Neonat., 11:310-327.

———— 1969. Unpublished data.

———— 1970. Kohlenhydrat- und Energiestoffwechsel bei chronischer Hypoxie neugeborener Kaninchen. *In* Joppich, G., and H. Wolf, eds. Metabolism of the Newborn. Stuttgart, Hippokrates-Verlag, pp. 285-306.

Štembera, Z. K., and J. Hodr. 1966. The relationship between the blood levels of glucose, lactic acid and pyruvic acid in the mother and in both umbilical vessels of the healthy fetus. Biol. Neonat., 10:227-238.

Stern, L., J. Leduc, and J. Lind. 1964. Hypoxia as a stimulus to catecholamine excretion in the newborn infant. II. The effect of exposure to 10% O_2. Acta Paediat. Scand., 53:13-17.

Strand, A. 1966. The function of the placenta and "placental insufficiency" with special reference to the development of prolonged foetal distress. Acta Obstet. Gynec. Scand., 45 (Suppl. 1):125-230.

Strang, L. B., and M. H. MacLeish. 1961. Ventilatory failure and right-to-left shunt in newborn infants with respiratory distress. Pediatrics, 28:17-27.

Stubbe, P., and V. Šabata. 1970. Wachstumshormonbestimmungen bei verschiedenen Gruppen von Neugeborenen. In Joppich, G., and H. Wolf, eds. Metabolism of the Newborn. Stuttgart, Hippokrates-Verlag, pp. 384-393.

———— and H. Wolf. 1969. Unpublished data.

———— and H. Wolf. 1970. The effect of death on growth hormone levels in prematurely born infants. J. Clin. Endocr. In Press.

Szabo, A. J., R. D. Grimaldi, and W. F. Jung. 1969. Palmitate transport across perfused human placenta. Metabolism, 18:406-415.

Taylor, P. M. 1960. Oxygen consumption in new-born rats. J. Physiol. (London), 154:153-168.

Thalme, B. 1967. Electrolyte and acid-base balance in fetal and maternal blood. Acta Obstet. Gynec. Scand., 45 (Suppl. 8).

Thomas, H. D., C. Gaos, and C. W. Vaughan. 1965. Respiratory oxygen debt and excess lactate in man. J. Appl. Physiol., 20:898-904.

Thorn, I. 1969. Cerebral symptoms in the newborn. Acta Paediat. Scand., (Suppl. 195):24.

Usher, R. 1961. The metabolic changes in respiratory distress syndrome of prematurity seen as a failure of somatic compensations for asphyxia. In Wolstenholme, G. E. W., and M. O'Connor, eds. Somatic Stability in the Newly Born. London, Churchill, Ltd., pp. 92-109.

VanDuyne, C. M., and R. J. Havel. 1959. Plasma unesterified fatty acid concentration in fetal and neonatal life. Proc. Soc. Exp. Biol. Med., 102:599-602.

———— H. R. Parker, and L. W. Holm. 1965. Metabolism of free fatty acids during perinatal life of lambs. Amer. J. Obstet. Gynec., 91:277-285.

VanLiere, E. J., and J. C. Stickney. 1963. Hypoxia. Chicago, University of Chicago Press, pp. 244-246.

Varga, F. 1967. Energy metabolism in infantile hypoxia. Acta Paediat. Acad. Sci. Hung., 8:279-294.

Vedra, B. 1963. "Partial anaerobiosis" in the human fetus. Amer. J. Obstet. Gynec., 86:1088-1092.

———— and J. Ulrych. 1960. Anaerobiosis in normal and asphyxiated premature newborns. Acta Paediat. (Uppsala), 49:129-134.

Villee, C. A. 1953. Regulation of blood glucose in the human fetus. J. Appl. Physiol., 5:437-444.

———— et al. 1958. The effects of anoxia on the metabolism of human fetal tissues. Pediatrics, 22:953-970.

Vízek, K., and P. Hahn. 1968. Lipolytic activity of mitochondria from brown adipose tissue. Physiol. Bohemoslov., 17:343.

Von Euler, U., Y. Larsson, and B. Persson. 1964. Glucose tolerance in the neonatal period and during the first six months of life. Arch. Dis. Child., 39:393-396.

Walpurger, G. 1967. Cytoplasmatische und mitochondriale Enzyme in der postnatalen Entwicklung des Rattenherzens. Klin. Wschr., 45:239-244.

Wang, C. S. C. et al. 1963. Relationship of blood lactate to acidosis and hypoxia in respiratory distress syndrome. J. Pediat., 63:732-733.

Warley, M. A., and D. Gairdner. 1962. Respiratory distress syndrome of the newborn—principles in treatment. Arch. Dis. Child., 37:455-465.

Weil, R. 1965. Pituitary growth hormone and intermediary metabolism. Acta Endocr. (Kobenhavn), (Suppl. 98).

Weisbrot, I. M. et al. 1958. Acid base homeostasis of the newborn infant during the first 24 hours of life. J. Pediat., 52:395-403.

Westin, B., R. Nyberg, J. A. Miller, Jr., and E. Wedenberg. 1962. Hypothermia and transfusion with oxygenated blood in the treatment of asphyxia neonatorum. Acta Paediat. (Uppsala), (Suppl. 139).

Westphal, O. 1968. Human growth hormone: A methodological and clinical study. Acta Paediat. Scand., (Suppl. 182).

Whaley, W. H., F. P. Zuspan, and G. H. Nelson. 1966. Correlation between maternal and fetal plasma levels of glucose and free fatty acids. Amer. J. Obstet. Gynec., 94:419-421.

Widdowson, E. M. 1961. Metabolic effects of fasting and food. In Wolstenholme, G. E. W., and M. O'Connor, eds. Somatic Stability in the Newly Born. London, Churchill, Ltd., pp. 39-49.

———— 1964. Changes in the composition of the body at birth and their bearing on function and food requirements. In Jonxis, J. H. P., H. K. A. Visser, and J. A. Troelstra, eds. Symposium on the Adaptation of the Newborn Infant to Extra-uterine Life. Springfield, Ill., Charles C Thomas, Publishers, pp. 1-13.

Wittels, B., and R. Bressler. 1965. Lipid metabolism in the new-born heart. J. Clin. Invest., 44:1639-1646.

Wolf, H. 1960. Blutzucker bei Neugeborenen. Klin. Wschr., 38:87-89.

———— 1969. Unpublished data.

————and V. Melichar. 1970. Die Elimination und der Umsatz von Triglyceriden bei reifen Neugeborenen und bei Frühgeborenen. In Joppich, G., and H. Wolf, eds. Metabolism of the Newborn. Stuttgart, Hippokrates-Verlag, pp. 203-230.

————V. Melichar, and R. Michaelis. 1968. Elimination of intravenously administered glycerol from the blood of newborns. Biol. Neonat., 12:162-169.

Zetterström, R. 1963. Neonatal chemistry. Ann. N. Y. Acad. Sci., 111:537-539.

Znamenáček, K., and H. Přibylová. 1964. Some parameters of respiratory metabolism in the first 3 days after birth. Acta Paediat. (Uppsala), 53:241-246.

Index

Page numbers in italic type refer to illustrations and tables.

Hoffman reflex 806, *807*
Homeostatic defense mechanisms 661-663
Human fetal activity 752-791
Human growth hormone 936-940
    treatment of premature infants 939
Hydramnios 652-653, 788
Hydrogen ion loads 670-672
Hydropenia 663-664
Hydroxyproline 890-891
Hyperbaria and hypoxia 1027
Hypercalcemia, intrauterine 707
Hypercorticism, maternal 924-925
Hyperglycemia
    and HGH response 937
    and hypoxia 1027
    resistance to anoxia *1028*
Hyperinsulinism 963
Hyperlactacidemia and hypoxia 1011, 1016-1017
Hypernatremia 667
Hyperparathyroidism 705-706, 708
Hyperphosphatemia 706-709
Hyperpotassemia 646, 803
Hyperthyroidism 945-946, 980
Hypertonic expansion of ECW 668
Hypocalcemia 709-710, 803, 810
    cesarean section 710
    in premature infants 709-710
Hypoglycemia
    and HGH response 937
    in newborns 1053-1056
Hyponatremia 663
Hypoparathyroidism 706, 708
Hypopituitarism 939
Hypothalamic-pituitary-adrenal axis 940, 943, 947
Hypothermia
    and hypoxia 1029, 1047
    and stagnant anoxia *1030*
Hypothyroidism 945-946, 980
Hypoxemia and L/P ratio 1059-1060
Hypoxia
    adenosine phosphates in tissues *1073*
    and adrenaline 1076
    biochemical changes
        in immature CNS *1011*
        in mature CNS *1012*
    biochemical responses of CNS 998-1013
    and blood gases 1048-1052
    and blood glucose *1054*, 1056, *1068*
    causes 993-994
    and central regulatory functions 1016
    characterization 994-995
    clinical prevention 1026
    duration 995, 1018
    from excessive O$_2$ consumption 993, 995
    functional 995
    functional responses of CNS 1013-1017
    and functions of the brain stem 1015
    and glycolytic enzymes 1071, *1072*
    intensity 995
    and liver glycogen 1055, *1070*
    and lowering of metabolic rate of CNS 1028-1029
    metabolic 995

Hypoxia (*cont.*)
    and metabolism of CNS 987-1032
    mortality 987
    and respiratory chain enzymes, 1074-1075, *1074*
    structural 995
    and tissue ATP 1072-1073
    tolerance 996-998, *998*, 1011-1013, *1013*, 1044
Hypoxia fetalis 1044
Hypoxia neonatorum, metabolic effects 1043-1077
Hypoxic brain damage 1015
Hypoxic changes, dynamics of 1017-1018
Hypoxic hypoxia *989*, 992-994
Hypoxic infants and oxygen consumption 1046-1047

Impulse conduction 799
Insensible perspiration 665
Insulin 959-968
    and blood glucose concentration 959-960
    and cell metabolism 960
    and fat synthesis from glucose 966-967
    in fetal metabolism 961-963
    in fetal plasma 961-963
    and gestational diabetic mother *965*, *967*, *968*
    and glucose utilization 966-967
    and human placenta 961-962
    measurements 960-961
    in neonatal metabolism 963-968
    in the neonatal period 966-968
    response to glucose in the neonate 963-966
Intracellular water 654-661, *656*, *666*
Intrafusal innervation 805
Intraocular pressure 882-883
Intrauterine fluids 643-653
Intrauterine pressure and bradycardia 865
Inulin clearance 681
Inulin space 654-655
Iodine transfer, placental 975-976
Ipsilateral flexion reflexes *760*, *761-766*
Islets of Langerhans 962
Isoenzymes in muscle 850-851

Keratin deposition 891-892
Kernicterus 725, *727*
Ketone bodies
    formation in liver 1064
    in plasma, postnatal changes 1060-1064, *1063*
17-ketosteroids in blood 917, 926-927
Kidney
    acid secretion 694-698
    carbonic anhydrase 694-695, 697
    concentrating mechanism 689-690
    diluting mechanisms 689-690
Krebs cycle reactions in muscle 849, *849*

Lacrimal system 883-884
Lactate
    in blood and tissue LDH 1059

1093